THE
AT-RISK INFANT

International Workshop on the "At Risk" Infant (2nd: 1983: Jerusalem)

THE
AT-RISK INFANT

Psycho/Socio/Medical Aspects

edited by

SHAUL HAREL, M.D.
Sackler School of Medicine, Tel Aviv University
Tel Aviv

and

NICHOLAS J. ANASTASIOW, PH.D.
Hunter College, City University of New York
New York

Associate Editors:

GALYA RABINOVITZ, M.A.
Tel Aviv University
Tel Aviv

YEHUDA SHAPIRA, M.D.
Hadassah University Hospital, Hadassah-Hebrew University Medical School
Jerusalem

Section Editors:

NICHOLAS J. ANASTASIOW, PH.D.
Hunter College, City University of New York
New York

LEO STERN, M.D.
Brown University, Rhode Island Hospital
Providence

ARTHUR H. PARMELEE, M.D.
UCLA School of Medicine
Los Angeles

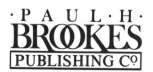

·P A U L·H·
BROOKES
PUBLISHING CO.

Baltimore • London

Paul H. Brookes Publishing Co.
Post Office Box 10624
Baltimore, Maryland 21204

Typeset by Brushwood Graphics, Baltimore, Maryland.
Manufactured in the United States of America by
The Maple Press Company, York, Pennsylvania.

This book has been developed from selected proceedings of the Second
International Workshop on the "At Risk" Infant held May 22–26, 1983, in
Jerusalem, Israel.

Library of Congress Cataloging in Publication Data
International Workshop on the "At Risk" Infant (2nd : 1983 : Jerusalem)
   The at-risk infant.

   "Selected proceedings of the Second International Workshop on the 'At Risk'
Infant held May 22–26, 1983, in Jerusalem, Israel"—T.p. verso.
   Includes bibliographies and index.
   1. Prenatal diagnosis—Congresses.   2. Fetus—Diseases—Etiology—Con-
gresses.   3. Infants (Newborn)—Medical examinations—Congresses.   4. Child de-
velopment—Congresses.   5. Children—Medical examinations—Congresses.   I.
Harel, Shaul.   II. Anastasiow, Nicholas J.   III. Title.
[DNLM: 1. Abnormalities, Drug-Induced—prevention & control—congresses.   2.
Child Development Disorders—prevention & control—congresses.   3. Child
Health Services—congresses.   4. Maternal Health Services—congresses.   5. Pre-
natal Diagnosis—congresses.   6. Primary Prevention—congresses.   W3 IN9327C
2nd 1983a / WS 350.6 I61   1983a]
RG628.I58   1983   618.92'01   84-9511
ISBN 0-933716-40-0

Contents

Contributors

Frank Ahern, Ph.D.
Assistant Professor
School of Public Health
University of Hawaii
1960 East-West Road, BIOMED C-105M
Honolulu, HI 96822

William A. Altemeier, III, M.D.
Professor of Pediatrics
Vanderbilt University Hospital
and
Department of Pediatrics
Metropolitan Nashville General Hospital
72 Hermitage Avenue
Nashville, TN 37210

Claudine Amiel-Tison, M.D.
Associate Professor of Pediatrics
Baudelocque Maternity Hospital
University of Paris V
Paris 75014
France

Nicholas J. Anastasiow, Ph.D.
Thomas Hunter Professor
Hunter College
695 Park Avenue
and
Program in Educational Psychology
Graduate Center
City University of New York
New York, NY 10036-8099

Janette Atkinson, Ph.D.
Medical Research Council Senior Scientist
Visual Development Unit
Kenneth Craik Laboratory
Department of Experimental Psychology
University of Cambridge
Cambridge CB2 3EB
Great Britain

Sue Atkinson, B.Sc., M.A., M.B., B. Chir., D.C.H.
Community Medicine
Bristol & Weston Health Authority
Bristol BS1 2
Great Britain

Dina Attias, M.D.
Hanna Khoushy Child Development Center
and
Departments of Pediatrics and Genetics
Haifa City Medical Center (Rothschild)
and
Faculty of Medicine
Technion-Israel Institute of Technology
Haifa
Israel

Célia Barbosa, M.D.
Pediatrician
Hospital de Crianças Maria Pia
Porto
Portugal

Moe Bergman, Ed.D.
Professor
Sackler School of Medicine
Tel Aviv University
Tel Aviv
Israel

Randall R. Blouin, M.D.
Department of Neurology
Vanderbilt University Medical Center and Children's Hospital
Nashville, TN 37232

Alfred W. Brann, Jr., M.D.
Professor of Pediatrics and of Gynecology and Obstetrics
Emory University School of Medicine
Atlanta, GA 30322

Rose M. Bromwich, Ed.D.
Department of Educational Psychology
California State University, Northridge
Northridge, CA 91330

Carol Browning, M.D.
Department of Pediatrics
Mt. Sinai Medical Center
950 North Twelfth Street
Milwaukee, WI 53201

Donna Bryant, Ph.D.
Frank Porter Graham Child Development Center
University of North Carolina at Chapel Hill
Chapel Hill, NC 27514

Monika Buchwald-Saal, M.D.
Division of Developmental Neurology and Child
    Development
Children's Hospital
Eberhard-Karls University
D 7400 Tuebingen
West Germany

Dale H. Bull, Ph.D.
Mailman Center for Child Development
Department of Pediatrics
University of Miami
Miami, FL 33101

**Neville R. Butler, M.D., F.R.C.P.,
    F.R.C.O.G., D.C.H.**
Department of Child Health
University of Bristol
Bristol BS2 8BJ
Great Britain

Paul Casaer, M.D.
Professor of Pediatrics-Neurology
Developmental Neurology Research Unit and
    Pediatric Neurology Section
Department of Pediatrics
University Hospital, Sint Rafaël-Gasthuisberg
B-3000
Leuven
Belgium

Sarale E. Cohen, Ph.D.
Assistant Professor of Pediatrics
UCLA School of Medicine
Los Angeles, CA 90024

Celia Cozakov, M.D.
Hanna Khoushy Child Development Center
Haifa City Medical Center (Rothschild)
and
Technion-Israel Institute of Technology
Faculty of Medicine
Haifa
Israel

Hannah Dar, D.Sc.
Department of Genetics
Haifa City Medical Center (Rothschild)
and
Faculty of Medicine
Technion-Israel Institute of Technology
Haifa
Israel

Lilly M.S. Dubowitz, M.D.
Department of Pediatrics
Post-Graduate Medical School
and
Hammersmith Special Health Authority

Hammersmith Hospital
Du Cane Road
London W12 OHS
Great Britain

Ephrem Eggermont, M.D.
Professor of Pediatrics-Neonatology
Developmental Neurology Research Unit and
    Department of Neonatology
Department of Pediatrics
University Hospital, Sint Rafaël-Gasthuisberg
B-3000
Leuven
Belgium

Rebecca E. Eilers, Ph.D.
Mailman Center for Child Development
Department of Pediatrics
University of Miami
Miami, FL 33101

Ilana Eli, D.M.D.
Department of Operative Dentistry
Sackler School of Medicine
and
School of Dental Medicine
Tel Aviv University
Tel Aviv
Israel

Patricia Ellison, M.D.
NIH Senior Research Fellow
Department of Psychology
University of Denver
2030 S. York Street
Denver, CO 80208

Moshe Feinsod, M.D.
Neuro-ophthalmology Unit and Laboratory of
    Clinical Sensory Physiology
Hadassah Medical Center
Jerusalem
Israel

Candice Feiring, Ph.D.
Department of Pediatrics
Academic Health Science CN-19
Rutgers Medical School
New Brunswick, NJ 08903

Gerald M. Fenichel, M.D.
Departments of Neurology and Pediatrics
School of Medicine
Vanderbilt University Medical Center and Chil-
    dren's Hospital
Nashville, TN 37232

Reuven Feuerstein, Ph.D.
Hadassah-WIZO-Canada
Research Institute
Jerusalem
Israel

Tiffany Field, Ph.D.
Associate Professor
Pediatrics and Psychology
University of Miami Medical Center
Mailman Center for Child Development (D-820)
P.O. Box 016820
Miami, FL 33101

Loretta P. Finnegan, M.D.
Director of Family Center
Associate Professor of Pediatrics, Psychiatry, and
    Human Behavior
Jefferson Medical College of the Thomas Jeffer-
    son University
111 S. 11th Street, Suite 6105
Philadelphia, PA 19107

Jeri E. Fitzpatrick, B.A., REEGT
Department of Neurology
Vanderbilt University Medical Center and Chil-
    dren's Hospital
Nashville, TN 37232

Nathan A. Fox, Ph.D.
Department of Human Development
University of Maryland
College Park, MD 20742

Joseph H. French, M.D.
New York State Office of Mental Retardation
    and Developmental Disabilities
Institute for Basic Research in Developmental
    Disabilities
1050 Forest Hill Road
Staten Island, NY 10314

Setsu Furuno, Ph.D.
Professor
School of Public Health
University of Hawaii
1960 East-West Road, BIOMED C-105M
Honolulu, HI 96822

Roseli Gomes, M.D.
Pediatrician
Hospital de Crianças Maria Pia
Porto
Portugal

Reena Greenberg, M.S.
Mailman Center for Child Development
University of Miami Medical Center
P.O. Box 016820
Miami, FL 33101

Gerhard Haas, M.D.
Division of Developmental Neurology and Child
    Development
Children's Hospital
Eberhard-Karls University
D 7400 Tuebingen
West Germany

Michael L. Hanes, Ph.D.
College of Education
University of South Carolina
Columbia, SC 29208

Shaul Harel, M.D.
Pediatric Neurology Unit and Child Development
    Assessment Center
Division of Pediatrics
Tel Aviv Medical Center
Sackler School of Medicine
Tel Aviv University
Tel Aviv
Israel

Mordechai Z. Himmelfarb, M.D.
Department of Otorhinolaryngology
Municipal Governmental Medical Center
Sackler Faculty of Medicine
Tel Aviv University
Tel Aviv
Israel

Moshe Holtzman, M.D.
Pediatric Neurology Unit and Child Development
    Center
Division of Pediatrics
Tel Aviv Medical Center
Tel Aviv University
Tel Aviv
Israel

Frances Degen Horowitz, Ph.D.
Department of Human Development and Family
    Life
University of Kansas
Lawrence, KS 66045

Michael Jaffe, M.B.Ch.B., M.R.C.P., D.C.H.
Head
Hanna Khoushy Child Development Center
Haifa City Medical Center (Rothschild)
and
Faculty of Medicine
Technion-Israel Institute of Technology
Haifa
Israel

Kurt Jagerman, B.D.S.
Department of Pediatrics
Haifa City Medical Center (Rothschild)
and
Faculty of Medicine
Technion-Israel Institute of Technology
Haifa
Israel

Herbert Judes, B.D.S. (Rand)
Department of Operative Dentistry
Sackler School of Medicine
and
School of Dental Medicine
Tel Aviv University
Tel Aviv
Israel

Michael Karplus, M.D.
Soroka University Hospital and Faculty of Health
    Sciences
and
Department of Neonatology
Soroka Medical Center
P.O. Box 151
Beer-Sheba 84-101
Israel

Pnina S. Klein, Ed.D.
School of Education
Bar-Ilan University
Ramat Gan
Israel

Janna G. Koppe, M.D.
Department of Neonatology
University of Amsterdam
Academic Medical Center
Meibergdreef 9
1105 AZ Amsterdam Zuidoost
The Netherlands

Jeanne-Claudie Larroche, M.D.
Maitre de Recherche au CNRS
Port-Royal Hospital
123 Port-Royal Boulevard
75674 Paris Cedex 14
France

Lewis A. Leavitt, M.D.
Infant Processes Section
Waisman Center on Mental Retardation and Hu-
    man Development
and
Department of Pediatrics
University of Wisconsin-Madison
Madison, WI 53706

Cyril Legum, M.D.
Director
Genetics Institute
Ichilov Hospital and Sackler Medical School
6 Weizman Street
Tel Aviv 64239
Israel

Diana C. Lewis, M.A.
Mailman Center for Child Development
Department of Pediatrics
University of Miami
Miami, FL 33101

Hans C. Lou, M.D.
The John F. Kennedy Institute
G1. Landevej 7
DK-2600 Glostrup
Denmark

Carlos H. Lozano, M.D., M.P.H.
Professor of Pediatrics and Perinatal Medicine
Universidad Nacional Autónoma de México
Chairman of Pediatrics
Instituto Nacional de Perinatología, SSA
México

Maria Maia, M.D.
Pediatric Neurologist
Hospital de Crianças Maria Pia
Porto
Portugal

Alexander Meijer, M.D.
Department of Child & Adolescent Psychiatry
Hadassah University Hospital
and
Hebrew University Medical School
Jerusalem
Israel

Richard Michaelis, M.D.
Division of Developmental Neurology and Child
    Development
Children's Hospital
Eberhard-Karls University
D 7400 Tuebingen
West Germany

David Wayne Mitchell, M.A.
Department of Human Development and Family
    Life
University of Kansas
Lawrence, KS 66045

Susan M. O'Connor, M.D.
Assistant Professor of Pediatrics
Vanderbilt University Hospital
Nashville, TN 37232

D. Kimbrough Oller, Ph.D.
P.O. Box 016820
Mailman Center for Child Development
Department of Pediatrics
University of Miami
Miami, FL 33101

Barbara J. Olson, M.D.
Departments of Neurology and Pediatrics
Vanderbilt University Medical Center and Chil-
    dren's Hospital
Nashville, TN 37232

Edgar Y. Oppenheimer, M.D.
Assistant Professor of Pediatrics and Neurology
Director of Pediatric EEG Laboratory
Boston University School of Medicine
Boston City Hospital
Boston, MA 02118

Katherine O'Reilly, R.P.T., M.P.H.
Coordinator, Physical Therapy
Kapiolani/Children's Medical Center
1319 Punahou Street
Honolulu, HI 96826

Arthur H. Parmelee, M.D.
Professor of Pediatrics
Head
Division of Child Development
UCLA School of Medicine
Los Angeles, CA 90024

David Prasse, Ph.D.
Department of Educational Psychology
University of Wisconsin-Milwaukee
Milwaukee, WI 53201

Galya Rabinovitz, M.A.
Child Development Assessment Center
Division of Pediatrics
Tel Aviv Medical Center
Tel Aviv University
Tel Aviv
Israel

Craig T. Ramey, Ph.D.
Frank Porter Graham Child Development Center
University of North Carolina at Chapel Hill
Chapel Hill, NC 27514

N. Paul Rosman, M.D.
Professor of Pediatrics and Neurology
Director of Pediatric Neurology
Associate Director of Pediatrics
Boston University School of Medicine
Boston City Hospital
Boston, MA 02118

Dana Schwartz, M.A.
Department of Otorhinolaryngology
Municipal Governmental Medical Center
Sackler Faculty of Medicine
Tel Aviv University
Tel Aviv
Israel

Susan F. Schwartz, M.S.
Department of Human Development and Family
   Life
University of Kansas
Lawrence, KS 66045

Eliahu Shanon, M.D.
Department of Otorhinolaryngology
Municipal Governmental Medical Center
Sackler Faculty of Medicine
Tel Aviv University
Tel Aviv
Israel

Yehuda Shapira, M.D.
Pediatric Neurology Unit
Department of Pediatrics
Hadassah University Hospital
and
Associate Professor of Pediatrics
Hadassah-Hebrew University Medical School
Jerusalem
Israel

Kathryn B. Sherrod, Ph.D.
Assistant Professor of Psychology
Peabody College/Vanderbilt University
Nashville, TN 37232

Linda S. Siegel, Ph.D.
Department of Special Education
Ontario Institute for Studies in Education
252 Bloor Street West
Toronto, Ontario M55 1V6
Canada

Julaine Siewert, M.A.
Department of Educational Psychology
University of Wisconsin-Milwaukee
Milwaukee, WI 53201

Susan B. Silverberg, M.S.
Waisman Center on Mental Retardation and Hu-
   man Development
and
Child and Family Studies Program
University of Wisconsin-Madison
Madison, WI 53706

Haim Sohmer, Ph.D.
Department of Physiology
Hebrew University—Hadassah Medical School
Jerusalem
Israel

Joseph J. Sparling, Ph.D.
Frank Porter Graham Child Development Center
University of North Carolina at Chapel Hill
Chapel Hill, NC 27514

Frieda Spivack, Ph.D.
Herbert H. Lehman College
City University of New York
Department of Specialized Services in Education
Division of Education
Bronx, NY 10468

Leo Stern, M.D.
Professor and Chairman of Pediatrics
Brown University
and
Pediatrician-in-Chief
Rhode Island Hospital
Providence, RI 02902

Marguerite B. Stevenson, Ph.D.
Waisman Center on Mental Retardation and Hu-
   man Development
and
Child and Family Studies Program
University of Wisconsin-Madison
Madison, WI 53706

Sherilyn Stoller, M.S.
Mailman Center for Child Development
University of Miami Medical Center
P.O. Box 016820
Miami, FL 33101

Dov Tamir, M.D.
Department of Health Care
Municipality of Jerusalem
44 Ha-Neviim Street
Jerusalem
Israel

Mary S. Thormann, Ed.D.
Professor of Education
Marymount College of Virginia
Arlington, VA 22207

Dorothy Tucker, B.A.
Research Assistant
Department of Pediatrics
Vanderbilt University Hospital
Nashville, TN 37232

James N. Ver Hoeve, Ph.D.
Infant Processes Section
Waisman Center on Mental Retardation and Human Development
and
Department of Pediatrics
University of Wisconsin-Madison
Madison, WI 53706

Peter M. Vietze, Ph.D.
Head
Mental Retardation Research Centers
National Institute of Child Health and Human Development
Bethesda, MD 20205

Barbara H. Wasik, Ph.D.
School of Education
University of North Carolina at Chapel Hill
Chapel Hill, NC 27514

David L. Webster, M.D.
Department of Neurology
Vanderbilt University Medical Center and Children's Hospital
Nashville, TN 37232

Susan Widmayer, Ph.D.
Mailman Center for Child Development
University of Miami Medical Center
P.O. Box 016820
Miami, FL 33101

Preface

T HE SECOND INTERNATIONAL WORKSHOP ON THE "AT-RISK" INFANT grew out of the positive responses of the participants who attended the First International Workshop in Tel Aviv in 1979 (Harel, 1980). The First International Workshop was designed to bring together persons from various disciplines who work toward prevention and/or amelioration of the factors contributing to the at-risk condition of many infants but who often do so in isolation. Assessment of the state of the art in 1979 levied a troublesome commentary: physicians—in particular, pediatricians and obstetricians—were frequently not in direct contact with neurologists and were even more distanced from allied professions such as psychology, speech/language therapy, audiology, nursing, and physical and occupational therapy. This gap was of major concern to the workshop organizers, but the segregation of allied professions was minor when compared to the lack of contact between the basic research worker in medicine and the medical practitioner. Even more disturbing was the gulf between researchers in medicine and professionals working in psychology and sociology.

The organizing committee, formed by Drs. N. Bogair, S. Harel, E. Chigier, and Y. Shapira of Israel, decided to initiate efforts to confront this isolation of disciplines by bringing together major research personnel in the fields of health science, psychology, sociology, and education with practitioners—pediatricians, obstetricians, neurologists, psychologists, nurses, day care workers, therapists, and teachers. It was a bold endeavor, yet the participants at the First International Workshop confirmed that it was successful.

Encouraged by the evaluation of the first workshop and letters from participants in many areas of the world stating that the workshop had planted the seeds for new collaborative efforts of research workers, practitioners, and service personnel, the International Advisory Committee members decided to go one step further. The aim of the Second International Workshop was similar to that of the first: encouraging communication among disciplines and between researchers and practitioners. However, in planning the second workshop, heavier emphasis was placed on presenting the results of efforts to ameliorate the at-risk state of the infant and efforts to prevent infants from becoming at-risk. Thus, the Second International Workshop was designed to emphasize preventive and therapeutic approaches as well as address basic research findings.

While the papers at the first workshop tended to be concerned with the early infancy period, the second workshop included more papers from the prenatal and perinatal periods and addressed the issue of the relationship between the at-risk condition of some infants and the at-risk state of their parents. This expanded focus is reflected in the contents of this book. Several chapters report on the effects of toxic substances such as alcohol, smoke, and anticonvulsants on the fetus, while others discuss genetic screening and parent education. Even the chapter arrangement underscores this emphasis on preventive and therapeutic approaches, with separate sections addressing the child's ecological environment, the events occurring during pregnancy and birth, and continued follow-up through infancy and early childhood.

Much of the success of the workshops lies in their generation of more questions than answers. The interactions arising from the exchange of information across disciplines will lead to new research and new practices. It is a growing experience, and one in which the reader can participate through the pages of this book. Researchers and practitioners alike should benefit from the diverse workshop reports, edited and updated for this text.

The editors wish to express thanks to the International and Israel Advisory committees whose efforts made the conference possible. Thanks also go to Tzipora Laxer, the workshop secretary who was untiring in her problem-solving before, during, and after the workshops, and to workshop chairpersons Drs. Leo Stern, Arthur Parmelee, and Nicholas Anastasiow. Finally, with great gratitude, the editors acknowledge all financial contributors, and especially acknowledge the personal and financial support of "International" Travel Ltd., which guaranteed that the conference could take place and provided a superb organization.

Shaul Harel
Nicholas Anastasiow
Galya Rabinovitz
Yehuda Shapira

REFERENCES

Harel, S. (ed.). *The at-risk infant*. Amsterdam: Excerpta Medica, 1980.

Dedicated to Dalia, Tali, Ronit, and Gil Harel, and
Roberta, Mary, and Jim Anastasiow, and Judy Smitheran.

THE
AT-RISK INFANT

Section I

ECOLOGICAL FACTORS THAT FOSTER DEVELOPMENT OF HIGH-RISK INFANTS AND CHILDREN

NICHOLAS J. ANASTASIOW, PH.D.
Hunter College, New York, New York

S ECTION I FOCUSES ON THE TOTAL ecological systems of children who are at risk and their families. For example, a child may be at risk medically due to prematurity, low birth weight, or perinatal complications; the infant's at-risk status has an impact on the family's ecological system by placing the family in a position of having to respond to the special needs of the at-risk infant. The situation is further complicated by parents and family systems who are at risk due to low socioeconomic status, medical disorders among one or more family members, or the isolation and stress endured by a single-parent family.

The work of Emmy E. Werner and her colleagues has been drawn upon to demonstrate the transactional nature of the at-risk infant's impact on the stable family, and/or the at-risk family's impact on the biologically normal and healthy infant. Werner, Bierman, and French's (1971) work clearly demonstrates that nurturing, responsive, and stimulating homes can help perinatal-stressed infants to survive the birth insult and, by age 10, to function normally in school settings. Conversely, these studies have shown that low-support homes tend to exacerbate the infant's risk condition so that, by age 10, these children are functioning poorly in school. Further, Werner and Smith's (1982) work has demonstrated that some children with as many as four risk factors have managed with inner and environmental supports to function relatively problem-free during their teenage years.

Section I further explores the transactional nature of the environmental and genetic-biological risk factors, and determines whether research in the years since 1979 has increased our knowledge of how to predict which children and families are at risk, how to modify the risk nature of the family and the child, and how to study the complexity of the transactions operating in the multivariate ecological setting. One risk group specifically focused on the young parent.

THE ADOLESCENT PARENT

One group that Section I focuses on is the adolescent parent. This group was chosen due to the continuing prevalence of adolescent pregnancies in many countries in the world. In the chapters that follow, Field (Chapter 4) and Thormann (Chapter 5) add to our knowledge of the nature of the young girl who becomes pregnant and of programs that enhance the outcomes of that pregnancy. Noted in the discussions during the plenary sessions at the 1983 International Workshop on the "At-Risk" Infant was the fact that not all adolescent parents have an increased chance of experiencing at-risk family environments. Research in the past 5 years has shown that older adolescents may have healthy-term infants, who grow into normal healthy children, particularly when the adolescent parent is provided with environmental supports from parents, marriage partners, or social service agencies (Anastasiow, 1982). The support of the family and larger culture provided to the adolescent and her child appears to be a critical ingredient in the healthy outcome of the pregnancy.

In some cultures, early social marriages are encouraged, and when the young couple is sexually mature and produces a child, the culture assists the young family in providing adequate pre- and postnatal care, as well as assists the young parents in child-rearing. The outcomes of these pregnancies produce well-functioning individuals as children and adults (Anastasiow, 1982; Werner & Smith, 1982). Less positive predictions can be made for parents under 15 years old and for adolescent women who have suffered isolation, loneliness, and neglect as children, who feel less in control of their destiny, and who have inadequate knowledge of child-rearing strategies (Anastasiow, 1982; Smith, 1980).

Hanes (Chapter 2) reviews the literature on parent impact on children through child-rearing practices. Field presents the results of her longitudinal study in working with adolescent parents, and Thormann presents an in-depth study of the knowledge of child-rearing strategies possessed by a sample of adolescents.

The adolescent's infant is but one potentially at-risk infant; therefore, this section addresses other at-risk infant groups and the problems of identifying and predicting at-risk infants.

PREDICTING THE AT-RISK CHILD AND/OR THE AT-RISK ENVIRONMENT

Several of the chapters that follow present research on instruments that measure infant and environmental stages and that have predictive power in identifying both positive and negative outcomes of children's intellectual and school functioning. Siegel's work (Chapter 7) offers support to the predictive power of selected infant and ecological measures. Fox and Feiring (Chapter 3) present data regarding the nature of the support system that facilitates the recovery of the at-risk and sick infant; the differential nature of the support system that they present sheds new light on the problem.

Altemeier's work (Chapter 10) in identifying the potentially abusive parent demonstrates the complexity of the prediction issue by identifying sources of abuse found in the childhood of the parent who is the abuser. Thus, increased knowledge of factors involved in predicting child abuse will require that research workers consider intervention strategies at earlier ages. Altemeier's chapter demonstrates the complexity of the problem and the growing trend of physicians who are becoming involved with social and psychological issues. Altemeier's research was conducted by a multidisciplinary team. It has been noted that there is a need for psychologists to make their tools and themselves available to physicians in their research efforts. Many psychologists have criticized the work of physicians without becoming involved in the complexities of this type of research.

INTERVENTION: TECHNIQUES AND METHODS

Furuno, in Chapter 6, discusses a team approach to working with at-risk infants in a hospital setting. Spivack (Chapter 11) offers a report on a multidisciplinary team working with teenage mothers. From a different perspective, Ramey (Chapter 8) presents data on the longitudinal study of prevention of mild retardation due to socially related causes.

Although these chapters present encouraging data, they further point to the complexity of the intervention issue. A handicapped child may have a major impact on an otherwise adequately functioning family system, with the process of grief and mourning being evoked by the presence of the handicapped child. In turn, the biologically healthy baby born into a disordered family may be abnormal by age 3 (see Siegel, Chapter 7). Transactional analyses are now possible utilizing newer statistical techniques of path analysis and causal modeling. Linear statistical models will not be appropriate statistical techniques for the issues involved with at-risk infants and their families, but the newer techniques mentioned above can handle complex reciprocal interactions. Research workers in the field may not have to invent new strategies but may have to modify (emulate) known strategies to meet the complexities of their research world.

Anastasiow, in Chapter 1, encourages interventionists to take a broad view of their efforts rather than to view intervention in the narrow spectrum of teaching a parent a single skill or set of skills. Intervention with parents, he argues, is essentially adult development—that is, the raising of the parents' level of emotional, personal, and cognitive functioning to higher levels of adult functioning. In essence, his position is that social change can be accomplished through the transformation of the individual.

PUBLIC POLICY

The effects of a disordered environment are long-lasting and powerful. Poverty, as Tolstoy wrote, is the world's worst prison. How does one free individuals from the vicious cycle of the various forms of abuse and deficiencies arising out of poverty? Although there are no simple solutions, some implications arising from the preparation of the chapters for this book need to be disseminated.

As the research in these chapters demonstrates, parenting practices can be so facilitating as to offset the high-risk status of the infant, whether that status is due to low birth weight, prematurity, or malnutrition (Richardson, 1976; Werner & Smith, 1982). Conversely, parenting practices can be so lethal as to magnify the risk factors and to create maladaptive behaviors in biologically sound infants from healthy genetic pools. These findings of the International Workshop on the "At-Risk" Infant in 1979 were reinforced and supported by additional research and practices presented at the 1983 Workshop and conveyed here in this volume. Training parents in facilitating child-rearing practices has been identified as a major means of minimizing the maleffects of risk factors, but the training must take place early in the preparent life of the individual or early in the child-rearing stage.

Education is a powerful tool in cultural evolution and a major factor in primary prevention. The mother's years of education play a critical role in her offspring's status. The role of the father is also critical, but, at present, is a very under-researched area.

Although there is still much to learn, a great deal is known. Decision-makers need to be aware that many of tomorrow's handicapped children could have lived normal lives if appropriate interventions had been made in the lives of their parents when the parents were children.

REFERENCES

Anastasiow, N.J. Adolescent pregnancy and special education. *Exceptional Children*, 1982, *49*(5), 396–401.

Richardson, S.A. The influence of severe malnutrition in infancy on the intelligence of children at school age. In: R.N. Walsh & W.T. Greenough (eds.), *Environments as therapy for brain dysfunction, Vol. 17, Advances in behavioral biology*. New York: Plenum Publishing Corp., 1976.

Smith, R. High risk families in rural communities: Characteristics of pregnant teenagers and their families. In: S. Harel (ed.), *The at-risk infant*. Amsterdam: Excerpta Medica, 1980.

Werner, E.E., Bierman, J.M., & French, F.E. *The children of Kauai.* Honolulu: University of Hawaii Press, 1971.

Werner, E.E., & Smith, R. *Vulnerable but invincible: A longitudinal study of resilient children and youth.* New York: McGraw-Hill Book Co., 1982.

The At-Risk Infant: Psycho/Socio/Medical Aspects
edited by Shaul Harel, M.D., and Nicholas J. Anastasiow, Ph.D.
Copyright © 1985   Paul H. Brookes Publishing Co., Inc.   Baltimore • London

Chapter 1

Parent Training
As Adult Development

Nicholas J. Anastasiow, Ph.D.
Hunter College, New York, New York

T HE RECENT IMPETUS TO TRAIN CHILDREN AT younger and younger ages can be seen as stemming from the pivotal work of J. Mc-Vicker Hunt, specifically in *Experience and Intelligence* (1961). Hunt challenged the notion that the IQ was genetically fixed at birth and suggested that intelligence was influenced by: 1) experience (initiated and under some control of the child), 2) training (the care-giver's responsiveness to the child's in-itiations), and 3) strategies that caregivers use in their responsiveness to and stimulation of their children, and the emotional support they provide (the amount of warmth and acceptance they show toward the child). Hunt grouped these factors into the construct ''environ-ment.'' Thus, environment is a cluster of fac-tors that facilitate or hinder the child's real-ization of his or her genetic potential. Hunt drew upon the work of Skodak (1966) and upon adoption literature; on Bowlby's (1969) and Spitz's (1959) speculations on maternal depri-vation and separation constructs, which were later embodied in the notions of attachment and attachment systems; and on Piaget's (1983) psychology and genetic epistomology.

In the era that followed Hunt's book, de-velopmental psychologists clarified the role that infants play in stimulating agents in the environment to care for them through operation of reflexes and fixed action patterns (Schaffer, 1977). Fixed action patterns (instincts) include the elicitation power of the social smile and infant eye contact. Furthermore, infant talents include the evolutionary-based communication system of emotions, as displayed in facial expressions and vocalizations through the cry, coo, and comfort sounds (Emde, Gaensbauer, & Harmon, 1976).

More recently, Werner and Smith (1982) have identified biological characteristics of the child (cuddly, warm, responsive infants) and ecological factors of caregivers (supporting grandparents, ministers, neighbors), which enable the severely high-risk infants (with four or more risk factors) to withstand a negative child-rearing environment and to function as healthy adolescents who display the capacity to love and to work.

Other researchers in the field, as sum-marized by Anastasiow (1982b) and Hunt (1979) have documented the impact of early environmental experiences on brain develop-ment and the necessity of enriched early envi-ronment and intervention if risk factors exist.

The cumulative effect of these trends has been to stimulate practitioners in a variety of professions (education, medicine, social work) to apply these findings by training parents in the knowledge of child growth and develop-

5

ment so as to facilitate their infants' development. Three large groups have been targeted to be trained to apply these findings through some type of intervention program.

The first group is the parent who resides in poverty. Children of these parents have traditionally done poorly in school, whether they reside in inner-city slums, canal boats, isolated hill regions, or the back seats of migrant-worker cars. Head Start in the United States is a program designed to have impact on the child who resides in poverty. Home intervention programs such as those of Gordon (1975) are attempts to change the debilitative education practices of the lower-class caregivers to more facilitative ones, should the change be necessary.

The second large group comprises young women who are having children during their early adolescent years. Evidence has been presented that these mothers are not knowledgeable in child development (Field, Thormann, and Siegel address this issue in their chapters).

The third group is composed of teachers of handicapped children, particularly teachers of preschool handicapped children, who are currently being pressed to become parent educators. These educators are attempting to teach parents of handicapped children to respond to the needs of their handicapped children. In addition, they are attempting to teach the principles of child development and to assist the parents through the grieving and loss process so commonly associated with having a handicapped child (Linder, 1983).

The curriculum developed for these three groups draws on knowledge of child growth and development, on parenting practices that facilitate development, and, in the case of the handicapped child, on the specialized knowledge of physical, occupational, and speech therapists, as well as on the skills of psychologists, social workers, and medical personnel. The current *zeitgeist* is to train parents in these knowledges and skills, on the premise that this is the most effective and economical way to reduce the impact of the high-risk state of the child, whether the state is related to perinatal stress, to ecological factors (which include parents at risk for abuse or neglect of the

infant), or to stress factors associated with low economic status. Psychologists in the field of child growth and development have argued that parenting education is more potent if delivered during the preparenthood period when values and attitudes are being formed (Anastasiow, 1982a), or during the early postpartum period when the specific child-care techniques can be put into practice as they are acquired (Badger, 1980; Field, 1980). This chapter contends that the missing ingredient in many programs is consideration of the maturity level of the person to be trained, regardless of the setting, timing, or state of the person. In addition, it considers the implications that this level of maturity has on the training program in terms of how training should occur and on the nature of the curriculum in terms of content focus.

Piaget's developmental theory offers suggestions about "when" (the age) that training can be most effectively conducted once the "how" and the "what" have been determined. In reverse terms, developmental theory can suggest what training can effectively achieve, and how it can be achieved, given the maturational level of the individual to be trained. Social learning theory (Bandura, 1977; Gagne, 1977) can specify the techniques and procedures for organizing and selecting curricula and make suggestions, once the developmental level of the individual has been determined, as to the context in which learning will occur. The combining of developmental and learning theories has come to be referred to as *cognitive learning* (Anastasiow, 1978), *contextualism* (Zimmerman, 1983), or *conceptual matching model* (Hunt & Sullivan, 1974).

It is assumed here that most parent-training programs attempt to have the parent act as a responsible adult, to utilize facilitating practices, and to reason and employ problem-solving strategies in raising their normal or at-risk child. These goals assume that the young adult is mature, has achieved the level of abstract reasoning defined by Piaget, and utilizes logical reasoning processes to solve problems. Both brain research and studies by Piaget confirm that, by age 15, the young adult should be capable of formal operation thought (Piaget's fourth developmental stage). It is argued that many young and older adults have not reached this stage of maturity and that the content of parent-training programs should be directed toward helping parents achieve higher levels of development while learning about the ways of facilitating their children's development. In essence, parent-training programs should be oriented to adult development.

MATURITY

Heath (1977) argues convincingly that the construct of maturity embodies the notions most commonly associated with the high point of adult development. To Heath, maturity implies competence in the R.H. White sense, self-actualization according to Maslow, and the psychoanalytical notions of ego strength (Loevinger, 1976). Heath perceives clusters of human functioning or principal sectors of human activity, which can be grouped as cognitive skills, self-concept, values, and personal relations, as composing the attributes of maturity. In each cluster, Heath postulates four interdependent dimensions: symbolization, allocentrism, integrated stability, and autonomy. Maturity is defined as increased potential and capacity to achieve symbolization, allocentrism, integration, and autonomy in each of the four sectors of human functioning (i.e., cognitive skills, self-concept, values, and personal relations).

In his work, Heath compared immature and mature American, Italian, and Turkish males. He found support on a cross-cultural basis for his notion that there is agreement on the term "maturity" as defined above. He found among the men nominated as mature that maturity per se predicts a multiple set of factors of psychological functioning that include: empathy toward others, ability to symbolize experience, possession of an integrated view of the self, and an ability to withstand probing and disturbing questions by responding reflectively. This set of behaviors was not mastered by the immature men in his study.

Other studies have demonstrated that physicians who are equally well trained differ markedly when identified as mature or immature. Mature physicians were markedly more empathetic with their patients, elicited their patients as colleagues, and were more flexible in their problem-solving as related to the nature of the illness. The less mature comparison group of physicians was more rigid and authoritarian and tended to perceive patients as stereotypes (Candee, 1977).

Other studies have demonstrated similar findings with school principals and supervisors (Sprinthall & Thies-Sprinthall, 1983). What is clear in these studies of maturity is that maturity per se does not have a direct relationship to the intelligence, age, or economic status of the adult. Maturity appears to be a product of training and is not achieved "naturally" by all human beings, as Piaget once proposed.

Neimark (1975) estimates that only 30% of the normal population functions at the abstract reasoning level. Bart (1977) suggests that abstract reasoning is obtained by these individuals in technological societies that require formal operations and have been trained through symbolically transmitted instruction. Piaget (1972) noted that not all individuals in all occupations achieved formal operations but felt that they could do so if instructed—a major concession for Piaget in reference to the sequence of his stage developmental theory, and reminiscent of the stance of Vygotsky (1978) and Luria (1982), who held that development of consciousness (a term including self, cognition, values, and perception) was dependent upon education.

Today it is commonly agreed among child development specialists that growth depends on appropriate interaction with the environment at the individual's level of development. A responsive environment takes the individual at his or her level of development and arranges events so as to further growth and acquisition of more complex skills.

It follows that if the goal of parent training is adult development—that is, the mature functioning of parents in Heath's sense—then some form of assessment of the maturation level of the parent-adult to be trained must be determined in order to define the level on which to build the training program. It becomes a problem of matching the program to the parents' maturity level (Hunt, 1974; Ulrey, 1981).

THEORIES OF STAGES
OF ADULT DEVELOPMENT

Cognitive Theories

There are several cognitive theories, the most widely known being that of Piaget. Piaget's theory has been well studied, and there is general agreement that the sequence of development follows that which he proposed: sensorimotor, preoperational, concrete operations, and formal reasoning or abstract thought. Agreement has not been reached on whether these are biologically timed stages (Zimmerman, 1983), but the order has not been challenged. Langer (1969) posits that 50% of the normal population of adults achieves the last stage. Arline (1975) has proposed a more advanced stage beyond formal operations, which she refers to as creative problem-finding. Neimark's (1975) work on the development of formal operations from a longitudinal perspective is also helpful.

The classic education model of cognition is found in the Taxonomy of Educational Objectives (Bloom, Krathwohl, & Masia, 1964), which provides a hierarchy of learning that implies a sequence but does not adhere to grade or age norms. Bloom's Taxonomy is classified as: mastery of subject matter (facts), comprehension, application, analysis, synthesis, and evaluation.

Hunt and Sullivan (1974) draw upon their earlier work and the work of Ausebel (1963) to propose an instructional stance in a conceptual matching model. Essentially, the model matches the person's development and learning style (P), with the learning environment (E), and assesses the outcome of the interaction of person and environment in terms of resulting behavior (B).

In the work of Hunt and Sullivan (1974), the levels of conceptual development are described as: a) an immature and unsocialized stage of dependent conforming, b) an independent self-reliant stage, and c) Hunt (1974) further proposed a more useful sequence for this chapter: unsocialized, impulsive, concrete dogmatic, dependent abstract, and self-directed abstract.

Duriv and Hughes (1982) present a perspective in which the parent is viewed as an information-seeker and learner. They believe that too many of the materials developed for parents do not meet their specific needs. They draw upon Hunt's (1974) conceptual model and speculation on the interaction parent's level of conceptual development and parent's child-rearing attitudes. In addition, they draw upon the Newberger (1982) proposed hierarchy of parental awareness—egotistic, conventional, subjective individualistic, and process interaction—to complete their model.

In recent work, Sameroff and Fiel (1982) have conceptualized four levels of parental constructions of the child: 1) symbiotic, 2) categorical, 3) compensating, and 4) perspective. The levels are hierarchical and, from level 1 to level 4, the parent moves from immediate here-and-now concerns in child care to viewing behavior as a result of an individual child's unique experience. The Sameroff and Fiel (1982) model is used in this chapter.

Self-Concept Ego Development

A major statement reqarding moral-ego development was made by Erikson (1963) in his eight stages of development. More recently, ego stages have been proposed by Loevinger (1976) as the presocial impulsive stage, the self-protective stage, the conformist stage, the conscientious stage, and the autonomous stage. Kohlberg's (1969) well-known sequence has been criticized for its liberal philosophy bent as truth, but support has been found for his sequence of obedience/punishment, naive/egotistic, social conformity, authority maintaining, and principles reasoning. Gilligan (1982) has presented evidence that Erikson's and Kohlberg's theories may apply to men but not to women.

A three-factor theory of interpersonal development was proposed by Schultz in the 1950s in his FIRO B scale. This scale measures the three dimensions of inclusion, exclusion, and desirability of relating to others (love) (Schultz, 1960).

There are a host of other scales to measure self-concept, values, and interpersonal relations too numerous to be mentioned here. What is clear is that a measure of psychological maturity can be assessed by using paper-and-pencil techniques as well as Heath's nomination procedure.

Models of Teaching

Joyce and Weil (1980) have presented a comprehensive set of models of teaching. These models range from didactic drill and practice to more advanced inquiry modes. Not all models have gained support, and the recent data on teaching/learning transactions support direct teaching for the comprehension of facts, and a higher ratio of indirect to direct teaching for the more advanced forms of functioning, such as analysis and synthesis. Sprinthall and Thies-Sprinthall (1983) propose that the procedures appropriate for learning school subject matter are also appropriate for the acquisition of more mature modes of independent functioning in the personal realm. Their position is the one adopted here.

The most commonly accepted principle of learning in education is to begin at the learner's level of development, and then provide instruction that matches that level. Glazer (1973) defines this notion as "assessing the entering level" of the student. D.E. Hunt (1974) proposes the same construct when he suggests the need to match the student to the instructional material. In the following section a model is constructed that attempts to match maturity level (cognitive, personal-social) and teaching styles. The scheme is presented in Table 1.

The generalization that can be made is that at lower levels of development, more direct teaching is required. Instructional techniques include lectures, reading, drill, recitation, tests, and homework. The student responds, absorbs, remembers, and rehearses. As the student acquires more sophisticated modes of functioning, the method of instruction should change to more indirect modes. At higher levels of functioning, the instructor demonstrates, questions, compares, contrasts, and examines. The student is asked to explain, demonstrate, translate, and interpret. At more advanced levels, the teacher does more observing and critiquing, while the student does more problem-solving and demonstrates his or her knowledge. At the most mature level, the teacher probes, guides, acts as a resource, reflects, extends, and analyzes. The pupil discusses, generalizes to detail, relates, compares, and abstracts. In the most advanced form, the student judges and disputes or challenges basic assumptions and makes a commitment to a mode of functioning. It should be clear that, as the student begins each high-level stage, the use of some lower-level techniques will be helpful, such as modeling, and providing examples to enable the student to move forward.

Goodlad (1983) found in his study of schools that teachers tend to use a limited set of techniques and grouping configurations, that is, they either listen or have the students work on assignments in large groups or as a total class. Teachers tend to talk and monitor. In the high schools Goodlad studied, there was little corrective feedback, less than 2%. There was also little guidance (3%), and a neutral tone was maintained 95% of the time. There was little student goal-setting, problem-solving, collaborative learning, autonomous thinking, or creativity. Given these data, it is not surprising that 30% (Neimark, 1975) to 50% (Langer, 1969) of the normal adult population does not consistently use abstract reasoning as a typical mode of thought. This fact is critically important if one accepts the notion that mature forms of functioning are a product of environmental transactions that facilitate growth.

Schooling is a powerful force in cultural evolution. Laosa (1981) has shown that the mother's years of schooling are the best predictor of the mother's child-rearing attitudes; when held constant, mother's years of schooling overrides the effects of birth order and cultural differences thought to be predictive of child-outcome variables. Years of schooling in these studies has been defined as 11 years, which has enabled these mothers to problem solve and deal with abstract modes of thought.

The Trainer's Stance

Hunt (1974) suggests that teachers adopt a three-R position: responsiveness, reciprocality, and reflexity. This allows the transfer to flow with the students' needs and development. Others, such as George Kelly (1955),

Table 1. Selected theories of adult development and implications for training adults

Bloom's Taxonomy	Cognitive skills and knowledge theorists		Self-concept ego strength theorists			Instructional stance	
	Piaget	Sameroff and Fiel	D.E. Hunt	Loevinger	Kohlberg	Teacher	Trainee
Mastery of the basic knowledge of the world	Sensorimotor	Symbiotic	Unsocialized	Presocial/impulsive	Obedience/punishment	Models, tells, and directs	Imitates, responds, explores, manipulates, and experiences
Comprehension	Preoperational	Categorical	Impulsive	Self-protective	Naive/egotistic	Lectures, drills, and provides rules/examples	Responds, absorbs, recognizes, and recalls
Application	Concrete operations	Compensating	Concrete/dogmatic	Conformist	Social conformity	Shows, facilitates, observes, and critiques	Solves and constructs
Analysis	Formal operations I	Perspective	Dependent abstract	Conscientious	Authority maintaining	Probes and guides	Discusses and uncovers
Synthesis	Formal operations II		Self-directed abstract	Autonomous	Principles reasoning	Reflects, extends, and analyzes	Generalizes, relates, and compares
Evaluation							

have postulated that the quality of our engagement in the world affects change. Thus, a supportive environment for change allows the individual to examine the set of personal constructs developed prior to entry into the class. Personal constructs provide both freedom of decision and limitation of action—freedom because the construct helps the individual deal with the meaning of events; limitation because the person can make no choice outside the system of constructs that he or she has developed. In essence, the trainer is attempting to assist the parent in adopting new personal constructs more fitting to the model of maturity that is appropriate for the culture in which the individual lives. One should be aware that giving up an old mode of thought is a painful process similar to grieving (Sprinthall & Thies-Sprinthall, 1983) or depression (Meshcheryakow, 1979). The grieving process of the parent of the handicapped child may have as much to do with the intellectual demands for new modes of operation as it has to do with the acceptance that the child is handicapped.

SUMMARY

It has been proposed that parent training is essentially a means to facilitate adult development. It has also been suggested that the construct "maturity" can serve as a guidepost for the assessment of the individual to be trained. This assessment can be made in the areas of cognitive skills, self-concept, personal values, and interpersonal skills, as a means of determining the level of functioning of the individual. Instructional strategies can then be implemented using a greater direct/indirect ratio for lower-level functioning adults and a greater indirect/direct ratio with higher-functioning individuals.

Growth is enhanced by a supportive environment that recognizes the difficulty of adopting new modes of operation (grieving/depression) and an environment that places the individual in significant role-taking responsibilities at the level of development (experience and the problem of the match). As growth proceeds, more difficult and more complex interactions can be planned, with pupils gaining new insights through the trainers' guided reflection of what has taken place (Dewey, 1938).

In any learning situation, time is a critical dimension. Parents of handicapped children will not only need the trainer's emotional support but will require time to learn, practice, and adopt new modes of thought. In mastery learning research, Bloom (1964) clearly indicated that to achieve 90%–100% mastery, the trainer must allow for a flexible time dimension for individuals to achieve the skills.

Utilizing this model, the parent trainer will not only assist parents in acquiring the skills that facilitate their children's growth, but will help these adults to develop higher levels of cognitive functioning. Both sets of skills should enhance the quality of life of the child and the adult, as well as the society in which they live.

REFERENCES

Anastasiow, N.J. Strategies and models for early childhood programs in integrated settings. In: M.J. Guralnick (ed.), *Early intervention of handicapped and nonhandicapped children*. Baltimore: University Park Press, 1978.

Anastasiow, N.J. *The adolescent parent*. Baltimore: Paul H. Brookes Publishing Co., 1982. (a)

Anastasiow, N.J. *The importance of early intervention for developmentally disabled children*. Chapel Hill, NC: Frank Porter Graham Child Development Center, 1982. (b)

Anastasiow, N.J. Adolescent pregnancy and special education, *Exceptional Children*, 1983, 49(5), 396–401.

Arline, V. Cognitive development in adulthood: A fifth stage. *Developmental Psychology*, 1975, *11*(5), 602–606.

Ausebel, D.P. *The psychology of verbal learning*. New York: Grune & Stratton, 1963.

Badger, E.D. Preparing teenage high-risk mothers. In: S. Harel (ed.), *The at-risk infant*. Amsterdam: Excerpta Medica, 1980.

Bandura, A. *Social learning theory*. Englewood Cliffs, NJ: Prentice-Hall, 1977.

Bart, W. *Piagetian cognitive theory and adult education*. Paper presented at the Adult Education Research Conference, Minneapolis, 1977.

Bloom, B. *Stability and change in human characteristics*. New York: John Wiley & Sons, 1964.

Bloom, B., Krathwohl, R., & Masia, B.B. *Taxonomy of educational objectives*. New York: John Wiley & Sons, 1964.

Bowlby, J. *Attachment and loss*, Vol. 1, Attachment. New York: Basic Books, 1969.

Candee, D. Role taking, role conception and moral reasoning as factors of good physicians' performance. *Moral Education Forum*, 1977, *2*, 14–15.

Dewey, J. *Experience and education*. New York: Colliers, 1938.

Duriv, H.F., & Hughes, R.H., Jr. Parent education: Understanding parents so that they can understand themselves and their children. In: S. Hill & B.J. Barnes (eds.), *Young children and their families*. Lexington, MA: Lexington Books, 1982.

Emde, R.N., Gaensbauer, T.J., & Harmon, R.J. *Emotional expression in infancy*. New York: International Universities Press, 1976.

Erickson, E. *Childhood and society*. New York: W.W. Norton & Co., 1963.

Field, T. Early development of infants born to teenage mothers. In: K. Scott, T. Field, & E. Robertston (eds.), *Teenage parents and their offsprings*. New York: Grune & Stratton, 1980.

Gagne, R.M. *The conditions of learning* (3rd ed.). New York: Holt, Rinehart & Winston, 1977.

Gilligan, C. *In a different voice*. Cambridge, MA: Harvard University Press, 1982.

Glazer, R. Educational psychology and education, *American Psychologist*, 1973, 557–566.

Goodlad, J.I. *A place called school*. New York: McGraw-Hill Book Co., 1983.

Gordon, I. *The infant experience*. Columbus, OH: Charles E. Merrill Publishing Co., 1975.

Heath, D.E. *Maturity and competence*. New York: Gardner, 1977.

Hunt, D.E. *Matching models in education*. Toronto: Ontario Institute for Studies in Education, 1974.

Hunt, D.E., & Sullivan, D.E. *Between psychology and education*. Hinsdale, IL: The Dryden Press, 1974.

Hunt, J.M. *Experience and intelligence*. New York: The Ronald Press, 1961.

Hunt, J.M. Psychological development: Early experience. In: M.R. Rosenzweig & L.W. Porter (eds.), *Annual review of psychology*, Vol. 30. Palo Alto, CA: Annual Reviews, Inc., 1979.

Joyce, B. & Weil, M. *Models of teaching*. Englewood Cliffs, NJ: Prentice-Hall, 1980.

Kelley, G. *The psychology of personal constructs*. New York: Norton, 1955.

Kohlberg, L. *Meaning and measurement of moral development*. Worcester, MA: Clark University Press, 1969.

Langer, J. *Theories of development*. New York: Holt, Rinehart & Winston, 1969.

Laosa, L. Maternal behavior: Sociocultural diversity in family interactions. In: R.W. Henderson (ed.), *Parent-child interaction*. New York: Academic Press, 1981.

Linder, T. *Early childhood special education: Program development and administration*. Baltimore: Paul H. Brookes Publishing Co., 1983.

Loevinger, J. *Ego development*. San Francisco: Jossey-Bass, 1976.

Luria, A.R. *Language and cognition*. New York: John Wiley & Sons, 1982.

Meshcheryakow, A. *Awakening to life*. Moscow: Progress, 1979.

Neimark, E. Intellectual development during adolescence. In: F. Horowitz (ed.), *Review of child development research*, Vol. 4. Chicago: University of Chicago Press, 1975.

Newberger, E.H. *Child abuse*. Boston: Little, Brown & Co., 1982.

Piaget, J. Intellectual evolution from adolescence to adulthood. *Human Development*, 1972, *15*, 1–12.

Piaget, J. Piaget's theory. In: P.H. Mussen (ed.), *Handbook of child psychology, Vol. 1: History, methods, and practices*. New York: John Wiley & Sons, 1983.

Sameroff, A., & Fiel, L.A. Parental concepts of development. In: I. Sigel (ed.), *Parental belief system*. Hillsdale, NJ: Lawrence Erlbaum Associates, 1982.

Schaffer, H.R. *Studies in mother-infant reaction*. New York: Academic Press, 1977.

Schultz, W.C. *FIRO B*. New York: Holt, Rinehart & Winston, 1960.

Skodak, H.M. Adult status of children with contrasting early life experience. *Monographs of the Society for Research in Child Development*, 1966, *31*(3), 1–65.

Spitz, R. *A genetic field theory of ego formation*. New York: International Universities Press, 1959.

Sprinthall, N.A., & Thies-Sprinthall, L. The teacher as an adult learner: A cognitive-developmental view. In: G. A. Griffin (ed.), *Staff development*. Chicago: National Society For The Study of Education, 1983.

Vygotsky, L.S. *Mind in society*. (M. Cole, V. John-Steiner, S. Scribner, & E. Souberman, eds.). Cambridge, MA: Harvard University Press, 1978.

Ulrey, G. Emotional development of the young handicapped child. In: N.J. Anastasiow (ed.), *Socioemotional development*. San Francisco: Jossey-Bass, 1981.

Werner, E.E., & Smith, R. *Vulnerable but invincible: A longitudinal study of resilient children and youth*. New York: McGraw-Hill Book Co., 1982.

Zimmerman, B.J. Social learning theory: A contextualist account of cognitive functioning. In: C.J. Brainerd (ed.), *Recent advances in cognitive developmental theory*. New York: Springer-Verlag, 1983.

The At-Risk Infant: Psycho/Socio/Medical Aspects
edited by Shaul Harel, M.D., and Nicholas J. Anastasiow, Ph.D.
Copyright © 1985   Paul H. Brookes Publishing Co., Inc.   Baltimore • London

Chapter 2

Parent Training
An Overview and Synthesis

MICHAEL L. HANES, PH.D.
University of South Carolina, Columbia, South Carolina

P ARENT TRAINING, PERHAPS MORE THAN ANY
other form of social or educational intervention, has gained widespread acceptance and
has become an important component in intervention programs focusing on the at-risk child.
The diverse body of literature on parent training ranges from descriptions of programs for
parents of poverty children (Gordon, Hanes, &
Lamme, 1975), and parents of high-risk infants
(Anastasiow, 1982; Goldberg, 1978; Scott,
Field, & Robertson, 1981), to programs for
abusive parents (Conger & Lahey, 1982). Four
questions guided the literature search and the
organization of this chapter.

1. What is the nature of the needs that parent-
   training programs try to address?
2. What is the content provided by these
   programs?
3. What are the developing trends in the
   delivery of parent-training services?
4. What are the long-term effects of parent
   training?

This chapter briefly summarizes the literature
related to each of these questions.

NEEDS FOR PARENT TRAINING

Over several generations, parent training has
served a variety of purposes (Gordon, 1977).
Longitudinal studies of school achievement

and the results indicating the significance of
home environment variables, as summarized
by Gordon (1976) and Goodson and Hess
(1975), are partially responsible for the increased interest in working with parents to
improve children's school achievement. In addition, growing interest in early intervention
with young children with identifiable developmental delays has led to the rapid expansion
and development of parent-training programs.
Cataldo (1980), Honig (1980), Levitt and
Cohen (1976), and Lillie and Trohanis (1976)
provide excellent reviews of early childhood
and special education parent-training programs.

A major factor distinguishing programs is
whether the programmatic focus is on the parent or the child or the family unit. The following sections discuss this distinction, and
compare the delivery system and preferred
content for each type of program.

Child-Centered Needs

The most common reason for initiating parent
training has been the recognition of a child-
centered need. Parent-training programs have
been developed to deal with a wide range of
child problems, including language disorders,
developmental delays, and behavior disorders.
Child-focused programs view the parent as the
primary recipient of program-directed training,

since the parent is seen as an important factor influencing the child's development. The most straightforward of these programs identify specific skills to be taught to the parent. In turn, the parent teaches the skill to the child. That is, the parent is an important conduit in the delivery system for the program to effectively intervene in the child's development.

In recent years, behavior analysis, behavior management, and behavior modification techniques have dominated the literature on child-focused parent-training programs. In a recent review of programs aimed at improving achievement of learning disabled children, Shapero and Forbes (1981) suggest that a behavioral orientation is a common approach to parent training in this area. They concluded, however, that the most effective behavior management training programs included components supporting parent development, i.e., counseling sessions. Examples include Patterson's (1980) work with aggressive children, and the work of Ward and Kellett (1982) with language disordered children.

A smaller number of studies have attempted to train parents in clinical strategies typically employed by professionals, such as play therapy (Ginsberg, 1976; McClannahan, Krantz, & McGee, 1982). As with behavioral management approaches, the parent is trained in a set of skills to be applied to a child-based problem.

Parent Needs

The movement to expand parent training is also reflected in the increased number of programs that focus directly on the parent. These programs attempt to modify the parent's behavior with an indirect effect on the child. The early work of the Parent Child Development Centers (Andrews, Blumenthal, Johnson, Kahn, Ferguson, Lasater, Malone, & Wallace, 1982) focusing on positive maternal behavior can be placed in this category. Other examples include work with adolescent mothers (Badger, 1981; Thompson, Cappleman, Conrad, & Jordan, 1982), abusive parents (Conger & Lahey, 1982; Wolfe, Stlawren, Graves, Brehony, Bradlyn, & Kelly, 1982), and drug dependent mothers (Lief, 1981).

Programs working with parents who are attempting to deal with a difficult or complex child problem are discovering that parents are likely to have personal adjustment problems that require specific attention (Parikh, 1981). In some cases, parent behaviors and attitudes may perpetuate dysfunctional behavior in the child (Conture, 1982). Canino and Reeve (1980) provide an excellent discussion of this last point.

Family-Oriented Needs

A third category of parent-training programs recognizes that parent-child interaction occurs within the context of a family environment. These programs focus on intrafamily processes and attempt to influence the behavior and attitudes of family members through parent-training strategies.

Both behaviorally oriented training (Rinn, Markle, & Wise, 1981) and training in counseling techniques (Euster, Ward, & Varner, 1982; Levant & Geer, 1981) have been equally effective in developing postive outcomes when working with foster parents. Schwebel, Moreland, Steinkohl, Lentz, & Stewart (1982) have reviewed programs for divorced parents and concluded that contingency management *and* communication skills are important content for training divorced parents. Hill, Raley, & Snyder (1982) argue for the need to include communication skills in programs for parents who are dealing with complex problems in the family.

CONTENT OF PARENT TRAINING

Skill-Oriented Programs

A wide range of programs and individual studies can be summarized in a broad category of *skill-oriented* programs. Included are programs that teach behavior management techniques such as observing and recording language behavior (Waters & Siegel, 1982) as well as the use of reinforcement and timeout techniques (Griest, Forehand, Rogers, Breiner, Furey, & Williams, 1982). A second subset of programs included in this category are those that attempt to teach the parent skills that are then taught to the child. These include programs training parents to teach the child self-help skills (Feldman, Manella, Apodaca, & Varni, 1982) or social and academic competencies (Firth, 1982; Johnson, 1981).

Several reviews of skill-oriented parent training are generally supportive of its efficacy (Berkowitz & Graziono, 1972; Forehand & Atkeson, 1977; Johnson & Katz, 1973; O'Dell, 1974). Treatment effects obtained through skill-oriented parent training, however, have proved difficult to generalize across behaviors, settings, and time (Forehand & Atkeson, 1977).

Process-Oriented Programs

Process-oriented programs are distinguished by an emphasis on interaction between parent and child, and an attempt to engage the parent in an analytic mode and to reflect on the interaction. A widely known program in this category is the Parent Effectiveness Training (PET) program (Gordon, 1975). The PET program trains parents in listening techniques, communication skills, and child-parent problem-solving. The Adlerian Approach to parent training and Systematic Training for Effective Parenting are also well-known process-oriented approaches.

Although practically no data are available on these specific programs, Eyberg and Robinson (1982) report significant effects for parents and children after an interaction-based training program. In addition, Eyberg and Robinson found significant results for untreated siblings.

Programs Oriented to Child Development

Child development-oriented programs emphasize training based on the notion that knowledge of the normally developing child is a necessary prerequisite for parenting. Included in this group are programs such as *Exploring Childhood* and *Footsteps: A Television Series on Parenting,* as well as Facilitating Early Environment for Development (Anastasiow, 1977). The available evidence suggests that child development knowledge can be effec-

tively disseminated to a wide range of audiences via a variety of methods. There may be periods when parents are more receptive to new information, and additional research is needed to determine if there are optimal periods for learning.

TRENDS IN SERVICE DELIVERY

While the traditional dichotomy of home-based versus center-based programs still holds true, the variations and combinations of these delivery strategies have been greatly expanded. Center-based programs now include programs that have been installed in pediatric practices, hospital settings, and community health agencies. Home-based programs have been expanded to include not only the professional parent educator as a home visitor, but also health care professionals, social workers, and other parents.

Perhaps the most significant development in parent-training delivery, however, is the implementation of parent-training programs within pediatric practices (Eastman & Mesibov, 1981; Koota, Kuritzke, Grijnszt, Rubin, & Teicher, 1982; and Petrie, Kratochwill, Bergan, & Nicholson, 1981). These programs range from teaching specific academic skills to comprehensive parent education classes.

EFFECTS OF PARENT TRAINING

Given the variety of parent education programs used to deal with the range of problems, it is probably safe to assume that there is much known about developing, implementing, and operating parent education programs. Unfortunately, there is much less empirical evidence to suggest that a given program will have a predictable, consistent effect. At the same time, parent training is attributed with producing short-term positive effects on a variety of parent and child measures. In fact, given the heterogeneous nature of the problems studied, it is somewhat surprising that parent training has been so successful with such a wide range of parent and child problems.

The fact that parents continue to develop and change, as well as the fact that the parent-child relationship changes and develops, seems to be clearly supported by the literature. For example, Maisto & German (1981) reported that maternal locus of control, which did not relate to child gains immediately after treatment, did relate to child cognitive and language gains that occurred after the treatment was completed. As another example, Ferland & Piper (1981) provided prenatal training on sensorimotor development and reported a significant impact on home environment at 3 months postnatal, but no significant impact at 8 months postnatal.

With this current knowledge of short-term outcomes of parent training, more appropriate questions about the nature of long-term impacts can now begin to be asked. The first priority should be the implementation of studies to examine a variety of potential long-term effects.

OUTCOMES AND THE FUTURE

After a number of years of providing parent-training services, the pieces of research findings are beginning to form an outline for future training programs and research studies.

Most importantly, the understanding of parents and the parenting process has grown immensely. Expanding the parenting behavior repertoire, for example, may be accomplished effectively through a series of modeling, shaping and feedback techniques. Maintaining these behaviors, however, may require on-going training and support in the form of small group discussions or seminar sessions.

In terms of information, the evidence from programs providing training in discrete, identifiable knowledge, principles, or techniques suggests that a variety of delivery modes are equally effective. With the broad and well-established information base on children's development, it seems most appropriate that all parent-training programs contain an extensive curriculum in child development.

Additional studies in the area of the timing and content of training are critical for the development of significant improvements in programming. Parallel to the need to examine the issues of timing and content is the recognition that parent training may have a multi-dimensional impact on the parent, child, and family unit. The recognition that a number of variables affect parent and child behavior leads to the recognition of a need for multi-dimensional measurements of parent-training program outcomes.

The important questions have only partial answers, but the questions are clear on what needs to be studied. There is general agreement that many parents/children/families need support to function effectively. Still to be determined are:

1. What needs to be provided in terms of support?
2. What are the most effective means of support?
3. Among the effective means, what are the most efficient means of providing support?

REFERENCES

Anastasiow, N.J. (ed.). *Preventing tomorrow's handicapped child today.* Bloomington: Institute for Child Study, Indiana University, 1977.

Anastasiow, N.J. *The adolescent parent,* Baltimore: Paul H. Brookes Publishing Co., 1982.

Andrews, S.R., Blumenthal, J.B., Johnson, D.L., Kahn, A.J., Ferguson, C.J., Lasater, T.M., Malone, P.E., & Wallace, D.B. The skills of mothering: A study of parent child development centers. *Monographs of the Society for Research in Child Development,* 1982, *47*(6), 83.

Badger, E. Effects of parent education program on teenage mothers and their offspring. In: K.G. Scott, T. Field, & E. Robertson (eds.), *Teenage parents and their offspring.* New York: Grune & Stratton, 1981.

Berkowitz, B.P., & Graziano, A.M. Training parents as behavior therapists: A review. *Behavior Research and Therapy,* 1972, *10,* 297–317.

Canino, F.J., & Reeve, R.F. General issues in working with parents of handicapped children. In: R.R. Abidin (ed.), *Parent education and intervention handbook.* Springfield, IL: Charles C Thomas, 1980.

Cataldo, C.Z. The parent as learner: Early childhood parent programs. *Educational Psychologist,* 1980, *15*(3), 172–186.

Conger, R.D., & Lahey, B.B. Behavioral intervention for child abuse. *Behavior Therapist,* 1982, *5*(2), 49–53.

Conture, E.G. Youngsters who stutter: Diagnosis, parent counseling, and referral. *Journal of Developmental and Behavioral Pediatrics,* 1982, *3*(3), 163–169.

Eastman, J.N., & Mesibov, G.B. Family interventions in a private pediatric practice. *Journal of Marital and Family Therapy,* 1981, *7*(4), 461–466.

Euster, S.D., Ward, V.P., & Varner, J.G. Adapting counseling techniques to foster parent training. *Child Welfare,* 1982, *61*(6), 375–382.

Eyberg, S.M., & Robinson, E.A. Parent-child interaction training: Effects on family functioning. *Journal of Clinical Child Psychology,* 1982, *11*(2), 130–137.

Feldman, W.S., Manella, K.J., Apodaca, L., & Varni, J.W. Behavioral group parent training in spina bifida. *Journal of Clinical Child Psychology,* 1982, *11*(2), 144–150.

Ferland, F., & Piper, M.C. Evaluation of a sensory-motor education program for "parents-to-be." *Child Care, Health and Development,* 1981, *7*(5), 245–254.

Firth, H. The effectiveness of parent workshops in a mental handicap service. *Child Care, Health and Development,* 1982, *8*(2), 77–91.

Forehand, R., & Atkeson, B.M. Generality of treatment effects with parents as therapists: A review of assessment and implementation procedures. *Behavior Therapy,* 1977, *8*, 575–593.

Ginsberg, B.G. Parents as therapeutic agents: The usefulness of filial therapy in a community mental health center. *American Journal of Community Psychology,* 1976, *4*(1), 47–54.

Goldberg, S. Prematurity: Effects on parent-infant interaction. *Journal of Pediatric Psychology,* 1978, *3*(3), 137–144.

Goodson, B., & Hess, R. *Parents as teachers of young children: An evaluative review of some contemporary concepts and programs.* Stanford, CA: School of Education, Stanford University, 1975.

Gordon, I. What are effective home learning environments for school age children? In: M. Hanes, I. Gordon, & B. Brievogel (eds.), *Update: The first ten years of life.* Gainesville: Division of Continuing Education, University of Florida, 1976.

Gordon, I.J. Parent education and parent involvement: Retrospect and prospect. *Childhood Education,* 1977, *54*(2), 71–79.

Gordon, I.J., Hanes, M.L., & Lamme, L. *Parent oriented homebased early childhood programs.* Gainesville: University of Florida, 1975.

Gordon, T. *Parent effectiveness training.* New York: New American Library, 1975.

Griest, D.L., Forehand, R., Rogers, T., Breiner, J., Furey, W., & Williams, C.A. Effects of parent enhancement therapy on the treatment outcome and generalization of a parent training program. *Behavior Research and Therapy,* 1982, *20*(5), 429–436.

Hill, B.M., Raley, J.R., & Snyder, D.K. Group intervention with parents of psychiatrically hospitalized children. *Family Relations: Journal of Applied Family and Child Studies,* 1982, *31*(3), 317–322.

Honig, A.S. Parent involvement and the development of children with special needs. *Early Child Development*

and Care, 1980, *6*(3–4), 179–199.

Johnson, C.A., & Katz, R.C. Using parents as change agents for their children: A review. *Journal of Child Psychology and Psychiatry,* 1973, *14,* 181–200.

Johnson, D.L. The influence of an intensive parent education program on behavioral continuity of mothers and children. *Child Study Journal,* 1981, *11*(4), 187–199.

Koota, I.R., Kuritzke, F. A., Grijnszt, J.M., Rubin, G.S., & Teicher, P.K. A parent education and support program in a private pediatric practice. *Journal of Developmental and Behavioral Pediatrics.* 1982, *3*(3), 159–162.

Levant, R.F., & Geer, M. F. A systematic skills approach to the selection and training of foster parents as mental health paraprofessionals: I. project overview and selection component. *Journal of Community Psychology,* 1981, *9*(3), 224–230.

Levitt, E., & Cohen, S. Educating parents of children with special needs: Approaches and issues. *Young Children,* 1976, *31*(4), 263–272.

Lief, N.R. Parenting and child services for drug dependent women. *National Institute on Drug Abuse: Treatment Research Monograph Series,* 1981, 455–498.

Lillie, D., & Trohanis, P. (eds.). *Teaching parents to teach.* New York: Walker Press, 1976.

McClannahan, L.E., Krantz, P.J., & McGee, G.G. Parents as therapists for autistic children: A model for effective parent training. *Analysis and Intervention in Developmental Disabilities,* 1982, *2*(2–3), 223–252.

Maisto, A.A., & German, M.L. Maternal locus of control and developmental gain demonstrated by high risk infants: A longitudinal analysis. *Journal of Psychology,* 1981, *109*(2), 213–221.

O'Dell, S. Training parents in behavior modification: A review. *Psychological Bulletin,* 1974, *81,* 418–433.

Parikh, J.K. An experiment with helping parents of developmentally handicapped children. *Child Psychiatry Quarterly,* 1981, *14*(3), 79–84.

Patterson, G.R. Mothers: The unacknowledged victims. *Monographs of the Society for Research in Child Development,* 1980, *45*(5), 64.

Petrie, P.A., Kratochwill, T.R., Bergan, J.R., & Nicholson, G.I. Teaching parents to teach their children: Applications in the pediatric setting. *Journal of Pediatric Psychology,* 1981, *6*(3), 275–292.

Rinn, R.C., Markle, A., & Wise, M.J. Positive parent training for foster parents: A one-year follow-up. *Behavioral Counseling Quarterly,* 1981, *1*(3), 213–220.

Schwebel, A.I., Moreland, J., Steinkohl, R., Lentz, S., & Stewart, J. Research-based interventions with divorced families. *Personnel and Guidance Journal,* 1982, *60*(9), 523–528.

Scott, K., Field, T., & Robertson, E. (eds.). *Teenage parents and their offspring.* New York: Grune & Stratton, 1981.

Shapero, S., & Forbes, C. R. A review of involvement programs for parents of learning disabled children. *Journal of Learning Disabilities,* 1981, *14*(9), 499–504.

Thompson, R.J., Cappleman, M.W., Conrad, H.H., & Jordan, W.B. Early intervention program for adolescent mothers and their infants. *Journal of Developmental and Behavioral Pediatrics,* 1982, *3*(1), 18–21.

Ward, S., & Kellett, B. Language disorder resolved. *British Journal of Disorders of Communication,* 1982, *17*(2), 33–52.

Waters, J.M., & Siegel, L.V. Parent recording of speech

production of developmentally delayed toddlers. *Education & Treatment of Children*, 1982, *5*(2), 109–120.

Wolfe, D.A., Stlawren, J., Graves, K., Brehony, K., Bradlyn, D., & Kelly, J.A. Intensive behavioral parent training for a child abusive mother. *Behavior Therapy*, 1982, *13*(4), 438–451.

The At-Risk Infant: Psycho/Socio/Medical Aspects
edited by Shaul Harel, M.D., and Nicholas J. Anastasiow, Ph.D.
Copyright © 1985   Paul H. Brookes Publishing Co., Inc.   Baltimore • London

Chapter 3

High-Risk Birth

Effects of Illness and Prematurity on the
Mother-Infant Interaction and the Mother's
Social Support System

NATHAN A. FOX, PH.D.
University of Maryland, College Park, Maryland
CANDICE FEIRING, PH.D.
Rutgers Medical School, New Brunswich, New Jersey

D URING THE LAST DECADE, NUMEROUS STUD-
ies have demonstrated the dynamic process whereby neonatal infant characteristics
affect either concurrent or subsequent caregiver behaviors to produce a unique interaction
relationship (Bell, 1968; Brazelton, 1978; Field,
1979; Lewis & Rosenblum, 1974; Osofsky &
Danzger, 1974). The relationship between
neonatal behavior and subsequent maternal
social-interactive behavior has been of particular interest to researchers studying high-
risk infants. Indeed, there has been a major
effort to examine the effect of certain high-risk
characteristics on subsequent maternal and infant behaviors (Bakeman & Brown, 1980;
DiVitto & Goldberg, 1979; Field, 1977).

In addition to examining the effect of neonatal characteristics on the mother-child interaction, researchers have recently underscored
the importance of the mother's social support
network and its influence on caretaking behavior (Bronfenbrenner, 1977; Cochran &
Brassard, 1979; Lewis & Feiring, 1979). Several investigators (Crnic, Greenberg, Ragozin,

Robinson, & Basham, 1983; Crockenberg,
1981; Lewis, Feiring, & Brooks-Gunn, in
press; Powell, 1979) have noted that the quality
of a child's socialization experiences is related
to the family's interaction with its social network, and that parental social support has the
potential for mediating stress. For example,
Crnic et al. (1983) found that mothers who
report greater support have infants who show
more responsiveness and affect expression,
while mothers who report more stress have less
responsive infants. Further, Crnic et al. (1983)
found that support acted as a moderator of the
effect of maternal stress on infant responsiveness and that social support was related to
positive maternal attitudes and behavior.

INFANT CHARACTERISTICS AND
THE MOTHER-CHILD INTERACTION

The birth of a preterm or sick infant is acknowledged as a stressful event (Beckwith & Cohen,
1978; DiVitto & Goldberg, 1979; Holmes,
Nagy, Slaymaker, Sosnowski, Prinz, & Pas-

The research reported on in this chapter was supported by a contract, #300-77-0303, awarded to Michael Lewis from
the Bureau for the Education of the Handicapped. The writing of this chapter was supported by a Graduate Research Board
Award to Nathan A. Fox from the University of Maryland.

ternak, 1982). Postnatal illness may contribute to the interactive difficulties between mothers and their infants and it may alter the mothers' caregiving behavior. For example, Field (1977) found that mothers of at-risk infants spent more time stimulating their infants during a face-to-face interaction than mothers of healthy infants. DiVitto and Goldberg (1979) found interactive differences between mothers of sick and healthy preterms, and Brachfeld, Goldberg, & Sloman (1980) reported that sick preterm infants were less responsive and more irritable than healthy preterms. Beckwith and Cohen (1978) observed preterm infants with varying degrees of medical complications at 1 month corrected age. They reported that infants who experienced a more hazardous medical course received more overall caretaking behavior. The authors interpret these results to indicate that mothers of sick preterm infants attempt to compensate for their infants' lack of responsiveness and early illness with greater caretaking behaviors.

The above studies demonstrate that postnatal illness and prematurity seem to affect the early mother-child interaction. What is not clear is whether the infant's illness, immaturity, or the mother-child interaction is responsible for differences in subsequent infant and caregiver behavior. It is important in high-risk infant research to sort out differences in infant and maternal behavior due to transient illness versus longer term organic problems. Infants who were ill in the postnatal period and who undergo no apparent handicap may recover behaviorally; mothers of infants who were sick, however, may continue to treat their infants differently because of the initial experience with postnatal illness. In this regard, the response of the social support system seems crucial. Relatives, friends, and neighbors may be hesitant or be unsure as to the type of support they can give to parents whose infant may or may not live or whose birth condition may lead to permanent handicap. The type of response of the social support system may provide the mother with the means to cope with the early

stress of the high-risk birth or it may isolate the mother even further. Clearly, the response of the network will have an effect on the mother's interactive behavior with her infant.

During the period of 1977–1981, data were collected on a sample of high-risk infants and their families in an attempt to answer some of the questions posed here and in the literature. The purpose of this chapter is to present some of the initial findings of this research with particular emphasis on the effect of neonatal characteristics on mother-child interaction as well as the response of the social support system to high-risk birth and possible implications of that support for social interaction.

Characteristics of the Study Group

The infants in the research study were born at a large, urban hospital in New York City. The infants were classified by their gestational age and postnatal medical outcome into four groups: healthy preterm; RDS preterm; sick term; and healthy term.

The healthy preterm group consisted of 29[1] babies whose gestational age was less than 37 weeks and whose birth weight was less than 2,200 grams. Gestational age was assessed by the Dubowitz exam (Dubowitz, Dubowitz, & Goldberg, 1970). All infants were appropriate for gestational age and singleton birth. These infants suffered no medical complications in the postnatal period.

Twenty-eight preterm infants made up the RDS preterm group. They had the same age and weight characteristics as the healthy preterm group, but were diagnosed as suffering from severe respiratory distress syndrome (RDS). RDS was defined by a positive chest X ray, and at least three of the following: 1) grunting, 2) flaring, 3) retractions, 4) necessity of mechanical ventilation (respirator) or continuous positive airway pressure (CPAP).

A third group of full-term infants (between 38 and 40 weeks gestational age, birth weight greater than 2,500 grams) experienced birth asphyxia during labor and delivery ($n = 20$). Asphyxia was defined by three criteria: 1) Ap-

---

[1]The number of subjects presented in this chapter varies from section to section due to certain selection criteria and missing data.

gar score of 4 or less at 5 minutes, 2) respiratory assistance for a minimum of 4 hours, and 3) evidence of metabolic acidosis (pH less than 7.2 in blood gas during the first hour of life).

Finally, a full-term healthy control group ($n = 28$) was selected. These infants were selected on several criteria: 1) 40 weeks gestational age, 2) birth weight greater than 2,500 grams, 3) Apgar score of 8 or greater at 5 minutes, and 4) no medical or neurological complications.

Table 1 presents the characteristics of the infants in the study. Male and female infants were equally distributed within each of the groups. Analyses of differences based on sex of the infant did not reveal any significant findings and the data were collapsed across sex of the child.

Mothers of the healthy term group were matched with mothers of the three risk groups according to income, occupation, and education of both parents, as well as family size and ethnicity. The families across the four groups were all poor, inner-city residents of New York City. Sixty-five percent were Hispanic, 28% were black and 7% were Caucasian. Most of the families were small in size and were comprised of a husband, wife, and two children (including the infant in the study). Between groups analyses of these characteristics indicated no differences across diagnostic group in parental education, age, marital status, occupation, income, or family size.

Mothers who had given birth to a preterm infant or a sick term infant were contacted 2–3 days after the birth of their child. At that time, the scope of the longitudinal study was presented to them and their signed consent was obtained. The staff of the project were all bilingual (Spanish and English) and interviews and testing took place in the mothers' language of choice.

The infants were seen first in the neonatal period as close to term (40 weeks conceptional age) as possible. At that time, they were assessed with the Brazelton Neonatal Behavioral Assessment Scale (NBAS) (Brazelton, 1973). Infants and their mothers were seen again at 3 months corrected or conceptional age, when they were videotaped together in a free-play situation. At that time, a detailed interview concerning each mother's social network took place.

The first set of data to be presented involved analysis of the infant's behavior on the NBAS and the relation of these responses to 3-month mother and infant interactive behavior. These relationships were analyzed in some detail on 62 infants by Jamie Greene (Greene, Fox, & Lewis, 1983).

NBAS at the Neonatal Period

The NBAS was administered to all infants by one of three trained examiners. Each of the examiners had been trained by a certified Brazelton trainer to ensure reliability ($r = .90$ across items) with both term and preterm infant samples. Testing was performed in an infant laboratory adjacent to the neonatal intensive care unit.

The preterm form of the NBAS was used in scoring the premature infants (Als, Tronick, & Brazelton, 1976). This form contains the original 27 behavioral items, the 13 reflex and

Table 1. Description of infant characteristics

Characteristics	Healthy preterm X̄ (S.D.)	Sick preterm X̄ (S.D.)	Sick full-term X̄ (S.D.)	Healthy full-term X̄ (S.D.)
Gestational age (weeks)	34.5 (1.8)	31.1 (3.0)	39.9 (1.6)	40 (.8)
Birth weight (grams)	1,921 (205)	1,363 (401)	3,443 (623)	3,594 (554)
Age at NBAS (days)	24 (8.5)	47 (27)	9 (4)	3 (2)
Conceptional age (weeks)	38 (1.83)	38 (2.65)	41 (1.93)	40 (.97)
Postnatal age at 3-month interaction (months)	3.70 (.82)	4.94 (1.12)	3.06 (.25)	3.12 (.34)
Corrected age for prematurity (months)	2.5	3	3	3

neurological items and, in addition, qualifying items that are scored along with the original NBAS material. In order to maximize the sensitivity of the NBAS in detecting behavioral differences, the data were analyzed with the seven-cluster approach suggested by Lester (Lester, Als, & Brazelton, 1978) using a seven- rather than a three-point scale (cf. Jacobson, Fein, Jacobson, & Schwartz, 1984). This approach reflects the pattern of most reported factor analytic solutions for both term (Sameroff, Krafchuk, & Bakow, 1978) and preterm (Sostek, Davitt, Renzi, Born, & Kiely, in press) infants.

Table 2 presents the data for each of the four groups for the clusters. Each of the Lester clusters was analyzed with a 2 (healthy/sick) by 2 (term/preterm) analysis of variance.

Three of the seven analyses revealed main effects for health: orientation ($F(1,58) = 3.81$, $p < .05$), state regulation ($F(1,58) = 7.61$, $p < .003$), and reflex ($F(1,58) = 10.94$, $p < .001$). Healthy infants displayed better orientation scores, state regulation, and fewer deviant reflexes than infants who were sick in the postnatal period. Three of the analyses revealed a significant main effect for maturity: motor ($F(1,58) = 3.75, p < .05$), autonomic regulation ($F(1,58) = 8.17, p < .001$), and reflex ($F(1,58) = 8.26, p < .006$). Preterm infants displayed poorer motor control, more abnormal reflexes, and less autonomic regulation than infants born at term. There were no significant interactions in any of the analyses.

Mother-Infant Interaction at 3 Months

As part of their 3-month assessment, mother and infant were videotaped together for 15 minutes in a playroom setting. The videotapes were coded with a behavioral checklist (Lewis & Lee-Painter, 1974). Analyses of variance with health (healthy/sick) and maturity (term/preterm) as factors were computed on a set of summary variables. Table 3 presents the means and standard deviations for each of these variables for all four groups. Results of these analyses revealed a main effect of health for infant look/gaze behavior ($F(1,58) = 4.06$, $p < .05$). Healthy infants looked longer at their mothers during the play session than sick infants. Significant main effects for maturity revealed that mothers of preterm infants were, overall, more responsive to their infants than mothers of term infants ($F(1,58) = 4.70$, $p < .03$) and, in particular, were more vocally responsive. Significant interactions of health and maturity revealed that sick-term infants received the most proximal ($F(1,58) = 4.43$, $p < .05$) and kinesthetic ($F(1,58) = 4.53$, $p < .05$) stimulation but also the least affective ($F(1,58) = 3.92, p < .05$) and distal stimulation ($F(1,58) = 3.34, p < .07$).

Relationship between Neonatal Characteristics and 3-Month Interaction

In order to identify the significant variance in maternal and infant behavior at 3 months that was accounted for by neonatal characteristics as measured by the NBAS, separate multiple regressions entering each of the six Lester clusters were computed on the infant and maternal summary behaviors. The orientation cluster was the only cluster that accounted for a significant portion of the variance in the outcome variables of infant fret/cry (18%:$F(1,58)$

Table 2. Measures of neonatal NBAS ratings and Postnatal Complications Scale for all four groups

	Healthy preterm (n = 14)	Sick preterm (n = 16)	Sick term (n = 16)	Healthy term (n = 16)	Total sample (N = 62)
Lester clusters					
Habituation	5.67 (.60)	6.42 (1.76)	5.77 (1.67)	5.20 (1.18)	5.76 (1.43)
Orientation	5.52 (1.87)	4.39 (1.35)	4.73 (1.60)	5.20 (1.52)	4.24 (1.60)
Motor	4.46 (1.15)	4.50 (1.10)	4.61 (1.12)	5.37 (.55)	4.74 (1.05)
State regulation	5.14 (1.39)	3.77 (1.09)	4.66 (1.55)	5.41 (1.23)	4.73 (1.43)
Autonomic regulation	5.96 (1.75)	6.72 (1.33)	4.28 (2.37)	5.50 (2.47)	5.60 (2.19)
Range	4.09 (.95)	4.39 (.54)	4.19 (.42)	4.17 (.89)	4.21 (.71)
Reflex	3.71 (3.14)	6.75 (2.74)	4.75 (3.32)	1.69 (1.49)	4.24 (3.27)
Postnatal Complications Scale	110 (35)	65 (11)	73 (12)	140 (30)	97 (31)

Table 3. Summary of infant-mother variables for all four groups

	Healthy preterm	Sick preterm	Sick term	Healthy term
General behavior				
Infant				
Fret/cry	20.21 (17.77)	23.50 (23.30)	16.12 (14.27)	16.31 (14.79)
Vocalize	27.57 (22.83)	27.81 (17.80)	17.87 (17.64)	27.62 (13.19)
Look/gaze	39.71 (17.19)	26.44 (17.38)	21.50 (18.01)	25.75 (19.75)
Mother				
General	231.28 (48.07)	228.75 (64.60)	239.12 (36.64)	246.25 (37.79)
Proximal	93.50 (42.52)	79.87 (42.80)	109.31 (38.97)	79.50 (38.02)
Distal	156.07 (52.52)	172.44 (47.85)	139.75 (44.82)	165.69 (36.28)
Kinesthetic	58.28 (44.24)	44.50 (41.75)	79.25 (35.40)	52.75 (25.69)
Affective	21.64 (23.29)	24.19 (24.86)	17.69 (18.60)	41.44 (34.63)
Proportion of responsivity				
Infant				
General	.10 (.23)	.12 (.19)	.12 (.27)	.17 (.23)
Mother				
General	.06 (.15)	.07 (.22)	.05 (.04)	.015 (.01)
Proximal	.02 (.03)	.018 (.01)	.06 (.03)	.08 (.01)
Vocal	.19 (.07)	.18 (.09)	.12 (.01)	.14 (.001)

$= 13.01$, $p < .01$), proportion of maternal general responsivity ($10\%:F(1,58) = 6.41$, $p < .03$), proportion of maternal proximal responsivity ($6\%:F(1,58) = 5.40$, $p < .03$), and proportion of maternal vocal responsivity ($8\%:F(1,58) = 4.06$, $p < .05$). None of the clusters by themselves or in combination accounted for a significant portion of the variance in any of the other summary mother or infant variables.

In order to determine the unique contribution of infant orientation behavior, a second set of multiple regressions was computed holding birth weight, gestational age, and infant postnatal complications score constant.

The results of these analyses revealed, first, that orientation accounted for a significant portion of the variance of the infant's fret/cry behavior at 3 months even while holding infant birth weight, gestational age, and PCS scores constant. Second, infant orientation behavior, measured on the NBAS, accounted for a significant portion of the variance in the mother's overall and proximal responsive behavior at 3 months even while holding birth weight, gestational age, and PCS constant.

These data, then, indicate that neonatal characteristics are related to the mother-child interaction at 3 months of age. The NBAS picked up differences in infant behavior due to maturity and illness. And, although few differences in infant behavior were found at 3 months of age, differences in maternal behavior were apparent. The most striking finding was that mothers of sick infants, and in particular sick-term infants, spent the least amount of time in social interaction and the most time in caretaking behavior as compared to the other groups. Infant alertness in the neonatal period seemed to be an important predictor of maternal behavior at 3 months. Mothers of alert infants used less proximal stimulation than mothers of infants who were rated as less attentive. And infants who were alert and attentive were less irritable in the interaction at 3 months of age. Of interest is the fact that maternal behavior continued to be influenced by the birth history of the child even though at 3 months few infant behavioral differences were found. It seems that mothers of high-risk infants continued to compensate for or be affected by the initial neonatal behavior of their infant and the stress of their infant's postnatal illness.

RESPONSE OF THE SOCIAL NETWORK

In addition to videotaping mother and infant at 3 months, the mother, at that visit, was interviewed concerning the nature of her social network and the type of support she had received. A standard questionnaire was administered, individually, to each mother. A series of questions was asked to provide information about who gave what kind of support. Specifically, within each of four categories of support (goods, services, advice, and financial), the mother was asked to name any person, describe his or her relationship to her (relative, friend, neighbor, coworker), and tell what was given. The mothers were given a description of the type of support for each category: goods, e.g., clothing, furniture, baby supplies; services, e.g., baby-sitting, household chores; advice, e.g., medical, parenting information, emotional; and financial, i.e., amount of money. The mother was free to list the identity of any person who may have provided assistance. After the mother had completed her list, she was always asked if there was anyone else she could think of who had provided assistance in a category. For subsequent data analysis, the lists of persons were classified into five groups: father, relatives (both father's and mother's relatives), close friends, neighbors, and coworkers.

Mothers were also asked to provide demographic information such as occupation, education, and income. In addition, information on the frequency of contact between mother and close friends both in close proximity and outside the neighborhood was obtained.

The interviews were not conducted to explore the mother's feelings or expectations regarding the assistance received. Instead, the interviews revolved around a standard set of questions that focused on the names and exact type of assistance that was provided. Rather than obtaining a global measure of the mother's sense of support, the focus was on the specific nature of assistance, which in turn provided a detailed description of assistance. (For a complete description of the methodology, see Feiring, Fox, Jaskir, & Lewis, in preparation.)

The data obtained from the social support questionnaire consisted of the number of relatives, friends, neighbors, and total number of people reported giving goods, services, advice, and money. These data on 105 subjects are presented in Table 4. A series of 2 (term/preterm) by 2 (healthy/sick) analyses of variance was conducted on the data.

The results of these analyses revealed a

Table 4. Mean number of people reported to give support by type of support by diagnosis and for total sample.

| | Goods | | | | | Services | | | | |
	HP	SP	ST	HT	Total sample	HP	SP	ST	HT	Total sample
Father	.03	.07	0	0	.03	.66	.57	.65	.57	.61
Relatives	2.59	2.07	2.85	3.25	2.68	1.14	1.00	.95	1.61	1.19
Friends	2.10	.68	2.85	1.43	1.69	.28	.18	.35	.21	.25
Co-workers	.10	.07	.10	.11	.10	0	0	0	0	0
Neighbors	.10	.11	.45	.29	.22	.14	.11	.10	.39	.19
Total people	4.86	3.21	7.10	4.96	4.88	2.41	1.96	2.15	3.07	2.42

| | Counseling | | | | | Money | | | | |
	HP	SP	ST	HT	Total sample	HP	SP	ST	HT	Total sample
Father	.31	.39	.30	.25	.31	.07	0	.10	0	.04
Relatives	.97	1.00	.80	.85	.91	1.24	1.45	1.70	1.75	1.53
Friends	.34	.39	.50	.21	.35	.62	.19	.50	.61	.48
Co-workers	0	0	0	0	0	.17	.07	0	.11	.10
Neighbors	.03	.07	.05	.07	.06	.03	.03	.20	.18	.11
Total people	2.07	2.29	2.10	1.50	1.98	2.31	1.48	2.75	2.71	2.29

HP = Healthy preterm (n = 26); SP = Sick preterm (n = 20); ST = Sick term (n = 20); HT = Healthy term (n = 24).

pattern relating health or immaturity of the infant to the type of support the mother reported. For example, mothers of term infants reported more people giving goods than mothers of preterm ($F(1,101)$ = 5.54, p < .02). A significant maturity/health interaction indicated that mothers of sick term infants reported the most people giving goods while mothers of sick preterm reported the least ($F(1,101)$ = 6.02, p < .02). Mothers of term infants reported more friends giving goods ($F(1,101)$ = 6.05, p < .04) and specifically mothers of sick term infants reported more friends giving goods whereas mothers of sick preterm infants reported the least number of friends ($F(1,101)$ = 13.45, p < .001).

Unlike the category of support with goods, which seemed to be highest with sick term infants, support offered with services revealed a pattern related to infant health. Mothers of healthy infants reported receiving more services than mothers of sick infants ($F(1,101)$ = 3.67, p < .05). In the final two categories, advice (counseling) and financial assistance (money), there were no significant main or interaction effects in the data for who gave what kind of support.

These data display an interesting pattern. They indicate that the response of the mother's social network is related to the diagnostic status of her infant. Having a premature infant affects the frequency with which people and, in particular, one's friends give goods. Since preterm infants remain in the hospital for a prolonged period of time after their birth, they may be less visible to a mother's friends who ordinarily would visit and acknowledge the infant's birth with gifts. Of all the support categories, goods probably represents the most common type of assistance. Hence, mothers of premature infants may feel more isolated from their friends as a result of not receiving as many goods (or presents) as mothers of term infants. Importantly, mothers whose sick preterm infants remained in the hospital the longest after birth reported receiving the fewest goods from friends.

Services may represent a more ongoing type of support that may require more interpersonal interaction than goods. In the current study,

health of the baby was related to total persons reported giving services, with mothers of sick infants reporting fewer people giving services than mothers of healthy infants. Sick infants may make more unusual caregiving demands and may also be perceived as more fragile. For example, DiVitto and Goldberg (1979) found that mothers of sick infants spent more time in caretaking activities and less time in playful interaction than mothers of healthy infants. Persons in the mother's social network may not have offered their services given the increased caregiving demands of the infant. Thus, mothers of sick infants may have received fewer services (e.g., baby-sitting) when in fact they may have needed help in order to adequately care for their infant.

THE RELATIONSHIP OF SOCIAL SUPPORT TO MOTHER-INFANT INTERACTION

Having demonstrated the effect neonatal behavior may have on the mother-infant interaction and the effect neonatal characteristics may have on the response of the social network, it now is of interest to examine the potential relationship between support and mother-infant behavior. As a first step in this investigation, correlations between social support variables and maternal behavior at 3 months were computed. Table 5 presents this correlation matrix. As can be seen, there is an interesting but different pattern for both goods and services in relation to maternal behavior. Mothers who reported receiving goods were the most proximal, least distal, and least engaged in toyplay or responsive vocalization. Note that mothers of sick term infants reported receiving the most goods. And, data from their 3-month infant interaction indicated that they were indeed more involved in caregiving and less involved in positive social interaction than the other mothers (cf. Greene et al., 1983). The correlations between number of persons offering services and maternal behavior offers another set of striking findings. Here, mothers who report receiving services (and they are mothers of healthy infants) engaged in more

Table 5. Correlation matrix of social support factors with maternal behavior at 3 months of age ($N = 90$)

						Responsivity			
Type of support	Who gave	Proximal stimulation	Distal stimulation	Positive affect	Toy play	Proximal	Distal	Vocal	Play
Goods									
	Father	.07	.02	−.04	.02	.31[a]	.06	.09	−.05
	Relatives	.17	−.17	0	.07	−.16	−.15	−.13	.07
	Friends	.31[b]	−.31[b]	0	−.32[b]	−.15	−.39[b]	−.23	−.03
	Total	.35[b]	−.36[b]	−.15	−.29[b]	−.17	−.22[a]	−.36[b]	.02
Services									
	Father	.21	.03	.01	.02	−.06	0	0	.24[a]
	Relatives	0	−.20	−.06	−.07	.07	.03	−.09	.25[a]
	Friends	.14	−.12	−.14	−.14	0	−.03	−.17	.24[a]
	Total	.06	−.14	−.16	−.11	.01	.02	−.18	.38[b]
Counseling									
	Father	−.10	.08	−.19	−.07	−.06	.10	.13	.11
	Relatives	.11	.02	.21	.13	.03	−.02	.02	.03
	Friends	.10	.02	.06	−.05	−.12	−.10	−.06	−.05
	Total	.08	−.02	.11	.06	−.08	−.08	−.03	−.07
Financial									
	Father	.13	−.01	.10	.11	0	.15	.01	−.05
	Relatives	.12	−.08	−.11	−.05	−.15	−.13	−.15	−.10
	Friends	0	−.08	.10	−.08	.10	−.10	−.20[a]	−.09
	Total	.18	−.18	−.05	−.22[a]	−.16	−.11	−.11	−.20

[a]$p < .01$.
[b]$p < .001$.

playful responsivity with their infant than mothers receiving few services.

While the overall correlations between counseling support and maternal behavior did not indicate any clear pattern, a coherent design did emerge when the data for maternal relatives were divided into two categories: mother's parents and father's parents. As can be seen in Table 6, there were significant but opposite correlations between advice given by the mother's parents or the father's parents and maternal interactive behavior at 3 months. When the mother's mother gave advice, a significant

positive relationship with maternal responsivity and vocalization emerged. When a mother-in-law gave advice, an equally strong but negative relationship with maternal responsivity existed.

Finally, mothers who reported a higher number of persons giving financial assistance were themselves less vocally responsive and played less with their infants than mothers reporting fewer instances of financial help.

SUMMARY AND CONCLUSIONS

These data argue for a complex relationship between infant diagnostic status at birth, response of the social network to the infant's birth, and subsequent maternal interactive behavior at 3 months of age. The birth of a premature infant or infant who is sick immediately after birth has a lasting effect upon the mother and on her social world. Preterm infants display less motor control and reflex behavior than term infants. They remain for a prolonged period in the hospital, and members of the mother's support group are less likely to

Table 6. Correlations between type of grandparent counseling and maternal behavior at 3 months ($N = 90$)

Advice from grandparents	
Mother's parents	
Maternal responsivity	.25[a]
Maternal distal responsivity	.23[a]
Maternal vocalization	.24[a]
Father's parents	
Maternal responsivity	−.27[a]
Maternal proximal responsivity	−.24[a]
Maternal distal responsivity	−.22[a]
Maternal vocalization	−.23[a]

[a]$p < .01$.

provide goods and gifts to the mother. This is particularly true of preterm infants who were also ill. Indeed, the probable perceived threat to a sick preterm infant's viability places them in the most at-risk status in terms of social network response and maternal interactive behavior.

On the other hand, if an infant is born at term and is ill, perceived viability of that child is probably higher and the social network will respond with gifts and goods to the mother. Mothers of sick term infants respond to their infants with a high degree of caretaking and proximal behavior. This type of maternal response may, in some sense, be compensatory for the level of arousal, or ability of the infant to maintain a high degree of arousal, during an interaction. One may even speculate that the support given to a mother of a sick term infant (gifts and goods) is a signal to her of her social world's acceptance of the child's viability. This signal could encourage the mother to continue to care for her infant as opposed to giving up or turning off to an irritable or nonreactive child.

The data also indicate that having a healthy preterm infant does not seem to affect either the social network's response or the mother's interactive behavior. Having a healthy infant, term or preterm, was associated with the provision of services to the mother (e.g., babysitting, housework). Provision of these services allowed the mother time to interact more freely with her child; hence, the increased toy play and positive affect in maternal behavior

associated with healthy infants and the provision of support services.

Finally, the delicate balance between who gives what kind of support and its effect on behavior is well illustrated with regard to the mother's report of advice. The fact that opposite patterns emerged in maternal behavior depending on whether one's own mother or one's in-law provided the advice underscores the sensitivity of the interactive, behavioral data to variations in social support. Provision of support whether it be goods, services, or advice occurs within a social context and the interpretation of the support seems to be subject to the relation between provider and recipient. Future work on the influence of support systems will have to take into account the psychological as well as the physical (genetic relative or geographic distance) relationships between network members.

In sum, the current data were an attempt to investigate the effects of diagnostic status (postnatal illness and immaturity) of newborn infants on the mother and her social world. Maternal behavior at 3 months as observed in a 15-minute interactive session was chosen as an outcome measure for this aspect of the study. The data indicated that illness and immaturity had different effects on maternal behavior as well as on the response of the mother's social support system. The results highlighted a complex interaction that underscored the powerful effect perinatal stress, and illness in particular, may have on the mother and infant's social world.

REFERENCES

Als, H., Tronick, E., & Brazelton, T.B. *Manual for the behavioral assessment of the premature and at-risk newborn.* (An extension of the Brazelton Neonatal Behavioral Assessment Scale.), 1976.

Bakeman, R., & Brown, J.V. Early interaction: Consequences for social and mental development at three years. *Child Development,* 1980, *51,* 437–447.

Beckwith, L., & Cohen, S.E. Preterm birth: Hazardous obstetrical and postnatal events as related to caregiver-infant behavior. *Infant Behavior and Development,* 1978, *1,* 403–411.

Bell, R.Q. A reinterpretation of the direction of effects in studies of socialization. *Psychological Review,* 1968, 75, 81–95.

Brachfeld, S., Goldberg, S., & Sloman, J. Parent-infant interaction in free play at 8 and 12 months: Effects of

prematurity and immaturity. *Infant Behavior and Development,* 1980, *3,* 289–305.

Brazelton, T.B. Neonatal Behavioral Assessment Scale. *Clinics in Developmental Medicine,* No. 50. London: Heinemann, 1973.

Brazelton, T.B. Introduction. In: A. Sameroff (ed.), Organization and stability of newborn behavior: A commentary on the Brazelton neonatal behavioral assessment scale. *Monographs of the Society for Research in Child Development,* 1978, 43 (5–6).

Bronfenbrenner, U. Toward an experimental ecology of human development. *American Psychologist,* 1977, *32,* 513–531.

Cochran, M.M., & Brassard, J.A. Child development and personal social networks. *Child Development,* 1979, *30,* 601–616.

Crnic, K.A., Greenberg, M.T., Ragozin, A.S., Robinson, N.M., & Basham, R.B. Effects of stress and social support on mothers and premature and full term infants. *Child Development.* 1983, *54,* 209–217.

Crockenberg, S.B. Infant irritability, mother responsiveness and social support influences on the security of infant-mother attachment. *Child Development,* 1981, *52,* 857–865.

DiVitto, B., & Goldberg, S. The effects of newborn medical status on early parent-infant interaction. In: T.M. Field, A.M. Sostek, S. Goldberg, & H.H. Shuman (eds.), *Infants born at-risk.* New York: Spectrum, 1979.

Dubowitz, L., Dubowitz, V., & Goldberg, C. Clinical assessment of gestational age in the newborn infant. *The Journal of Pediatrics,* 1970, *72,* 1–10.

Feiring, C., Fox, N.A., Jaskir, J., & Lewis, M. The relation of social support to mother-infant interaction in high risk infants. In preparation.

Field, T.M. Effects of early separation interactive deficits, and experimental manipulations on infant-mother face-to-face interaction. *Child Development,* 1977, *48,* 763–771.

Field, T. Interaction patterns of preterm and term infants. In: T. Field, A. Sostek, S. Goldberg, & H.H. Shuman (eds.), *Infants born at-risk.* New York: Spectrum, 1979.

Greene, J.G., Fox, N.A., & Lewis, M. The relationship between neonatal characteristics and 3 month mother-infant interaction in high risk infants. *Child Development,* 1983, *54,* 1286–1296.

Holmes, D.L., Nagy, J.N., Slaymaker, F., Sosnowski, R.J., Prinz, S.M., & Pasternak, J.F. Early influences of prematurity, illness and prolonged hospitalization on infant behavior. *Developmental Psychology,* 1982, *18,* 744–750.

Jacobson, J.L., Fein, G.G., Jacobson, S.W., & Schwartz, P.M. Factors and clusters for the Brazelton Scale: An investigation of the dimensions of neonatal behavior. *Developmental Psychology,* 1984, *20,* 339–353.

Lester, B.M., Als, H., & Brazelton, T.B. *Scoring criteria for seven clusters of the Brazelton Scale.* Unpublished manuscript, Child Development Unit, Children's Hospital Medical Center, Boston, 1978.

Lewis, M., & Feiring, C. The child's social network: Social object, social functions and their relationship. In: M. Lewis & L. Rosenblum (eds.), *The child and its family: The genesis of behavior,* Vol. 2. New York: Plenum Publishing Company, 1979.

Lewis, M., Feiring, C., & Brooks-Gunn, J.B. The social network of normal and handicapped children. In: S. Landesman-Dwyer & P. Vietze (eds.), *The environments of handicapped children.* New York: Plenum Publishing Corp., in press.

Lewis, M., & Lee-Painter, S. An interactional approach to the mother-infant dyad. In: M. Lewis & L. Rosenblum (eds.), *The effect of the infant on its caregiver.* New York: John Wiley & Sons, 1974.

Lewis, M., & Rosenblum, L.A. *The effect of the infant on its caregiver.* New York: John Wiley & Sons, 1974.

Osofsky, J.D., & Danzger, B. Relationships between neonatal characteristics and mother-infant interaction. *Developmental Psychology,* 1974, *10*(1), 124–130.

Powell, D.R. Family-environment relations and early child bearing: The role of social networks and neighborhoods. *Journal of Research and Development in Education,* 1979, *13,* 1–11.

Sameroff, A.J., Krafchuk, E.E., & Bakow, H.A. Issues in grouping items from the neonatal behavioral assessment scale. In: A. Sameroff (ed.), Organization and stability of newborn behavior: A commentary on the Brazelton neonatal behavioral assessment scale. *Monographs of the Society for Research in Child Development,* 1978, *43,* (5–6).

Sostek, A.M., Davitt, M.K., Renzi, J., Born, W.S., & Kiely, S.C. Factor analysis of behavioral assessments of preterm neonates. *Infants Behavior and Development,* in press.

The At-Risk Infant: Psycho/Socio/Medical Aspects
edited by Shaul Harel, M.D., and Nicholas J. Anastasiow, Ph.D.
Copyright © 1985   Paul H. Brookes Publishing Co., Inc.   Baltimore • London

Chapter 4

Home- and Center-Based Intervention for Teenage Mothers and Their Offspring

TIFFANY FIELD, PH.D.
SUSAN WIDMAYER, PH.D.
REENA GREENBERG, M.S.
SHERILYN STOLLER, M.S.
University of Miami Medical Center, Miami, Florida

MOST OF THE RESEARCH ON THE PROBLEM OF teenage pregnancy has focused on the undesirable socioeconomic outcomes of the mother. Investigations of teenage offspring have typically reported only neonatal outcomes, noted to be similar to the outcomes for neonates of adult women when the teenage mothers have received prenatal intervention (McLaughlin, Sandler, Sherrod, & Vietze, 1979; Osofsky and Osofsky, 1970). The longer-term outcomes of teenage offspring are uncertain since in most cases both the intervention and investigative efforts have ceased at the neonatal period.

The literature on teenage mothers fairly consistently shows negative long-term socioeconomic consequences of early childbearing such as lower levels of education and greater dependency on public assistance (cf. Furstenberg, 1976). Some of the more widely cited retrospective studies of teenage offspring suggest that as infants, teenage offspring are subjected to less educated parents who have relatively limited knowledge and unrealistic expectations regarding developmental milestones, and relatively punitive child-bearing attitudes (DeLissovoy, 1973). As preschoolers, a number of teenage offspring have been described as "unable to complete the preschool inventory because of severe physical and psychological handicaps" (Furstenberg, 1976), and later, as school-age children, they are unable to maintain grade-appropriate reading levels (Oppel & Royston, 1971). Data from large-scale studies in New York City (Dryfoos & Belmont, 1978), the National Collaborative Perinatal Project (Broman, 1978), and Great Britain (Record, McKeown, & Edwards, 1969) suggest that holding socioeconomic status constant, maternal youth is a significant contributor to deflated later childhood IQ scores. In most of these studies, factors including the lesser education of the teenage mother, her less viable socioeconomic status,

This research was funded by grants #OHD90C1358 and OHD90C1764 from the Administration of Children, Youth and Families. The authors are grateful to the infants and mothers who participated in this study and to Ann Colavecchio, Mary Chen, Carol Eshelman, Jackie Zagursky, Sharon Stringer, Ed Ignatoff, and Mercedes de Cubas for their assistance.

and negative attitudes toward child-rearing have been implicated as correlates of the unfavorable developmental outcomes of her offspring.

Most intervention programs relating to teenage pregnancy risk factors have been directed at the prenatal and neonatal course of the mothers and infants. Although the teenage mother is physiologically immature relative to the adult mother, the prenatal programs designed to prevent obstetrical complications common to youth have apparently minimized these complications. Prenatal intervention studies (McLaughlin et al., 1979; Osofsky & Osofsky, 1970) report no biological disadvantage to teenage offspring whose mothers have received comprehensive prenatal services. However, they do find that teenage mothers are less verbal in interactions with their infants and suggest that mother-infant interactions may well be an important problem area. Despite the uneventful neonatal outcomes following prenatal intervention, the long-term negative outcomes suggest that intervention is ceasing at the point at which the need for intervention appears to be most critical.

Programs that have continued intervention for teenagers and their offspring following delivery report a reduction in high school drop out rates and recidivism (Hardy, King, Shipp, & Welcher, 1981) as well as more optimal developmental outcomes for the teenage offspring (Badger, 1981). A recent biweekly home-based parent training program in infant stimulation for premature offspring of teenage mothers by the authors suggests a number of positive effects as follows: 1) at 4 months, the intervention infants showed more optimal growth, developmental test performance, and face-to-face interactions; 2) their mothers rated their infants' temperament more optimally, expressed more realistic developmental milestones and child-rearing attitudes, and received higher ratings on face-to-face interactions; and 3) at 8 months, the intervention group received more optimal Bayley Mental (Bayley, 1969), home stimulation, and infant temperament scores.

A number of problems appeared to persist for the mothers of this home-based intervention program despite the positive effects of the program on early infant development and mother-infant interactions. These included: 1) the failure of mothers to return to school or seek job training or employment, 2) continuing poor financial status of the teenage mothers, and 3) conflicts in the home between the teenager and her mother regarding child-rearing responsibilities and attitudes. In an attempt to address these problems, a center-based intervention program was organized to provide: 1) free nursery care for the infants of teenage mothers, and 2) paid job training for the mothers as teacher aide trainees in the same nursery. The authors hoped that this program would improve the mothers' socioeconomic status by giving them financial support, job training, incentives to return to school or seek postschool employment, a stimulating place to leave their infants while in school or at work, education in child-rearing and early stimulation, and additional time and experience with their own and others' infants. This program would offer the same parent training in infant stimulation, developmental milestones, and child-rearing attitudes as had been offered in the home-based intervention program, but in addition would provide day care, paid job training, and counseling and thereby have an effect on the mothers' socioeconomic problems. This center-based intervention program was then compared with the following programs: 1) a biweekly home-based intervention program providing parent training in infant stimulation, 2) a free day care program, and 3) a control group receiving no intervention. To control for self-selection factors, all mothers were randomly assigned to these groups following their volunteering for intervention. All groups were seen at 4-month intervals for assessments of the intervention effects.

METHOD

Subjects

The recruitment of neonates and their mothers began in November-December, 1978, and the intervention programs in January, 1979. Forty mothers and infants were enrolled in each of the intervention and control groups.

The mothers were black, lower-class teenagers ranging in age from 13 to 19 years ($\overline{X} = 16.9$) and their infants were delivered at term without perinatal complications. All of the mothers lived at home with their parent(s) and siblings. None of the infants' grandmothers were employed, and thus they served as caregivers for the infant during the teenage mother's absence. Some of the girls were completing their schooling, some were gainfully employed, and some were only participating in the program.

Procedure

Center-Based Intervention The center-based intervention program was attended by one-third of the mothers and infants who spent 20 hours weekly in the infant nursery (a space provided by the Mailman Center that is large enough to serve 20 infants and mothers and consists of a sleep room with cribs and play-feeding room). The mothers and their infants attended the program for 4 hours per day either after their morning school hours or before their evening school hours if they were attending school. The city of Miami's CETA consortium provided minimum wage salaries for the mothers on an hourly basis only for the hours worked and up to 20 hours per week. The CETA contract for paid training was a six-month contract, after which time the mothers were assisted in finding employment.

The program was initially staffed by two black women who were professionals with teaching experience both in early childhood and with teenagers and who had been mothers themselves.

During the 4 hours of paid training per day, the mothers participated in the following program: 1) child-care skills and techniques for stimulating and interacting with their infants (the same developmentally age-referenced caretaking, sensorimotor, and interaction exercises are photographically illustrated on cards and accompanied by homemade toys originally prepared for the home-based intervention group; a list of these exercises appears in the chapter appendix); 2) lectures by Mailman Center and Medical School professionals as well as films on nutrition, child develop-

ment, behavior management, etc.; 3) group counseling sessions on school, work, home, child-rearing, boyfriend, and money problems; 4) modeling of parenting and child-care techniques by the staff; and 5) actual child care of their own and others' infants in the nursery program.

The positive features of this program were manifested in the data reported in the results section of this chapter, in the peer group camaraderie and support system (which is not directly reflected by the data given their somewhat immeasurable qualities), and by the steady attendance of the teenage girls.

Problems that emerged in this program included the following:

1. Enrollment in the CETA program was difficult for these girls because they were considerably more unmotivated than the typical CETA program enrollee, and the enrollment process for the CETA program involved 2 days of paper processing including securing all Social Security numbers of all family members and notarized affidavits, all of which required very close supervision and support by the staff.

2. Because of this previous problem, a number of teenagers failed to complete the enrollment process, necessitating recruitment of more teenagers than the program actually enrolled.

3. Also, related to the extremely low socioeconomic status of the mothers (lower than that of other groups, e.g., Hardy et al. and Badger intervention groups as manifested by the unemployed grandmothers) were other behavior management problems that occurred. For example, a teenage mother recently released from prison stole money from staff and occasionally appeared in the infant nursery during a drugged state.

4. Since the unemployed grandmothers were more convenient caregivers for the infants of the teenage mothers, only a few of the mothers agreed to enroll their infants in 40 hours per week nursery care, while the majority of mothers had their infants in nursery care for only their 20 hours of paid training per week.

5. Role and personality conflicts developed between the black infant nursery teachers who had been teenage mothers and the teenage mothers. These conflicts appeared to take the form of the teachers assuming mother surrogate roles and the teenage mothers playing rebellious adolescents. This latter problem resulted in the black staff members resigning and being replaced by white female professionals who appeared to be assuming more teacher- and less parent-like roles, thus reducing conflicts between teachers and trainees.

Home-Based Intervention The home-based intervention program was provided for one-third of the mother-infant dyads. This program of biweekly home visits trained the mothers in infant stimulation exercises (caretaking, sensorimotor, and interaction exercises). The home visits were made by a developmental psychologist and a trained CETA (black teenager) aide who demonstrated the exercises to the mother (6 exercises per visit), provided the illustrated cards and toys, asked the mother to demonstrate the exercises to ensure her understanding of them, and then asked the mother to practice each of these for 5 minutes daily and record the time of day the exercise was completed and whether it was successfully performed by the infant. At the subsequent visit, the mother was asked to demonstrate these exercises and show the psychologist and CETA aide her completed exercise cards as an index of whether she actually performed the exercises. During these intervention sessions, the CETA aide observed and played with the teenage mother's siblings or interacted with family members in order to minimize interruptions of the intervention session.

The positive aspects of this program were expected to be less than those of the center-based program, but equivalent to those previously reported for the home-based program for preterm infants (Field, Widmayer, Stringer, & Ignatoff, 1980). The effects may not be as dramatic as those reported for the preterm infants, given that the infants in this program were term infants, and thus did not require intervention to the same extent, but were ex-

pected to fare more optimally than the control-term infants not receiving intervention.

The problems with the home-based intervention were consistent with those reported for the home-based intervention program for preterm infants, including missed and rescheduled appointments, discomfort associated with slum visits (and frightening incidents such as the theft of a purse), and the impossibility of knowing with any confidence whether the mothers were actually performing the exercises. (A future control group with social visits alone is planned to assess the potential Hawthorne effect, or the treatment effect of merely visiting the mothers.) Another problem that emerged in this particular home-based intervention program may relate to the previously mentioned problem of staffing black women who had been teenage mothers as interventionists. Thinking that a woman who had experienced the same cultural background, a teenage pregnancy, and had surmounted these hardships to become a professional might serve as a more appropriate model in addition to developing better rapport with the lower-class black teenage mothers, such a woman was hired. This staffing pattern was in contrast to using white middle-class graduate students in psychology as interventionists in an earlier home intervention program (accompanied by CETA aides in both home intervention programs). The authors' experience with the use of the black adult woman professional versus the white graduate student was that more apparent compliance and fewer missed appointments occurred with the latter arrangement. This may relate again to the black adult woman assuming a more surrogate mother-like role than a teacher role with the teenage mothers as was noted in the center-based nursery program. However, the dynamics of this problem are somewhat confounded given that the home-based program staffed by graduate student interventionists involved intervention for preterm infants and their mothers, while the black woman interventionist was serving term infants and their mothers. Previous longitudinal studies with this population have shown that the attrition and noncompliance rate is much greater among mothers of term infants who are considered healthy and relatively less difficult babies than preterm infants. Thus, the relative motivation of the mothers appears to differ as a function of the babies' health and developmental status, and the task of motivating the mothers of term babies to perform the exercises might have been greater irrespective of the characteristics of the interventionist.

Free Day Care A third comparison group provided free day care for the infants of teenage mothers. This consisted of the same infant stimulation program for the infants, thus freeing the mother of her caretaking responsibilities during school or work hours. Following recruitment of volunteer intervention mothers, the authors were unable to recruit mothers specifically for the free day care program. Since several teenage intervention programs have noted the need for free day care (Badger, 1981; Hardy et al., 1981), the authors' experience may not generalize to other programs and area needs. There are a number of factors that appear to differentiate this program population from that of Badger and Hardy. First, this program apparently has an even lower-class sample, as manifested by the grandmothers being unemployed, unlike the grandmothers of the Badger and Hardy programs. Second, the Miami public transportation system is reputedly much less efficient than that of Badger's location (Cincinnati) or Hardy's (Baltimore). The buses have very sporadic schedules, long and indirect routes, and the taxis are prohibitively expensive. When the mothers were interviewed about their unwillingness to participate in the free day care program, they suggested that it was too inconvenient transportation-wise and school schedule–wise, and much more convenient to leave their infants with the grandmother.

Control Group The control group received no intervention except the positive effects that could be attributed to having periodic assessments. Although an immediate attrition was anticipated in this sample as a function of not providing any intervention, the expected attrition was not experienced.

Assessments

Demographic data, prenatal and obstetric data, as well as attitudes of the mother were rated during the neonatal period. The infants were assessed at the neonatal period, at 4 months, and at 1 year.

Prenatal/Obstetrical Data Included in the prenatal/obstetrical data were the mother's age, number of school years completed, number of months enrolled in the local prenatal intervention program, first prenatal visit and total number of prenatal visits, parity, length of labor, type of delivery, type of delivery medication, and an Obstetric Complications Scale rating (Littman & Parmelee, 1978).

Neonatal Data Neonatal data included: a) the traditional birth measures (gestational age, birth weight, birth length, head circumference, 5-minute Apgar scores); b) the Ponderal Index (weight/length^3 × 100)(Miller & Hassanein, 1971); c) the Postnatal Complications Scale (Littman & Parmelee, 1978); d) the infant's systolic and diastolic blood pressure measured by arteriosonde; and e) the Brazelton Neonatal Behavioral Assessment Scale (Brazelton, 1973), summarized by the four a priori scoring dimensions: interaction, motor, state, and stress (Als, Tronick, Lester, & Brazelton, 1977).

Maternal Stress and Attitude Measures Measures of maternal stress and attitude included: a) maternal systolic and diastolic blood pressures (measured by arteriosonde); b) the State-Trait Anxiety Scale (Spielberger, Goursuch, & Lushene, 1970); and c) the Perinatal Anxieties and Attitudes Scale (PAAS) (Field, 1979), an assessment of attitudes and anxieties of the mother about herself or her infant during the pregnancy, labor, delivery, and postpartum periods.

Maternal Assessments of Infants Maternal assessments of infants included: a) the Mother's Assessment of the Behavior of her Infant (MABI)(Field, Dempsey, Hallock, & Shuman, 1978), an adaptation of the Brazelton Neonatal Behavioral Assessment Scale designed to tap the mother's assessment of her infant's behaviors; and b) the Maternal Developmental Expectations and Childrearing Attitudes Survey (MDECAS) (Field, 1979), an assessment of the mother's knowledge of the average age that developmental milestones are achieved, including smiling, crawling, walking, and talking, as well as her attitudes toward child-rearing, including feeding, early stimulation, teaching, and disciplinary practices used to evaluate the degree to which maternal expectations are realistic and child-rearing attitudes are nonpunitive.

Four-Month Assessments Four-month assessments were made at the mother's home and included: a) growth measurements (weight, length, and head circumference); b) the Denver Developmental Screening Test (Frankenburg & Dodds, 1967); c) the Carey Infant Temperament Questionnaire (Carey, 1970); and d) videotaped mother-infant feeding (Field, 1977a) and face-to-face play interactions (Field, 1977b), coded on a number of variables including the amount of infant gaze aversion and fussiness, and the amount of mother attentiveness and stimulation, rated according to the criteria of an Interaction Rating Scale (IRS) (Field, 1979).

One-Year Assessments One-year assessments were also made at the mother's home and included: a) growth measurements (weight and length), b) Bayley Mental and Motor Scales (Bayley, 1969), and c) the Caldwell Home Scale (Caldwell, Heider, & Kaplan, 1966).

RESULTS

Neonatal Data

As can be seen in Table 1, the groups (control, home intervention, and nursery intervention) did not differ at birth as would be expected since the teenage mothers were randomly assigned from the same population. The mothers averaged 17 years of age, made their first prenatal visit at approximately 4 months, and attended a prenatal intervention program for only 1 month. The late prenatal visits combined with a moderate number of obstetrical complications suggest that the prenatal care of the mothers was less than optimal.

However, their infants experienced only a minimal number of postnatal complications, and although they were somewhat small for date (birth weight/length^3 × 100), their Apgar

Table 1. Means for prenatal/obstetrical and neonatal measures

Measures	Control	Home intervention	Nursery intervention
Prenatal/obstetrical			
Maternal age	17	17	17
Prenatal intervention (months)	02	01	01
First prenatal visit (months)	03	05	04
Obstetrical complications	104	114	100
Neonatal			
Gestational age (days)	277	280	282
Birth weight (grams)	3,133	3,258	3,098
Birth length (cms)	51	51	51
Head circumference (cm)	34	34	34
Apgar—1 minute	08	09	08
Apgar—5 minutes	09	09	09
Ponderal Index	2.36	2.45	2.33
Brazelton			
Interaction	2.4	2.4	2.5
Motor	2.0	2.4	2.2
State	2.2	2.0	2.0
Stress	1.7	1.3	1.5
Postnatal complications	147	160	160
Maternal			
State anxiety	38	33	38
Trait anxiety	41	37	41
PAAS	20	21	19
Child-rearing attitudes	05	06	07

scores and Brazelton scores were in the normal range except for Brazelton interaction scores which were less than average. Mothers' levels of state and trait anxiety were relatively high, and more than the average number of perinatal anxieties were expressed by these teenage mothers. Similarly, their child-rearing attitudes were somewhat punitive or less than optimal, and their developmental expectations unrealistic.

There were no reliable group differences among any of the above measures. This suggests that the random assignment of volunteer intervention mothers to the various intervention and control groups resulted in a fairly even distribution across these measures and equivalent status at birth against which to measure the effects of intervention. The non-optimal scores on various prenatal and neonatal measures were not surprising given similar findings from the authors' previous study that included term infants of teenage mothers (Field, 1979).

Four-Month Assessments

At 4 months, both the infants of the home visit and nursery intervention groups were greater weight and received better Denver Developmental Screening Test scores than the control-group infants. The mothers of the infants receiving intervention assigned less "difficult" temperament ratings to their infants on the Carey Infant Temperament Questionnaire, which is a 67-item scale that taps temperament qualities including rhythmicity, distractibility,

mood, threshold, intensity, approach, and activity of the infants. The infants' ratings on these temperament dimensions are then summarized on a scale of 1 (easy) to 4 (difficult).

Face-to-face interactions of the infants and their mothers were videotaped at this assessment. The videotaped interactions were coded using an interaction rating scale designed by the authors and standardized on 150 infants. This scale included 3-point ratings of the mothers' and infants' alertness, eye contact, facial expressions, vocalizations, and the sensitivity and contingency of each other's behaviors. The ratings were then averaged for a face-to-face interaction score for the mother and infant with a 3 being an optimal score. In addition, the proportion of time the mothers talked and the infants gaze-averted was quantified since these measures have been noted to differentiate normal and disturbed interactions. As can be seen in Table 2, the interaction ratings for both mothers and infants of each of the intervention groups were better than those of the control group. Mothers of the intervention groups, but particularly the nursery intervention group, talked to their infants a greater percentage of the interaction time and their infants gaze-averted a lesser proportion of the time as compared to the control-group mother-infant dyads.

One-Year Assessments

The data analyses at 1 year revealed greater weight and superior Bayley scores for the intervention as compared to the control infants,

Table 2. Four-month assessments[a]

| | Means | | |
	Control	Home	Nursery
Weight (grams)	6,237	6,772[c]	6,774[c]
Length (cms)	67	67	68
Denver Developmental Screening Test	30	35[c]	36[c]
Temperament rating	3.8	3.4[b]	3.1[d]
Interaction—Infant rating	2.2	2.5[b]	2.6[b]
—Mother rating	2.3	2.5[b]	2.7[c]
—Mother talking (%)	41	49 $<$[e]	72[e]
—Infant gaze aversion (%)	64	54 $>$[b]	33[c]

[a]All significance levels refer to comparisons between the control group and the specific intervention group (home or nursery). $<$ or $>$ denotes direction of differences between intervention groups.
[b]$p < .05$.
[c]$p < .01$.
[d]$p < .005$.
[e]$p < .001$.

Table 3.   One-year assessments[a]

	Means		
	Control	Home	Nursery
Weight (grams)	9,307	10,020[b]		11,066[c]
Length (cms)	74	76		76
Bayley Mental (MDI)	105	112[b]		119[c]
Bayley Motor (PDI)	102	109[c]	$<^b$	119[c]
Caldwell Home Scale	27	32		34[e]
Return to work/school (%)	21	39[b]	$<^c$	74[e]
Repeat pregnancy (%)	19	09[b]	$>^d$	01[e]

[a]All significance levels refer to comparisons between the control group and the specific intervention group (home or nursery). $<$ or $>$ denotes direction of differences between intervention groups.
[b]$p < .05$.
[c]$p < .01$.
[d]$p < .005$.
[e]$p < .001$.

with the nursery intervention infants receiving better motor scores than the home-visit intervention infants. In addition, the percentage of mothers returning to work or school during the first year was greater for the nursery group than the home-visit group, which, in turn, was greater than the control group. The incidence of repeat pregnancy during the first year was significantly lower for the nursery than the home-visit group mothers, which, in turn, was lower than for the control-group mothers (Table 3).

DISCUSSION

The growth and development of the infants of both intervention groups exceeded that of the control-group infants over the first year of life. The infants weighed more, their interactions were better, and their motor skills were more developed during the early assessment periods. At 1 year, the Bayley scale scores were better for the intervention infants. Their weights and more advanced motor skills may have been mediated by the greater amounts of infant stimulation provided for the intervention infants.

Although the home-visit and nursery intervention infants did not differ during the early assessments, except that the nursery group mothers talked more and their infants gaze-averted less during early interactions, they did differ at later assessments. Only the nursery group infants received better temperament ratings, which may have been related to those

mothers spending more time and interacting more with their infants. The developmental scores of the nursery intervention group first exceeded those of the home-visit infants at 1 year on the Bayley Motor scale. The more intensive stimulation program of the nursery may have facilitated more advanced motor skills. Thus, significant growth and development gains were noted for infants of both intervention groups, with the infants of the nursery group eventually showing a greater advantage than the home-visit group.

The mothers clearly benefited most from the nursery intervention based on their greater rate of return to work or school and their lesser incidence of repeat pregnancy. Although it is not clear which of the additional benefits for the nursery group mothers "made the difference" (for example, the pay check, the job training, the additional time with their infants, or the modeling of parenting skills by the teachers on a daily basis), the course of these mothers following their training suggested "hidden benefits." Even though these mothers were being trained as teacher aides, 82% of those seeking additional schooling entered nurses' aide or medical technology training programs. They appeared, then, to have developed an interest in paramedical professions, perhaps because their nursery was located in a medical school and perhaps because they were inspired by the medical faculty and staff parents of the infants they cared for as they frequented the nursery in their white coats.

The nursery intervention may be the most cost-effective of the programs inasmuch as it provided a service to medical faculty and staff and facilitated both the socioeconomic status of teenage mothers and the development of their infants at a very low cost. Since the literature suggests that the most severe consequences to the teenage mother are socioeconomic dependency which is noted to mediate developmental delays in their infants, a program that not only facilitates infant development but also improves socioeconomic status of the mother may have longer-term benefits for both the teenage mother and her infant.

Some general concerns deriving from the authors' experience establishing these intervention programs and observing these mother-infant dyads merit further discussion. First, the problem of sampling from a relatively noncompliant population results inevitably in a self-selection problem. There were a number of teenage mothers who would not volunteer for the intervention project (approximately 10% of those invited). Of those who did volunteer and were randomly assigned to the free day care group, no mothers were willing to participate due to the already mentioned inconvenience of transportation and greater convenience of grandmother caretaking. Of those randomly assigned to the center-based nursery intervention group, only two-thirds managed to complete the CETA enrollment process. Of those assigned to the home-based intervention, approximately one-third dropped out almost immediately due to a number of factors such as the program's inability to locate the new residence of mothers, legal entanglements such as indictments for child abuse or neglect, and

family conflicts such as the grandmother claiming primary care of the infant and essentially removing the teenage mother from the situation.

Despite the self-selection problem resulting in the recruitment of the most motivated of this relatively unmotivated group, the teenage mothers were a very impoverished, noncompliant, difficult group of girls who presented considerable problems including depression, learned helplessness, noncompliance, drug abuse, irresponsibility and threatened abuse of their infants, truancy from high school, and legal problems such as petty theft and assaultive behaviors. A number of the girls were victims of physical abuse themselves and although no evidence of physical abuse toward infants was observed, the mothers frequently related incidents of having abused their infants. These reports, as well as observed drug abuse and violations of parole in the case of one of the mothers presented conflicts about the program's own legal responsibilities. Knowing that these may be the very mothers who might benefit most from an intervention of this kind posed the conflict of whether to continue or terminate the involvement of mothers if and when they presented problems of this kind. Certainly, the intervention program had some positive effects on infant development and maternal attitudes, and the school enrollment rates (a 40% return to high school and a 20% enrollment in community colleges) suggested that the program also had positive effects on the educational and socioeconomic goals and activities of the mothers.

REFERENCES

Als, H., Tronick, E., Lester, B.M., & Brazelton, T.B. The Brazelton Neonatal Behavioral Assessment Scale (BNBAS). *Journal Abnormal Child Psychology*, 1977, 5, 215–231.

Badger, E. Effects of parent education program on teenage mothers and their offspring. In. K.G. Scott, T. Field, & E.G. Robertson (eds.), *Teenage parents and their offspring*. New York: Grune & Stratton, 1981.

Bayley, N. *Manual for the Bayley Scales of Infant Development*. New York: The Psychological Corporation, 1969.

Brazelton, T.B. *Neonatal Behavioral Assessment Scale*. London: Spastic International Medical Publications, 1973.

Broman, S. *Seven year outcome of 4,000 children born to teenagers in the U.S.* Unpublished manuscript, National Institute of Nervous Diseases and Stroke, Bethesda, MD, 1978.

Caldwell, B.M., Heider, J., & Kaplan, B. *The inventory of home stimulation*. Paper presented at the annual meeting of the American Psychological Association, New York, September, 1966.

Caputo, D.V., Goldstein, K.M., & Taub, H.B. The development of prematurely born children through middle childhood. In: T. Field, A. Sostek, S. Goldberg, & H.H. Shuman (eds.), *Infants born at risk*. New York: Spectrum, 1979.

Carey, W.B. A simplified method of measuring infant

temperament. *The Journal of Pediatrics*, 1970, *77*, 188–194.

DeLissovoy, V. Child care by adolescent parents. *Children Today*, 1973, *2*, 22–25.

Dryfoos, J., & Belmont, L. *Long term development of children born to New York City teenagers*. Unpublished manuscript, Columbia University, New York, 1978.

Field, T. Effects of early separation, interactive deficits and experimental manipulations on infant-mother face-to-face interaction. *Child Development*, 1977, *48*, 763–771. (a)

Field, T. Maternal stimulation during infant feeding. *Developmental Psychology*, 1977, *13*, 539–540. (b)

Field, T. Interaction patterns of preterm and term infants. In: T. Field, A. Sostek, S. Goldberg, & H.H. Shuman (eds.), *Infants born at risk*. New York: Spectrum, 1979.

Field, T., Dempsey, J., Hallock, N., & Shuman, H.H. Mothers' assessments of the behavior of their infants. *Infant Behavior and Development*, 1978, *1*, 156–167.

Field, T., Widmayer, S., Stringer, S., & Ignatoff, E. Teenage, lower-class, Black mothers and their preterm infants: An intervention and developmental follow-up. *Child Development*, 1980, *51*, 426–436.

Frankenburg, W.K., & Dodds, J.B. The Denver Developmental Screening Test. *The Journal of Pediatrics*, 1967, *71*, 181–191.

Furstenberg, F.F. The social consequences of teenage pregnancy. *Family Planning Perspectives*, 1976, *8*, 148–164.

Hardy, J., King, T.M., Shipp, D.A., & Welcher, D.W. A comprehensive approach to adolescent pregnancy. In: K.G. Scott, T. Field, & E.G. Robertson (eds.), *Teenage parents and their offspring*. New York: Grune & Stratton, 1981.

Littman, B., & Parmelee, A.M. Medical correlates of infant development. *Pediatrics*, 1978, *61*, 470–474.

McLaughlin, J., Sandler, H.M., Sherrod, K., & Vietze, P.M. *Social-psychological characteristics of adolescent mothers and behavioral characteristics of their first-born infants*. Unpublished manuscript, Peabody College, Nashville, 1979.

Miller, M.C., & Hassanein, K. Diagnosis of impaired fetal growth in newborn infants. *Pediatrics*, 1971, *43*, 511–515.

Myers, J. *Fundamentals of experimental design*. Boston: Allyn and Bacon, 1972.

Oppel, W., & Royston, A.B. Teenage births: Some social, psychological and physical sequelae. *American Journal of Public Health*, 1971, *61*, 751–756.

Osofsky, H., & Osofsky, J. Adolescents as mothers: Results of a program for low-income pregnant teenagers with some emphasis upon infants' development. *American Journal of Orthopsychiatry)*, 1970, *40*, 825–834.

Record, R.G., McKeown, T., & Edwards, J.G. The relation of measured intelligence to birth order and maternal age. *Annals of Human Genetics*, 1969, *33*, 61–69.

Spielberger, C.D., Goursuch, R.L., & Lushene, R.E. *The State-Trait Anxiety Inventory*. Palo Alto, CA. Consulting Psychologist Press, 1970.

The At-Risk Infant: Psycho/Socio/Medical Aspects
edited by Shaul Harel, M.D., and Nicholas J. Anastasiow, Ph.D.
Copyright © 1985   Paul H. Brookes Publishing Co., Inc.   Baltimore • London

APPENDIX
Intervention Exercises

Age	Title of exercise (minutes per day)	Age	Title of exercise (minutes per day)
2 weeks	Sponge bath and lotion rub (10) Feeding (10) Rocking and singing lullaby (10)	7 months	Hand feeding Walking on hands (10) Lying and sitting on the ground (5) Banging toys (5)
2–4 weeks	Face and voice play (5) Toy play (5) Looking for toy (5) Voice play (5)	8 months	Handing baby toys (5) Holding things (5) Hiding a squeak toy (5) Sound game (5)
4 weeks	Talking and smiling (5) Crying Mobile and crib toys Relaxing the body (5)	9 months	Playing ball (5) Finding toys (5) Showing baby pictures (5) Sitting and crawling (10)
4–6 weeks	Exercising baby's legs (5) Exercising baby's arms (5)	10 months	Ringing a bell (5) Follow the leader (5) Bathing (10) Calling attention to sounds
6 weeks	Blowing and whispering (5) Plate puppet (5) Feeling things (5)	11 months	Reading (10) "Give me the toy" game (5) Feel game (5) Game on the stool (5)
6–8 weeks	Grasping (5) Singing and dancing (5)	12 months	Crouching/standing (10) Coloring with crayon (10) Putting blocks in a can (5) Shopping
8 weeks	Cup clapper (5) Listening for sounds (5) Wrist bands Tour of the house (5)	13 months	Emptying containers (5) Learning new words (5) Creeping game (10) Playing catch (10)
8–10 weeks	Leg stretch (5) Arm stretch (5)	14 months	Handing objects to mommy (10) Imitating animals (5) First steps (5) Turning pages (10)
10 weeks	Ankle bells Pull toy (5) Body massage (5)	15 months	Baby feeds you (5) Learning commands (10) Opening and closing containers (10) Where did it go? (10)
10–12 weeks	Imitating baby's sounds (5) Lifting head up (5)	16 months	Sniffing and touching (10) Drinking from a cup (5) Learning body parts: the face (5) Meeting another baby two times per week
12 weeks	Cradle gym Splash in warm water (5) Different heights Finding sounds (5)	17 months	Matching like objects (5) Getting dressed (10) Building a tower (5) Learning to follow directions (5)
12–14 weeks	Rolling from side to side (5) Strengthening muscles (5)	18 months	Opposites (10) Points to objects and pictures (5) Climbing into a chair (5) Ring around the rosey (10)
14 weeks	Standing on lap (5)		
14–16 weeks	Sit up game (5) Face-to-face game (5)		
16 weeks	Hide & go seek around the crib (5) Face sock Peek-a-boo (5) Holding toys (5)		
5 months	Strengthening the buttocks (5) Bath time (10) Lifting head and back (5) Baby's slide (5)		
6 months	Pedaling (5) Getting ready to crawl (5) Bouncing baby (5) Balloon (5)		

39

Chapter 5

Attitudes of
Adolescents toward
Infants and Young Children
A Developmental Approach

MARY S. THORMANN, ED.D.
Marymount College of Virginia, Arlington, Virginia

MATERNAL PERSONALITY AND ATTITUDINAL variables in relation to the occurrence of disturbances in child-rearing and/or the presence of mental illness in the mother have been the object of recent research. Studies of maternal personality organization, exploring the mother's inability to integrate the experience of pregnancy and child-rearing into her overall world view, have examined the subsequent occurrence of child abuse and neglect (Brunnquell, Crichton, & Egeland, 1979; Egeland & Brunnquell, 1979) and the hospitalization of the mother for severe emotional disturbance during the first years following childbirth (Cohler, Weiss, & Grunebaum, 1970a; Grunebaum, Weiss, Cohler, Hartman, & Gallant, 1982). Little empirical research has been devoted, however, to the examination of attitudinal variables of the *teenage* mother. This chapter is concerned with the study of child-rearing attitudes of pregnant teenagers and the relationship of those variables to selected sociodemographic variables. The research findings are presented within a developmental context.

It is the assumption of this study that child-rearing attitudes, knowledge, expectations, and perceptions are important sources of ad-ditional data for the interpretation of observed mother-child interactions (Parke, 1978; Parke & Tinsley, 1982) and that these data are critical to a multivariate approach to the conceptualization of the environment in which children are born and reared (Sameroff, 1982). Child-rearing attitudes are values (Anastasiow, 1981), and they are an important part of the general culture in which a child is raised (Parke & Tinsley, 1982).

CHILD-REARING ATTITUDES AND DEVELOPMENTAL ISSUES

Motherhood can be viewed as a series of developmental tasks (Grunebaum et al., 1982), and child-rearing attitudes, as they are discussed in this chapter, are seen as indices of the mother's ability to adapt to the parenting role. Successful adaptation is dependent not only on the developmental status of the child and the needs he or she presents to the mother but also on the mother's own maturational status. There needs to exist a match, a synchronization, between maternal and child initiations and responses in the interaction process. This synchronization is, in part, a function of the mother's own personality and her ability to adapt to the needs of the developing child. This ability represents the "contextual plasticity" (Sameroff, 1982) of child-rearing. Both the adolescent mother's level of progress with respect to the major developmental tasks of adolescence and her psychosocial status in general are important variables to consider in this context of mother-child interaction.

Constituting the developmental tasks of motherhood are the major child-rearing issues (see Table 1), as delineated by Sander (1962, 1964) on the basis of longitudinal observations of mother-child pairs. These issues form the basis for the assessment of child-rearing attitudes (Cohler, Weiss, & Grunebaum, 1970b) for the present study. As seen in Table 1, each of the issues is characterized by the emergence of a prominent, or modal, feature, which is related to the age and developmental status of the child. The resolution, or successful negotiation (Sander, 1962), of a particular issue is dependent upon how appropriately the mother responds to the needs the child presents to her. As shown in Figure 1, the issues constitute the continuum of development during the first 3 years of the child's life.

ADOLESCENT PREGNANCY AND THE CAREGIVING ENVIRONMENT

Efforts to understand the environment in which children of teenage mothers are born and reared have come from a number of sources over the past decade. The inquiry has been extensive, in part, because childbearing in adolescence is an important phenomenon in the United States. In 1979, the last year for which statistics are available (Moore & Burt, 1982), 16% of all births and 29% of all first births were to women 19 years of age or younger. Moreover, a large proportion of these young women keep their babies rather than give them up for adoption, with estimates ranging as high as 97% (Zelnik & Kantner, 1978).

Research has examined consequences of early childbearing from various perspectives. Sociocultural correlates have been identified, including lower educational attainment, single parenthood and marital instability, higher fertility or large family size, poverty, and, as a function of level of educational attainment, welfare dependency (for review, see Moore & Burt, 1982). The results of a large, prospective, epidemiological study indicated that mother aloneness, as a family structure variable, is associated with childbearing in adolescence as well as long-term psychological effects such as increased sadness and tension (Brown, Adams, & Kellam, 1980; Kellam, Adams, Brown, & Ensminger, 1979; Kellam, Ensminger, & Turner, 1977).

Developmental effects for the children of adolescent mothers have been found in the areas of intellectual development, socioemotional development, and achievement in school (Belmont, Cohen, Dryfoos, Stein, & Zayac, 1981; Broman, 1981; Hardy, King, Shipp, & Welcher, 1981; Marecek, 1979), although it is clear that effects attributed to maternal age need to be seen as interacting with environmental effects. The findings from these and other studies indicate that the subsequent development of children is jeopardized by early parenthood (Baldwin & Cain, 1980). Determination of how these effects can be mediated is critical to planning and implementing intervention programs. The assumption is made that parents provide the final causal pathway through which culture and environmental factors affect the development of the young child (Ramey & Gowan, 1979).

The mechanisms by which parents influence the developmental process are, of course, multifaceted. Results of the few studies that have explored mother-infant interaction patterns, using teenage mothers as subjects, suggest that the mother-child relationship is an area that needs to be further explored (Epstein, 1980; Osofsky & Osofsky, 1970; Sandler, 1978; Sandler, Vietze, & O'Connor, 1981). For example, it has been shown that, on measures of verbal interaction, scores are significantly lower for teenage mothers and their infants (Osofsky & Osofsky, 1970). Data indicate that parental expectations and knowledge of child development, with respect to the cognitive and language areas, are inadequate (Epstein, 1980). One investigator has suggested that there may be some subtle influence of the mother-child relationship, comparable to that of birth order

Table 1. Schematic description of the developmental tasks of motherhood[a]

Major mother-child interaction issues	Modal feature	Caregiving probes
Period of initial adaptation	Establishing biological rhythm	Does the mother read the baby's cues regarding feeding, elimination, sleep, wakefulness? Does she respond to cues appropriately?
Period of reciprocal exchange	Smiling response	Is mother able to provide stimulation to which baby can respond? Is stimulation appropriate to baby's state (neither over- nor under-stimulation)? Is there a back and forth sequence of smiling play? Does mother know baby is capable of communicating with her?
Period of early directed infant activity	Meshing of mother-infant behaviors	Does mother perceive baby's efforts to initiate interaction? Are her responses appropriate to baby's initiatives (such as holding a spoon while being fed)? Can mother perceive and does she accept the baby's curiosity about the world?
Period of focalization on the mother	"Stranger anxiety"	How does the mother deal with separation from her baby? Is she able to perceive the baby's desire to have her to herself or himself? Can she maintain appropriate distance between herself and her baby? How does she deal with the ambivalence of the baby's crying when she leaves him or her?
Period of self-assertion	Toilet training	Does the mother recognize the basic struggle of this period? Does she understand that the child needs to show autonomy and a sense of will? Does she respond appropriately?
Period of destructive action	Autonomy and selfhood: Showing anger and destroying things	Does the mother understand the child's *intent* when she or he is angry and destroys things? Is the mother able to channel, rather than suppress, the child's angry feelings?
Period of challenge to the mother	Autonomy and selfhood: Negatives and refusals	How does the mother deal with the child's refusal to do things and his or her negativistic behavior in general? Is she too controlling and/or too permissive? Is she able to demonstrate flexibility in her responses? Is she able to set limits when needed? Does she understand what the child is saying through his or her behavior?
Period of widening reciprocal exchange	Exploring the environment through play	Does the mother provide opportunities for the child's need to explore the environment? Does she understand the importance of play to the child's development? Does she provide opportunities for solitary play? For play with others?

[a]Adapted from Sander's formulations (1962, 1964) and work of Cohler et al. (1970b).

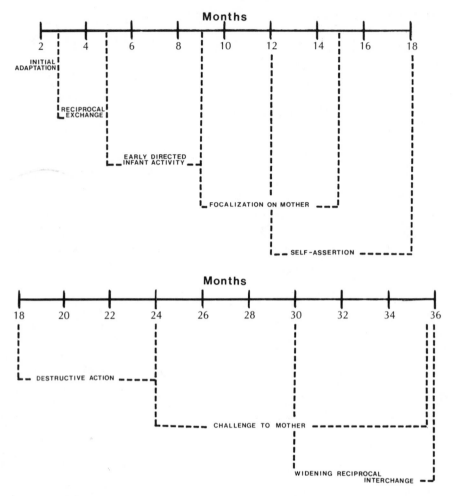

Figure 1. Mother-child interaction issues—issues for the maternal attitude scale. (Cohler et al., 1970b; based on Sander's formulation, 1962, 1964.)

(Belmont et al., 1981), found to be associated with the mental development of children.

The extent to which the maternal personality of the adolescent mother, as expressed through basic beliefs or attitudes toward child-rearing, is able to mediate the impact of sociocultural and environmental factors on the development of young children remains to be demonstrated. It is the purpose of this chapter to present findings from an exploratory study that investigated child-rearing attitudes in a population of pregnant teenagers, as well as the relationship between assessed attitudes and selected sociodemographic variables, such as education of the mother and wantedness of the baby. The study used an age-specific design, and con-

trolled for marital status, parity, and trimester of pregnancy.

METHODS

Sample Group

The sample consists of 50 women from black ($n = 29$), white ($n = 19$), and Hispanic ($n = 2$) ethnic groups ranging in age from 14 to 17 years, and selected from four sites located in the Washington, D.C., and Baltimore, Maryland, areas. Three of the sites were homes for unwed mothers; the fourth site was the outpatient clinic of a large, general hospital serving a low-income population. Thirty-eight percent of the sample was selected from the outpatient clinic. All of the subjects were un-married, primaparous, and in the last trimester of pregnancy. All who met those eligibility requirements were recruited and were part of the sample population.

Norm Group

For purposes of comparison, the norm group was comprised of a sample ($n = 48$) of mentally well mothers ranging in age from 20 to 45 years. This group is described in a recent publication by Cohler, Gallant, Grunebaum, Weiss, and Gamer (1980).

Measures

The Maternal Attitude Scale (MAS) developed by Cohler et al. (1970b), and the Demographic/Descriptive Data Form, developed by Epstein (1980) and adapted for use in this study by the investigator, were the two instruments used to collect data.

Attitudes toward child-rearing were assessed using the Maternal Attitude Scale, a 233-item instrument using the Likert technique of summated ratings and developed as a result of extensive pretests of over 700 mothers. It yields five independent factors and is computer scored. For the present study, the Short-Form of the MAS, consisting of 45 items, as adapted by Egeland, Deinard, Brunnquell, Phipps-Yonas, and Crichton (1979) was used. The format of the MAS was adapted by the investigator for this study. The five factors of the MAS and sample statements are schematically portrayed in Table 2.

The Demographic/Descriptive Data Form was used to gather information in four general areas: 1) sociodemographics of the respondent (age, race, education), 2) social indices of the respondent's family (marital status, parental and maternal education and occupation), 3) anticipated sources of financial support, and 4) personal history of the respondent (age at menarche, feelings about menarche, prevention of pregnancy, and wantedness of the baby). The variables derived from this form were self-scoring.

Statistical analyses of the data were planned to answer the following questions:

1. Were the child-rearing attitudes of the study population maladaptive, compared to the norm group, with respect to: a) appropriate versus inappropriate control of the child's (aggressive) impulses, b) encouragement versus discouragement of reciprocity, c) appropriate versus inappropriate closeness, d) acceptance versus denial of the emotional complexity in child-rearing, and e) comfort versus discomfort in perceiving and meeting the baby's (physical) needs?

2. Was there a significant relationship or difference, as appropriate, between child-rearing attitudes of the study population and a) the research site, b) subjects' age,

Table 2. Schematic description of the five factors of the maternal attitude scale (MAS) and sample statements[a]

MAS Factor	Sample statements
I: Appropriate versus inappropriate control of the child's (aggressive) impulses	A child should be punished for breaking his (her) own toys in a fit of anger. A child should be permitted to say "I hate you" to his (her) parent.
II: Encouragement versus discouragement of reciprocity	Most of the time, babies don't even understand it when their mothers smile at them. A 3-month-old baby can't really tell you what he (she) is thinking by a smile.
III: Appropriate versus inappropriate closeness with the child	A woman's body can never look quite the same once she has given birth to a child.
IV: Acceptance versus denial of the emotional complexity in child-rearing	Mothers have no difficulty in bringing up children. Parents always tell the truth to their children.
V: Feeling of competence versus lack of competence in perceiving and meeting the baby's (physical) needs	A mother's milk is bad for her infant. Babies are frequently so demanding that their mothers have no time for anything else.

[a]Based on work of Cohler et al. (1970b).

race, and educational status, c) parents' educational level and marital status, and d) wantedness of the baby?

RESULTS

Child-Rearing Attitudes of Adolescent Mothers

Findings derived from the statistical analyses of the data, using the *t* test, indicated that there were significant differences ($p = .05$) between scores for the adolescent mothers (study group) and the norm group on four of the five factors of the Maternal Attitude Scale. These findings are summarized in Table 3.

As can be seen, the adolescent mothers obtained scores indicating maladaptive attitudes regarding control of the child's aggressive impulses, encouragement of reciprocity, and acceptance of the emotional complexity in child-rearing. Scores indicating adaptive attitudes were obtained regarding being able to perceive and meet the baby's physical needs. On the basis of these findings, study group mothers would have difficulty understanding the reasons underlying aggressive behaviors of their children and would have difficulty setting limits for the child's behavior (either too restrictive and/or too controlling). While the adolescent mothers would feel comfortable about meeting the physical needs of their children, they would not recognize their role in eliciting behaviors from their infants nor would they appreciate the baby's efforts to communicate with them, and would, perhaps, see the infant's attempts to reach out and explore the environment as bothersome. Finally, the findings indicate that the adolescent mothers

have a tendency, to a significant extent, to deny any concerns about the complexity of child-rearing and are not able to deal effectively with the ambivalence and stress inherent in becoming a mother. This finding indicates a lack of personal integration in this area.

Child-Rearing Attitudes and Selected Sociodemographic Variables

The findings indicate that there are within-group differences in child-rearing attitudes in this study group of adolescent mothers. A significant relationship ($p = .05$) was found between certain sociodemographic variables and attitudes toward child-rearing. Three variables emerged as the most important: educational level of the adolescent mother's father, educational level of her mother, and the adolescent mother's desire to have a baby, termed "wantedness of the baby."

Specifically, those subjects who had more facilitative attitudes toward control of the child's (aggressive) impulses had fathers whose educational level was higher, who themselves were older (within the 14- to 17-year age range), and who wanted to have a baby. The adolescent mothers who believed in the importance of developing a relationship with their infants had mothers whose educational level was higher, and who themselves wanted to have a baby. Being able to admit to having concerns about caring for a child and having less ambivalence about the pregnancy experience were related to the educational level of both of the subjects' parents. Finally, the adolescent mothers' feelings of competence regarding the physical care of the baby were related to having not dropped out of school and wanting to have a baby. In sum, wantedness of

Table 3. Comparison of study group and norm group on five factors of the Maternal Attitude Scale

| MAS factor | Study group | | Norm group | | |
	X̄	S.D.	X̄	S.D.	t
Appropriate control of child's impulses (I)	−0.611	1.38	0.148	1.37	−2.73[a]
Encouragement of reciprocity (II)	−0.158	1.64	0.462	0.74	−2.43[a]
Appropriate closeness (III)	0.484	1.35	0.115	0.83	1.63
Acceptance of complexity (IV)	−0.762	1.37	−0.163	1.08	−2.41[a]
Comfort in meeting baby's needs (V)	0.691	1.48	0.192	0.86	3.55[a]

[a]Significant at the .05 level.

the baby emerged as the most important variable related to within-group differences of this population of adolescent mothers.

DISCUSSION

Although the interpretation of the data presented above is somewhat difficult because of the paucity of research assessing personality and attitudinal variables with this population of mothers, the findings seem to support the evidence from studies that have examined mother-child interaction (Epstein, 1980; Osofsky & Osofsky, 1970; Sandler, 1978; Sandler et al., 1981), child abuse and neglect (Brunnquell et al., 1979; Egeland et al., 1979), and mental illness of mothers (Cohler et al., 1970a; Grunebaum et al., 1982). As mentioned previously in this chapter, the assessment of attitudinal variables provides additional sources of data for understanding the mother-child relationship. In fact, research that does not take into account these variables, which represent the cultural context for understanding development, has been called into question (Sameroff, 1982).

In the present study, the finding of maladaptive attitudes among adolescent mothers regarding the encouragement of reciprocity supports Epstein's (1980) findings that teenage subjects' most characteristic interactive style was nonverbal, or the "no talking" style. This is consistent with the belief that babies are passive beings and cannot communicate with their mothers. Also, findings indicating maladaptive attitudes toward the resolution of the issue of appropriate control of the child's aggressive impulses lend support to other research that has assessed the social and emotional development of children of teenage mothers. Results from Broman's (1981) and Marecek's (1979) studies have shown that the children of teenage mothers have a significantly higher frequency of deviant behavior, although differences were found based on race and favoring the children of black mothers (Broman, 1981), a result again underscoring the importance of attention to variables in addition to maternal age.

In American society, childbearing in adolescence is seen as an interruption of the life course rather than a normal part of it, which may be true in more traditional societies (Pebley, Casterline, & Trussell, 1982); it is a "role more appropriate to adulthood than to adolescence" (Kellam et al., 1979, p. 23). Thus, the premature assumption of the role of motherhood in American society can be expected to be associated with certain conflicts and concerns such as remaining in school, working out child-care arrangements, supporting another person, and continued dependence on others. These are in addition to the stresses imposed by the normal developmental tasks of adolescence. To deal with these issues effectively, they must be acknowledged and confronted. The findings from the present study indicate that these young women are less able to recognize and deal with these feelings. The denial of child-rearing concerns has been shown, in other studies, to be associated with mental illness in the mothers (Cohler et al., 1980) and disturbances of child-rearing, specifically child abuse and neglect (Brunnquell et al., 1979; Egeland et al., 1979).

In sum, it is possible to identify a child-rearing profile, albeit a tentative one, of adolescent mothers in this study. These mothers would be likely to experience difficulties in establishing a reciprocal relationship with their children and may have serious problems in their responses to their children's aggressive and destructive actions. Furthermore, these mothers would be unlikely to seek help from others or even to acknowledge that they do need assistance in child-rearing. Their "psychological profile" could be characterized as defensive and inhibited.

IMPLICATIONS

The implications of these findings suggest that attitudinal variables are important for identifying risk situations and for intervening in the lives of these mothers. In addition, it is clear that motivational factors, such as the desire to have a baby, should be considered when planning intervention efforts. There appears to be a high-risk group within a high-risk group.

Intervention efforts must not only address the adolescent's role as parent in the global sense but must be directed toward incorporating approaches specific to the population being served. In this regard, conceptualization of intervention as operating on various levels is useful. Newberger's (1979) approach is illustrative. Three levels of intervention were identified: structural, facilitative, and caretaking. *Structural intervention* would facilitate in the parent a more mature conception of the child as a person, of the maternal role, and of the parent-child relationship in general, while personal and environmental stresses that inhibit the mother's understanding of the child would be addressed through *facilitative intervention.* These could include legal aid, medical care, and employment counseling. *Caretaking intervention* addresses parental practices. The emphasis at this level would be on techniques and strategies to assist the mother to respond to the child's physical, cognitive, and emotional needs.

The ability of the adolescent mother to benefit from intervention may not only be a function of specific needs, as described above, but of her psychosocial status, including level of cognitive development. For instance, how a parent interprets the behavior of his or her child is related to the level at which the parent views development (Sameroff, 1982), which, in turn,

is a function of abstractive ability. "At progressively higher levels, parents are able to place the elements of the interaction into an increasingly broader context . . . and eventually are able to take perspective and separate the child from the particular environment in which he or she was raised" (Sameroff, 1982, p. 148).

Whatever particular intervention approach is used with this population, it seems clear that it must be an interactive approach that incorporates the mother's feelings about child-rearing issues. Child-rearing attitudes are a product of a long family history and orientation on "how to raise children" and are resistent to simple intervention strategies (Anastasiow, 1981). The mother needs to be supported so that she is able to provide nurturance to another person. It has been said that a mother is able to invest in her infant to the extent that someone has invested in her. Parent education that stresses only techniques and strategies would not only be ineffective with this population of mothers, but it would also preclude an opportunity to invest in the mother through communicating the value and importance of her own feelings.

REFERENCES

Anastasiow, N.J. The needs of early childhood education for the handicapped: A song for the 80's. *Journal of the Division for Early Childhood,* 1981, *2,* 1–7.

Baldwin, W., & Cain, V.S. The children of teenage parents. *Family Planning Perspectives,* 1980, *12,* 34–43.

Belmont, L., Cohen, P., Dryfoos, J., Stein, Z., & Zayac, S. Maternal age and children's intelligence. In: K.G. Scott, T. Field, & E. Robertson (eds.), *Teenage parents and their offspring.* New York: Grune & Stratton, 1981.

Broman, S.H. Longterm development of children born to teenagers. In: K.G. Scott, T. Field, & E. Robertson (eds), *Teenage parents and their offspring.* New York: Grune & Stratton, 1981.

Brown, C.H., Adams, R.G., & Kellam, S.G. A longitudinal study of teenage motherhood and symptoms of distress: The Woodlawn community epidemiological project. In: R. Simmons (ed.), *Research in community and mental health,* Vol. 2. Greenwich: JAI Press, 1980.

Brunnquell, D., Crichton, L., & Egeland, B. *Maternal personality and attitude in disturbances of child-rearing.* Paper presented at the annual meeting of the American Psychological Association, New York, September, 1979.

Cohler, B.J., Gallant, D.H., Grunebaum, H.U., Weiss, J.L. & Gamer, E. Child-care attitudes and development of young children of mentally ill and well mothers. *Psychological Reports,* 1980, *46,* 31–46.

Cohler, B.J., Weiss, J.L., & Grunebaum, H.U. Child-care attitudes and emotional disturbance among mothers of young children. *Genetic Psychology Monographs,* 1970, *82,* 4–47. (a)

Cohler, B.J., Weiss, J.L., & Grunebaum, H.U. *The maternal attitude scale* (preliminary manual). Unpublished manuscript, Harvard University, Cambridge, MA, 1970. (b)

Egeland, B. & Brunnquell, D. An at-risk approach to the study of child abuse: Some preliminary findings. *Journal of the American Academy of Psychiatry,* 1979, *18,* 219–235.

Egeland, B., Deinard, A., Brunnquell, D., Phipps-Yonas, S., & Crichton, L. *A prospective study of the antecedents of child abuse* (final report). Washington, DC: Department of Health, Education, and Welfare, September, 1979.

Epstein, A.S. *Assessing the child development information needed by adolescent parents with very young children* (final report). Washington, DC: January, 1980.

Grunebaum, H., Weiss, J.L., Cohler, B.J., Hartman, C.R., & Gallant, D.H. *Mentally ill mothers and their children*. Chicago: University of Chicago Press, 1982.

Hardy, J.B., King, T.M., Shipp, D.A., & Welcher, D.W. A comprehensive approach to adolescent pregnancy. In: K.G. Scott, T. Field, & E. Robertson (eds.), *Teenage parents and their offspring*. New York: Grune & Stratton, 1981.

Kellam, S.G., Adams, R.G., Brown, C.H., & Ensminger, M.E. *The long-term evolution of the family structure of adolescent and older mothers*. Paper presented at the annual meeting of the Society for Research of Social Problems, Boston, August, 1979.

Kellam, S.G., Ensminger, M.E., & Turner, R.J. Family structure and the mental health of children. *Archives of General Psychiatry*, 1977, *34*, 1012–1022.

Marecek, J. *Economic, social and psychological consequences of adolescent child rearing: An analysis of data from the Philadelphia collaborative perinatal project* (Final Report). Washington, DC: National Institute of Child Health and Human Development, September, 1979.

Moore, K.A., & Burt, M.R. *Private crisis, public cost*. Washington, DC: The Urban Institute Press, 1982.

Newberger, C.M. *Child abuse and the development of a parental consciousness*. Paper presented at the annual meeting of the Society for Research in Child Development, San Francisco, March, 1979.

Osofsky, H.J., & Osofsky, J.D. Adolescents as mothers. Results of a program for low-income pregnant teenagers with some emphasis upon infant development. *American Journal of Orthopsychiatry*, 1970, *40*, 825–835. (a)

Parke, R.D. Parent-infant interaction: Progress, paradigms, and problems. In: G.P. Sackett, (ed.), *Observing behavior, Vol. 1: Theory and application in mental retardation*. Baltimore: University Park Press, 1978.

Parke, R.D., & Tinsley, B.R. The early environment of the at-risk infant: Expanding the social context. In: D.D. Bricker, (ed.), *Intervention with at-risk and handicapped infants*. Baltimore: University Park Press, 1982.

Pebley, A.R., Casterline, J.B., & Trussell, J. Age at first birth in 19 countries. *International Family Planning Perspectives*, 1982, *8*(1), 2–7.

Ramey, C.T., & Gowan, J.W. *Maternal characteristics and intellectual development: Implications for parent education to prevent sociocultural mental retardation*. Paper presented at the annual meeting of the American Psychological Association, New York, September, 1979.

Sameroff, A.J. The environmental context of developmental disabilities. In: D.D. Bricker, (ed.), *Intervention with at-risk and handicapped infants*. Baltimore: University Park Press, 1982.

Sander, L. Issues in early mother-child interaction. *Journal of the American Academy of Child Psychiatry*, 1962, *2*, 141–166.

Sander, L. Adaptive relationships in early mother-child interactions. *Journal of the American Academy of Child Psychiatry*, 1964, *3*, 221–263.

Sandler, H.M. *Effects of adolescent pregnancy on mother-infant relationships: A transactional model* (progress report). Washington, DC: National Institute of Child Health and Human Development, May, 1978.

Sandler, H.M., Vietze, P.M., & O'Connor, S. Obstetric and neonatal outcomes following intervention with pregnant teenagers. In: K.G. Scott, T. Field, & E. Robertson (eds.), *Teenage parents and their offspring*. New York: Grune & Stratton, 1981.

Zelnik, M., & Kantner, J. First pregnancies to women aged 15–19: 1976 and 1971. *Family Planning Perspectives*, 1978, *10*, 11–20.

Chapter 6

Transdisciplinary Teamwork
with Parents of
Premature Infants

SETSU FURUNO, PH.D.
University of Hawaii, Honolulu, Hawaii
KATHERINE O'REILLY, R.P.T., M.P.H.
Kapiolani/Children's Medical Center, Honolulu, Hawaii
FRANK AHERN, PH.D.
University of Hawaii, Honolulu, Hawaii

THE EFFICACY OF SOME FORM OF EARLY intervention as a means of ameliorating the long-term effects of prematurity is now generally accepted. Still under debate, however, are many issues having to do with the relative effectiveness of different methods, types, patterns, or temporal arrangements of intervention, as well as the relative roles of parents versus professionals as intervening agents.

Among the earliest modern studies of intervention with premature infants was that of Hasselmeyer (1964), who found that extrasensory tactile and kinesthetic stimulation resulted in quiet behavior in the infant before feeding, in contrast to a group normally handled who exhibited crying behavior. Other studies have shown that gentle rocking, vestibular stimulation, and stroking have each shown positive effects for weight (Freedman, Boverman, & Freedman, 1966), motor development

and respiratory functioning (Korner & Thoman, 1972; Neal, 1977), as well as cardiac functioning during active sleep (Rose, Katalin, Riese, & Bridger, 1980). Tactile, auditory, and visual stimulation during and after hospitalization resulted in significant gains in cognitive development (Powell, 1974; Scarr-Salapatek & Williams, 1973). Visual, tactile, kinesthetic, and auditory stimulation by nurses during each feeding resulted in significantly higher 6-month Bayley Mental and Motor scores for treated infants (Leib, Benfield, & Guidubald, 1980).

Barnard and Bee (1981), in testing the efficacy of temporally patterned kinesthetic and auditory stimulation for premature infants immediately following birth, found immediate positive changes in infant activity and long-term changes in cognitive development. Barnard and Bee (1981) describe the intervention as an effort to offset "*inappropriate* stimu-

Funded by the Education of the Handicapped Act, 1970 (PL 91-230), U.S. Department of Education, Grant No. G008000208.

51

lation," e.g., lack of a predictable daily schedule. "*Insufficient* stimulation" has been the theoretical basis for most intervention studies, e.g., lack of normal tactile, kinesthetic, social, and auditory input. Mothers have also been encouraged to visit and care for their infants in the nursery and this practice has been shown to result in significantly higher Stanford-Binet scores (Kennell, Jerault, & Wolfe, 1974).

One study that showed that infant development was not affected by intervention programs was similar to the Parent Intervention Group (to be described later), but differed in that intervention occurred later, between ages 10 months and 2 years (Sigman & Parmelee, 1979).

Some projects such as the Education for Multi-handicapped Infants (EMI) at the Children's Rehabilitation Center and Newborn Intensive Care Unit of the University of Virginia Medical Center (Wallens, Elder, & Hastings, 1979) provided standard stimulation procedures for all infants. These activities were not based on individual infant assessment, but efforts were taken to avoid overstimulation and to ensure that the infant's state was appropriate before activities were initiated.

The use of transdisciplinary teams became widespread in infant development programs through the efforts of the United Cerebral Palsy Association's National Collaborative Infant Project (Haynes, 1976). The transdisciplinary team is one that reduces handling of an infant by many professionals, but requires that team members collaborate and trust each other enough to share their professional skills. Only one team member, the care manager, works directly with the infant and the family, using others as consultants. This reduction in fragmentation benefits parents as well as infants by reducing the possibility of conflicting advice, and fostering the concept of the parent as the most important caregiver for the infant.

The studies cited, as well as many others, have suggested, first, that intervention per se requires careful and comprehensive professional assessment and planning that takes into consideration the unique attributes of the infant as well as the family, and second, that intervention may best be based on the "deficit" model. This deficit model holds that premature infants, having had to emerge from the uterus without the protection of the uterine environment for the expected length of time, need not only assistance based on precise assessment to reduce possible deviant movement patterns and abnormal postural tone, but also sensory input provided with sensitive regard for the baby's state.

This chapter presents results obtained from the Family Centered Care Project (FCCP) which was designed to study the relative effectiveness of three models of intervention: 1) a transdisciplinary model in which a team of professionals works with parents *and* their premature infant (family intervention), 2) a more traditional model whereby a nurse specialist works with only the parents (parent intervention), and 3) a model whereby only regular medical and nursing care are provided by the hospital (control).

The present results are directed toward three primary hypotheses:

1. Precise assessment of motor, language, tactile, auditory, and oral functioning in the premature infant, followed by an individually planned multisensory treatment program, will enhance development as evidenced by Bayley (Bayley, 1969) and Gesell (Knobloch & Pasamanick, 1974) scores.

2. Teaching the parent(s) specific activities to do with their infants will enhance parent-infant bonding and interaction, and promote infant development.

3. Promotion of early contact by the parent(s), including educating them about the preterm infant's development and behavior, and allowing them to observe their infant's performance on the Neonatal Behavioral Assessment Scale (Brazelton, 1974) will enhance parent-infant bonding and interaction as measured by the Nursing Child Assessment Feeding and Teaching Scales (Barnard, 1978).

The parent intervention group, when compared with the control group, tested only hypothesis three, whereas the family intervention group tested all three hypotheses.

STUDY SAMPLE

All infants in the FCCP were those who were consecutively admitted to the Kapiolani/ Children's Medical Center's Neonatal Intensive Care Unit (NICU) who met either of two conditions: 1) birth weight under 1,500 grams, or 2) birth weight under 2,000 grams *and* being on a ventilator for at least 48 hours, were eligible for the FCCP. Infants with central nervous system (CNS) dysfunction and those with specific defects such as Down syndrome or spina bifida were excluded.

The FCCP covered the period of January 1981 through July 1983. At admission to the Neonatal Intensive Care Unit (NICU), infants who were eligible were randomly assigned to each of the three groups, and informed-consent procedures were initiated. Due to infant deaths and differential parental acceptance into the study groups, the number of infants was not equally distributed; there were 36 infants in the family intervention group, 32 in the parent intervention group, and 32 in the control group for a total of 100 infants.

PROCEDURE

Family Intervention Group

Assignment to the family intervention group involved a set of procedures that encompassed the project staff's interpretation of the transdisciplinary model. This included individualized assessment of the infant and a treatment program designed by the team of physical, occupational, and speech therapists, and educator.

The assessment covered the oral, tactile, motor, social-behavior, auditory, and language domains. In addition to standardized assessment instruments, e.g., the Neonatal Behavioral Assessment Scale (NBAS) (Brazelton, 1974) and the Bayley Scales of Infant Development (1969), various special purpose assessment instruments were developed by each member of the professional team.

Following the initial assessments, long-term goals and short-term objectives were developed based on each infant's identified needs. Activities designed to meet these objectives were developed and taught to the parents. Assessments were done when infants reached a state of stability as defined by the neonatologist. Intervention was provided daily by the care manager and/or a parent.

Assessments were ongoing during each intervention session. The infant's state was carefully assessed in order to decide how much intervention and what type was appropriate for the infant at that moment. Responses of the infant to the intervention were also carefully monitored so that the caregiver could be alert to signs of stress or of readiness for interaction.

Activities were designed to assist the infants in achieving an optimal state for interaction, and in fostering skills appropriate to the infant's developmental level. For example, an irritable baby might need consoling before an alert state was achieved for presentation of auditory or visual stimuli. A drowsy baby might require tactile, vestibular, and kinesthetic stimulation to assist arousal. Motor skills such as beginning head control or preweight bearing on hands and feet were facilitated when appropriate to gestational age, and when the infant was in a receptive state. Attention to oral development included activities to prevent tactile hypersensitivity during gavage feeding and to encourage nonnutritive sucking, and techniques to facilitate coordinated sucking and swallowing during nippling.

Intervention by the team began when the babies were medically stable. Infants received an activity program lasting 15–30 minutes, 5 days per week by either the parent or the care manager. Following discharge from the hospital, weekly visits were planned, but they actually occurred approximately two times per month, and were combinations of home visits and outpatient hospital visits.

Parent Intervention Group

Assignment to the parent intervention group involved a set of activities that was subsumed under the model of intervention through parent education. The basis of this model was that by instructing the parents about premature behavior and development and the importance of interacting early with the infant and by supporting their caretaking efforts, they would be able to provide effective intervention in appropriate amounts for the infants. This education was provided to these parents primarily through the clinical nurse specialist with input from the other professional staff.

The nurse met with parents one to two times per week during the hospital phase and approximately twice per month following hospital discharge on a home visiting basis.

The social worker worked with families in both family and parent intervention groups from the time an infant was admitted until discharge. The activities of the social worker varied from case to case. Within 24 to 48 hours after admission, fathers were usually already visiting in the NICU. The social worker not only met with the father, but also tried to arrange a conference with the neonatologist if he or she had not yet spoken to the father. The social worker familiarized the father with the unit, helped him work out financial details, and provided him with a glossary of technical terms. The social worker also called the mother, or the social worker at the referring hospital if the infant had been flown in from a hospital on a neighbor island. The social worker served as an advocate to the family and tried to remove as many barriers as possible so that the family could focus on the baby.

Additionally, the social worker maintained contact with the family throughout the hospital course by facilitating the financial situation, supporting the family emotionally, and helping them with community resources. The care manager and the nurse specialist worked with the families more specifically in relation to increasing the interaction with the infant.

Another important feature of the intervention process for both treatment groups was the parental opportunity to observe the Brazelton assessment (NBAS) by the clinical nurse specialist. The NBAS was used rather than the Assessment of Preterm Infant Behavior (APIB) (Als, Lester, Tronick, & Brazelton, 1982),

because the APIB was not available at the current time. Dr. Brazelton authorized use of the NBAS after the infant reached 38 weeks gestational age if the infant was medically stable. Having parents view the infant's performance on this scale has been demonstrated to act as a powerful intervention tool. Parents can focus on the infant's skills and model their interaction on what they observe with the tester (Brazelton, 1982).

Control Group

Assignment to the control group involved the usual set of activities available in a standard hospital care and treatment regime. This care included all the medical and nursing expertise that would be expected in a regional perinatal center. Social work and occupational and physical therapy services were available only as requested by the physician. The follow-up performance and capabilities of infants in this group thus served as a baseline for comparison to the more involved and distinct intervention models.

Assessment Phases

Data were obtained from infants at various occasions during the course of intervention and in relation to the phases of the infants' hospital experience. Briefly, these data collection periods were:

Acute Phase (AP)—the period during which the infant required ventilation

Subacute Phase (SP)—the period during which the infant required supplemental oxygen

Recovery Phase (RP)—the period from the time the infant no longer required oxygen until hospital discharge

Discharge Phase (DP)—the period of about 1 week prior to discharge when final testing was done

1-Month Outpatient Follow-up (OP1)—the first 4 weeks following hospital discharge, which usually corresponded to 1 month corrected age

3-Month Outpatient Follow-up (OP3)—the period up to 3 months corrected age

9-Month Outpatient Follow-up (OP9)—the period up to 9 months corrected age

Not all infants were assessed at each period. Control group infants were not assessed during the hospital recovery, outpatient 1-month, or outpatient 3-month phases.

Assessment Instruments

A large variety of assessment instruments and procedures were used in the FCCP. Only those that pertain to the results reported in this chapter are described.

Brazelton Neonatal Behavioral Assessment Scale (Brazelton, 1974) Items of the Brazelton were clustered to form scales related to the infant's: a) ability to shut out disturbing stimuli (habituation), b) responsiveness to auditory and visual stimuli (orientation), c) muscle tone and activity level (motor performance), d) irritability and level of excitement (range of state), e) capacity to cuddle and self-console (regulation of state), f) tremor, startles, and skin color (autonomic regulation), and g) reflexes. The Brazelton was used at the hospital recovery phase, at discharge weeks, and at 1 month following discharge.

Nursing Child Assessment Feeding Scales (NCAF) (Barnard, 1978) The NCAF includes a series of items describing a mother's sensitivity to and clarity of cues, her cognitive and emotional growth-fostering capacity, her response to distress, and the infant's responsiveness to parents. Assessment was done during a feeding session at recovery phase, discharge week, outpatient 3 months, and 9 months.

Nursing Child Assessment Teaching Scales (NCAT) (Barnard, 1978) The NCAT tests for the same areas as described for the NCAF, but parent-infant interaction is assessed through a teaching task. This assessment was used at outpatient 3- and 9-month phases.

Maternal Developmental Expectations and Childrearing Attitudes Scale (MDECAS) (Field, 1980) The MDECAS measures the mother's knowledge and attitudes about child-rearing. The scale takes the form of a questionnaire for mothers but has also been used in interview style when there are language difficulties. This scale was used at hospital discharge and outpatient 9-month phases.

Parent Satisfaction Scale The Parent Satisfaction Scale is an unpublished scale developed by the project to assess parents' reactions to their participation in the project, and to give them an opportunity to provide staff with feedback regarding procedures that need to be changed. This scale was given at the hospital discharge and at the outpatient 9-month stage.

The Bayley Scales of Infant Development (Bayley, 1969) The Bayley Mental Developmental and Perceptual Developmental Index provides scores relative to cognitive and perceptual motor development of infants. This index was used as a major outcome variable at the 9-month outpatient stage.

Receptive-Expressive Emergent Language Scale (REEL) (Bzoch & League, 1971) The REEL scale includes observation and parent interview items designed to assess an infant's developing language abilities. It was given only at the 9-month outpatient stage.

Gesell Developmental Schedules (Knobloch & Pasamanick, 1974) The Gesell Developmental Schedules are the standard developmental assessment, measuring a child's abilities in personal-social, language, fine motor, gross motor, and adaptive domains. They also provide a developmental quotient as a summary score. This test was done at outpatient 3- and 9-month stages.

Morbidity Scale (Lubchenco, 1973) The Morbidity Scale assesses the potential risk of an infant's problems based on items surrounding the birth and delivery and initial characteristics of the infant. This assessment was done during the acute phase.

ANALYSES OF RESULTS

Assignment of the at-risk infants to the three groups was made without consideration of characteristics of either the parents or infants other than those criteria mentioned previously in the study sample section. In order to examine the possibility of bias, a series of tests was developed to distinguish differences between groups for infant and parent characteristics. Table 1 presents the breakdown of the

Table 1. Ethnicity of infants by treatment group

Ethnicity	Family intervention	Parent intervention	Control
Caucasian	3	6	2
Japanese	5	2	5
Chinese	2	0	0
Filipino	4	1	1
Mixed Oriental	5	7	5
Mixed Hawaiian	11	7	14
Other	6	8	4
Missing	0	1	1
Total:	36	32	32

infants' ethnicity by intervention group. There is no significant association between ethnicity and group (chi-square = 29.7, df = 24, p = 19). Analyses of variance were also carried out for clinical characteristics of infants with no significant group effects. Selected demographic characteristics of the parents by intervention group were also analyzed with no significant group effects, although there was a suggestion of paternal age being higher for the parent intervention group (F = 3.02, p = .054) and maternal education being higher for the parent intervention group (F = 2.8, p = .064).

Since maternal education has been known to be associated with outcome variates such as cognitive and language development, when significant tests of group effects were found, a subsequent test of group effects was always done using Analysis of Covariance (ANCOVA) with both maternal age and maternal education as covariates.

Gesell Developmental Schedules

Table 2 presents means and standard deviations of Gesell scores for the 3- and 9-month follow-up periods by intervention group. There were no group differences in Gesell scores. Analyses of covariance were done for the 3-month follow-up scales and no significant group effects were noted. Some interesting patterns of mean scores did, however, emerge. Control group means were lowest in 5 out of 6 comparisons at 3 months. Both the family and parent intervention groups' infants scored better than did control group infants. The parent intervention group showed higher means and reduced variation when compared to the family

intervention group. This pattern of results was not seen for the 9-month Gesell means.

Bayley Scales

Bayley Scale scores administered at 9 months are also presented in Table 2. Both intervention groups' means were higher than the controls. For the Psychomotor Developmental Index (PDI), p = .10, and for the Mental Developmental Index (MDI), p = .05. Parent intervention group means were higher than family intervention group means for both the Mental Development Index and the Psychomotor Development Index.

Receptive-Expressive Emergent Language Scale (REEL)

REEL Scale scores are presented at the 9-month follow-up in Table 3. Intervention groups show significantly higher scores for expressive and combined language quotients.

Nursing Child Assessment Feeding (NCAF) and Teaching (NCAT) Scales

Means and standard deviations for NCAF scales at the 3-month follow-up were obtained for only the family and parent intervention groups (Table 4). At the 9-month follow-up, both intervention group means tended to be higher than the control group on all but one of the NCAF subscales and were significantly higher on the total scores and for the subscales measuring response to distress (p = .02), and clarity of cues (p = .02). The direction and significance of these group differences did not change after adjusting for covariates. Means and standard deviations for the NCAT scales at the 3-month assessment showed no differences between parent and family intervention groups (Table 5).

The contrast between the results for NCAF and NCAT scores suggests that interaction between parents and infants is different during teaching and feeding, and that differences that might be due to intervention may be unique to specific occasions. These same scales were administered again at the 9-month follow-up to both intervention groups as well as the control group.

Table 2. Gesell and Bayley Scale scores by intervention group

	3-Month follow-up			9-Month follow-up		
	N	Mean	S.D.	N	Mean	S.D.
Gesell						
Personal-social						
Family	20	92	20	19	94	12
Parent	20	98	16	19	95	11
Control	17	88	21	20	93	11
Language						
Family	20	101	31	19	90	11
Parent	20	108	27	19	93	10
Control	17	93	26	20	91	9
Fine motor						
Family	20	91	21	19	95	11
Parent	20	100	14	19	94	12
Control	17	94	26	20	92	18
Gross motor						
Family	20	93	30	19	108	23
Parent	20	100	16	19	110	22
Control	17	86	26	20	96	24
Adaptive						
Family	20	91	19	19	101	12
Parent	20	96	17	19	99	9
Control	17	90	22	20	101	21
Overall Development Quotient						
Family	20	94	21	19	98	13
Parent	20	99	15	19	98	11
Control	17	90	23	20	94	14
Bayley Psychomotor Index						
Family				18	93	19[a]
Parent				16	102	14
Control				10	85	26
Bayley Mental Index						
Family				18	92	20[b]
Parent				16	105	16
Control				10	86	26

[a]p = .10.
[b]p = .05.

Table 3. REEL Scale scores by intervention group

	9-Month follow-up		
	N	Mean	S.D.
REEL			
Receptive			
Family	18	88	14[a]
Parent	17	95	13
Control	10	83	16
Expressive			
Family	18	82	13[b]
Parent	17	88	14
Control	10	69	17
Language			
Family	18	85	13[b]
Parent	17	92	12
Control	10	76	16

[a]p = .10.
[b]p = .01

Maternal Developmental Expectations and Childrearing Attitudes Scale (MDECAS)

The MDECAS was administered at the discharge and the 9-month phases. No group differences were noted for any of the parent measures, including this scale designed by Field (1980) to test knowledge and attitude of child growth and development. All groups of parents performed poorly in knowledge, but did well in attitudes. Parent satisfaction measures were obtained from the family and parent groups only and no differences were noted. Both groups tended to be overwhelmingly positive in their response to the project.

Table 4. NCAF scores by intervention group

	3-Month follow-up			9-Month follow-up			p
	N	Mean	S.D.	N	Mean	S.D.	
Total							
Family	13	56.6	9.1	15	62.3	4.0	
Parent	14	61.8	9.0	13	62.2	4.8	p = .03
Control		NA		6	54.3	12.5	
Sensitivity to cues							
Family	13	12.8	1.8	15	12.9	1.7	
Parent	14	14.1	1.5	13	12.8	1.0	p = .06
Control		NA		6	11.3	1.6	
Response to distress							
Family	13	10.0	1.1	15	9.8	1.2	
Parent	14	9.6	1.8	13	9.0	2.1	p = .02
Control		NA		6	6.8	3.8	
Social-emotional growth fostering							
Family	13	11.0	2.5	15	12.1	1.5	
Parent	14	11.7	1.8	13	11.5	2.0	
Control		NA		6	10.5	3.1	
Cognitive growth fostering							
Family	13	6.2	2.1	15	6.5	1.2	
Parent	14	7.2	1.9	13	6.5	1.8	
Control		NA		6	7.0	1.8	
Clarity of cues							
Family	13	10.9	2.3	15	13.1	1.7	
Parent	14	12.4	2.2	13	13.9	1.6	p = .02
Control		NA		6	11.2	2.9	
Responsiveness to Parent							
Family	13	5.8	2.1	15	7.9	1.7	
Parent	14	7.5	1.9	13	8.6	1.5	
Control		NA		6	7.5	2.7	

Correlations among Measures: Brazelton, Gesell, and Bayley Scales

Relationships between infant-parent interaction measures and the cognitive and perceptual motor development of the child were also studied as a possible means of predicting the infant's later competence. Table 6 shows the correlations between Brazelton scores at hospital discharge and Gesell scores at 3 months. Table 7 shows the correlations of Brazelton scores at discharge with Gesell and Bayley scores obtained during the follow-up assessments at 9 months.

High scores on the Gesell gross motor, adaptive, overall developmental quotient (DQ) and DQ less than 80 and the Bayley Mental Development scores appear to be negatively related to infants' ability to habituate to the environment. This may be explained by the possibility that when a baby is able to control his or her responses by shutting out excessive stimulation, he or she may also be giving fewer cues to the caretaker for a need for appropriate stimulation.

In contrast, the ability of the infant to orient to auditory and visual stimuli appears to be strongly related to all items except language on the Gesell at 3 months. These relationships are not all continuous at the 9-month level, but there is a relationship with Gesell gross motor scores. High orientation scores appear to be predictive of the Bayley Mental and Psychomotor Development at 9 months.

Motor performance on the Brazelton was highly correlated with all of the Gesell measures at 3 months and also with mental development on the Bayley.

The infant's capacity for state regulation (defined as his or her ability to quiet himself or herself and to be consoled) was highly correlated with cognitive and motor functioning at 3 months based on the Gesell (Table 6).

Table 5. NCAT scores by intervention group

	3-Month follow-up			9-Month follow-up			p
	N	Mean	S.D.	N	Mean	S.D.	
Total							
Family	22	48.5	8.5	16	56.1	7.6	
Parent	14	50.3	5.3	13	57.0	5.9	
Control		NA		7	54.8	7.4	
Sensitivity to cues							
Family	22	8.4	1.8	16	8.4	1.7	
Parent	14	8.9	1.0	13	8.2	1.5	
Control		NA		7	8.7	1.5	
Response to distress							
Family	22	9.7	1.6	16	10.2	1.3	
Parent	14	10.0	1.2	13	9.2	1.3	p = .09
Control		NA		7	9.2	1.3	
Social-emotional growth fostering							
Family	22	8.5	1.9	16	8.9	1.5	
Parent	14	8.9	1.5	13	9.0	1.6	
Control		NA		7	9.7	1.0	
Cognitive growth fostering							
Family	22	8.8	3.4	16	10.6	3.0	
Parent	14	8.6	2.4	13	11.1	2.9	
Control		NA		7	10.6	2.2	
Clarity of cues							
Family	22	7.5	1.6	16	9.1	1.0	
Parent	14	7.9	1.2	13	9.5	1.1	
Control		NA		7	9.0	1.1	
Responsiveness to Parent							
Family	22	5.6	2.3	16	8.9	2.5	
Parent	14	6.1	2.1	13	13.5	12.6	
Control		NA		7	8.7	3.9	

Infant Behavior and Parent-Infant Interaction

Another set of relationships examined was that between infant organization at discharge and parent-infant interactions, obtained during feeding (Table 8) and teaching (Table 9) at 9 months. It was noted that cognitive growth fostering is negatively related to habituation on the NCAT (Table 9) and to the range of state on the NCAF (Table 8). In other words, the better the ability of the infant to quiet and console himself or herself and to shut out the environment, the less likely is provision by the mother of cognitive stimulation. Should the infant also show considerable range in behavior (e.g., irritability, peak of excitement), the less likely will be the engagement of the mother during feeding in cognitive growth-fostering activities.

Autonomic regulation, motor performance, and regulation of state are negatively related to clarity of cues and responsiveness to parent by infant (see Table 9). These results suggest possibly that a well-regulated infant does not find it necessary to provide clear cues. As a consequence, the infant at 9 months does not respond to the parent during the teaching sequence. In contrast, during feeding, perhaps because the infant is receiving food, he or she tends to be more responsive and to provide cues clearly.

Orientation of the infant to auditory and visual stimulation again demonstrates a strong relationship with overall maternal interaction and mother's sensitivity to cues of the infant.

The infant's motor performance appears to relate positively to maternal sensitivity to cues, but relates negatively to the infant's capacity to provide clear cues during the teaching sequence (Table 9). During the feeding sequence, however, motor performance is positively related to the infant's capacity to provide cues clearly (see Table 8).

Table 6. Correlations of Brazelton scores at discharge with Gesell scores at 3 months

	Brazelton scores						
	Habituation	Orientation	Motor performance	Range of state	Regulation of state	Autonomic regulation	Reflexes
Gesell: 3 months							
Personal-social		.30[a]	.30[a]		.30[a]		
Language		.29[a]					
Fine motor	.31[a]	.29[a]			.39[a]		
Gross motor	.28[a]	.26[a]			.28[a]		
Adaptive	.37[b]	.39[a]			.39[b]	.26[a]	
Overall DQ	.27[a]	.31[a]			.37[b]		
DQ less than 80					.45[b]		

[a]$p = <.05.$
[b]$p = <.01.$

DISCUSSION

The goal of the study reported in this chapter was to test intervention procedures related to precise assessment of the infant's state and needs, and to develop a program of environmental modification that would be applied consistent with and appropriate to the baby's capacities.

Three study groups were formed to test three intervention models. *Family intervention* involved direct intervention with infants and parent(s) through a care manager, who demonstrated and taught activities appropriate to the babies' needs. *Parent intervention* involved educational intervention with the parent(s) to promote interaction, attachment, and caregiving skills. The *control group* involved all the medical and nursing expertise available in a regional perinatal center.

Results suggest that infants in treatment groups have done much better than those in the control group. The investigators are fully aware, however, that standard infant psychometric tests show poor predictive validity, and that test scores up to 18 months of age account for only a fractional portion of the variance in later IQs. The long-term effects of treatment will become evident as these families will be followed at the hospital until 6 years of age.

Assessment data were obtained from infants at various times during the intervention. A large variety of assessment instruments and procedures, including the Brazelton, Gesell, Bayley, REEL, NCAF, and NCAT were used. The relationship evidenced between the Brazelton items and the outcome variables will be examined over the years to assess their predictive quality. Of interest also is the rather curious finding of the negative relationship between habituation of the infant during the teaching session, and the caretaker's cognitive growth fostering and high scores on the Gesell and Bayley at 9 months. This finding, if rep-

Table 7. Correlations of Brazelton scores at discharge with Gesell and Bayley scores at 9 months

	Brazelton scores						
	Habituation	Orientation	Motor performance	Range of state	Regulation of state	Autonomic regulation	Reflexes
Gesell: 9 months							
Personal-social							
Language						−.28[a]	
Fine motor							
Gross motor	−.55[b]	.28[a]					
Adaptive	−.51[b]						
Overall DQ	−.52[b]						
DQ less than 80	−.41[b]						
Bayley							
Psychomotor Index	−.59[b]	.33[a]					
Mental Index	−.73[b]	.46[b]	.47[b]				

[a]$p = <.05.$
[b]$p = <.01.$

Table 8. Correlation of Brazelton at discharge with parent-infant interaction scales at 9 months

	Brazelton scores						
	Habituation	Orientation	Motor performance	Range of state	Regulation of state	Autonomic regulation	Reflexes
Nursing Child Assessment Feeding Scale (NCAF)							
Total		.40ᵃ					
Sensitivity to cues							
Response to distress				.44ᵇ			
Social-emotional growth fostering							
Cognitive growth fostering				−.41ᵃ			
Clarity to cues			.36ᵃ				
Responsiveness to parent							

ᵃp = <.05.
ᵇp = <.01.

licated, would suggest that professionals can utilize such information to work with mothers to have them observe more closely their interactions with their infants.

A significant result in relation to environmental modification is the strength of the orientation items on the Brazelton as related to positive behavior on the part of the caretaker. These results continue to verify the significance of careful intervention efforts. The extent of relationships between motor behavior and outcome variables is also of interest and suggests the former's importance in overall development.

At 3 months, all Gesell subtests except fine motor were better in experimental than control groups, but significance was not demonstrated. Nine-month scores were better in gross motor, fine motor, and overall DQ. The lack of significant differences may be due to the small sample size at the 9-month stage. Another possible reason for lack of differences is that control group families at times received intervention from other sources. If a need for intervention was identified for inpatient control infants by the medical or nursing staff, referral was made to the occupational and physical therapy departments. When discharged from the hospital, high-risk infants are typically referred by physicians to the community infant development programs and therefore would have received some type of intervention.

Table 9. Correlation of Brazelton at discharge with parent-infant interaction scales at 9 months

	Brazelton scores						
	Habituation	Orientation	Motor performance	Range of state	Regulation of state	Autonomic regulation	Reflexes
Nursing Child Assessment Teaching Scale (NCAT)							
Total							
Sensitivity to cues		.39ᵃ	.38ᵃ		.46ᵇ		
Response to distress		.36ᵃ					−.46ᵇ
Social-emotional growth fostering							
Cognitive growth fostering	−.61ᵃ						
Clarity of cues			−.41ᵃ		−.36ᵃ	−.42ᵃ	
Responsiveness to parent						−.40ᵃ	.44ᵇ

ᵃp = <.05.
ᵇp = <.01.

Bayley and REEL scores at 9 months were higher in both of the intervention groups.

Mother-infant interaction scores as measured at 3 months on the NCAF were done only for the two intervention groups. In total scores and mother's sensitivity to cues, the parent intervention group did significantly better than the family intervention group. The reason for this is not clear. At 9 months, when all three groups were again tested, both intervention groups surpassed the control group on all items except cognitive growth fostering. Significance was achieved in overall interactions ($p = .03$), response to distress ($p = .02$), and clarity of cues ($p = .02$), with sensitivity to cues approaching significance ($p = .06$).

DIRECTIONS AND IMPLICATIONS FOR FUTURE RESEARCH

The unequal numbers and the minimal number of clear control subjects suggest that it would be useful to use the population who are already part of the hospital's follow-up study as the control population. A group of infants born and discharged prior to the FCCP study may provide a contrast group who had no early planned intervention.

Despite the fact that the project terminated in August of 1983, the physical and occupational therapists will continue to be called on by physicians to work with certain infants who may be suspect for motor problems. By using covariate analysis to control for the possibly sicker population with whom these therapists are typically requested to work, the number of subjects to test out the treatment process may be increased as was done in the family intervention group of this study. Follow-up of these samples at 3 and 6 years to examine cognitive function and motor development, is anticipated.

Very little was done in the present study to differentiate neighbor island families from Oahu families—an analysis that may be useful to differentiate between local or long-distance care.

In summary, some evidence has been demonstrated to support the usefulness of early family intervention when a premature infant is born.

REFERENCES

Als, H., Lester, B., Tronick, E.Z., & Brazelton, T.B. Manual for the Assessment of Preterm Infants' Behavior (APIB). In: H.E. Fitzgerald, B.M. Lester, & M.M. Yogman (eds.), *Theory and research in behavioral pediatrics*. New York: Plenum Publishing Corp., 1982.

Barnard, K. *Nursing Child Assessment Feeding Scales (NCAF) and Nursing Child Assessment Teaching Scales (NCAT)*. Seattle: University of Washington, 1978.

Barnard, K., & Bee, H.L. *Premature infant refocus*. Final report of project supported by the Maternal Child Health (MCH) and the Crippled Children's Services (CCS) Research Grants Program. Washington, DC, September, 1981.

Bayley, N. *The Bayley Scales of Infant Development*. New York: The Psychological Corporation, 1969.

Brazelton, T.B. Neonatal Behavioral Assessment Scale. *Clinics in Developmental Medicine*, No. 50. Philadelphia: J.B. Lippincott, 1974.

Brazelton, T.B. Early intervention, what does it mean? In: H.E. Fitzgerald, B.M. Lester, & M.M. Yogman (eds.), *Theory and research in behavioral pediatrics*. New York: Plenum Publishing Corp., 1982.

Bzoch, K., & League, R. *Receptive-Expressive Emergent Language Scale*. Baltimore: University Park Press, 1971.

Field, T. Early development of infants born to teenage mothers. In: K. Scott, T. Field, & E. Robertson (eds.), *Teenage parents and their offspring*. New York: Grune & Stratton, 1980.

Freedman, D., Boverman, H., & Freedman, N. *Effects of kinesthetic stimulation on weight gain and on smiling in premature infants*. Paper presented at the annual meeting of the Orthopsychiatric Association, San Francisco, April, 1966.

Hasselmeyer, F.G. The premature neonate's response to handling. *American Nurses Association, Convention Clinical Sessions* 1964, *11*, 15–24.

Haynes, U.E. The National Collaborative Infant Project. In: T.D. Tjossem (ed.), *Intervention strategies for high-risk infants and young children*. Baltimore, University Park Press, 1976.

Kennell, J., Jerault, R., & Wolfe, H. Maternal behavior one year after early and extended post-partum contact. *Developmental Medicine and Child Neurology*, 1974, *16*, 172–179.

Knobloch, H., & Pasamanick, B. (eds.). *Gesell and Amatruda's developmental diagnosis* (3rd ed.). New York: Harper & Row, 1974.

Korner, A.F., & Thoman, E. The relative efficacy of contact and vestibular proprioception stimulation in soothing neonates. *Child Development*, 1972, *43*, 443–453.

Leib, S., Benfield, D.G., & Guidubald, J. Effects of early intervention and stimulation on the preterm infant. *Pediatrics,* 1980, *66,* 83–90.

Lubchenco, L. Appendix 5. In: M.H. Klaus & A.A. Fanaroff (eds.), *Care of the high risk neonate.* Philadelphia: W.B. Saunders, 1973.

Neal, M.V. Vestibular stimulation and development of the small premature infant. *Community Nursing Research,* 1977, *8,* 291–302.

Powell, L.F. The effect of extra stimulation and maternal involvement on the development of low birth weight infants and on maternal behavior. *Child Development,* 1974, *45,* 106–113.

Rose, S.A., Katalin, S., Riese, M., & Bridger, W. Effects of prematurity and early intervention on responsivity to tactual stimuli: A comparison of preterm and full-term infants. *Child Development,* 1980, *51,* 416–425.

Scarr-Salapatek, S., & Williams, M.L. The effects of early stimulation on low birth weight infants. *Child Development,* 1973, *44,* 94–101.

Sigman, M. & Parmelee, A.H. Longitudinal Evaluation of the Preterm Infant. In: T.M. Field, A.M. Sostek, S. Goldberg, & H.H. Shuman (eds.), *Infants Born At Risk.* Jamaica, NY: SP Medical and Scientific Books, 1979.

Wallens, P., Elder, W., & Hastings, S.N. *From the beginning: The EMI high risk nursery intervention program manual.* Charlottesville: Department of Pediatrics, University of Virginia Medical Center, 1979.

The At-Risk Infant: Psycho/Socio/Medical Aspects
edited by Shaul Harel, M.D., and Nicholas J. Anastasiow, Ph.D.
Copyright © 1985   Paul H. Brookes Publishing Co., Inc.   Baltimore • London

Chapter 7

Biological and Environmental Variables as Predictors of Intellectual Functioning at 6 Years of Age

LINDA S. SIEGEL, PH.D.

Ontario Institute for Studies in Education, Toronto, Ontario, Canada

O NE OF THE IMPORTANT ISSUES IN IMPROVING the physical and mental health of children is the formulation of screening techniques to predict which children will subsequently show problems. Of particular interest are the high-incidence, low-severity problems such as learning disabilities, behavior difficulties, and mild delays in intellectual functioning that are economically and psychologically costly but that may be ameliorated if remediation is provided early in development.

Systems that have been proposed to meet this goal of improving the physical and mental health of children have met with varying degrees of success. Studies using data from the Collaborative Perinatal Project have achieved relatively good prediction of IQ and achievement test scores in childhood but have used a complex system with many variables to accomplish this prediction (e.g., Broman, Nichols, & Kennedy, 1975; Smith, Flick, Ferriss, & Sellman, 1972). A relatively simple system has been developed by Ramey, Stedman, Borders-Patterson, and Mengel (1978), but information about the ability of this system to predict the outcome for an individual child has not been reported.

A number of systems have been relatively successful in predicting outcome early in development (e.g., Caputo, Taub, Goldstein, Smith, Dalack, Pursner, and Silberstein, 1974; Field, Hallock, Ting, Dempsey, Dabiri, & Shuman, 1978; Littman & Parmelee, 1978), but the efficacy of these systems for predicting development in older children is not known.

This author has developed a risk index, involving a relatively small set of reproductive, perinatal, and demographic variables, which has been relatively successful in predicting aspects of cognitive and language development in children at 2 (Siegel, Saigal, Rosenbaum, Morton, Young, Berenbaum, & Stoskopf, 1982), 3 (Siegel, 1982a), and 5 (Siegel, 1982b, 1983c) years. This chapter examines the ability of this risk index to predict intellectual functioning, as measured by the Wechsler Intelli-

The author wishes to thank Lorraine Hoult, Denise Marshall, and Wendy McHugh for their help with the data collection and analyses. This research was supported by grants from the Ontario Mental Health Foundation and the March of Dimes Birth Defects Foundation.

gence Scale for Children–Revised (WISC-R) (Wechsler, 1974). On the basis of the past studies on the effectiveness of this risk index, it was expected that the index would successfully predict scores and be useful in detecting children with low scores.

The ability of infant tests to predict intelligence test scores at 6 years was also examined. In previous studies, this author has found that the Bayley Scales (Bayley, 1969) and the Uzgiris-Hunt Scale (Uzgiris & Hunt, 1975) predict subsequent scores and discriminate children who will show developmental delay (Siegel, 1979, 1981, 1982c, 1983a, 1983b, 1983c). With heterogeneous samples, others have also found moderate correlations with tests of intellectual functioning in middle childhood (e.g., Ramey, Campbell, & Nicholson, 1973; Wilson, 1978a,b). It was expected that the prediction of developmental functioning and delay based on the risk index could be improved with the use of infant tests. In addition, a measure of the environment, the Home Observation for the Measurement of the Environment (HOME) (Bradley & Caldwell, 1976), was used to assess environmental influence on development. In summary, it was expected that developmental outcome would not be determined by a single factor but that measurement of a variety of biological and environmental factors would be necessary for the successful prediction of developmental outcome.

METHOD

Subjects

All the infants whose birth weights were under 1,500 grams and who were born and/or treated at the McMaster University Health Sciences Centre Neonatal Intensive Care Unit in the period of July 1, 1975 to June 30, 1976 were enrolled for longitudinal prospective study. The preterm infants were separated into groups of appropriate-for-gestational-age (AGA) or small-for-gestational-age (SGA) infants. The SGA group was composed of preterm infants under 1,501 grams whose birth weight was 2 standard deviations or more below the mean weight for their gestational age based on the

Usher-McLean (Usher & McLean, 1969) norms for a Canadian sample.

The comparison group of full-term infants consisted of demographically similar infants who were born after uncomplicated singleton deliveries and who experienced a normal perinatal course. The preterm and full-term infants were matched on socioeconomic level, parity, sex, and age of the mother at the birth of the infant. The demographic characteristics of the entire sample have been reported previously (e.g., Siegel et al., 1982).

There were 44 full-term and 42 preterm children available for testing at 5 years. Most of the children who were not available from the original sample had moved outside the area. However, 10 preterm children and 1 full-term child had sequelae (blindness, severe retardation, and/or cerebral palsy) such that it was not meaningful to administer developmental tests. Four of the preterm infants died in the first 12 months following their discharge from the Neonatal Intensive Care Unit.

The demographic characteristics of the children who were available for study at 6 years were as follows: Hollingshead socioeconomic status (SES), % class 3-5, preterm = 81.0%, full-term = 63.2%; % male, preterm = 50.0, full-term = 60.5; % firstborns, preterm = 37.5, full-term = 40.5. The groups were not significantly different on these variables (χ^2). The mean maternal age for both groups was 26.1 years. The preterm children had a mean birth weight of 1.20 kilograms and a mean gestational age of 30.5 weeks.

Developmental Testing

The children were seen at 4, 8, 12, 18, 24, 36, 48, 60, and 72 months. Chronological age was used as the basis for developmental testing, although scores corrected for the degree of prematurity were also considered when it was possible to do so. They were administered the Bayley Scales of Infant Development (Bayley, 1969) at 4, 8, 12, 18, and 24 months, a modified version of the Uzgiris-Hunt Scale (Uzgiris & Hunt, 1975) at 4, 8, 12, and 18 months, the Reynell Developmental Language Scales (Reynell, 1969) at 24, 36, and 48 months, a battery designed to predict learning disabilities (Satz, Taylor, Friel, & Fletcher, 1978) at 48 and 60 months, and the Wechsler Intelligence Scale for Children–Revised (WISC-R) (Weschler, 1974) at 72 months.

Risk Index Variables

Reproductive, perinatal, and demographic variables were used for each child. The reproductive variables were birth order (gravidity), amount of maternal smoking during pregnancy (none, less than 10, 10–20, over 20 cigarettes per day), and number of previous spontaneous abortions. The perinatal variables included birth weight, 1-minute and 5-minute Apgar scores, and, for the preterm infants, gestational age, severity of respiratory distress (RDS), birth asphyxia, and apnea. The following definitions for RDS were used: a) severe = assisted ventilation, X-ray evidence of RDS, and/or oxygen levels higher than 80%; b) moderate = assisted ventilation, continuous positive airway pressure (CPAP), and/or oxygen between 40% and 80%; and c) mild = oxygen less than 40%. A 1-minute Apgar score less than 5 was defined as asphyxia. For apnea, a record of the number of days in which apneic spells lasted longer than 20 seconds was kept. Hollingshead socioeconomic status, sex, and maternal and paternal educational levels were also included as demographic variables in the analyses.

RESULTS

IQ Scores at 6 Years

The scores of the preterms and full-terms on the WISC-R and the subtests are shown in Table 1. As can be seen from the table, the full-terms had significantly higher Verbal, Performance, and Full Scale IQ scores, and significantly higher scores on all the subtests with the exception of Picture Completion. Typically, the full-term children performed slightly above average while the preterm children performed slightly below average. While the mean scores provide an indication of the group performance, a critical question involves the number of children in each group with scores in the problem range. A score below 80 is classified as indicative of a significantly below average mental functioning. A score below 90 is

Table 1. Mean scores of preterm and full-term groups on the WISC-R at 6 years

	Full-term (N = 44)	Preterm (N = 42)
WISC-R IQ		
Verbal IQ	106.30	96.78[c]
Performance IQ	110.37	100.36[c]
Full Scale	108.93	98.29[c]
Subtests		
Verbal		
Information	11.37	10.12[a]
Similarities	10.51	8.86[a]
Arithmetic	11.33	9.71[b]
Vocabulary	11.67	9.66[b]
Comprehension	10.58	9.05[a]
Digit Span	10.60	9.17[a]
Performance		
Picture Completion	11.33	10.64
Picture Arrangement	11.30	9.98[a]
Block Design	11.90	9.81[c]
Object Assembly	11.79	10.38[a]
Coding	11.26	9.66[b]
Mazes	11.40	9.48[c]

[a] $p < .05$.
[b] $p < .01$.
[c] $p < .001$.

also typically associated with special educational intervention. The percentages of preterm and full-term children who attained scores in this range in these groups are shown in Table 2. As can be seen in Table 2, there were significantly more preterms with Performance IQ scores less than 90, but no differences between the percentage of preterms and full-terms with IQ scores less than 80, perhaps because there were so few children in this category.

Prediction of IQ Scores Using a Risk Index

Stepwise linear multiple regression analyses were conducted with the risk index variables described previously. The results of these analyses are shown in Table 3. As can be seen in Table 3, in all cases, the risk index variables were significantly correlated with the WISC-R IQ scores. For the Performance and Full Scale scores, the multiple correlations were higher for the preterm than the full-term group. While demographic variables, SES (socioeconomic status), and maternal education were obviously important factors, reproductive factors (e.g., a history of previous spontaneous abortions, birth order, maternal smoking) and factors

Table 2. Percentage of children with WISC-R scores below 80 and 90

	Below 80		Below 90	
	Full-term	Preterm	Full-term	Preterm
Verbal IQ	4.7	14.6	9.3	24.4[a]
Performance IQ	2.3	4.8	2.3	16.7[a]
Full Scale IQ	0	9.8	7.0	24.4[a]

[a]$p < .05$.

reflecting the severity of the perinatal insult (e.g., apnea, asphyxia) were important also.

Stepwise linear discriminant function analyses were conducted with the risk index variables to predict which of the children would have IQ scores of less than 90. The following classification system was used: the true negatives were children with scores in the normal range who were predicted as being normal; the true positives were children with low scores who were predicted as having low scores, the false negatives were children with low scores who were predicted as being normal, and false positives were children for whom low scores were predicted but who, in fact, had scores in the normal range. The results of these analyses are show in Table 4. As can be seen from Table 4, the variables in the risk index were quite successful in predicting which children would be delayed. In all cases, there were few false negatives, that is, children who were predicted as being normal but, in fact, had scores in the

problem range. There were more false positives, that is, children with scores in the normal range who would have been predicted as being delayed on the basis of the variables in the risk index. Including the scores from the Bayley Scales did not add significantly to the risk index. For example, the multiple correlation of the risk index variables, SES, maternal smoking, maternal education, sex, and apnea, with the WISC-R verbal IQ was .58 for the preterms. Adding the 12-month Bayley Mental Developmental Index (MDI) increased the correlation to .63.

Infant Tests as Predictors of WISC-R Scores

The correlations of the Bayley Scales administered in infancy and the WISC-R IQ at 6 years are shown in Table 5. As can be seen from Table 5, there were statistically significant correlations between the WISC-R scores at 6 years and the Bayley scales. At 4 and 8 months,

Table 3. Results of the multiple regressions of analyses of risk index predictions

Full-term		Preterm	
Verbal IQ			
SES		SES	
Previous spontaneous abortions		Maternal education	
Sex	.58	Apnea	.58
Birth order		Sex	
Apgar, 1 minute		Maternal smoking	
Performance IQ			
Maternal education		SES	
Previous spontaneous abortions		Apnea	
Sex	.44	Sex	.76
Maternal smoking		Maternal education	
Birth order		Asphyxia	
		Maternal smoking	
Full Scale IQ			
Maternal education		SES	
Previous spontaneous abortions		Apnea	
Sex	.59	Maternal education	.71
Apgar, 1 minute		Sex	
Birth order		Asphyxia	

SES = socioeconomic status.

Table 4. Results of the discriminant function analyses of the prediction of WISC-R IQ at 6 years

	True negative	True positive	False negative	False positive	% Correct prediction
		Verbal IQ			
Full-term	32	4	0	2	94.7
Preterm	23	7	3	8	73.2
		Performance IQ			
Full-term	39	1	0	3	93.0
Preterm	28	6	1	4	87.2
		Full Scale			
Full-term	33	3	0	7	83.7
Preterm	15	10	0	16	61.0

the Psychomotor Developmental Index (PDI), the scale that measures motor functions, was more highly correlated with the WISC-R scores while this trend was reversed at 12 months. The correlations of the PDI administered at 18 months with the WISC-R are low possibly because the scale does not sample a wide enough variety of functions at that age.

The Bayley MDI can be separated into subscales according to a system developed by Kohen-Raz (1967). The correlations of the Kohen-Raz subscales with the WISC-R are shown in Table 6. As can be seen in Table 6, perceptual-motor abilities are particularly important predictors early in development, conceptual abilities become more important later on, and language items begin to become important at 12 months and are the significant ones at 2 years. However, in some cases, the language items are not correlated with the Performance IQ because the items on the performance scale are more dependent on per-

ceptual motor and spatial abilities than on language abilities. At 2 years, the eye-hand coordination items were more highly correlated than the language items with the Performance Scale, while at the same point in time, the language items were more highly correlated than the eye-hand coordination items with the Verbal Scale. The scores on the Uzgiris-Hunt Scales were also significantly correlated with the WISC-R 6-year IQ scores, but typically, the correlations were of a lower magnitude than the correlations between the Bayley Scales and the 6-year scores.

Preschool Tests as Predictors of WISC-R IQ Scores

The correlations of the Reynell Language Scales and the Stanford-Binet with the WISC-R scores are shown in Table 7. With the exception of the Language Comprehension Scale at 2 years and the WISC-R Performance Scale, all the correlations were statistically significant.

Table 5. Correlations of the Bayley Scales administered in infancy with the WISC-R scores at 6 years

Bayley Scales	Time of administration of Bayley (months)				
	4	8	12	18	24
		WISC-R Verbal IQ			
MDI[a]	NS	.24[c]	.44[d]	.43[d]	.56[d]
PDI[b]	.35[d]	.36[d]	.39[d]	NS	.36[d]
		WISC-R Performance IQ			
MDI[a]	.26[c]	.22[c]	.39[d]	.43[d]	.40[d]
PDI[b]	.41[d]	.37[d]	.37[d]	.22[c]	.27[c]
		WISC-R Full Scale IQ			
MDI[a]	.23[c]	.27[c]	.48[d]	.50[d]	.56[d]
PDI[b]	.42[d]	.42[d]	.42[d]	.21[c]	.37[d]

[a]MDI = Mental Developmental Index.
[b]PDI = Psychomotor Developmental Index.
[c]$p < .05$.
[d]$p < .001$.

Table 6. Correlations of the Kohen-Raz Subscales with the WISC-R IQ scores at 6 years

Kohen-Raz Subscales	Time of administration of the Bayley (months)				
	4	8	12	18	24
	Verbal IQ				
Eye-hand coordination	.21[a]	.23[a]	.42[c]	.31[b]	.43[c]
Manipulation	.32[b]	NS	.34[c]	.28[b]	*
Conceptual abilities	NS	.32[b]	.34[c]	.28[b]	*
Imitation-comprehension	*	NS	.39[c]	.37[c]	.54[c]
Vocalization-social	*	.20[a]	.30[b]	.24[b]	.54[c]
	Performance IQ				
Eye-hand coordination	.31[b]	.39[c]	.37[c]	.46[c]	.55[c]
Manipulation	.33[b]	.34[c]	.32[b]	.44[c]	*
Conceptual abilities	.25[b]	.39[c]	.37[c]	.47[c]	*
Imitation-comprehension	*	.29[b]	.43[c]	.33[b]	.47[c]
Vocalization-social	*	.21[a]	NS	NS	.43[c]
	Full Scale IQ				
Eye-hand coordination	.28[b]	.34[c]	.44[c]	.43[c]	.53[c]
Manipulation	.37[c]	.28[b]	.34[c]	.40[c]	*
Conceptual abilities	.19[a]	.39[c]	.39[c]	.41[c]	*
Imitation-comprehension	*	.26[b]	.39[c]	.41[c]	.57[a]
Vocalization-social	*	.23[a]	.36[c]	.40[c]	.54[c]

[a] $p < .05$.
[b] $p < .01$.
[c] $p < .001$.
NS = not significant.
*Cannot calculate.

Not surprisingly, the correlations of the language measures are not as high with the Performance scale as they are with the Verbal scores.

The correlations of the elements of the Satz Battery (Satz et al., 1978) with the WISC-R IQ are shown in Table 8. The Beery VMI and the Recognition Discrimination were the best predictors, the Peabody Picture Vocabulary Test (PPVT) was more highly correlated with the Verbal Scale, and the Alphabet Recitation and Finger Localization were the least highly correlated.

Correlations of the HOME with the WISC-R

The correlations of the HOME scale with the WISC-R are shown in Table 9. The correlations later in development are higher than those early in development. Because only a

Table 7. Correlations of the Reynell Language Scales and Stanford-Binet with the WISC-R at 6 years

	Verbal	Performance	Full Scale
Reynell			
2 years			
Comprehension	.44[a]	NS	.38[a]
Expression	.53[a]	.36[a]	.51[a]
3 years			
Comprehension	.51[a]	.45[a]	.55[a]
Expression	.52[a]	.42[a]	.54[a]
4 years			
Comprehension	.62[a]	.29[b]	.51[a]
Expression	.55[a]	.28[b]	.51[a]
Stanford-Binet			
3 years	.47[a]	.41[a]	.53[a]

[a] $p < .001$.
[b] $p < .01$.
NS = not significant.

Table 8. Correlations of the 4-year Satz Battery with the WISC-R at 6 years

Satz Battery	Verbal	Performance	Full Scale
PPVT IQ	.56[a]	.23[b]	.49[a]
Beery VMI	.39[a]	.46[a]	.49[a]
Recognition Discrimination	.43[a]	.45[a]	.52[a]
Finger Localization	.23[b]	NS	.23[b]
Alphabet Recitation	.28[c]	NS	.25[b]

[a] $p < .001$.
[b] $p < .05$.
[c] $p < .01$.
NS = not significant.

limited portion of the sample was administered the HOME due to a limitation of grant funds, it was not possible to add the HOME to the risk index to calculate the additional predictive power gained by this information.

DISCUSSION

It is possible to predict intellectual performance with some reasonable amount of precision and to specify which children are likely to develop difficulties. Variables that are a reflection, at least in part, of environmental factors were important components of the risk index. However, variables reflecting reproductive factors (previous spontaneous abortions, birth order) and biological factors (e.g., apnea, asphyxia) were important also. While variables reflecting the degree of insult during the perinatal period have been found to moderately correlate with subsequent development, environmental factors are important also (e.g., Smith et al., 1972; Willerman, Broman, & Fiedler, 1970). The correlations of a measure of the environment, the HOME scale, with the 6-year IQ scores became increasingly stronger with development. A similar result has been noted by Bee, Barnard, Eyres, Gray,

Hammond, Spietz, Snyder, and Clark (1982). It may be that the biological factors are more significant determinants of early scores but the influence of the environment appears to be greater for functions that mature later, especially language.

Infant and preschool test scores were correlated with subsequent test scores. There appear to be significant continuities in development. Even infant tests administered as early as 4 months predicted WISC-R scores at 6 years. There even seems to have been some specificity on the relationships; language items were more highly correlated with the Verbal Scale score, and perceptual motor items were more highly correlated with the Performance Scale scores. Infant test scores did not provide as accurate predictions as the risk index. The relative success of this risk index depends on several factors. It is relatively simple, and the information can easily be collected in the perinatal period. Furthermore, the system uses several classes of factors. As Bee et al. (1982) have noted, no single isolated factor can account for much of the variance in outcome.

While this system was successful at detecting virtually all the children who would attain scores in the range, there were also a number of

Table 9. Correlations of the HOME total score with the WISC-R at 6 years

WISC-R	Time of administration of the HOME (months)		
	12	36	60
Verbal	NS	.42[c]	.35[c]
Performance	.31[a]	.27[b]	.33[c]
Full Scale	.26[b]	.45[c]	.42[c]

[a] $p < .05$.
[b] $p < .01$.
[c] $p < .001$.
NS = not significant.

false positives, children who were predicted as having below average scores but who achieved scores in the normal range. The evaluation of these results depends on the consequences of being "positive," that is, detected as being "at risk." The consequences of this detection might involve being placed in an infant stimulation program that may have a significant ameliorative effect on development and is certainly not harmful. Failure to receive adequate remediation may have harmful consequences so the errors in this risk system do not seem to be as serious as if there were a higher proportion of false negatives. In any case, the use of a risk index such as this one appears to be a promising technique for the detection of developmental problems.

SUMMARY

The purpose of this study was to develop a risk index that would predict developmental problems. A prospective longitudinal study of very low birth weight preterm (<1,500 grams) and full-term children was conducted. A risk index composed of perinatal, reproductive, and demographic variables was successful in predicting 6-year WISC-R IQ scores and in determining which children would have low scores. Scores on the Bayley Scales and measures of the home environment were also related to outcome. Developmental outcome is not determined by a single factor; a variety of biological and social factors are important for the prediction of developmental difficulties.

REFERENCES

Bayley, N. *The Bayley Scales of Infant Development*. New York: The Psychological Corporation, 1969.

Bee, H.L., Barnard, K.E., Eyres, S.J., Gray, C.A., Hammond, M.A., Spietz, A.L., Snyder, C., & Clark, B. Prediction of IQ and language skill from perinatal status, child performance, family characteristics, and mother-infant interaction. *Child Development*, 1982, *53*, 1134–1156.

Bradley, R.H., & Caldwell, B.M. The relation of infants' home environment to mental test performance at 54 months: A follow-up study. *Child Development*, 1976, *47*, 1172–1174.

Broman, S.H., Nichols, P.L., & Kennedy, W.A. *Preschool IQ: Perinatal and early developmental correlates*. Hillsdale, NJ: Lawrence Erlbaum Associates, 1975.

Caputo, D.V., Taub, H.B., Goldstein, K.M., Smith, N., Dalack, J.D., Pursner, J.P., & Silberstein, R.M. An evaluation of the parameters of maturity at birth as predictors of development at one year of life. *Perceptual and Motor Skills*, 1974, *39*, 631–652.

Field, T.M., Hallock, N., Ting, G., Dempsey, J., Dabiri, C., & Shuman, H.H. A first year follow-up of high risk infants: Formulating a cumulative risk index. *Child Development*, 1978, *49*, 119–131.

Kohen-Raz, R. Scalogram analysis of some developmental sequences of infant behavior as measured by the Bayley Infant Scale of Mental Development. *Genetic Psychology Monographs*, 1967, *76*, 3–21.

Littman, B., & Parmelee, A.H. Medical correlates of infant development. *Pediatrics*, 1978, *61*, 470–474.

Ramey, C.T., Campbell, F.A., & Nicholson, J.E. The predictive power of the Bayley scales of infant development and the Stanford-Binet intelligence test in a relatively constant environment. *Child Development*, 1973, *44*, 790–795.

Ramey, C.T., Stedman, D.J., Borders-Patterson, A., & Mengel, W. Predicting school achievement from information available at birth. *American Journal of Mental Deficiency*, 1978, *82*, 525–534.

Reynell, J. *Reynell Developmental Language Scales*. Windsor, Berkshire, England: NFER, 1969

Satz, P., Taylor, H.G., Friel, J., & Fletcher, J. Some developmental and predictive precursors of reading disabilities: A six year follow-up. In: A.L. Benton & D. Pearl (eds.), *Dyslexia: An appraisal of current knowledge*. New York: Oxford University Press, 1978.

Siegel, L.S. Infant perceptual, cognitive, and motor behaviours as predictors of subsequent cognitive and language development. *Canadian Journal of Psychology*, 1979, *33*, 383–395.

Siegel, L.S. Infant tests as predictors of cognitive and language development at two years. *Child Development*, 1981, *52*, 545–557.

Siegel, L.S. Reproductive, perinatal and environmental factors as predictors of the cognitive and language development of preterm infants. *Child Development*, 1982, *53*, 963–973. (a)

Siegel, L.S. Reproductive, perinatal, and environmental variables as predictors of development of preterm (<1501 grams) and fullterm children at 5 years. *Seminars in Perinatology*, 1982, *6*, 274–279. (b)

Siegel, L.S. Early cognitive and environmental correlates of language development at 4 years. *International Journal of Behavioral Development*, 1982, *5*, 433–444. (c)

Siegel, L.S. Correction for prematurity and its consequences for the assessment of the very low birthweight infant. *Child Development*, 1983, *54*, 1176–1188. (a)

Siegel, L.S. Home environmental influences on cognitive development in preterm and fullterm children. In: A.W. Gottfried (ed.), *Home environment and early mental development*, New York: Academic Press, 1983. (b)

Siegel, L.S. Predicting possible learning disabilities in preterm and fullterm children. In: T. Field & A. Sostek (eds.), *Infants born at risk: Physiological and perceptual processes*. New York: Grune & Stratton, 1983. (c)

Siegel, L.S., Saigal, S., Rosenbaum, P., Morton, R.A., Young, A., Berenbaum, S., & Stoskopf, B. Predictors of development in preterm and fullterm infants: A model for detecting the "at risk" child. *Journal of Pediatric Psychology*, 1982, *7*, 135–148.

Smith, A.C., Flick, G.L., Ferriss, G.S., & Sellman, A.H. Prediction of developmental outcome at seven years from prenatal, perinatal, and postnatal events. *Child Development*, 1972, *43*, 495–507.

Usher, R., & McLean, F. Intrauterine growth of live-born caucasian infants at sea level. *Journal of Pediatrics*, 1969, *74*, 901–910.

Uzgiris, I., & Hunt, McV. *Assessment in infancy: Ordinal scales of psychological development*. Urbana: University of Illinois Press, 1975.

Wechsler, D. *Wechsler Intelligence Scale for Children— Revised*. New York: The Psychological Corporation, 1974.

Willerman, L., Broman, S., & Fiedler, M. Infant development, preschool IQ, and social class. *Child Development*, 1970, *41*, 69–77.

Wilson, R.S. Sensorimotor and cognitive development. In: F.D. Minifie & L.L. Lloyd (eds.), *Communicative and cognitive abilities: Early behavioral assessment*. Baltimore: University Park Press, 1978. (a)

Wilson, R.S. Synchronies in mental development: An epigenetic perspective. *Science*, 1978, *202*, 939–948. (b)

The At-Risk Infant: Psycho/Socio/Medical Aspects
edited by Shaul Harel, M.D., and Nicholas J. Anastasiow, Ph.D.
Copyright © 1985   Paul H. Brookes Publishing Co., Inc.   Baltimore • London

Chapter 8

Educational Interventions
to Enhance
Intellectual Development
Comprehensive Day Care versus Family Education

Craig T. Ramey, Ph.D.
Donna Bryant, Ph.D.
Joseph J. Sparling, Ph.D.
Barbara H. Wasik, Ph.D.
University of North Carolina at Chapel Hill, Chapel Hill, North Carolina

I N THE LATE 1960s, EDUCATORS, PSYCHOLO-gists, and pediatricians began to conduct educational intervention programs that were designed to prevent retarded cognitive development with socially defined high-risk infants. Typically, the infants were judged to be at risk for mild mental retardation due to their families' severely disadvantaged socioeconomic and educational status. On average, children from such families have consistently been shown to have lowered levels of cognitive development relative to children from more advantaged families. (See Ramey & Finkelstein, 1981, for a review of these findings.) Furthermore, the cognitive differences between children from advantaged and severely disadvantaged families typically begins during the second year of life (e.g., Knobloch & Pasamanick, 1953; Ramey & Haskins, 1981). Thus, many of the intervention programs designed to prevent retarded intellectual development have been implemented sometime during the first year of life.

The target of the intervention has sometimes been the child only, at other times, the mother only (as teacher of the child), and with increasing frequency, both mother and child as an educational dyad. The forms of the intervention have been innovative and varied. There have been day care programs such as the Children's Center in Syracuse, New York (Caldwell & Richmond, 1968), and the Abecedarian Program in Chapel Hill, North Carolina (Ramey & Haskins, 1981); and home-visit programs such as the Florida Parent Education Project (Gordon & Guinagh, 1978) and the Ypsilanti-Carnegie Infant Education Project in Michigan (Epstein & Weikart, 1979). There have been studies of the efficacy of parent group meetings by Badger (1981) and studies of center-based parent-training programs such as the ones conducted at the Parent Child Development Centers (Andrews, Blumenthal, Johnson, Kahn, Ferguson, Lasater, Malone, & Wallace, 1982). There have also been intervention programs that combined

This research has been supported by grants from the Special Education Program of the Office of Education, The Administration for Children, Youth, and Families, and the National Institute for Child Health and Human Development.

various treatment forms, such as the Milwaukee Project (Garber & Heber, 1981), which used educational day care, home visits, and job training for the mothers.

What all these early intervention programs had in common was that they began with at-risk infants from low-income families and tried to induce positive developmental outcomes in the children. An area in which these early intervention programs differed was the amount and types of contact that the program staff had with family members and the target child. Based on a recent review of prevention-oriented studies that used random assignment to treatment or control groups, Ramey and Bryant (1982) have advanced the hypothesis that the intensity of the educational treatment (as measured by time and types of contact with the target child) is directly and positively related to the level of intellectual development attained by high-risk children. Although intensities of various treatment programs can be compared across studies, no studies to the authors' knowledge have attempted to experimentally manipulate the level of intervention received by the children and their families. The project to be described in this chapter, Project CARE (Carolina Approach to Responsive Education), includes two treatment groups that vary in intensity of educational programs, as well as a randomly assigned control group.

In its educational program and evaluation strategies, Project CARE has been guided by a version of General Systems Theory as proposed by Ramey, MacPhee, and Yeates (1982) and applied to the concept of developmental retardation. One of the assumptions of the general systems approach to retardation is that development is a process by which the child is continuously changed by the constant interaction of his or her genotype with the ever-changing environment. Environment is construed to include the child's family system and the broader network of financial resources, cultural milieu, sources of stress, and sources of support that impinge on family functioning. It follows from the general systems theory that developmental change will be positively related to the number of causally related developmental factors that are influenced by a particular program and by the sum of the intensities of the causally related interventions. For example, an intervention program that provides educational and social support to the parents in addition to educational day care for the child is more likely to produce developmental change than a program that provides only one of those services.

Because of this general systems perspective, the authors have attempted to measure growth and change in many areas of family functioning, in addition to measuring the child's intellectual, social, and emotional development. However, this chapter concentrates primarily on the relationship between variations in intensity of educational programs and the children's intellectual response to those interventions during the first 3 years of life.

METHOD

Beginning in November, 1978, 64 families were identified (including two sets of twins) whose infants were at risk for developmental delay. To do this, the High-Risk Index reported by Ramey and Smith (1977) was used to screen for eligible families in the local area (see Table 1). Eligible families were randomly assigned to one of three experimental conditions—day care plus family education, family education alone, or an educationally untreated control group. Children entered the study in two cohorts, one group of infants in the fall of 1978 and another group in the fall of 1979. The oldest children were about 5 years old as of March, 1983, and the youngest had just turned 3 years old. A comparison group of 18 families from the general population who wanted day care for their same-age infants was also recruited to participate in Project CARE.

The initial demographic characteristics of the three high-risk groups and the 18 more advantaged families from the General Population Sample (GPS) are presented in Table 2. For the three high-risk groups, the average age of the mothers at their child's birth was about 22 years, and of the fathers, about 25. Mothers' and fathers' educations varied from an average of 10.5 to 11.4 years of schooling across high-risk groups. Mothers' Full Scale Wechsler Adult Intelligence Scale scores were in the mid-80s. The families' risk status and income

Table 1. High-Risk Index

Factor							Weight
Mother's educational level (last grade completed)							
6							8
7							7
8							6
9							3
10							2
11							1
12							0
Father's educational level (last grade completed)							
6							8
7							7
8							6
9							3
10							2
11							1
12							0

Family income (per year)

Size	1–2	3–4	5–6	7–8	9–10	11–12	
Annual	2,000	4,500	7,000	7,500	8,000	8,500	8
gross	3,000	5,500	8,000	8,500	9,000	9,500	7
income	4,000	6,500	9,000	9,500	10,000	10,500	6
	5,000	7,500	10,000	10,500	11,000	11,500	4
	6,000	9,500	12,000	12,500	13,000	13,500	1

Factor	Weight
Father absent for reasons other than health or death	2
Any member of mother's or father's immediate family required special services in school (special class placement, repeated school failure)	3
Any member of mother's or father's immediate family required special community services provided for mentally disabled persons (training school, disability payments, institutionalization, sheltered workshop)	3
Siblings of school age who are one or more grades behind age-appropriate grade or who score equivalently low on school administered achievement tests	3
Payments received from welfare agencies within past 5 years	3
Record of father's work indicates unstable and unskilled or semiskilled labor	3
Records of mother's or father's IQ indicate scores of 85 or below	3
Records of siblings' IQ indicate scores of 85 or below	3
Relevant social agencies in the community indicate that the family is in need of assistance	3
One or more members of the family has sought counseling or professional help in the past 5 years	1
Special circumstances not included in any of the above that are likely contributors to cultural or social disadvantage	2

Criterion for inclusion in High Risk sample is a score ≥ 11.

were also comparable across groups as can be seen in Table 2. The high-risk families were quite different from the families in the GPS who were more representative of the predominantly well-educated and affluent parents of young children in the university town where the project was located.

Treatment Programs

Day Care Plus Family Education The day care component of the day care plus family education treatment group was derived from its predecessor at the Frank Porter Graham Center known as the Carolina Abecedarian Project (Ramey & Haskins, 1981). The primary curriculum resources, *Infant Learningames* and *Learningames for the First Three Years* (Sparling & Lewis, 1979), emphasized activities that stimulate both the social/emotional domain and the intellectual/creative domain of child development. The day care program was developed with the hypothesis that relative inferiority in the areas of language development and motivation to learn are par-

Table 2. Demographic characteristics of Project CARE families at time of child's birth

	High-risk			GPS[a]
	Family education plus day care (N = 15)	Family education (N = 24)[b]	Control (N = 23)	Family education plus day care (N = 18)
Age of mother	22	20	22	28
Age of father	25	24	24	29
Education of mother	10.9	10.6	11.3	14.6
Education of father	11.4	11.1	10.9	16.6
Mother's Wechsler Adult Intelligence Scale Scores				
Full Scale	86.8	86.8	87.5	105.06
Verbal	84.8	85.8	85.7	106.17
Performance	90.9	90.0	92.4	103.18
High-Risk Index	20.0	21.0	20.3	4.8
Income[c]				
Mother's	$4,079	$2,796	$2,641	$10,486
	(n = 8)	(n = 14)	(n = 10)	(n = 12)
Family's	$5,173	$7,514	$6,388	$18,541
	(n = 14)	(n = 23)	(n = 23)	(n = 18)
% single, never married	56%	84%	70%	12%
% single, separated, & divorced (combined)	75%	84%	83%	15%
Characteristics of target				
Target child				
% boys	56%	63%	65%	53%
% black	94%	96%	83%	41%

[a]GPS = General Population Sample.
[b]There are 2 sets of twins in the Family education group for a total of 24 mothers and 26 children in the group.
[c]Mothers and/or families with no incomes or no reported incomes were not included.

ticularly detrimental to normal development (Ramey & Gallagher, 1975). The experiences of the day care group children were planned to foster cognitive/linguistic development and to promote appropriate and adaptive social behavior.

The goal of the treatment program was not an abstract improvement in social or intellectual growth, but a specific goal of improving those adaptive skills that would enhance the child's ability to adapt to the educational setting when he or she reached school age. This was also a strongly stated goal of the families as well. The day care setting was operated with this goal in mind so as to provide environments that, as Harms and Cross (1978) have described, were predictable and promoted self-help; were supportive and facilitated socioemotional adjustment; were reflective of child's age, ability, and interests; and varied in activities.

Children began attending the center as young as 6 weeks of age; attendance began by age 3 months in most of the cases. The center operated from 7:45 A.M. to 5:30 P.M. each weekday for 50 weeks per year. Transportation to and from the center was provided for those children who needed it. The center cared for children on one floor of a four-story research building. The settings for the children were structured to be age- and developmentally appropriate. Generally, children were grouped according to age, with sections for infants, toddlers, and so on. Throughout the day, teachers participated actively with and talked to the infants. The goals of the educational environment were to promote independence and self-help while enriching relevant developmental domains including language and concept acquisition.

The typical teacher/child ratio was between 1:3 and 1:4 during the first 3 years. Teaching staff varied in their level of formal training (averaging 7 years of direct experience), but all had demonstrated skill and competence in working with young children. Staff development was a critically important and ongoing process. Of particular importance was the language training program that sought to help teachers develop children's communication skills through strategies based on current research in adult-child verbal interaction.

The focus of the authors' efforts was to promote a particular *kind* and *amount* of verbal interaction between teacher and day care pupil. Much of the curriculum language work was derived from the educational frameworks developed by Tough (1976) and Blank (1973). The encouraged verbal interaction was largely modeled on what a middle-class mother establishes with her child. Since the day care effort was competing with extensive experience in another type of linguistic environment (the home), it was assumed that the effort could not be as casual and diluted as in normal family interaction. To foster certain types of linguistic functioning in the child's repertoire, the authors tried to provide a large number of practice opportunities for communication and for social, representational, syntactic, and semantic competence. The theoretical framework and a more detailed treatment of the language experiences and inservice training are described by Ramey, McGinness, Cross, Collier, and Barrie-Blackley (1982).

In addition to this day care educational experience, the children in the day care plus family education group also received the same family education curriculum that is described below.

Family Education The family education treatment component and its rationale has been described by Ramey, Sparling, and Wasik (1981). The principal method of parent education was person-to-person contact in parents' homes with a paraprofessional family educator about every 10 days. Approximately 92% of the visits were with the mother, although on a few occasions the fathers and grandparents were the participants. As of June, 1983, 4,585 home visits had been conducted with families, including families in both treatment groups. The focus of the home visit in a majority of instances (77%) was a child-learning activity derived from *Learningames* which acted as the entree to an exchange of information on child development, family problem-solving, or the teaching of parenting skills. These visits typically lasted about an hour (64% were between 30 and 60 minutes; 21% were longer than 1 hour) in the parent's

home, although other kinds of contacts were used when necessary to accommodate the parent's scheduling needs.

A basic part of the family education program was a curriculum designed to teach parents problem-solving skills germane to the family. The conceptual framework for problem-solving was a modification of Spivack and Shure's (1974) Problem Solving System. The rationale for such training was based upon a conceptualization of problem-solving ability as necessary for effective parenting and for handling day-to-day problems, and that this ability can be enhanced by specific training. To implement the parent training, family educators were taught to help the mothers further develop their problem-solving skills. The training consisted of teaching the mother the steps of a problem-solving model and how to use this model in dealing with ongoing family concerns. The specific steps of the model were: 1) problem identification, 2) generation of solutions, 3) evaluation of solutions, 4) decision-making, 5) implementation, and 6) evaluation of decision outcomes.

Ongoing weekly sessions with the family educators were the main means of training them in helping the parents learn problem-solving skills. These weekly meetings also served as an opportunity for the family educators to discuss with the project's directors their interactions or concerns with specific mothers. The curriculum is described in a manual concerning the home-visiting program (Wasik & Ramey, 1982) and in a manual describing the procedures used to teach parents problem-solving (Wasik, 1982).

As noted earlier, families with children participating in the day care program also received weekly family education home visits from a family educator. Often, this person was the child's teacher. Families in the family education only group received only home visits from a family educator. It is important to note that the frequency of visits was very similar for both groups (averaging about 2.5 visits/month), and that the family educators underwent the same training and used the same curriculum items. Parent workshops were scheduled about one evening a month and parents from both groups were invited to attend and did attend in approximately equal proportions. The authors are confident that the family education component was the same for both groups. Both received the home-visit program and the test of the intensity hypothesis comes with the addition of day care for one group.

RESULTS

Figure 1 contains a summary of mean Mental Developmental Index (MDI) (Bayley, 1969) and Stanford-Binet (Terman & Merrill, 1973) IQ results from the three high-risk experimental groups and the GPS comparison group for the first 36 months of age. Children were given the Bayley test at 6, 12, 18, and 24 months of age, and the Stanford-Binet at 36 months.

Table 3 contains the numbers of children for whom complete tests were available at each assessment occasion, the means and standard deviations of the Bayley MDI and Stanford-Binet IQ scores, analysis of variance results comparing performance across each of the five

assessment occasions separately, and a summary of pairwise comparisons among the four groups. The results indicate that none of the four groups differed from one another at 6 months of age when the four groups considered together received an overall mean Bayley MDI score of 107. This score indicates that the four groups as a whole were approximately one-half of a standard deviation above the national average at that assessment occasion.

The four groups began to differ significantly at the 12-month assessment occasion and continued to differ at each assessment occasion thereafter. At 12 months, the GPS and day care plus family education groups were equal and superior to the control group which was, in turn, superior to the family education only group. This pattern of results was replicated in both the 18- and 24-month Bayley MDI performances. At 24 months, the GPS group and the day care plus family education group obtained normatively superior scores of 120 and 114 respectively. The control and family education only groups both showed a decline from previous test scores, with the family education

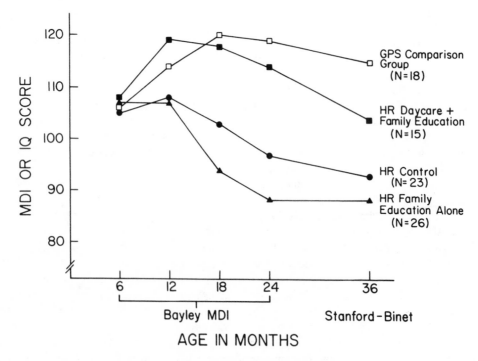

Figure 1. Mean Bayley MDI and Stanford-Binet IQ scores for High-Risk (HR) children in treatment groups of varying intensity in relation to a General Population Sample (GPS) comparison group.

Table 3. Mean Bayley MDI and Stanford-Binet IQ results with ANOVAs and pairwise comparisons

Test administered	Age (months)	Day care plus family education			Family education only			Control			GPS[a]			F	p	Pairwise comparison
		n	M	S.D.	n	M	S.D.	n	M	S.D.	n	M	S.D.			
Bayley Scales of Infant Development Mental Development Index (MDI)	6	14	108.7	10.8	26	107.5	16.8	23	105.0	12.8	18	106.2	14.0	$F_{(3,77)} = 0.24$	.87	
MDI	12	15	119.3	9.1	26	107.8	13.6	22	108.5	13.6	18	116.9	11.1	$F_{(3,77)} = 4.30$	.0075	GPS = DC+FE > CON > FE
MDI	18	15	118.7	12.0	25	94.3	13.6	22	103.1	13.3	17	121.1	15.6	$F_{(3,75)} = 17.35$	<.0001	GPS = DC+FE > CON > FE
MDI	24	15	114.1	13.7	26	88.9	13.9	22	97.4	12.3	16	120.2	13.1	$F_{(3,75)} = 23.46$	<.0001	GPS = DC+FE > CON > FE
Stanford-Binet Intelligence Scale IQ	36	14	104.5	7.0	25	88.6	14.8	22	92.9	12.6	15	115.3	16.2	$F_{(3,72)} = 14.66$	<.0001	GPS > DC+FE > CON = FE

[a]GPS = General Population Sample.

only group receiving the lower score of 90 and the control group receiving an MDI of 97.

At 36 months, the children were administered the Stanford-Binet Intelligence Scale, which was scored using the 1972 norms. For the first time, the mean performance of the day care plus family education group was significantly lower than that of the GPS group (115 vs. 105); this difference was due primarily to a 10-point drop from the MDI 24-month performance for the day care plus family education group compared to a 5-point drop for the GPS group. However, both of these groups were developmentally superior to the family education and control groups which did not differ from one another.

DISCUSSION

The developmental trends shown in Figure 1 are strikingly different. Several points can be made about these results. First, at 6 months, the three high-risk groups had Bayley MDI scores that were quite similar. This finding was expected because random assignment should have made the groups initially comparable, and no data exist to predict that early intervention should have a beneficial effect by this age. The MDI scores of the GPS group were also quite similar to the high-risk groups and the mean of each of the groups was above the national average of 100 by 5–12 points.

By 12 months, the groups began to diverge, with the scores of the GPS group and the day care plus family education group increasing substantially, with means of 117 and 119, respectively. The scores of the other two high-risk groups remained about the same, still somewhat above the average of 100. There are two types of advantages that may explain the superior performance of the GPS and high-risk day care plus family education groups. Relative to the high-risk groups, children in the GPS sample experienced more advantaged, enriched environments and the correlates that accompany such environments (e.g., broader exposure to language). Relative to the children in the other two high-risk groups, children in the high-risk day care plus family education group experienced the advantage of a daily

systematic educational treatment at the Frank Porter Graham Center. This advantage was reflected in high MDI scores, scores that were no different from those of the GPS comparison group.

The MDI scores at 18 and 24 months remained high for the GPS group and the high-risk day care plus family education group. However, it was during this time period that a relatively steep decline occurred in the scores of the other two high-risk groups. The scores of the high-risk control group dropped to 103 at 18 months and 97 at 24 months, while the scores of the high-risk family education alone group dropped to 94 and 89 at those same ages. Project CARE included two sets of twins who happened to both be assigned to the family education alone group; at 18 and 24 months the very low scores of these children pulled the group mean 3–4 points lower than it would have been without the twins included. Nevertheless, the treatment group that received only family education showed no positive intellectual effects at these ages. The decline of both the high-risk control and family education children might be explained by the increasingly important role of language skills in the Bayley test and their corresponding lack of skills in that area in particular. The decline might also be explained by the cumulative negative effects of being reared in impoverished environments.

At 36 months, when tested with the Stanford-Binet Form L-M (using 1972 standardization norms), the GPS comparison group and the high-risk day care plus family education group scored well above average. The high-risk control and family education alone groups continued to score much lower, with their scores averaging around 90. The mean scores of these two lower groups were still not at the level that would be considered mildly mentally retarded, but there were several individual children in both of these groups who would be so diagnosed. There were no children in either the GPS comparison or high-risk day care plus family education groups who scored below 85 on the 36-month Stanford-Binet, and the means of both groups were still well above normal. The GPS comparison group performed significantly higher than the high-risk day care plus family education group. Essentially, the pattern evident in the 18-month scores continued at 24 and 36 months.

There are several conclusions that can be drawn from these results. First is that an intense intervention that provided full time day care for high-risk children and parent education for their families did prevent the decline in the children's intellectual development that was evidenced in the two groups that did not receive as intense an intervention. The mean difference score across testing times between the high-risk day care and control groups was 11.7 points. The mean difference score between the high-risk day care and family education alone groups was 15.6 points. The standard deviation of the tests given was also 15 points. It is interesting to note that the difference between the most intensively treated high-risk group and the other two high-risk groups is about the same (approximately 15 points) as the difference usually reported between the IQ scores of black and white children.

The second conclusion to be drawn from

these results is that an intervention consisting of parent education alone is not an intervention of enough intensity to have an impact on these scores. This is not to say that the intervention has had no effect because there may be changes occurring in the family in domains that were not measured. It also may be the case that this form of intervention may take longer to manifest its effects. These results are seen as developmental in nature, and all children will be followed until they are 5 years old.

CARE Results in Relation to Other Studies

The authors have recently completed a review of 18 compensatory education programs that reported random assignment to groups (Ramey, Bryant, & Suarez, in press). Table 4 presents data on Stanford-Binet scores at age 3 for the 10 studies that intervened with high-risk children during infancy. The studies have been rank-ordered based on the magnitude of the differences in the Experimental (E) and Control (C) group scores. In relation to these other

Table 4. Early childhood results at age 3

	E-C difference	Stanford-Binet scores		Norms used
		E	C	
Milwaukee Project (Garber & Heber, 1981)	32	126[a]	94	1960
Abecedarian Project (Ramey & Haskins, 1981)	7	101[a]	84	1972
Project CARE (Ramey et al., 1981)	12	105[a]	93	1972
Mobile Unit for Child Health (Gutelius, Kirsch, MacDonald, Brooks, & McErlean, 1977)	8	99[a]	91	1960
Family-Oriented Home Visiting Program (Gray & Ruttle, 1980)	8	93[a]	85	1972
PCDC-Birmingham (Andrews et al., 1982)	7	98[a]	91	1960
PCDC-New Orleans (Andrews et al., 1982)	6	105[a]	99	1960
PCDC-Houston (Andrews et al., 1982)	4	108	104	1960
Florida Parent Education Program (Gordon & Guinagh, 1978)	4	95	91	1960
Ypsilanti-Carnegie (Lambie, Bond, & Weikart, 1974)	3	104	101	1960

[a]Difference between the E and C group significant at the .05 level or better.

projects, Project CARE was among the most intense in terms of treatment and showed a large difference between the day care and control groups.

The studies summarized in Table 4 seem to cluster into four groups. The Milwaukee Project showed the largest E-C difference, 32 points, and forms a category of its own. The Milwaukee Project included day care, parent training and job training—a very comprehensive treatment. The other two full-day day care projects, the Abecedarian Project and Project CARE, showed E-C differences of about one standard deviation, 17 and 12 points, respectively, and they form a second cluster. These three most intense studies, taken together, produced the strongest treatment effects.

The third cluster of studies includes four programs that had significant, although modest, group differences—6, 7, or 8 IQ points, approximately one-half standard deviation. Two of these were PCDC center-based, parent-focused interventions (Andrews et al., 1982). The other two were home-visit, parent-focused studies (Gray & Wandersman, 1980; Gutelius, Kirsch, MacDonald, Brooks, & McErlean, 1977). Compared on the basis of intensity, the Mobile Unit for Child Health seemed more

intense and lasted for twice as long as the Family-Oriented Home Visiting Program, yet both had E-C differences of 8 points. The Family-Oriented Home Visiting Program was the least intense of the seven studies that showed significant treatment effects.

The fourth cluster of studies with results through age 3 included the three projects with no significant E-C group differences. They were the Houston PCDC program, the Florida Parent Education Program, and the Ypsilanti-Carnegie Infant Education Program. In two of these three studies, (Houston and Ypsilanti) both the E and C groups had mean Stanford-Binet scores greater than 100. In the Florida Parent Education Program, experimental subjects who had participated in all 3 years of intervention were performing significantly higher than controls, but when all E groups were combined (including 1- and 2-year treatment groups) the difference was not significant.

In summary, the 3-year Stanford-Binet results presented in Table 4 tend to support an intensity hypothesis. Programs that have many hours and years of contact with the families and particularly many hours of direct contact with the children are likely to have the most positive effect on children's intellectual outcome.

REFERENCES

Andrews, S.R., Blumenthal, J.B., Johnson, D.L., Kahn, A.J., Ferguson, C.J., Lasater, T.M., Malone, P.E., & Wallace, D. B. The skills of mothering: A study of Parent Child Development Centers. *Monographs of the Society for Research in Child Development*, 1982, *47*(6).

Badger, E. Effects of parent education program on teenage mothers and their offspring. In: K.G. Scott, T. Field, & E. Robertson (eds.), *Teenage parents and their offspring*. New York: Grune & Stratton, 1981.

Bayley, N. *The Bayley Scales of Infant Development*. New York: The Psychological Corporation, 1969.

Blank, M. *Teaching learning in the preschool: A dialogue approach*. Columbus, OH: Charles E. Merrill Publishing Co., 1973.

Caldwell, B.M., & Richmond, J.B. The Children's Center in Syracuse, New York. In: L.L. Dittmann (ed.), *Early child care: The new perspectives*. New York: Atherton Press, 1968.

Epstein, A.S., & Weikart, D.B. *The Ypsilanti-Carnegie Infant Education Project: Longitudinal follow-up*. Ypsilanti, MI: High/Scope Educational Research Foundation, 1979.

Garber, H., & Heber, R. The efficacy of early intervention with family rehabilitation. In: M. Begab, H.C. Haywood, & H.L. Garber (eds.), *Psychosocial influences in retarded performance: Strategies for improving competence*, Vol. 2. Baltimore: University Park Press, 1981.

Gordon, I.J., & Guinagh, B.J. *Middle school performance as a function of early stimulation*. (Final report to the Administration for Children, Youth and Families, Project No. NIH-HEW-OCD-90-C-908). Gainesville: University of Florida, Institute for Development of Human Resources; and Chapel Hill: University of North Carolina, School of Education, March, 1978.

Gray, S., & Ruttle, K. The Family-Oriented Home Visiting Program: A longitudinal study. *Genetic Psychology Monographs*, 1980, *102*, 299–316.

Gray, S.W., & Wandersman, L.P. The methodology of home-based intervention studies: Problems and promising strategies. *Child Development*, 1980, *51*, 993–1009.

Gutelius, M.G., Kirsch, A.D., MacDonald, S., Brooks, M.R., & McErlean, T. Controlled study of child health supervision: Behavioral results. *Pediatrics*, 1977, *60*, 294–304.

Harms, T., & Cross, L. *Environmental provisions in day care*. Chapel Hill: Day Care Training and Technical Assistance System, Frank Porter Graham Child Development Center, University of North Carolina, 1978.

Knobloch, H., & Pasamanick, B. Further observation on the behavioral development of Negro children. *Journal of Genetic Psychology*, 1953, *83*, 137–157.

Lambie, D.Z., Bond, J.T., & Weikart, D.P. *Home teaching with mothers and infants: The Ypsilanti-Carnegie Infant Education Project—An experiment*. Ypsilanti, MI: High/Scope Educational Research Foundation, 1974.

Ramey, C.T., & Bryant, D.M. Evidence for prevention of developmental retardation during infancy. *Journal of the Division for Early Childhood*, 1982, *5*, 73–78.

Ramey, C.T., Bryant, D.M., & Suarez, T.M. Preschool compensatory education and the modifiability of intelligence: A critical review. In: D. Detterman (ed.), *Current topics in human intelligence*. Norwood, NJ: Ablex Publishing Corporation, in press.

Ramey, C.T., & Finkelstein, N.W. Psychosocial mental retardation: A biological and social coalescence. In: M. Begab, H. Garber, & H.C. Haywood (eds.), *Causes and prevention of retarded development in psychosocially disadvantaged children*. Baltimore: University Park Press, 1981.

Ramey, C.T., & Gallagher, J.J. The nature of cultural deprivation: Theoretical issues and suggested research strategies. *North Carolina Journal of Mental Health*, 1975, *7*, 41–47.

Ramey, C.T., & Haskins, R. The causes and treatment of school failure: Insights from the Carolina Abecedarian Project. In: M. Begab, H.C. Haywood, & H. Garber (eds.), *Psychosocial influences and retarded performance: Strategies for improving competence*, Vol. 2. Baltimore: University Park Press, 1981.

Ramey, C.T., McGinness, G.D.. Cross, L., Collier, A.M., & Barrie-Blackley, S. The Abecedarian approach to social competence: Cognitive and linguistic intervention for disadvantaged preschoolers. In: K. Borman (ed.), *Socialization of the child in a changing society*. London: Pergamon Press, 1982.

Ramey, C.T., MacPhee, D., & Yeates, K.O. Preventing developmental retardation: A general systems model. In: L.A. Bond & J.M. Joffee (eds.), *Facilitating infant and early childhood development*. Hanover, NH: University Press of New England, 1982.

Ramey, C.T., & Smith, B.J. Assessing the intellectual consequences of early intervention with high-risk infants. *American Journal of Mental Deficiency*, 1977, *81*, 318–324.

Ramey, C.T., Sparling, J.J., & Wasik, B. Creating social environments to facilitate language development: An early education approach. In: R. Schiefelbusch & D. Bricker (eds.), *Early language intervention*. Baltimore: University Park Press, 1981.

Sparling, J., & Lewis, I. *Learningames for the first three years: A guide to parent-child play*. New York: Walker and Co., 1979.

Spivack, G., & Shure, M. *Social adjustment of young children: A cognitive approach to solving real-life problems*. San Francisco: Jossey-Bass, 1974.

Terman, L.M., & Merrill, M.A. *Stanford-Binet Intelligence Scale: 1972 Norms Edition*. Boston: Houghton Mifflin Co., 1973.

Tough, J. *Listening to children talking*. London: Ward Lock Educational, 1976.

Wasik, B.H. *A manual for teaching parents problem solving skills*. Chapel Hill, NC: Frank Porter Graham Child Development Center, 1982.

Wasik, B.H., & Ramey, C.T. (eds.). *Manual of home visiting in Project CARE*. Chapel Hill, NC: Frank Porter Graham Child Development Center, 1982.

The At-Risk Infant: Psycho/Socio/Medical Aspects
edited by Shaul Harel, M.D., and Nicholas J. Anastasiow, Ph.D.
Copyright © 1985   Paul H. Brookes Publishing Co., Inc.   Baltimore • London

Chapter 9

A Comparison of the Behaviors
of Preterm and Full-Term Infants
Implications for Mother-Infant Interaction

Susan F. Schwartz, M.S.
Frances Degen Horowitz, Ph.D.
David Wayne Mitchell, M.A.
University of Kansas, Lawrence, Kansas

THE NEONATAL BEHAVIORAL ASSESSMENT Scale (NBAS) administered at the time of hospital discharge provides a description of the infant's emerging behavioral repertoire (Brazelton, 1973). The scale allows the examiner to interact with the infant in a systematic manner to reveal the infant's responses to auditory and visual stimulation, to being handled, and to being upset. The tester also has the opportunity to evaluate the infant's motoric organization, state regulation and range, and variability of behavior. Its use over the last decade in documenting the behavioral organization of full-term infants has been widespread (for review, see Horowitz & Linn, 1982). More recently, modified versions of the NBAS have been used to describe the behavioral responses of the preterm infant. In comparison to full-term infants, it has even been found that at comparable conceptional ages, the preterm infant's responses are different and usually less optimal (DiVitto & Goldberg, 1979; Ferrari, Grosoli,

Fontana, & Cavazzuti, 1983; Field, Hallock, Ting, Dempsey, Dabiri, & Shuman, 1978; Telzrow, Kang, Mitchell, Ashworth, & Barnard, 1982).

The performance of normal infants on the NBAS has been related to subsequent maternal behavior in mother-infant interactions. In two studies, Osofsky (Osofsky, 1976; Osofsky & Danzger, 1974) reported a positive correlation between maternal attention and NBAS measures of infant responsiveness to auditory and visual stimulation during the exam. But absolute levels of performance may not be the most important dimension of neonatal behavior. Linn & Horowitz (1983) found that mothers were more contingently responsive to infants whose scores during the Brazelton examination were more variable day-to-day than infants whose scores were more stable day-to-day. It has also been noted that the mothers of preterm infants are less active with them compared to mothers of full-term infants when the obser-

This research was supported in part by the National Institutes of Child Health and Human Development in a grant to the second author (HD 10608) and a grant to the Department of Human Development and Family Life at the University of Kansas (5-T32HD07173).

The authors wish to express their appreciation to Howard A. Fox, M.D., Department of Newborn Medicine, Kansas University Medical Center, for his continued support of our research; to the nursing staff of the Newborn Special Care Unit for their help and cooperation; to Patricia L. Linn, Ph.D., for her help and encouragement in the early development of the NBAS-KAPI; and to Madelyn Moss who helped collect data throughout the study.

vations take place during the preterm infant's hospitalization (DiVitto & Goldberg, 1979; Klaus & Kennell, 1970; Leifer, Leiderman, Barnett, & Williams, 1972). And, preterm infants continue to appear to be generally more difficult to engage in a reciprocal interaction throughout the early months (Field, 1980). However, in contrast to in-hospital data, parents of the preterm infant subsequently appear to work more actively than the parents of the full-term infant to involve their offspring in an interaction (Beckwith & Cohen, 1978; DiVitto & Goldberg, 1979; Field, 1977), presumably to compensate for, or to overcome, the infant's difficulties in interacting. Although differences are somewhat less apparent as the infant becomes older, some differences in interactive patterns continue to be evident (Goldberg, Brachfeld, & DiVitto, 1980).

Mother-infant interaction patterns contribute significantly to the developmental outcome of the preterm infant. While prenatal and perinatal risk factors contribute to developmental outcome (Siegel, 1982), it has been found that maternal caregiving variables and correlates of these are stronger predictors (Beckwith & Cohen, 1980). In order to better understand the dynamics involved in the development of preterm infants, it is necessary to further delineate both the organismic (infant) and environmental (including maternal behavior) aspects of the transactional model. In this, model, both organismic and environmental factors are considered to contribute to developmental outcome with environmental factors playing a particularly important role for preterm and high-risk infants (Sameroff & Chandler, 1975).

In this chapter, the authors describe the preterm infant's contribution to subsequent mother-infant interaction. The behavior of a sample of preterm infants was studied using a variant of the Brazelton Scale called the NBAS-Kansas Assessment of the Preterm Infant (KAPI). The KAPI involves the NBAS plus the supplementary items of the NBAS-K (Neonatal Behavioral Assessment Scale with Kansas Supplements) (Horowitz, Sullivan, & Linn, 1978; Lancioni, Horowitz, & Sullivan, 1980a, b) and the special qualifier items for stressed and preterm infants developed by

Brazelton and Als and their colleagues (Als, Lester, Tronick, & Brazelton, 1980). The NBAS-K includes items to assess the infant's overall responsiveness, the amount of examiner persistence required to test the infant, the infant's overall irritability, and whether the infant was reinforcing to the examiner. The supplement also allows for assessment of the infant's "modal" or typical behavior whereas the original NBAS looks only at the infant's best behavior. The NBAS-KAPI was administered to each preterm infant a minimum of four times—twice just prior to hospital discharge, 2 weeks following hospital discharge, and 4 weeks following hospital discharge. It was of special interest to compare the preterm infants when they reached 40 weeks conceptional age with a term sample. Therefore, an exam was scheduled when the infant was 40 weeks conceptional age. If this exam did not coincide with one of the four scheduled administrations of the NBAS-KAPI, then the total number of NBAS-KAPI evaluations was increased to five.

METHOD

Subjects

This chapter is a preliminary report on a subsample of preterm infants from a larger sample of preterm infants. The completed study will eventually provide a normative report on preterm infant behavior in comparison to a normative database on term infant behavior. This chapter presents data on 45 preterm infants born between February, 1981 and May, 1982, who were admitted to the Newborn Special Care Unit at Kansas University Medical Center. Criteria for inclusion in the study included a birth weight less than or equal to 2,500 grams and a gestational age less than or equal to 36 weeks as determined by the Ballard assessment (Ballard, Novak, and Driver, 1979). All infants were appropriate weight and length for their gestational age. Infants who had any of the following conditions were excluded from the sample: diagnosed CNS disorders, recognized chromosomal disorders, severe metabolic disorders, mental retardation, or respiratory distress requiring more than 5 days of assisted ventilation. All infants in the sample were discharged to their parents and did not require special medical care at home. At birth, the preterm infants averaged almost 33 weeks gestational age; at discharge, the mean conceptional age was approximately 36 weeks. The mean length of hospital stay was 23.53 days ($SD = 14.44$) with a range of 3–66 days.

A group of 45 full-term infants matched on the variables of sex, race, and mother's educational level provided a comparison group. These normal full-term infants, born either at Lawrence, Kansas, Memorial Hospital or the University of Kansas Medical Center, were part of a larger study of normal term infants conducted between September, 1976 and December, 1977. The full-term infants were also appropriate weight and length for their gestational age. A further description of the sample can be seen in Table 1.

Examiners

All examiners were trained to an interrater reliability of 90% or above on the NBAS-K (Horowitz et al., 1978) with at least two different reliable trained examiners. In addition, the examiners for the preterm infants were trained to an interrater reliability of 90% or above on the NBAS-KAPI.

Setting

For both groups of infants, the setting for the tests done at hospital discharge was a small, quiet room adjacent to their respective nur-

series. Tests done after hospital discharge were performed in the infant's home.

Assessment Tool

The assessment tool used in this study for the full-term infants was the Neonatal Behavior Assessment Scale with Kansas Supplements (NBAS-K) (Horowitz et al., 1978). For the assessment of the preterm infants, the NBAS-Kansas Assessment of the Preterm Infant (NBAS-KAPI) was developed (Schwartz & Horowitz, in preparation). The NBAS-KAPI is basically a modified NBAS-K. The modifications involved the omission of several items that during pilot work did not fit the preterm response, and the addition of nine qualifier scores. The items from the NBAS-K *not* scored on the NBAS-KAPI are: 1) response decrement to pinprick, 2) alertness, 3) general tonus, 4) motor maturity, 5) skin color, 6) quality of infant responsiveness, and 7) examiner persistence. The nine qualifier items (developed by Als et al., 1980) include: 1) quality of responsivity, 2) cost of attention, 3) balance of tone, 4) range and flexibility of states, 5) regulatory capacity, 6) examiner facilitation, 7) robustness and endurance, 8) control over input, and 9) interfering variables.

Procedure

For the full-term infants, repeated assessments were made on each of the first 3 days of life. A fourth and a fifth evaluation were performed at

Table 1. Description of preterm and full-term infant groups

Clusters	Preterm		Full-term	
	Mean	S.D.	Mean	S.D.
Gestational age	32.8 weeks	(2.30)	All full-term	
Birth weight	1,857.60	(324.90)	3,408.10	(463.23)
Length	43.20	(3.23)	51.30	(3.03)
Mothers' age	26.78	(5.28)	25.06	(5.94)
Gravida	2.57	(1.48)	2.46	(1.79)
Parity (live children)	2.18	(2.94)	2.11	(1.60)
Apgar at 1 minute	6.09	(2.09)	8.07	(1.34)
Apgar at 5 minutes	7.68	(1.70)	9.30	(.83)
Conceptional age at discharge	36.16	(1.45)		
Mothers' education:				
12 years or less	n = 24		n = 24	
More than 12 years	n = 21		n = 21	
Mothers' race:				
Black	n = 11		n = 11	
White	n = 34		n = 34	
Infants' sex:				
Female	n = 25		n = 25	
Male	n = 20		n = 20	

2 and 4 weeks postdischarge. These infants were tested by at least three different examiners. Only the scores from the evaluations done on the third day of life and 4 weeks postdischarge were analyzed for this report. The examination done on the third day of life served as the infant's 40-week conceptional age exam as well as the discharge exam. For the preterm infants, assessments were made on two different occasions after the infant weighed at least 2,000 grams, had been transferred out of an isolette for at least 12 hours to an open crib, and was free of medical problems. Most assessments took place within 1 to 3 days prior to hospital discharge. Care was made not to do an examination immediately following such procedures as a physical examination. Most of the NBAS-KAPI evaluations were done about 1 hour after the infant completed a feeding. A third and a fourth evaluation were done at 2 and 4 weeks postdischarge. As has been noted, an additional examination was done for preterm infants if the infant's conceptional age of 40 weeks did not coincide with one of the four scheduled tests. The infants were tested by at least two different examiners. This chapter reports only on the results from the second examination done in the hospital, the examination at 4 weeks postdischarge, and the examination at 40-weeks conceptional age.

Data Analysis

The data were analyzed according to an adaptation of the cluster reduction scheme suggested by Lester (Lester, in press). Because the analysis included only items that were scored for both the full-term and preterm groups, the clustering scheme used was a modification

including the appropriate items from the NBASK and omitting the items from the standard NBAS that were not scored. Also, it should be noted that, for this analysis, the habituation and reflex items were not included although these items were scored during the NBAS-KAPI. The resulting clusters were defined as: 1) best orientation—inanimate visual, inanimate auditory, animate visual, animate auditory, inanimate visual and auditory, and animate visual and auditory; 2) modal orientation—same items except scored for modal responses; 3) motor maturity—pull to sit, defensive movements, and activity; 4) range of state—peak of excitement, rapidity of build-up, irritability, lability of state; 5) regulation of state—cuddliness, consolability with intervention, self-quieting activity and hand-to-mouth facility; and 6) autonomic regulation—tremulousness and startle.

RESULTS

The cluster means were calculated and compared using a t test for matched pairs with degrees of freedom adjusted appropriately. The means, standard deviations, and t values for the comparisons between the two groups at hospital discharge, at 4 weeks postdischarge, and at 40 weeks conceptional age, are presented in Tables 2, 3, and 4, respectively. Differences on cluster scores were revealed for each set of comparisons. At the time of hospital discharge (see Table 2), significant differences were found on the best orientation, the modal orientation, the range of state, and the regulation of state clusters. At hospital discharge, full-term infants showed superior orientation on the best score as well as superior orientation

Table 2. Preterm and full-term infants at hospital discharge

Clusters	Preterm		Full-term		
	Mean	S.D.	Mean	S.D.	t value
1. Best orientation	6.05	(1.14)	6.90	(0.99)	4.01[a]
2. Modal orientation	5.04	(1.37)	5.69	(1.35)	2.28[b]
3. Motor maturity	5.43	(0.78)	5.49	(0.85)	0.33
4. Range of state	3.59	(0.62)	3.91	(0.78)	2.31[b]
5. Regulation of state	4.61	(1.13)	5.26	(1.08)	2.80[c]
6. Autonomic regulation	6.92	(1.14)	6.71	(1.11)	0.85

[a] $p < .001$
[b] $p < .05$.
[c] $p < .01$.

Table 3. Preterm and full-term infants at 4 weeks posthospital discharge

Clusters	Preterm		Full-term		t value
	Mean	S.D.	Mean	S.D.	
1. Best orientation	6.85	(0.91)	7.36	(0.77)	2.68[a]
2. Modal orientation	6.25	(1.23)	6.06	(1.13)	0.67
3. Motor maturity	5.94	(0.57)	5.87	(0.72)	0.44
4. Range of state	3.64	(0.82)	3.65	(0.89)	0.07
5. Regulation of state	4.21	(1.19)	4.58	(1.13)	1.34
6. Autonomic regulation	6.81	(1.52)	7.76	(1.33)	3.13[b]

[a]$p < .05$
[b]$p < .01$.

on the modal score. Full-term infants at discharge also had higher range of state scores and better regulation of state scores.

At 4 weeks posthospital discharge (see Table 3), the groups differed on the best orientation and the autonomic regulation clusters. The full-term infants had superior orientation for the best score, and better autonomic regulation than the preterm infants.

At 40 weeks conceptional age (see Table 4), significant differences were found on scores in the regulation of state cluster. The full-term infants had better regulation of state scores.

DISCUSSION

The purpose of this chapter was to document the behavioral organization of the preterm infant throughout the neonatal period and compare it to that of the full-term infant. The comparison yielded results similar to those of previous investigations. However, whereas other investigators have compared preterm and full-term infants either at 40 weeks conceptional age (Ferrari et al., 1983; Telzrow et al., 1982) or at hospital discharge (Field et al., 1978; DiVitto & Goldberg, 1979), this study, with its repeated measures, did both. In addition, it allowed examination of the influence of

home environment (4-week posthospital discharge measure) as well as biological maturation (40-week conceptional age measure). Differences were revealed for each comparison.

At hospital discharge, when the preterm infants were approximately 36 weeks conceptional age and the full-terms 40 weeks conceptional age, there was a difference on four of the six cluster scores, with the full-term infants performing significantly better than the preterm infants. Thus, a mother took home a behaviorally different infant if the infant was preterm as compared to full-term, and the immediate interactive opportunities were likely different in those initial home experiences for both groups. Four weeks later, when the mean conceptional age of the preterm group was 40 weeks, behavioral differences had modulated with significant differences only on best orientation and on autonomic regulation, though the autonomic regulation cluster score at discharge was not one of the four significant differences. The full-term infants were still performing better on best orientation and now showed significantly better autonomic regulation. When conceptional age of 40 weeks was used to match the preterm and term infant comparisons (i.e., every preterm infant was approximately 40 weeks conceptional age rather

Table 4. Preterm and full-term infants at 40 weeks conceptional age

Clusters	Preterm		Full-term		t value
	Mean	S.D.	Mean	S.D.	
1. Best orientation	6.62	(0.97)	6.91	(1.00)	1.27
2. Modal orientation	5.87	(1.42)	5.76	(1.28)	0.37
3. Motor maturity	5.70	(0.80)	5.48	(0.87)	1.16
4. Range of state	3.65	(0.70)	3.95	(0.70)	1.87
5. Regulation of state	4.34	(1.18)	5.25	(1.11)	3.45[a]
6. Autonomic regulation	6.75	(1.18)	6.69	(1.11)	0.26

[a]$p < .01$

than the group mean being 40 weeks), only one significant difference was found: regulation of state. Thus, the number of behavioral differences was reduced by controlling for conceptional age. This is an important qualification related to the use of a group mean in looking at the effect of conceptional age on behavior.

Mothers of preterm and term infants took home behaviorally different infants. By 4 weeks postdischarge, the behavioral differences of infants had diminished but were present in two areas (best orientation and autonomic regulation clusters). These behavioral changes were likely mediated by both maturational and environmental factors. It is interesting to speculate that the initial differences in the preterm behavioral repertoire affect early mother-infant interaction and, as others have

noted, mothers compensate. From this study, it would appear that this early compensation contributes to the reduction of behavioral differences. As far as can be determined, this is the first documentation of early behavioral changes in the preterm infant population after 4 weeks of home experience. However, maturational factors also play a role as evidenced by the even fewer differences when conceptional age was carefully controlled.

Additional analyses will permit researchers to look further at individual differences within the preterm population and to investigate the character of behavioral variability and stability over time. Such analyses along with other research being carried out with preterm infants have the power to illuminate the processes that are at work in the very early development of high-risk infants.

REFERENCES

Als, H., Lester, B.M., Tronick, E., & Brazelton, T.B. Manual for the Assessment of Preterm Infant Behavior (APIB). In: H.E. Fitzgerald, B.M. Lester, & M.M. Yogman (eds.), *Theory and research in behavioral pediatrics*, Vol. 1. New York: Plenum Publishing Corp., 1980.

Ballard, J.L., Novak, K.K., & Driver, M. A simplified score for assessment of fetal maturation of newly born infants. *The Journal of Pediatrics*, 1979, 95, 769–774.

Beckwith, L., & Cohen, S.E. Preterm birth: Hazardous obstetrical and postnatal events as related to caregiver-infant behavior. *Infant Behavior and Development*, 1978, 1, 403–411.

Beckwith, L., & Cohen, S.E. Interactions of preterm infants with their caregivers and test performance at age two. In: T.M. Field, S. Goldberg, D. Stern, & A.M. Sostek (eds.), *High risk infants and children: Adult and peer interactions*. New York: Academic Press, 1980.

Brazelton, T.B. *Neonatal Behavioral Assessment Scale*. Philadelphia: J.B. Lippincott, 1973.

DiVitto, B., & Goldberg, S. The effects of newborn medical status on early parent-infant interaction. In: T. Field, A. Sostek, S. Goldberg, & H.H. Shuman (eds.), *Infants born at risk*. New York: SP Medical and Scientific Books, 1979.

Ferrari, F., Grosoli, M.V., Fontana, G., & Cavazzuti, G.B. Neurobehavioral comparisons of low-risk preterm and fullterm infants at term conceptional age. *Developmental Medicine and Child Neurology*, 1983, 25, 450–458.

Field, T.M. Effects of early separation, interactive deficits and experimental manipulations on mother-infant face to face interaction. *Child Development*, 1977, 48, 763–771.

Field, T.M. Interactions of preterm and term infants with their lower and middle-class teenage and adult mothers.

In: T.M. Field, S. Goldberg, D. Stern, & A.M. Sostek (eds.), *High-risk infants and children: Adult and peer interactions*. New York: Academic Press, 1980.

Field, T.M., Hallock, N., Ting, G., Dempsey, J., Dabiri, C., & Shuman, H.H. A first year followup of high risk infants: Formulating a cumulative risk index. *Child Development*, 1978, 49, 119–131.

Goldberg, S., Brachfeld, S., DiVitto, B. Feeding, fussing, and play: Parent-infant interaction in the first year as a function of prematurity and perinatal medical problems. In: T.M. Field, S. Goldberg, D. Stern, & A.M. Sostek (eds.), *High risk infants and children: Adult and peer interactions*. New York: Academic Press, 1980.

Horowitz, F.D., & Linn, P.L. The Neonatal Behavioral Assessment Scale: Assessing the behavioral repertoire of the newborn infant. In: M. Wolraich (ed.), *Advances in developmental and behavioral pediatrics*. Greenwich, CT: JAI Press, 1982.

Horowitz, F.D., Sullivan, J.W., & Linn, P.L. Stability and instability in newborn behavior: The quest for elusive threads. In: A. Sameroff (ed.), Organization and stability of newborn behavior: A commentary on the Brazelton Neonatal Behavioral Assessment Scale. *Monographs of the Society for Research in Child Development*, 1978, 43, 29–45.

Klaus, M.H., & Kennell, J.H. Mothers separated from their newborn infants. *Pediatric Clinics of North America*, 1970, 17, 1015–1037.

Lancioni, G., Horowitz, F.D., & Sullivan, J. NBAS-K: I. A study of its stability and structure over the first month of life. *Infant Behavior and Development*, 1980, 3, 341–359. (a)

Lancioni, G., Horowitz, F.D., & Sullivan, J. NBAS-K: II. Reinforcement value of the infant's behavior. *Infant Behavior and Development*, 1980, 3, 361–366. (b)

Leifer, A.D., Leiderman, P.H., Barnett, C.R., & Williams, J.A. Effects of mother-infant separation on maternal attachment behavior. *Child Development* 1972, *43*, 1203–1218.

Lester, B. M. The NBAS: Data analysis, prediction, and a glimpse at the future. In: T.B. Brazelton (ed.), *The Neonatal Behavioral Assessment Scale* (2nd ed.). Philadelphia: J.B. Lippincott, in press.

Linn, P. L., & Horowitz, F. D. The relationship between infant individual differences and mother-infant interaction during the neonatal period. *Infant Behavior and Development*, 1983, *6*, 415–427.

Osofsky, J. D. Neonatal characteristics and mother-infant interaction in two observational situations. *Child Development*, 1976, *47*, 1138–1147.

Osofsky, J. D., & Danzger, B. Relationships between neonatal characteristics and mother-infant interaction. *Developmental Psychology*, 1974, *10*, 124–130.

Sameroff, A. J., & Chandler, M. J. Reproductive risk and the continuum of caretaking casualty. In: F. D. Horowitz (ed.), *Review of child development research*, Vol. 4. Chicago: University of Chicago Press, 1975.

Schwartz, S. F., & Horowitz, F. D. The preterm infant: Behavioral development in the early months. In preparation.

Siegel, L. S. Reproductive, perinatal, and environmental factors as predictors of the cognitive and language development of preterm and fullterm infants. *Child Development*, 1982, *53*, 963–973.

Telzrow, R. W., Kang, R. R., Mitchell, S. K., Ashworth, C. D., & Barnard, K. E. An assessment of the behavior of the preterm infant at 40 weeks conceptional age. In: L. P. Lipsitt & T. M. Field (eds.), *Perinatal risk and newborn behavior*. Norwood, NJ: Ablex Publishing Corp., 1982.

The At-Risk Infant: Psycho/Socio/Medical Aspects
edited by Shaul Harel, M.D., and Nicholas J. Anastasiow, Ph.D.
Copyright © 1985   Paul H. Brookes Publishing Co., Inc.   Baltimore • London

Chapter 10

Working with Parents to Prevent Child Abuse

WILLIAM A. ALTEMEIER, III, M.D.
SUSAN M. O'CONNOR, M.D.
DOROTHY TUCKER, B.A.
Vanderbilt University Hospital, Nashville, Tennessee
KATHRYN B. SHERROD, PH.D.
Peabody College/Vanderbilt University, Nashville, Tennessee
PETER M. VIETZE, PH.D.
Mental Retardation Research Centers, NICHD, Bethesda, Maryland

THE INCIDENCE OF CHILD ABUSE HAS IN-creased rapidly over the past 2 decades. According to recent estimates, between 1% and 2% of all children in this country will sustain nonaccidental injury at the hands of their parents at some point during childhood (Krug & Davis, 1981). This high incidence and the profound physical and emotional damage that result make prevention a high priority. Professionals in medicine, nursing, and social services have the opportunity to reduce this problem during three critical phases in the evolution of abusive tendencies: 1) at the first display of abusive tendencies, 2) immediately after abuse occurs, and 3) during long-term follow up. The first phase takes place when parents who have not yet abused their children behave in a manner that suggests they could develop this problem. This phase could be managed most ideally by predicting which parents are at highest risk for becoming abu-sive, and intervening to alleviate their prob-lems before injuries are inflicted. Although work has begun on predictive instruments, a practical and reliable method to select families at high risk is not yet available, and testing of intervention methods in this situation has barely begun. In the meantime, it is still possi-ble to be alert to parents with high-risk charac-teristics like those discussed in this chapter and offer general social support and counseling.

The second phase of abusive tendencies occurs immediately following the non-accidental injury of a child. Here, the first priority is to protect the child from immediate danger. This usually means hospitalization for several days while injuries are treated; sub-clinical bone trauma is identified by longbone, chest, and skull X rays; decisions are made about whether or not abuse has occurred; and long-term management is planned. When ad-mitting the child, the physician may not wish to

Research for this chapter was supported by the National Center on Child Abuse and Neglect; Children's Bureau Administration on Children, Youth and Families; Office of Human Development Services/Department of Health, Education and Welfare Grant No. 90-C-419 and 90-CA-2138; William T. Grant Foundation; and the National Institute of Mental Health, Grant No. RO1 MH31195-01.
The authors wish to express their thanks to Mrs. Claudia Stewart for assistance in preparing this manuscript.

mention abuse, but instead indicate global concern about the injuries and a desire to investigate them further. Even if the injuries are minor, parents usually agree to hospitalization, perhaps because they sense things are out of control at home. After the child is hospitalized and the family has calmed down somewhat, it seems prudent to tell parents that they will be investigated by protective services. This can be softened to some extent by indicating that this is routine and required by law for injuries such as those sustained by the child, and that the investigation will be confidential. If the injuries are minor and not obviously the result of abuse, parents may be advised that the investigation could consist of nothing other than an interview unless other reasons to suspect abuse are uncovered. Throughout this phase, it is important to be as honest and sympathetic as possible toward these parents in order to maintain rapport for long-term intervention and follow-up. In addition, hostility and aggression from any source may play a role in developing or maintaining abusive tendencies.

The third phase involves the long-term follow-up and rehabilitation of the family after a diagnosis of child abuse has been made. Here, the primary goal is to make the home as safe as possible for return of the child, and to follow him or her carefully for reoccurrence of nonaccidental injury. The following discussion is directed toward developing a strategy to rehabilitate abusive parents and prevent parents who exhibit high-risk characteristics from becoming abusive.

ETIOLOGY OF ABUSE

In order to stop abuse or prevent it from starting, it is necessary to understand the characteristics of individuals and their environments that lead to this condition. Two approaches have been used to uncover parental characteristics that are associated with abuse: retrospective and prospective.

The Retrospective Approach

In retrospective studies, a group of families known to have abused their children are interviewed for characteristics, and these results are compared to similar data obtained from a control group matched for socioeconomic status. It is important that both the abuse and comparison groups come from the same economic population because, otherwise, it is difficult to determine whether characteristics of abusive families are related to the abuse or to their low socioeconomic strata. Retrospective studies have indicated that abusive families: 1) are more likely to have been battered during their own childhood, 2) have low self-esteem, 3) are socially isolated, 4) distrust others, 5) have increased life stress, and 6) freely express aggressive impulses (Milner & Wimberly, 1979; Parke & Collmer, 1975; Steele & Pollock, 1968). Unemployment of the father, poor and overcrowded housing, large family size, high mobility, and alcohol or drug abuse (Baldwin & Oliver, 1975; Fontana, 1973; Parke & Collmer, 1975) have also been implicated as risk factors.

Most of the information about the etiology of abuse is derived from retrospective studies. When the study is objective, includes a broad degree of severity of abuse, and carefully matches control and abuse groups, it aids in the understanding of this problem. However, one deficiency is inherent in the retrospective approach. In order to be included in the abuse group, a parent must have abused a child and been discovered, reported, and investigated. The honesty, social relationships, and self-perceptions of parents are likely to change after experiencing this sequence of events. For example, abusing one's child and being investigated could decrease self-esteem, increase life stress, promote isolation and distrust of others, and possibly lead to alcohol abuse. Thus, it is difficult to be certain whether characteristics identified retrospectively preceded the abuse, and therefore might have contributed to it, or whether they were actually produced by the abuse and its discovery.

The Prospective Approach

One approach to sorting pre- from post-abuse characteristics is to study families before the abuse has occurred. This requires interviewing a large number of parents and following them for subsequent abuse. The characteristics of those who go on to abuse their children are then compared to those who do not. The problem with this approach is that the low incidence of abuse necessitates collecting prospective data from a large number of subjects. The high cost of this approach makes it difficult, especially now when funding is so limited. Nevertheless, a few prospective studies have been reported (Altemeier, O'Connor, Vietze, Sandler, & Sherrod, 1982; Egeland, Breitenbucker, & Rosenberg, 1980; Egeland & Brunnquell, 1979; Hunter, Kilstrom, Kraybell, & Loda, 1978).

The following is a description of a project started in 1975 at Nashville General Hospital, an inner-city hospital that serves indigent people from the Nashville area. Details of methods may be found elsewhere (Altemeier et al., 1982; Altemeier, Vietze, Sherrod, Sandler, Falsey, & O'Connor, 1979). Informed consent was obtained from all mothers who registered for prenatal clinic during a 15-month period; 94% agreed to participate and each of these received a 35-minute interview while waiting to see an obstetrician. The interviews were stopped after 1,400 expectant mothers were recruited. These mothers were then followed for abuse of the children they were carrying at the time of interview (target infants), or for abuse of siblings that had not previously been reported. Abuse was defined as a report to protective services of an injury, with the subsequent investigation indicating substance of this report. Reports of neglect and instances of growth failure due to inadequate feeding of infants (nonorganic failure to thrive, or NOFT) were also monitored. The families were followed until the beginning of 1980 at which time the average age of target infants was 40 months. Among the 1,400 families, a search of all protective services reports throughout the state of Tennessee indicated that 30 had been reported for child abuse during the 5 years of the study. The data suggested that it was possible to predict high risk for child abuse to a degree that was statistically significant. However, accuracy was too low for practical application and extended for only 2 years following the interview (Altemeier et al., 1982). The following data are based upon a comparison of 23 of the 30 families reported for abuse within 2 years versus the remaining 1,377 families. These results, reported previously (Altemeier et al., 1982; Altemeier et al., 1979; Altemeier, Vietze, Sherrod, Sandler, Tucker, & O'Connor, 1980), indicated that many characteristics determined retrospectively were also evident prospectively, although some characteristics evident in the former were not found when viewed prospectively. The results further suggested that aberrant nurture during childhood may form the foundation for subsequent child abuse.

The interview was divided into eight major sections:

1. Mother's perception of her nurture as a child
2. Positive and negative feelings about her pregnancy
3. Knowledge of parent skills and philosophy about discipline
4. Social support available from others
5. Personality factors of self-image, isolation, and tolerance to stress
6. Alcohol, drug, and health problems in the family
7. Expectations of child development
8. A revised Life Stress Inventory for both the mother and father (Holmes & Rahe, 1967)

Nurture during Childhood Important differences among the 23 families reported for abuse compared to the remaining families were found for the first three of these eight categories. Fifteen questions involved the mother's perception of her own nurture during childhood; significant differences were seen in four questions. For example, 17% of mothers in the abuse category reported that they had lived in foster care homes at some time during childhood compared to 2% of the remaining families ($p \leq .0001$). Mothers in the abuse category were more likely to be estranged from their own mothers ($p \leq .01$), to feel their parents were displeased with them ($p \leq .01$), and to have received severe punishment during their childhood that was considered unfair ($p \leq .01$). Mothers in the abuse category answered other nurture questions in the expected direction, but these did not reach significance. These answers were: mothers rejected their own mother as models ($p = .09$), felt they were unloved as children ($p = .11$), reported repeated beatings by parents ($p = .13$), received beatings severe enough to be seen by a physician ($p = .14$), were raised in two-parent homes ($p = .14$), had unhappy childhoods ($p = .19$), and were punished by abuse ($p = .19$). There were no appreciable differences among families ($p > .2$) in feeling that children made their parents nervous, let their parents down, had negative attitudes toward their fathers, or had ever been beaten (one or more times) by their parents. Thus, there was a relationship between aberrant nurture during childhood and becoming an abusive parent, but it was interesting that being beaten or physically abused did not seem as important as being unwanted or unloved. It was also interesting that 29% of the 1,400 women in the study received punishment by parents that would generally be considered abusive.

Negative Feelings about Pregnancy
The mothers' feelings about the pregnancies they were carrying at the time of the interview also differed in the two groups. Mothers in the abuse category were significantly more likely to reject this pregnancy when it was first recognized ($p \leq .05$), and at the time of interview ($p \leq .05$), to have had an unplanned pregnancy ($p \leq .01$), and to report that their mood had been adversely affected by the pregnancy ($p \leq .05$). Although these findings were not surprising, other reports indicating that unwanted pregnancy is an antecedent of child abuse are rare. Perhaps this is because it is more difficult to document these attitudes retrospectively.

Knowledge of Parent Skills Parenting attitudes, knowledge, and behavior also differed significantly in the abuse and comparison groups. Twenty-six percent of the abusive mothers had lost a child (other than the one abused in this study) to foster care or an "avoidable" death compared to 2% of the controls ($p \leq .0001$). It was not known whether these children had been voluntarily surrendered to foster care or whether they were forcefully removed because of maltreatment. The other major difference between the abusive and comparison families concerned tendencies toward violence. Those in the abuse group were significantly more likely to fear they might hurt one of their other children ($p \leq .01$) and to report that they had violently attacked someone recently ($p \leq .05$). Significantly more in the abuse group also reported that screaming babies made them feel angry ($p \leq .05$). This supported what was found in many other retrospective studies; namely, that parents of abusive children tend to express violent tendencies and to have experienced violence from others (Kempe, Silverman, Steele, Droegemueller, & Silver, 1962).

Other Characteristics Table 1 summarizes the important demographic characteristics of the abuse versus comparison families. These were either extracted from the life stress section of the interview or were collected immediately before initiating the interview. It was concluded from this information that age, race, and education were not significant antecedents of child abuse. An observation not previously reported in the literature was that mothers in the abuse category tended to be either below the fifth percentile (less than 100 pounds) or above the 95th percentile (greater than 180 pounds) in their usual prepregnancy weights. Almost half of the mothers in the abuse category had abnormal weights, and these were about equally divided between those who were unusually light and unusually heavy. Several types of information from this table also suggest that increased exposure between parents and children, or stress related to the parent-child interaction, may put a family at risk for abuse. As has also been found in retrospective studies, the abusive families tended to have more children, and especially more young children (Parke & Collmer, 1975). Inadequate spacing (another infant in the home below 1 year of age at the time of prenatal interview) was also more prevalent in the abuse category. It was surprising to find that mothers who had married at some point seemed to be at higher risk for abuse than those who had never been married. Although no relationship was found between being divorced or separated from a husband and abuse, mothers who had always been single were less likely to have a

Table 1. Mothers' demographic data

		Percentage of each group	
	p value	Abuse (n = 23)	No abuse (n = 1,377)
Usual weight below the fifth or above the ninety-fifth percentile[a]	<.0001	48	9
More than one child under 5 years old	.0008	39	12
More than one child any age	.001	52	21
Moved more than once per month	.001	9	0.1
More than one pregnancy in past year	.002	30	6
Usual weight below the fifth percentile[a]	.007	22	3
Usual weight above the ninety-fifth percentile[a]	.007	26	6
Left job in past year	.01	9	38
Married at some time	.03	91	67
Changed jobs in past year	.06	13	33
Age greater than 20 years	.20	65	50
Race	>.2		
Education	>.2		

[a]Prepregnancy weights were determined from maternal medical charts for all 23 in the abuse category and a sample of 83 women selected randomly from the remaining 1,377. All other percentages were calculated from the full 1,377 comparison group.

child reported for abuse then those who had married at any time. This could be a chance observation that just happened to reach significance. The only other explanation for this is that perhaps being married increases parent-child exposure and stress because two parents are available instead of one. In view of the fact that many but not all studies (Gaines, Sandgrund, Greene, & Power, 1978; Hunter et al., 1978) have found higher rates of unmarried mothers in the abuse group, further studies will be necessary to clarify this observation. It was also surprising to find that mothers who had left a job in the past year had a significantly lower incidence of abuse, and those that had changed jobs in the past year also tended to have a lower incidence. These questions related to employment were initially included in the stress inventory, but after further examination, they did not seem to represent stresses that increased risk for abuse. However, on analyses of these and related questions, it was concluded that positive responses seemed to indicate that less women in the abuse category were "working mothers" who sought employment away from the home. Again, having a job outside the home may decrease parent-child exposure and therefore decrease opportunities for abuse. Retrospective studies have described an as-

sociation between paternal unemployment and abuse, and exposure may play a similar role here. Finally, both prospective and retrospective studies suggest that parents who abuse their children are more likely to change residence frequently. Two of the 23 in the abuse category moved more than once per month for the preceding year (17 and 23 times per year), while only one from the 1,377 comparison group moved with this frequency (13 times).

Several characteristics often mentioned in retrospective studies were not evident in the prospective approach. There was minimum evidence that mothers who would be in the abusive category had low self-esteem, and no evidence that they were more isolated, or that they had less support from family, friends, or the father of the infant they were carrying at interview. Family, alcohol, and drug problems were not more prevalent among the abuse group. An extensive investigation of the mother's expectations for child development revealed no differences. Although it is risky to draw conclusions from negative data, the authors speculate that these characteristics may have been present retrospectively because they resulted, at least in part, from the abuse and its discovery. As such, they would not be true antecedents. However, once abuse has occurred and these characteristics have developed, they might contribute to the continuation of an abusive pattern.

THE RELATIVE IMPORTANCE OF VARIOUS ANTECEDENTS FOR ABUSE

This prospective study suggests that unwanted pregnancy, increased family exposure and stress, aggressive or violent tendencies, excessive changes of residence, overweight or underweight body habitus, and aberrant nurture during childhood all seem to be true antecedents of child abuse. Each of these antecedents could be addressed to a greater or lesser degree by intervention. In fact, the current strategy to prevent recurrent abuse within a family involves searching for factors that seem to predispose to this condition, and devising intervention to deal with each problem individually. Because of the number and diversity of these conditions, a multidisciplinary team consisting of protective service workers, nurses, physicians, social workers, and legal professionals is often utilized to plan and expedite the program. This is a relatively expensive approach, and would be particularly impractical for families who were judged to be at risk for abuse but had not yet begun to injure their children.

An alternative approach would be to determine whether one of the conditions that predisposes to nonaccidental trauma might be more important than the others in forming a foundation for abusive behavior. That is, one risk factor (or a limited number) may be primary in causing abuse, and may make the

family susceptible not only to the abuse but to the development of other characteristics associated with this condition. These secondary conditions could then act in concert with the primary characteristic in leading to nonaccidental injuries of children. If this were true, the most efficient long-term strategy would be to direct intervention resources toward the primary risk factor. Although there was no direct way to address this objective several indirect approaches were tried. The first approach asked which of the original eight interview categories was related to NOFT and neglect. The reasoning was that if one was most important, it might also be most consistently related to all three types of maltreatment. The data of Table 2 and that reported above indicate that aberrant childhood nurture was the only category that correlated significantly with all three forms of maltreatment (abuse, neglect, and NOFT). To approach this in a different way, forty-two questions were selected from the interview that were significantly associated with abuse, neglect, or NOFT. These questions were subjected to principal axis factor analysis using data from all 1,400 subjects. The strongest factor, that is, the factor that shared the greatest variance with all of the 42 variables, was made up of the majority of childhood nurture questions. Finally, it was postulated that if aberrant nurture during childhood were the foundation for the development of other risk factors for abuse, it should also be strongly related to the other risk factors. Table 3 summarizes the correlation of childhood nurture with each of the other eight interview categories. Relatively low but sig-

Table 2. Correlation of neglect and NOFT with interview categories

Interview Category	Neglect ($n = 117$)	NOFT ($n = 101$)
1. Childhood nurture	−.265[a]	−.328[a]
2. Pregnancy attitude	.001	−.095
3. Parenting attitude and skills	−.274[a]	−.152
4. Support	−.120	−.139
5. Personality, self image	−.111	−.135
6. Alcohol, drug, health problems	−.107	−.122
7. Child development expectations	.076	−.104
8. Life stress inventory		
Mother	−.089	.338[a]
Father	.008	.270[a]

[a]$p < .01$.

Table 3. Correlation of childhood nurture with other interview categories

	Correlation (N = 1,400)
1. Childhood nurture	1.000
2. Pregnancy attitude	.139[a]
3. Parenting attitude and skills	.209[a]
4. Support	.210[a]
5. Personality, self-image	.368[a]
6. Alcohol, drug, health problems	.304[a]
7. Child development expectations	.006
8. Life stress inventory	
Mother	−.286[a]
Father	−.086[b]

[a] $p < .01$.
[b] $p < .05$.

nificant correlations were observed in all categories except for the mother's expectations of child development. This category was also the one that was least related to any of the three types of maltreatment and the authors have concluded that it is of little or no importance as an antecedent of abuse, neglect, or NOFT. Correlations were also set up for an overall score of all childhood nurture questions and each of the other interview questions. These correlations were significant at $p \leq .05$ in the expected direction for 56 of the 102 questions. Taken together, these data suggest that childhood nurture may form the foundation for becoming an abusive parent. One should keep in mind that when conditions are associated with each other, it is very difficult to sort out cause and effect so that the above is primarily speculation. On a conceptual basis, aberrant nurture would also seem to be the most logical candidate to predispose to the development of other factors for abuse. It precedes their development temporally in individuals and would be expected to change many aspects of personality and parenting behavior.

SPECULATIONS ABOUT STRATEGY TO PREVENT CHILD ABUSE

Classical theories of etiology of child abuse generally require that a series of events must come together in order to produce an incident of nonaccidental child injury. The prevailing theory is that at least three types of problems must all occur at the same time. These involve a special parent, a special child, and some stressful precipitating event. According to this prevailing theory, the special parent is likely to have experienced abuse as a child, be isolated from society, have a low income, a poor self-image, little support from others, violent tendencies, and excessive expectations of children. The special child may be portrayed as a premature infant, a child who is handicapped with developmental deficiency or physical disabilities, or one who is particularly noxious to parents for whatever reason. The precipitating stress may be a sudden loss of job or any other disturbing life event. This theory predicts that child abuse will only occur if all three of these things happen to be operating at the same time in the same family.

The data presented here suggest a somewhat different sequence of events. The authors speculate that aberrant nurture during childhood lays the foundation for subsequent child abuse. Furthermore, feeling unwanted or unloved seemed to be a stronger antecedent than outright abuse at the hands of parents. If children are reared under these conditions, the authors postulate that they may have a greater chance for developing other antecedents in the years that follow. They are more likely to have unwanted pregnancies, increased life stresses, aggressive and violent tendencies, and other antecedents of child abuse as identified in this prospective study. After the onset of child abuse, parents may then develop lowered self-esteem, isolation from friends and family, a lack of support from others, alcohol and drug problems, and excessive expectations of their children (or dissatisfaction with the performance of their abused offspring). The authors realize that this sequence of events is at best an oversimplification. All of these characteristics will obviously interact with each other, and the environment must have an impact on the parents regardless of nurture. However, the major implication is that prevention of aberrant childhood nurture may be the single most effective way to prevent child abuse over the long run. That is to say, if aberrant nurture or its effects can be decreased, child abuse should be reduced in the next generation. Furthermore, the reduction of aberrant nurture in one generation may have far-reaching effects that involve many generations thereafter. If experiencing an aberrant nurture predisposes a person to becoming a parent who provides similar nurture to his or her children, intervention to break this cycle at one point may benefit several subsequent generations without additional intervention.

Unfortunately, preventing or reducing the effects that follow aberrant nurture will be a difficult goal to achieve. The most direct manner of doing this might be to predict high risk in prospective parents and offer intervention before abuse begins as discussed in the introduction of this chapter. In addition, this intervention might be specifically directed at promoting desirable parenting behaviors and minimizing the effects produced by aberrant nurture during childhood. This raises the question of what type of intervention might be effective in compensating for aberrant nurture. Some clues may be evident in what is known about prevention of child abuse irrespective of the above theory. Cohn (Cohn, 1978, 1980) has provided the most comprehensive review of this subject thus far by collecting 3 years of data from 11 demonstration projects that involved 1,724 parents. The effectiveness of various intervention approaches to improve parenting function and reduce recidivism for abuse and neglect during treatment were compared in the different programs. None of the approaches was highly effective, but in general, lay workers were somewhat more useful than professional workers, and the best approach was an initial phase in which protective service employees managed these families immediately after abuse had occurred, followed by a longer-term phase in which lay individuals supplied support and counseling. The most effective of the latter seemed to be Parents Anonymous. This observation is not inconsistent with the theory of causation presented above. It may be that lay workers, especially those affiliated with organizations like Parents Anonymous, perform a nurturing function for abusive mothers and fathers, and act as substitute parents.

Therefore, it may be possible to at least partially compensate for aberrant nurture during childhood if some of the following conditions are considered. First, an individual (or group) could serve as a "substitute parent" for mothers and fathers who have either abused their children or who appear to be at high risk for subsequent abuse. This individual could be a social worker, a physician who provides pediatric care for the children or obstetrical care for the mother, a nurse practitioner or nurse midwife who maintains long-term contact with the families, or perhaps a clergyman. Candidates for lay substitute parents might also include the type of substitute grandparent utilized by Kempe and co-workers in their original intervention programs developed in Denver (Kempe & Helfer, 1972). The authors further suggest that it might be detrimental for the "substitute parent" to play the same type of role as that which the mother and father of the high-risk abusive parents played when the latter were children. That is, the nurturing worker should be separated from the law enforcement agency that identifies or investigates and punishes guilty parents, and this individual should be as sympathetic toward the parents as possible. Second, the intervention worker should develop as strong a relationship with the family as possible. There should be continuity in this relationship in that the worker should change as infrequently as possible, and should be as accessible as possible, especially in times of stress. The intervention worker must also be accepted by the parents to some degree. Since it is necessary for such an individual to form a nurturing relationship with the parents, every attempt should be made to get the parents to agree to this type of help voluntarily instead of using a court order to force compliance. The activities of the intervention worker could be modeled after those of the grandparent to the child at risk. Such a substitute grandparent would be available to hear out the problems of the high-risk or abusive parents, offer them support and sympathy, give them suggestions and advice, and be advocates of both the parents and the child.

Of course, all of the above remains theory not yet subjected to a controlled study. An experiment that would test the above would require a group of either known abusive parents or those predicted to be at high risk for subsequent abuse. These families could then be randomly divided into experimental and control groups, and the former might receive intervention modeled after the above scheme, while the control group should receive the followup and management that is currently practiced within that community. A comparison of subsequent abuse, as determined by an independent agency blind to which individuals were assigned to experimental or control groups could then determine outcome. Although such experiments will be difficult, costly, and fraught with ethical questions, they will be necessary in order to obtain clear information about the effectiveness of various intervention programs.

REFERENCES

Altemeier, W., O'Connor, S., Vietze, P., Sandler, H., & Sherrod, K. Antecedents of child abuse. *The Journal of Pediatrics,* 1982, *100,* 823–829.

Altemeier, W., Vietze, P., Sherrod, K., Sandler, H., Falsey, S., & O'Connor, S. Prediction of child maltreatment during pregnancy. *Journal of the American Academy of Child Psychiatry,* 1979, *18,* 205–218.

Altemeier, W., Vietze, P., Sherrod, K., Sandler, H., Tucker, D., & O'Connor, S. Prediction of child maltreatment in pregnancy. In: S. Harel (ed.), *The at risk infant.* Amsterdam: Excerpta Medica, 1980.

Baldwin, J. & Oliver, J. Epidemiology and family characteristics of severely abused children. *British Journal of the Preventive Society of Medicine,* 1975, *29,* 205–221.

Cohn, A. *Essential elements of successful child abuse and neglect treatment.* Paper presented at the Second International Congress on Child Abuse and Neglect, London, September, 1978.

Cohn, A. The pediatrician's role in the treatment of child abuse: Implications from a national evaluation study. *Pediatrics,* 1980, *65,* 358–361.

Egeland, B., Breitenbucker, M., & Rosenberg, D. Prospective study of the significance of life stress in etiology of child abuse. *Journal of Consulting and Clinical Psychology,* 1980, *48,* 195–205.

Egeland, B. & Brunnquell, D. An at-risk approach to the study of child abuse: Some preliminary findings. *Journal of the American Academy of Child Psychiatry,* 1979, *18,* 219–235.

Fontana, V. The diagnosis of the maltreatment syndrome in children. *Pediatrics,* 1973, *51,* 780–782.

Gaines, R., Sandgrund, A., Greene, A., & Power, E. Etiological factors in child maltreatment: A multivariate study of abusing neglecting and normal mothers. *Journal of Abnormal Psychology,* 1978, *87,* 531–540.

Holmes, T., & Rahe, R. The social readjustment rating scale. *Journal of Psychosomatic Research,* 1967, *11,* 213.

Hunter, R., Kilstrom, N., Kraybell, E., & Loda, F. Antecedents of child abuse and neglect in premature infants: A prospective study in a newborn intensive care unit. *Pediatrics,* 1978, *61,* 629–635.

Kempe, C., & Helfer, R. Innovative therapeutic approaches. In: C. Kempe & R. Helfer (eds.), *Helping the battered child and his family.* Philadelphia: J. B. Lippincott, 1972.

Kempe, C., Silverman, F., Steele, B., Droegemueller, W., & Silver, H. The battered child syndrome. *Journal of the American Medical Association,* 1962, *181,* 17–24.

Krug, D., & Davis, P. Study findings. *National study of the incidence and severity of child abuse and neglect.* DHHS Publication N. (OHDS) 81-30325, 41–43, 1981.

Milner, J., & Wimberly, R. An inventory for the identification of child abusers. *Journal of Clinical Psychology,* 1979, *35,* 95–100.

Parke, R., & Collmer, C. Child abuse: An interdisciplinary analysis. In: E. Hetherington (ed.), *Review of child development research,* Vol. 5. Chicago: University of Chicago Press, 1975.

Steele, B., & Pollock, C. A psychiatric study of parents who abuse infants and small children. In: R. Helfer & C. Kempe (eds.), *The battered child.* Chicago: University of Chicago Press, 1968.

The At-Risk Infant: Psycho/Socio/Medical Aspects
edited by Shaul Harel, M.D., and Nicholas J. Anastasiow, Ph.D.
Copyright © 1985   Paul H. Brookes Publishing Co., Inc.   Baltimore • London

Chapter 11

At-Definite-Risk Infants
and Their Adolescent Mothers

Frieda Spivack, Ph.D.
Herbert H. Lehman College, City University of New York, Bronx, New York

HILDREN BORN TO TEENAGE MOTHERS DIS- play intellectual deficits, largely because of the economic and social impact of early childbearing upon their young parents. Such children are more likely to spend part of their childhood in one-parent households. Many authors have noted that these children when mature will also have children themselves while still adolescents and that they will be worse off in terms of physical health, social-emotional development and later school achievements than children of older mothers (Belmont, Cohen, Dryfoos, Stein, & Zayac, 1981; Chilman, 1980; Nelson, 1973; Osofsky & Osofsky, 1970; Ramey & Bryant, 1982; Sameroff & Chandler, 1975; Sandler, Vietze, & O'Connor, 1981).

Additionally, teenage mothers of infants born with genetic and medical problems are often too overwhelmed by these responsibilities to manage their infants' extra needs. These infants are "at definite risk" as a result of their compounded problems. Their teenage mothers find it difficult to provide for their own physiological needs, let alone those of their infants. Hospitals such as Kingsbrook Jewish Medical Center have provided special services for these infants and their teenage mothers. At-definite-risk infants and their mothers, in addition to needing clinic and therapy ap-

pointments for medical complications, have basic housing, welfare, and social network problems. To ameliorate these problems, home-care provider units and a continuum of medical, therapy, and special education services have been funded through the Developmental Disabilities Assistance and Bill of Rights Act of 1975 (Public Law 94-103).

Egeland and Sroufe (1981), in identifying their sample of adequate and inadequate child-care mothers, found that "the inadequate caring group are younger, less well educated, unmarried at the time of the child's birth. All these factors tend to be correlates of mal-adaption" (p. 45). Egeland and Sroufe found that some of the inadequate young mothers' patterns of mothering and/or rejection created baby reactions of either anxious resistance or anxious avoidance patterns toward their mothers. "A sizeable percentage of infants change toward a more secure attachment with their mothers between ages 12 and 18 months with intervention from child protection and other child care agencies" (p. 46). Attachment relationships can change, and they are affected substantially by stabilizing influences in the lives of mother and infant. In fact, Vaughn, Egeland, Sroufe, and Waters (1979) report that the presence of adults other than the young mother in some way mitigates the deleterious health and other effects on the child often associated with teenage childbearing. Therefore, home-care units were created with a home-care provider especially trained to model positive mothering patterns for teenage mothers.

HOME-CARE SERVICES TO PARENTS AND CHILD

Although the purpose of the continuum of services and home-care provider units program was to provide resources to the parent and direct services to children, the actual day-to-day work demanded that direct services be provided for teenage mothers as well. This program began in September, 1982, and will continue until September, 1985. Twenty mothers and their handicapped children were identified and placed in home-care provider units. Mothers are ages 17–21 and children are 10 days old to age 4. This program provides developmental stimulation in the home-care provider unit and pediatric and rehabilitative care in the hospital. In addition, the home-care provider unit gives training in parenting and supportive social services for parents.

The most vulnerable mothers (five out of a population of 15 mothers) were ambivalent regarding the help they received, at times accepting, other times defensive, and sometime separating from the program when the program demands could not be met. When the family was separated from the program, the consequences were severe. Over the summer vacation, one of the severely handicapped children died as a result of his own serious problems and parent neglect. Another mother, when allowed to her own devices, began to drink alcohol heavily, and left a supportive extended family environment with her young babies for the "street." It was found that a number of professional persons are needed to help maintain the teenage mothers when monitoring and daily involvement with the home-care unit is temporarily discontinued. (During the last 3 weeks of August, 1983, this program was closed for staff vacations.)

Objective Outcomes of the Kingsbrook Continuum of Services and Home-Care Provider Units Program

The convenience of having rehabilitative clinics, pediatric and adult emergency care, and a child-caring agency under one roof helps adolescent mothers to bring their infants and themselves for treatment at Kingsbrook Jewish Medical Center. The home-care providers within the Kingsbrook catchment community are additionally used for modeling correct parenting behaviors such as daily care routines, developmental stimulation, preparation of proper foods for young children, etc. In addition, respite care is provided for mothers who go for job training or clinic appointments. The achievement outcomes for the first year of the program are described below.

Child Progress   As a result of the Kingsbrook program, positive growth and development for at-definite-risk infants have been promoted. All infants were able to progress from 5 to 10 months developmental age according to the Bayley Scales of Infant Development (Bayley, 1969) during the first year of the program. Multidisciplinary intervention from a team of specialists including special education teachers and therapeutic and medical personnel resulted in each child receiving the requisite individual therapy to facilitate his or her motor and sensorimotor development.

Teenage Mothers' Progress   As a result of consistent direct training and supervision given to teenage mothers, their understanding of developmental milestones and activity training for their children has been enhanced. Mothers who attended 90% of the sessions increased their positive interaction with their infants as demonstrated by significantly higher scores on the mother-child interaction checklist developed by the program.

Lower socioeconomic families have been given the opportunity for job training as a result of respite care provisions for the child. In addition, individual and family needs have been met due to positive parent modeling given to teenage mothers, and regular supportive services provided through the hospital. Teenage parents' understanding and acceptance of their handicapped infants have been facilitated and positive changes have been effected.

Elimination of Child Abuse Child abuse is common for the difficult and erratic group of teenage mothers. Interference in this behavior is regarded as an infringement upon their "rights" as a mother, and creates a rift between professionals and parents. Child neglect is apparently more common among teenage parents because they desire to satisfy their own personal needs above their infants' needs. Not understanding daily care routine and scheduling for infants, the mothers fail to provide the minimum nourishment and grooming.

The home-care provider staff, with the support of other at-definite-risk families, has become the teenage mothers' social network, case manager, friend, transporter, and reinforcer of doctors' orders.

The hospital program provides a 12-point evaluation for neurologically impaired infants and a pediatric walk-in clinic for these infants. In addition, the hospital offers individual therapy: occupational, physical, and speech therapy. However, hospitals don't become involved when individual appointments made by teenage mothers for their handicapped infants are broken. These cases are simply dropped. However, the home-care staff, in developing a close relationship with the mothers, makes it the mission of the agency to follow through with broken appointments through rescheduling and monitoring of future appointments.

Young teenage mothers need to be helped and counseled regarding the treatment of their babies. Ignorance of their own or their infants' needs leads to malnourishment and neglect. Not understanding the developmental se-

quence of infants' abilities, they demand too much from a defenseless and vulnerable baby. Most difficult for the Kingsbrook staff is the task of teaching mothers to provide basic nourishment for themselves and their babies. Daily, the home-care provider prepares a three-course lunch to demonstrate good nutritional practices and to teach cooking skills. Ordinarily, the teenage mother buys hot dogs, potato chips, and sodas for herself and her baby. This behavior typifies the lack of knowledge of a nourishing diet and a lack of understanding of babies' developmental feeding needs.

The experiences of the Kingsbrook project lead to the conclusion that the cycle of child abuse can be broken and eradicated. Numerous other studies support the same conclusion. The results of one such study are reported in the article "Breaking the Cycle in Abusive Families" (Hunter & Kilstrom, 1979). The subjects of the study were 282 premature infants (premature babies are often delivered by teenage mothers and prone to abuse). Forty-nine of the infants' families had a history of child abuse. Characteristics associated with child abuse were used to evaluate the parent and child. After 12 months, nine of the babies were maltreated. The remaining 40 family members did not abuse their children. Both groups (nonrepeating and repeating families) had similar characteristics. The mothers in both groups were teenagers, they had money problems, and their infants were premature. However, there were some salient differences (see Table 1).

In this study, as in other studies, the most significant factor in reducing child abuse relates to the social resources of the teenage parent. The mothers involved in their extended families do not repeat the child-abuse syn-

Table 1. Differences among families with a history of child abuse

Characteristics	Nonrepeating families (n = 40)	Repeating families (n = 9)
Current social resources:		
1. Married	60%	78%
2. Parents living together	58%	67%
3. Mother living with extended family	30%	0%
4. Social network involvement	73%	22%
5. Adequate child-care arrangements	73%	22%

Adapted from Hunter and Kilstrom (1979).

drome. The home-care unit staff and family became the extended family for the teenage mothers. Through their support and concern, teenage mothers in the Kingsbrook project have been able to become nonrepeaters of child abuse. Mother-child interaction and consistency of involvement as promulgated by the Kingsbrook project, also lead to a non-repetition of child abuse. Monitoring and providing ongoing child-care services help stabilize the family's life and reduce child abuse. In Table 2, the figures for parent-infant contact prove this point.

ILLEGITIMATE BIRTHS

Adolescent motherhood is actually not a new problem at all. The change of attitude toward adolescent mothers is the result of sharp increases of illegitimacy. Presently, 49% of pregnant teens choose to have their babies; 1.3 million children are now being raised by teenage mothers, more than half of whom are unmarried. The father makes arrangements with more than one teenage paramour, often without real interest in his progeny. Immature, poverty-stricken teenage mothers feel defenseless and often despair that their lives cannot become normal again. Most often they decide not to abort because they think that by having the baby, they can maintain contact with the baby's father and, through public assistance, support a nuclear family arrangement. Unfortunately, the latter arrangement tends to be short-lived, replete with financial problems and misdemeanors and felonies perpetrated by aggression, eventually souring the relationship.

The rate of illegitimate births to single teenage girls living alone has remained quite high in spite of a greater utilization of birth control and the marked increase in abortion. To some extent, these changes represent a change in attitude and in life-style.

An additional factor related to illegitimate births is discussed by Vinovskis (1981) in her research on the epidemic of adolescent pregnancy. The fact that the government administration and Congress have only concentrated their attention on the prevention of adolescent childbearing or the care of the pregnant teen-

agers has not done enough to solve the illegitimacy problem. Nothing has been done to force young fathers to support their children or to marry the adolescent mothers as was done 40 years ago. One would think that to be eligible for enrollment in the Aid for Families with Dependent Children (AFDC) program, the father of the child of the teenage mother should be present to determine eligibility, whether or not he is employed. Presently, this is not the case. Instead, the father who accepts responsibility loses the financial support for his child. If the parent is employed, by law he is compelled to contribute to the support of his unborn child and the mother, according to his income.

Whether the father is employed or unemployed, the experiences of the Kingsbrook project found that the fathers are receiving welfare funds and food stamps from their unmarried spouses. In demanding his "just half" or more, he creates a problem of accountability of the monies for the Bureau of Social Services Welfare Department.

Presently, for many of these families, legal aid attorneys are used to adjudicate these problems. In the Kingsbrook project, a legal consultant serves to litigate problems that could be resolved.

ISSUES AND PROBLEMS FOR THE LEGAL CONSULTANT WORKING WITH TEENAGE FAMILIES

Some of the legal problems that Kingsbrook became involved with are related to marriage and family and the teenage parent. Some general issues that it addresses are marriage and divorce, child support, and separation. Others are more specific, such as custody and adoption, rights of natural fathers and mothers, fostercare and child-care agencies, and aid to dependent children and child-protection agencies.

A few of the families who sought help from Kingsbrook are in the United States on a tourist visa. Therefore, the legal consultant is faced with problems related to immigration such as citizenship and naturalization, permanent residency, rights of employment, and deportation.

Having a handicapped child creates legal educational issues such as mandated edu-

Table 2. Parent-infant contact

Parent-infant contact in nursery	Nonrepeating families (n = 40)	Repeating families (n = 9)
1. Mother visited more than once a week	95%	44%
2. Mother visited within 4 days of admission	80%	22%
3. Father visited	80%	67%
4. Extended family visited	85%	22%

Adapted from Hunter and Kilstrom (1979).

cation, treatment of the handicapped child, petitioning for tuition aid, and understanding the concepts of labeling, classifying, and testing handicapped children. Explaining the complexities of procedural hearings such as the hearing officer's determination is another responsibility of the legal consultant.

Some of the teenage parents are involved in criminal actions and needed an understanding of defense, bail, probation, juvenile delinquency, visitation rights, criminal association, etc. Many of the parents who are in the Kingsbrook project are substance abusers, with alcohol and marijuana being the most prevalent drugs. They need to understand the work of addiction agencies and services and how addiction cases are litigated.

Many of the teenage parents do not have appropriate housing and need to know about Section 8 housing and project housing for the indigent, as well as tenant eviction and/or other landlord/tenant dispute ramifications.

Most of the teenage parents are on public assistance and need help in comprehending welfare benefits, Medicaid, Supplementary Social Security, disability, and financial assistance and benefits. Many teenage parents have consumer problems relating to their installment credit buying.

Also lacking among most teenage parents is an understanding of laws that provide constitutional mandates, due process, privacy and equality, and constitutional protection of human rights, whether this had to do with legal defense for specific racial and national groups (NAACP), or laws that expand and delimit rights and provisions for handicapped persons.

STRUGGLERS FOR SURVIVAL

Mothers who fared most poorly in the Kingsbrook project are those who could not confront the realities of their situations. The problems of being unable to accept the handicapped infant or his or her disability are for some parents related to their own poor sense of identity and a self-critical awareness of their own life-styles. The Kingsbrook staff has found that it needs to be in constant touch with teenage mothers so that immediate intervention might forestall major problems. Living on the fringes of society, parents surviving without protection or familial support are in danger of being taken advantage of by others. Their day-to-day existence without real knowledge of the "ropes" impairs their ability to deal with imminent dangers and their own fears and anxiety. They stumble into treatment and programming, with limited involvement, not accepting their problems. Some are teenage mothers who deliver babies with fetal alcoholic syndrome; some do not know they are pregnant until the last trimester. They nourish their bodies so poorly that they sustain prenatal and perinatal complications including prematurity, difficult labor, difficult postlabor recuperation, and severely involved infants. Often, the newborn remains for further testing at the hospital. The teenage mother does not return too soon. Sometimes she is not capable of understanding the directions of the doctor. Isolated, alone, feeling overwhelmed and incapable of acting on her own or her child's behalf, her distress is often multiplied.

Dora

Dora, a 16-year-old mother of two, said that she had to leave Mary at the hospital for further examination. Mary was born with fetal alcoholic syndrome resulting in a seizure disorder. Dora's grandmother (with whom Dora was living) made sure her granddaughter picked up the baby, albeit 2 days after the baby was medically discharged. This "pick-up" was also urged by the social worker. One week later, the baby was returned to the hospital severly dehydrated, with welts on her behind, as a result of poor care. Again, Dora came later than expected to pick up the baby and, again, the previous episode was repeated. This time, Dora blamed the hospital for discharging her baby too soon.

Dora enjoyed talking about "soaps" and the new baby in "This Is Your Life," as her own jittery and highly irritable baby was left on the sofa whimpering to unresponsive ears. The mother refused to accept that drinking beer had anything to do with her baby's problems. She said she plans to return to school to become a receptionist, but she has already been out of school for 3 years. In questioning Dora further about what she would do in the future, she answered firmly, "I must watch my soaps, no matter what."

Dora was receiving AFDC monies, which she shared with her grandmother. A symbiotic relationship developed between them that sometimes created anger and hostility and resulted in a falling out. The Kingsbrook staff was able to assist Dora's grandmother in helping Dora raise her children, while Dora received counseling on a regular basis to help her get along with her grandmother. Dora's grandmother needed to become less authoritarian with Dora and Dora needed to be able to understand her grandmother's needs without becoming insulting and abrasive. Twice during the summer, Dora left the safety of her grandmother's home with her two babies for the street after many arguments and back-and-forth accusations of parent neglect. It took a lot of support for Dora and her grandmother to finally come together again and to become better related to each other.

Tanya

At age 15, Tanya was already over 5'7" and enjoyed frolicking with much older men. Her own mother had a number of "husbands," and had been pregnant more than 10 times, and Tanya was not sure of the name of her own father. Blissfully unconcerned, she endeared herself to an auto mechanic at the neighborhood garage. She found herself pregnant, growing exceedingly larger each day. She felt undaunted; she flaunted her condition before her schoolmates and family. The mechanic mentioned the possibility of living together, and Tanya was pleased. She didn't like living with her mother and her many siblings. She wanted an independent life. The natural father lived with Tanya intermittently, providing no support, but eager to use Tanya's welfare money and food stamps.

Twin sons were born to Tanya after a full-term pregnancy. Tanya felt she had been given *two* gifts. Unfortunately, after 2 days of life, one son was doing poorly and was thought to be both physically and medically involved. Tanya was sure the nurse had done something "bad to her baby." The other twin developed well. After 6 months, Tanya became pregnant again. Nine months later, Lonnie was born with septic arthritis as a result of Tanya's untreated gonorrhea. Tanya was sure that Lonnie's condition was the result of hospital malpractice. One day, she presented herself at the clinic with no appointment and screamed curses at the amazed staff. She refused to go to "that" hospital anymore, although it was just around the corner from where she lived, and her sons needed emergency hospital care. Her Medicaid cards for her children gained acceptance to another hospital and she falsified information regarding her previous problems and medication. Thus, Tanya was often questioned by the Bureau of Social Services for the many episodes of forging records of entitlements.

Tanya's welfare and her child Supplementary Security Income checks were discontinued as a result of her manipulations. It took 6 months for Tanya to receive monetary help for herself and her children from various social agencies.

Tanya was in serious trouble with the police when her landlord accused her of destroying the refrigerator and stove in the apartment. But it was not until the experience last summer, when her very handicapped baby died and she could not find money for a decent burial, that she finally returned to her own mother for support and comfort. After this juncture, Tanya was able to pull herself together and relate better to her problems, her situation, and her two surviving children. The legal consultant of the Kingsbrook project was often needed to help Tanya with many of the above offenses against her.

Raffaelina

Raffaelina appeared at the rehabilitation hospital demanding to take home her 2-year-old son, Bobby, an involved spastic quadriplegic child hospitalized as a result of child abuse and neglect. Bobby's father was with her, and she carried a newborn precariously on her back.

At the time Raffaelina had given birth to her second child, she was already well known to the Bronx Women's Agencies and Child Welfare and Protection Agencies. Raffaelina's "husband" had wanted her to have more children. Both man and wife considered themselves permanent welfare recipients. They both know that more money was coming to them if they had more children.

Later that summer, when the second child was then 9 months old, Raffaelina found shelter in an abandoned tenement, hiding from the natural father who was abusive to her. At age 18, she continued to need protection from the abuse she had suffered since childhood, only now it was her mate who was the persecutor.

She had no idea that her own two children were being neglected by her disorganized lifestyle. She refused homemaker services and a decent place to live. She didn't know how to prepare meals and wasn't aware of how to handle babies. Bobby's condition was the result of her lack of providing him with food. Tired of the shelter for abused women, she struck out on her own.

The check for Bobby's welfare had already been taken away, since his long-term hospital placement was approved. It occurred to Raffaelina that if her "husband" knew she was pregnant for a third time, he would be more eager to find her. Raffaelina was not aware that child protection agents were also looking for her and her baby. One day she brought the baby to a leaking water hydrant to wash the child and herself. Cold water was splashed on the baby. The baby's screams alerted the police and the child was brought to a Bronx hospital with a high fever and seizure activity, a result of dehydration and undernourishment.

More permanent arrangements were made for Raffaelina's second child. When her mate found that the second check would be taken away, he brutally assaulted his wife, causing her to miscarry her third pregnancy and leaving her alone and deserted.

MEANS OF SURVIVAL

When parents don't understand the problems of their handicapped children, and find their social problems to be too difficult to handle, they fantasize other worlds—Dora's soap operas, Tanya's outrageous blaming of the hospital, or Raffaelina's incredibly negligent behavior. As a result of their irresponsibility, treatment does not proceed properly. Confronting these parents about their wrongdoings is useless. They do not realize that their actions are causing harm rather than solving problems. Therefore, learning from the consequences of their behavior is not always possible. Kingsbrook mainly helps those mothers in their day-to-day trials and tribulations, and in so doing, helps them to function, albeit precariously.

When teenage mothers are able to come through a full year of the Kingsbrook program they are better candidates for parent learning the second year. The second year of treatment could concentrate upon family counseling, vocational development, and achievements of their child's learning.

REFERENCES

Bayley, N. *Bayley Scales of Infant Development.* New York: The Psychological Corporation, 1969.

Belmont, L., Cohen, P., Dryfoos, J., Stein, Z., & Zayac, S. Maternal age and children's intelligence. In: K. Scott, T. Field, & E. Robertson (eds.), *Teenage parents and their offspring.* New York: Grune & Stratton, 1981.

Chilman, C.S. Social and psychological research concerning adolescent childbearing: 1970-1980. *Journal of Marriage and the Family,* 1980, *3,* 378–812.

Egeland, B., & Sroufe, L.A. Attachment and early maltreatment. *Child Development,* 1981, *52,* 45–48.

Hunter, R.S., & Kilstrom, N. Breaking the cycle in abusive families. *American Journal of Psychiatry,* 1979, *136,* 1321–1334.

ECOLOGICAL FACTORS THAT FOSTER DEVELOPMENT

Nelson, S. Schoolage parents. *Children Today*, 1973, *2*, 22–24.

Osofsky, H.J., & Osofsky, J.D. *Adolescents as mothers: Results of a program for low income pregnant teenagers with some emphasis upon infants' development*. Paper presented at the American Orthopsychiatric Association Convention, San Francisco, March, 1970.

Public Law 94-103, *Developmental Disabilities Assistance and Bill of Rights Act*, June 26, 1975.

Ramey, C.T., & Bryant, D.M. Evidence involving prevention of developmental retardation during infancy. *Journal of the Division of Early Childhood*, 1982, *5*, 6–12.

Sameroff, A.J., & Chandler, M.J. Reproductive risk and the continuum of caretaking causality. In: F.D. Hor-

owitz (ed.), *Review of child development research*. Chicago: University of Chicago Press, 1976.

Sandler, H.M., Vietze, P.M., & O'Connor, C. Obstetric and neonatal outcomes following intervention with pregnant teenagers. In: K. Scott, T. Field, & E. Robertson (eds.), *Teenage parents and their offspring*. New York: Grune & Stratton, 1981.

Vaughn, B.E., Egeland, B., Sroufe, L.A., & Waters, E. Individual differences in infant mothers' attachment at 12 and 18 months: Stability and change in family under stress. *Child Development*, 1979, *50*, 971–975.

Vinovskis, A. An "epidemic" of adolescent pregnancy? Some historical considerations. *Journal of Family History*, 1981, *30*, 220–229.

Section II

PREGNANCY AND
THE PERINATAL PERIOD

Leo Stern, M.D.
Brown University, Providence, Rhode Island

T HE ANTENATAL, INTRAPARTUM, AND POSTPARTUM factors that ultimately may influence both immediate and long-term neurological outcome are ones that have already been previously defined, and although there is clearly room for additional specific items to be included, the broad outlines of these and their categorization have already been well established.

In reviewing this area for the present volume, the authors in this section have concentrated on in-depth exploration of some of these specific factors utilizing both more recent studies and databases as well as a number of newer concepts that have emerged as a result of a more specific, detailed appreciation of individual pathogenetic mechanisms. An excellent example of such alterations in this context can be seen in this section which examines our pathological knowledge of fetal brain damage of circulatory origin, perinatal hypoxic-ischemic encephalopathy and its relationship to the autoregulation of cerebral blood flow, and the elaboration of the concept of periventricular injury.

In addition to more and newer knowledge, some tentative steps have been taken toward two further alterations in approaches to the relationship of perinatal events and future outcome. Both of these involve a change in how specific events and/or databases are approached.

The first of these approaches effectively signals an alteration in the previously considered, almost sacrosanct but curiously static, appreciation of long-term evaluation of neurological and developmental outcomes. With the experience of time, newer diagnostic and imaging techniques, and alterations in socioeconomic conditions, the rationale for and the necessity to alter the criteria and their relative value scales for neonatal outcomes have become increasingly apparent. Both the changing predictive features of neurological assessment and the specific approaches toward altering the criteria themselves are reported in this section.

The second change is a deeper and more detailed appreciation of the relationship of measured neonatal parameters and future outcomes. Here it is not the database but the understanding of its significance that needs to be changed. Some examples of commonly used neonatal events may serve to illustrate this problem.

Thus, both neonatal hypoglycemia and hyperbilirubinemia are known to carry prognostic significance for future central nervous system (CNS) and developmental outcome. Yet in both cases, what is measured is a concentration of a substance (glucose or bilirubin) in the blood, and what is anticipated is the effect on the brain. Clearly, the plasma level by itself is of no prognostic value without a better understanding of its cellular and/or tissue effects. Glucose is the primary fuel for oxidative phosphorylation in the central nervous system, and a significant reduction in its supply to the brain would result in impairment of oxygen-dependent energy synthesis. Yet, the factors that govern CNS uptake, utilization, and disposition of glucose are only vaguely understood and not yet amenable to easy measurement or determination. A dynamic understanding of these events, as well as glucose sparing or substitution mechanisms under adverse circumstances, would materially enhance the understanding of this relationship. The newer, about to be implemented, imaging techniques (nuclear magnetic resonance and positron emission tomography) may afford such opportunities for study.

The relationship of bilirubin elevation in plasma to its cellular deposition in the brain and the mechanisms of CNS injury are currently beginning to be better understood. The factors involved include the phenomenon of bilirubin-albumin binding and its dissociation or displacement, the integrity of the vascular tight endothelial junctions that govern vascular permeability, and the function of the bilirubin oxidase system that may normally operate to neutralize the effects of any bilirubin that does penetrate the central nervous system. The role of Pa_{CO_2} dependent blood flow (carbon dioxide is a cerebral vasodilator) as well as the precise mechanism of CNS injury (e.g., an intracellular effect as opposed to impairment of the integrity of the cell membrane) will further govern how the significance of such elevated plasma levels that accompany the visual appearance of the jaundiced newborn will come to be appreciated.

Other parameters of neonatal biochemical and physiological disturbances need to be similarly approached. Thus, both hypocalcemia, with its known resultant CNS irritability and potential for convulsive disturbances, and acidosis, particularly that which occurs in the preterm infant under a variety of adverse circumstances, need to be explored for their specific cellular and interactive effects. In connection with the latter, there is considerable evidence that both extra- and intra-cellular drug metabolism may be remarkably affected by pH changes and that, therefore, drugs and other therapeutic agents administered for valid specific indications may be either ineffective or potentially toxic under such conditions.

Finally, there is the question of the interaction of multiple disordered events, a relatively common occurrence in the sick newborn infant. Improved computerized evaluation by such means as multivariant analysis will be helpful but must also be preceded by a specific understanding of the biological interactions of such events in their multiple simultaneous or sequential presentation.

In examining its objectives, this section was intended both to be current for what is known and explorative for what needs to be done in the future. To the extent that these goals are realizable, we may anticipate a more in-depth and specific understanding of this increasingly complex and ever-fascinating relationship.

The At-Risk Infant: Psycho/Socio/Medical Aspects
edited by Shaul Harel, M.D., and Nicholas J. Anastasiow, Ph.D.
Copyright © 1985   Paul H. Brookes Publishing Co., Inc.   Baltimore • London

Chapter 12

Antenatal Screening
for Fetal Malformations
and Genetic Disorders

CYRIL LEGUM, M.D.
Ichilov Hospital and Sackler Medical School, Tel Aviv, Israel

T HE COMPOSITION OF THE AMNIOTIC FLUID of Rhesus immunized human fetuses was described over 30 years ago (Bevis, 1950). Since then, antenatal screening for genetic and other disorders has come a long way (Brock, 1982; Galjaard, 1982; Milunsky, 1980). At present, there are several hundred centers, mainly in the western world, offering amniocentesis as a routine procedure (Lynch, Kimberling, Pellettera, & Paul, 1983). In some countries, mass screening programs for detecting carriers of certain deleterious Mendelian genes are offered to certain ethnic groups with a relatively high gene frequency for a particular disease (Committee for the Study of Inborn Errors of Metabolism of the U.S. National Academy of Sciences, 1975; Gitzelmann, 1982; Kaback, 1977; Scriver, in preparation, Simpson, Dallaire, Miller, Hamerton, & Miller, 1976). The financial cost of such programs is considerable but this is offset by the cost of caring for, hospitalizing, and institutionalizing severely handicapped and usually incurable children.

This chapter outlines some of the methodology employed in establishing a screening program and in monitoring its proficiency. Programs for detecting Down syndrome, Tay-Sachs disease, and neural tube disorders cur-

rently in progress in Israel are compared and future trends are briefly mentioned.

DEFINING THE AIM OF THE PROGRAM

The first step in establishing an antenatal screening program is to define the aim of the program. This aim may be treatment, selective abortion, or research.

Treatment

For programs with treatment as their main objective, most of the techniques are applied during the final trimester. Palliative procedures are employed to tide the fetus over until more definite measures can be carried out after the birth. Examples of such programs are:

1. *Fetal Rh isoimmunization* in which the diagnosis of an affected fetus in a high-risk mother is followed by an intrauterine blood transfusion of the fetus.
2. *Fetal hydrocephaly* in which sonographic detection of the lesion provides the possibility, in some situations, of inserting a catheter, *in utero,* from the fetal brain ventricle into the amniotic fluid. Postpartum shunt procedures may then make it

possible to achieve normal or nearly normal function.

3. *Fetal hydronephrosis* in which sonographic detection of the anomaly will permit placement of a shunt between the fetal bladder and the amniotic fluid. Definitive surgery postpartum may result in normal function.

These procedures carry considerable risk to the fetus but are certainly acceptable to some families. Intrauterine treatment should obviously only be undertaken in the setting of a hospital team and with great attention to detail.

Selective Abortion

The most common aim of antenatal screening is the detection of a fetus with an incurable disease in order to offer the parents the alternative of selective abortion. In order to be eligible for such a program, the mother must be at relatively high risk for the condition. To qualify for the Down syndrome program in Israel, the mother needs to be at a risk greater than 1:250 for bearing such a child. Therefore, only mothers older than 37 years or who have previously borne a child with a chromosomal disease or who have been identified as translocation carriers are eligible for the test. As this covers less than 10% of the pregnant population in any one year and as the frequency of Down syndrome in Israel is about 1:600 live births, only a minority of affected fetuses are, in fact, diagnosed and aborted during the second trimester of pregnancy. In monogenic disorders such as Tay-Sachs disease, β-thalassemia and sickle cell anemia, preliminary mass screening programs are used to identify high-risk couples. Only those couples with a high (1:4) risk who demonstrated the carrier state prior to the eighteenth week of pregnancy are offered amniocentesis. The preventative effectiveness of such programs is usually high provided that the target population is willing to comply. A different situation is encountered when screening for a neural tube defect, which is a polygenically determined embryonic developmental lesion. The test employed, maternal serum alpha fetoprotein (ms-AFP),

which is inexpensive and simple to do, has a high rate of false positive results. This creates much maternal anxiety and requires a finely coordinated team to minimize the problem. Ultrasonography can be used as a screening test in the second trimester and is particularly useful in screening pregnancies of mothers at risk for the recurrence of renal agenesis. Screening for selective abortion has to be achieved during the second trimester before the fetus becomes viable.

Research

A third possible aim of antenatal screening is research. In such programs it is mandatory for the parents to sign informed consent forms explaining the nature of the research being carried out; the risks to the fetus, the mother, and to the continuation of the pregnancy; and of the chances of a misdiagnosis. The antenatal diagnosis of two of the more common and most burdensome genetic diseases, cystic fibrosis and Duchenne muscular dystrophy, still belong in this category. For mothers at risk of having a fetus affected by Duchenne muscular dystrophy, an X-linked recessive disorder affecting only males, their best alternative for ensuring unaffected children is still fetal sexing and the abortion of male fetuses, even though statistically half are unaffected.

MINIMAL REQUIREMENTS

Antenatal screening should be carried out only within the framework of an integrated program. The minimal requirements for such an integrated program include:

1. Facilities for the dissemination of information about the program to the target population being screened, the rest of the community, medical and paramedical personnel, government agencies, and religious groups

2. A reliable laboratory with a special interest in the test and sufficient staff and equipment to ensure regular and uninterrupted testing throughout the year

3. An obstetrics department and genetic counseling service with a special interest

in the program and the ability to handle crisis situations around the clock

4. A program coordinator whose duties include the rapid retrieval of women with positive test results, the follow-up of the outcome of all pregnancies, and the promotion of a smooth and rapid flow of information between the laboratory, the patients being screened, and the medical attendants

5. A suitable target population for screening (Not all populations will comply with the program to the same extent. The reasons for noncompliance are varied. Religious and political beliefs, economic factors, an unreliable test, and poor delivery of the program may all have profound effects on the compliance rate of a specific population being screened.)

6. Quality control, which is an essential and a critical requirement for any antenatal screening program

In evaluating the test, several parameters should be observed. These are readily calculated by comparing the results of the screening test with the outcome of the pregnancies (Table 1). These values can then be used to estimate the ability of the test to detect abnormal fetuses (sensitivity), to exclude normal fetuses (specificity), and to predict efficiency (Table 2). A program for which there is a limit on eligibility or a poor rate of compliance may have a poor overall preventative effectiveness in spite of an efficient test. Preventative effectiveness is measured by multiplying sensitivity by eligibility by compliance (Table 2). A test with a low false negative rate will be highly sensitive, whereas a test with a high false positive rate will not be specific. In areas where the condition being screened for is relatively common, there are relatively more true positives and therefore a higher predictive efficiency for the test.

A COMPARISON OF THE CAPABILITY OF DIFFERENT SCREENING TESTS

Israel is populated by Jews, Muslims, and Christians. In the Tel Aviv area, there are over 12,000 Jewish births and over 4,000 non-Jewish births each year. Of the Jewish births, about 60% are to Sephardi parents and about 60% to Ashkenazi parents. Three major antenatal screening programs have been running concurrently in the Tel Aviv area since 1979. Table 3 compares these programs in terms of the parameters mentioned previously.

The Down syndrome prevention program had a near perfect test in terms of sensitivity, specificity, and predictive efficiency. Nevertheless, less than half of the Down syndrome children were detected by the program. This is because only 10% of pregnant women are eligible for the test due to the cutoff point in the program which states a woman must be 37 years of age or older at the time of the last menstrual period to qualify for the testing. As there is often less willingness in North America to bear children at a later age, it may well be that the decline in the incidence of Down syndrome in recent years is more a result of the relaxation of antiabortion laws than a direct consequence of the amniocentesis programs that have become so commonplace in North America.

A few babies with Tay-Sachs disease are still being born in Israel in spite of an excellent test system. The reasons for this are probably those of diminished compliance because of religious objection to abortion and failure to refer the parents for testing before the sixteenth week of pregnancy. In the United States, increasing numbers of Jews of the present generation are marrying nonJewish partners. This may turn out to be no less an important reason for the reduction in the birth of Tay-Sachs infants in America as are the well-publicized programs currently popular in the United States.

Table 1. Comparison of test results with outcome of pregnancy

	Positive test	Negative test
Abnormal outcome	True positives (tp)	False negatives (fn)
Normal outcome	False positives (fp)	True negatives (tn)

Table 2. Estimating the capability of the test

Sensitivity (Se)	$\dfrac{tp}{tp + fn}$
Specificity (Sp)	$\dfrac{tn}{tn + fp}$
Predictive efficiency (Pe)	$\dfrac{tp}{tp + fp}$
Eligibility (E)	
Compliance (C)	
Preventative effectiveness	Se × E × C

In contrast to the above two programs, the neural tube defect prevention program has a relatively poor screening test. Maternal serum alpha fetoprotein testing has a rather high false negative as well as a high false positive rate but ends up with a much superior preventative effectiveness because of 100% eligibility and better compliance than in the other two programs. An interesting observation in the Tel Aviv program has been the fact that Jewish mothers of Yemenite origin have a significantly higher median value for serum alpha fetoprotein than do other Jewish ethnic groups. A difference in alpha fetoprotein medians has also been noticed between black and white mothers in the United States (Crandall, Schroth, & Lebherz, 1982). Neural tube defect prevention programs in Great Britain are more effective than in Israel or the United States because of the greater incidence of this birth defect there. As previously mentioned, a high incidence improves the predictive efficiency of the test and thus increases the effectiveness of the entire program. Although the problems of methodology, expense, and maternal anxiety associated with these programs are considerable, nevertheless they seem to have "caught on" and become an integral part of the public health and preventative medicine programs of many western countries.

FUTURE TRENDS

Much effort is currently being expended in the search for new, quicker, more accurate, and safer techniques of antenatal screening (Brock, 1982; Galjaard, 1982). A simple method of obtaining trophoblastic tissue via the vagina was described by Kazy, Rozovsky, and Bakharev in 1982. This method may, in the future, prove to be superior to amniocentesis as a means of examining fetal tissue. Chromosomal and biochemical tests can be carried out, using this method, as early as the tenth week of pregnancy. The automation of karyotyping using a dual laser sorter in a bivariate flow apparatus may, in the future, speed up amniocentesis, enabling the test to be offered to younger mothers as well (Dean & Dinkel, 1978). An inexpensive, rapid, and relatively simple alternative to amniocentesis will become available when researchers learn how to isolate fetal lymphocytes from the maternal bloodstream without interfering with their ability to multiply in tissue culture. Gene mapping and the use of gene splicing technology has already made it possible to diagnose some fetal hemoglobinopathies without having to resort to fetoscopy (Old, Ward, Petrou, Karagotzu, Modell, & Weatherall, 1982). Fetoscopy is becoming a safer procedure and is useful when a blood sample or a skin biopsy must be obtained. Some centers have recommended ultrasonography as a routine screening test. However, even though there have been noteworthy improvements in resolution, fetal imaging is often not detailed enough, except in an-

Table 3. Comparison of the capability of different screening tests in Israel

	Down syndrome (DS) (1:600)	Tay-Sachs (TS) (1:2,500)	Neural tube disorders (NTDs) (1:600)
Sensitivity	1.00	1.00	0.80
Specificity	1.00	1.00	0.61
Predictive efficiency	1.00	1.00	0.03
Eligibility	0.10	0.40	1.00
Compliance	0.50	0.75	0.75
Preventative effectiveness	0.05	0.30	0.60

encephaly and renal agenesis, to allow a definitive diagnosis of a malformation to be made with certainty.

CONCLUSION

In order to operate an antenatal screening program for the diagnosis, treatment, and research of fetal disorders, it is of paramount importance to have the necessary resources and to pay meticulous attention to detail. Poorly executed programs with ill-defined aims are bound to do more harm than good. It is hoped that better funding, newer technology, and program accreditation will all contribute to making these programs more widely accessible and acceptable to the general public.

REFERENCES

Bevis, D.C.A. Composition of liquor amnii in hemolytic disease of the newborn. *Lancet,* 1950, *2,* 443.

Brock, D.J.H. *Early diagnosis of fetal defects.* Edinburgh: Churchill Livingstone, 1982.

Committee for the Study of Inborn Errors of Metabolism, National Research Council. *Genetic Screening programs, principles and research.* Washington, DC: U.S. National Academy of Sciences, 1975.

Crandall, B.F., Schroth, P.C., Lebherz, T.B. Racial differences in maternal serum alpha fetoprotein levels. *Human Genetics,* 1982, *34,* 85A.

Dean, P.N., & Dinkel, P. High resolution dual laser flow cytometry. *Journal of Histochemistry and Cytochemistry,* 1978, *26,* 622–627.

Galjaard, H. (ed.). *The future of prenatal diagnosis.* Edinburg: Churchill Livingstone, 1982.

Gitzelmann, R. Rationales for genetic screening. In: B. Bonne-Tamir, T. Cohen, & R.M. Goodman (eds.), *Human genetics Part B: Medical aspects.* New York: Alan R. Liss, Inc., 1982.

Kaback, M.M. (ed.). *Tay Sachs disease: Screening and prevention.* New York: Alan R. Liss, Inc., 1977.

Kazy, Z., Rozovsky, I.S., & Bakharev, V.A. Chorion biopsy in early pregnancy; a method for early prenatal diagnosis of inherited disorders. *Prenatal Diagnosis,* 1982, *2,* 39–45.

Lynch, H.T., Kimberling, W., Pellettera, K.M., & Paul, N.W. *International directory of genetic services* (7th ed.). White Plains, NY: March of Dimes Birth Defect Foundation, 1983.

Milunsky, A. *Genetic disorders and the fetus: Diagnosis, prevention and treatment.* New York: Plenum Publishing Corp., 1980.

Old, J.M., Ward, R.H.T., Petrou, M., Karagotzu, F., Modell, B., Weatherall, D.J. First trimester fetal diagnosis for hemoglobinopathies: 3 cases. *Lancet,* 1982, *2,* 1413–1416.

Scriver, C.R. (ed.). Report of a workshop on population screening held in Strasbourg, France in 1982. In preparation.

Simpson, N.E., Dallaire, L., Miller, J.R., Hamerton, J.L., & Miller, J. Prenatal diagnosis of genetic disease in Canada, report of a collaborative study. *Canadian Medical Association Journal,* 1976, *115,* 739–746.

Chapter 13

Maternal Drinking
and the Fetal Alcohol Syndrome

N. Paul Rosman, M.D.
Edgar Y. Oppenheimer, M.D.
Boston University School of Medicine and Boston City Hospital, Boston, Massachusetts

Henry Fielding, the eighteenth-century social reformer, wrote in 1751, "What must become of an infant who is conceived in Gin? With the poisonous distillations of which it is nourished, both in the Womb and at the Breast" (Fielding, 1751). In the years since this inquiry the same question has been asked repeatedly, though interest in this subject has waxed and waned. References suggesting an ill effect of maternal alcohol ingestion on the development of offspring abound in antiquity. In the Old Testament, an angel appears to Samson's mother saying, "Behold, thou shalt conceive and bear a son; and now drink no wine or strong drink ..." (Judges 13:7). Later, laws in both Carthage and Sparta prohibited alcohol use by newly married couples to prevent conception while intoxicated. From 1720 to 1750, England was swept by a "gin epidemic" (Warner & Rosett, 1975). In order to help aristocratic farm interests by providing new markets for grain, the government lifted the traditional restrictions on the distillation of liquor. As a result, cheap and plentiful gin flooded the country creating a social crisis. In 1726, during this period of crisis, the College of Physicians petitioned Parliament to reinstate control of the distilling trade, citing gin as a cause of "weak, feeble and distempered children" (Beaumont, 1841–1842, pp. 340–343). In one of the largest studies ever to examine alcohol as a cause of mental retardation, MacNicholl surveyed school children in New York City (MacNicholl, 1905). He found that 53% of 6,624 children of drinking parents were "dullards," whereas of 13,523 children of abstainers, only 10% were "dullards." Interest in the effects of alcohol dropped dramatically in the 1920s when prohibition went into effect in the United States. In the 1940s, the long-held view that alcohol was harmful was refuted. Authorities in the field asserted that there was no acceptable evidence to show that acute alcoholic intoxication had any effect on the human germ or had any influence in altering heredity. They attributed damaged offspring to the poor nutrition of the alcoholic mother and the bad influence of the home of the alcoholic (Haggard & Jellinek, 1942). Reports of adverse effects of alcohol reappeared in the 1950s, especially from France, and a resurgence of medical interest was sparked by reports of the injurious effects of alcohol on unborn offspring by Jones and Smith (1973), who were probably the first to coin the term "fetal alcohol syndrome" (FAS), and by

Lemoine, Harousseau, Borteyru, and Menuet (1968), and Ulleland, Wennberg, Igo, and Smith (1970).

CRITERIA FOR DIAGNOSIS OF THE FETAL ALCOHOL SYNDROME (FAS)

Based on a review of the principal and associated features of FAS in 245 cases from around the world (Clarren & Smith, 1978), the Fetal Alcohol Study Group of the Research Society on Alcoholism (Rosett, 1980) concluded that the diagnosis of FAS should be made only when the patient has signs in each of three categories:

1. Prenatal and/or postnatal growth retardation (weight, length, and/or head circumference below the 10th percentile when corrected for gestational age)
2. Central nervous system involvement (signs of neurological abnormality, developmental delay, or intellectual impairment)
3. Characteristic facial dysmorphology with at least two of three signs:
   a. Microcephaly (head circumference below the third percentile)
   b. Microophthalmia and/or short palpebral fissures
   c. Flat or absent philtrum, thin upper lip, and/or flattening of the maxillary area

In the absence of signs in all three categories, the term "possible fetal alcohol effects" is used.

STUDIES AT THE BOSTON CITY HOSPITAL

A collaborative prospective study of the FAS was undertaken at the Boston City Hospital in 1974. In the initial pilot study (1974–1976) (Ouellette, Rosett, Rosman, & Weiner, 1977), the outcome in 322 babies born to a cohort of 633 women was analyzed. In a subsequent extension of the study (1977–1979), an additional 1,690 mother/child pairs were investigated (Hingson, Alpert, Day, Dooling, Kayne, Morelock, Oppenheimer, & Zuckerman, 1982).

The results of these studies are outlined below.

Pilot Study

Of 685 women eligible, 633 (92%) voluntarily participated in the pilot study conducted by Ouellette et al. (1977). The women were interviewed with a structured questionnaire. Nutritional status was evaluated based on replies to the questions, "What did you eat yesterday?" and "Were yesterday's meals typical?" Information was also obtained regarding the use of tobacco, narcotics, sedatives, amphetamines, hallucinogens, and marijuana. Alcohol intake was assessed both in terms of volume and variability. A "drink" was defined as that quantity that contained 3/4 ounce of absolute alcohol. The women were categorized in three drinking groups:

Group I—abstinent or rare drinkers (never drink or drink less than once per month and never consume five or more drinks on an occasion)

Group II—moderate drinkers (drink more than once a month but do not meet drinking criteria for heavy drinkers)

Group III—heavy drinkers (consume an average of more than one-and-a-half drinks per day and sometimes consume five or more drinks on an occasion)

On the second or third day following delivery, a pediatric neurologist carried out a detailed pediatric, neurological, and developmental examination on each child in the study, without prior knowledge of the prenatal or delivery history or of the mother's drinking status. Gestational age was assessed by Dubowitz criteria (Dubowitz, Dubowitz, & Goldberg, 1970). Length, weight, and head circumferences were plotted by percentiles using standardized anthropometric charts for Boston newborns, and the Lubchenco Tables (Lubchenco, 1970). Congenital anomalies were recorded and classified as major (such as microcrania) or minor (such as malformed ears). Each infant's functional state was recorded, with particular attention paid to tone, jitteriness, and sucking response. Additional his-

Table 1. Mothers and babies by drinking categories

Group I	Group II	Group III
	Mothers interviewed ($N = 633$)	
326 (52%)	249 (39%)	58 (9%)
	Babies examined ($N = 322$)	
152 (47%)	128 (40%)	42 (13%)

torical information concerning the pregnancy and delivery was obtained by the examining physician only after coding of the data obtained on physical examination was completed.

Results Mothers and babies were categorized on the basis of the mother's drinking history as seen in Table 1.

Most of the women interviewed were poorly nourished, but diets reported by the heavy-drinking women were not significantly different from those of the total clinic population. Thus, at registration in the clinic, few of the diets met the daily requirements for pregnant women recommended by the National Research Council. The percentages of recommended dietary constituents consumed were: vitamin A—22%, vitamin C—58%, vitamin D—24%, thiamine—57%, riboflavin—46%, niacin—56%, calcium—35%, iron—7%, and protein—82%. Heavy drinking was associated with heavy smoking; 60% of mothers in Group III were heavy smokers consuming more than one package of cigarettes per day, while only 20% of mothers in Group II and approximately 15% of those in Group I smoked heavily.

Infants were classified as abnormal if they had an abnormal neurological examination or if growth retardation or congenital anomalies were present. Of the infants born to heavy-drinking women (Group III), only one-third

were considered normal at the time of the newborn examination. By contrast, two-thirds of infants born to abstinent, rare, or moderately drinking women (Groups I and II) were normal (Table 2).

Neurological examination showed that hypotonia was seen somewhat more frequently and jitteriness was seen three times more frequently in Group III infants than in those in Groups I and II (Table 2). Major differences were found in specific growth parameters among the three groups of babies. Birth weight and body length were lower in Group III offspring than in those in Groups I and II. In addition, smaller head circumferences were more often found among Group III offspring than in children born to abstinent, rare, or moderate drinkers. (Five of 42 infants born to heavy drinkers were microcephalic as compared to one of 274 infants in the lesser-drinking groups.) Congenital abnormalities were found in the offspring of women in all three drinking groups but were significantly more frequent in children in Group III (Table 2). None of the infants was diagnosed as having the complete FAS when examined in the Newborn Nursery. (At follow-up examination, however, two of the children were found to demonstrate signs of the full syndrome.)

Thus, the pilot study indicated an increased

Table 2. Maternal drinking categories and clinical status of 322 babies

Infant status	Group I ($n = 152$)	Group II ($n = 128$)	Group III ($n = 42$)
Any abnormality	35%	36%	69%
Hypotonic	13%	9%	17%
Jittery	10%	11%	29%
Growth abnormality	18%	19%	52%
Congenital anomaly			
Any	9%	14%	31%
Cardiac	<1%	5%	12%
Limb	6%	5%	10%
Other noncraniofacial	2%	5%	7%
Craniofacial	6%	8%	33%
Multiple	3%	5%	19%

frequency of neurological abnormalities, growth retardation, and congenital anomalies in Group III offspring, suggesting that heavy alcohol intake during pregnancy posed a significant risk to the unborn child.

Extended Study

Of 3,222 mother/child pairs at the Boston City Hospital eligible for the extended study conducted by Hingson et al. (1982), 2,514 (78%) newborns were examined. Each infant received a detailed neurological, morphological and growth assessment by one of four study pediatricians, one of whom was a developmentalist and three of whom were pediatric neurologists. Seventy-five percent of the newborns were examined before the third day of life. As with the pilot study, the examinations were conducted without prior awareness of maternal drinking history or other interview data. Of the mothers whose babies were examined, 1,690 (67%) received a 30–40-minute structured interview by one of five English or Spanish-speaking interviewers. These 1,690 mother/child pairs comprised the study group.

  Results Of the 1,690 mother/child pairs, only one infant showed the full FAS, while 38 (2%) had congenital abnormalities, and 36 (2%) exhibited features compatible with the FAS. Prior to pregnancy, 6% of the mothers drank two or more drinks daily; 2.8% drank that much during at least one trimester of the pregnancy (during which the mean consumption was 6 drinks per day).

  Demographic composition of the study group, as well as the reported consumption of alcohol, coffee, meals and dietary supplements, tobacco, marijuana and psychoactive drugs, are indicated in Table 3.

  In order to assess the relative contributions of multiple variables on fetal outcome and, in particular, on birth weight and gestational age, multiple regression analyses were performed (Table 4). This statistical analysis indicated that the level of maternal drinking prior to pregnancy was significantly related to shorter gestation, but neither level of drinking prior to pregnancy nor level of drinking during pregnancy was significantly related to infant growth measures, congenital abnormalities, or features compatible with the FAS. On the other

Table 3. Selected characteristics of mothers interviewed at Boston City Hospital after delivery, February, 1977 to October, 1979 (N = 1,690)

age < 18 yr	12%
Black	59
Hispanic	22
White/other	19
Family income < $500/month	88
Education < 8th grade	15
Primiparous	32
No prenatal care	3
Average daily consumption of drinks during pregnancy	
0	65
0.01–0.99	28
1.00–1.99	5
2.00+	3
Coffee (cups/week during pregnancy)	
0	58
0–6.99	24
7–13.99	9
14–20.99	5
21+	5
Meals/day during pregnancy	
1	2
2	18
3	80
Use of vitamin and iron supplements	90
Cigarette smoking during pregnancy	
Never	58
<Half a pack daily	16
One-half to one pack daily	12
>One pack daily	14
Frequency of marijuana use during pregnancy	
Never	86
<Once/month	3
Once/month but < once/week	3
1–2 times/week	6
3+ times/week	2
Psychoactive drug use ever	
Heroin	2
Amphetamines	7
LSD	3
Sedatives/barbiturates	9
Psychoactive drug use during pregnancy	1

From Hingson et al. (1982); reprinted by permission.

hand, women who used marijuana during pregnancy delivered smaller infants as well as infants who were five times more likely to have features compatible with the FAS.

DISCUSSION

Although the pilot study showed an adverse effect of drinking during pregnancy on growth and development of offspring, the later extended study did not. The latter findings must be interpreted cautiously, however, since heavy drinking was reported infrequently in the population assessed in the extended study.

Table 4. Multiple regression analyses on birth weight and gestational age using data from hospital interviews

Dependent variable	Independent variables[a]	Increase in R^2	Beta coefficient
Birth weight	Gestational age	.29	.474
	Age at pregnancy	.03	.111
	Weight change during pregnancy	.03	.194
	Weight prior to pregnancy	.02	.187
	Black/not black	.02	.141
	Cigarettes/day	.01	−.058
	Infant sex	.008	.086
	Marijuana use	.003	−.069
	$(N = 1,343, R = .65, R^2 = .43)$		
Gestational age	Weight change during pregnancy	.02	.163
	Weight prior to pregnancy	.02	.128
	History of maternal illnesses	.01	−.086
	Infant sex	.004	.064
	Iron supplement consumption	.004	.058
	Father's drinking	.003	.072
	Average daily drinks prior to pregnancy	.005	−.073
	$(N = 1,365, R = .29, R^2 = .08)$		

[a]Variables significant at $p < .05$.

Nonetheless, these results do underscore the need to account for numerous variables, each potentially injurious, that might be operative in a given case. For example, had the study examined cigarette smoking and birth weight without consideration of confounding variables, it would have been concluded that women who smoked at least one package of cigarettes per day during pregnancy ($n = 177$) delivered babies whose mean birth weight was 194 grams less than that of babies whose mothers never smoked. Controlling for confounding variables, the actual impact of cigarette smoking becomes a weight reduction of 83 grams. Similarly, marijuana use during pregnancy ($n = 181$) examined in isolation is associated with infants who were 300 grams lighter than infants of nonmarijuana users, but controlling for confounding variables reduces the difference to 105 grams. Finally, women who had two or more alcoholic drinks per day during pregnancy ($n = 30$) had babies 228 grams lighter when confounding variables are not considered. When confounding variables are considered, however, the difference becomes nonsignificant at 51 grams.

SUMMARY AND CONCLUSION

For many centuries, it has been suggested that alcohol consumed during pregnancy may ad-

versely affect the unborn child. The accepted clinical features of the FAS have been derived largely from data gathered from 245 cases reported from around the world, and such data have suggested strongly an association between excessive alcohol intake during pregnancy and abnormalities in the offspring. Such was also indicated by the Boston City Hospital pilot study, a prospective study that showed an association between heavy alcohol usage during pregnancy and the occurrence in newborns of neurological abnormalities, growth retardation, and congenital anomalies. However, in a larger, more comprehensive prospective study at the Boston City Hospital in which multiple variables were considered, growth retardation and features compatible with the FAS were found to occur as a result of several adverse features: lower maternal weight change, maternal illness, cigarette smoking, and marijuana use.

Present data certainly warrant continuing public awareness of the potential hazard to the fetus of heavy alcohol intake during pregnancy. The result of the extended study and the known higher frequencies of tobacco, marijuana, and drug usage in heavy drinkers emphasizes that multiple factors must be carefully considered before abnormalities in a child can be ascribed solely to alcohol use during pregnancy.

REFERENCES

Beaumont, T. Remarks made in opposition to the views of Dr. Clutterbuck. *Lancet,* 1841–1842, *2,* 340–343.

Clarren, S.K., & Smith, D.W. The fetal alcohol syndrome. *New England Journal of Medicine,* 1978, *298,* 1063–1067.

Dubowitz, L.M., Dubowitz, V., & Goldberg, C. Clinical assessment of gestational age in the newborn. *The Journal of Pediatrics,* 1970, *77,* 1–10.

Fielding, H. *An enquiry into the causes of the late increase of robbers etc. with some proposals for remedying this growing evil.* London: A. Millar, 1751.

Haggard, H.W., & Jellinek, E.M. *Alcohol explored.* Garden City, NY: Doubleday & Co., 1942.

Hingson, R., Alpert, J.J., Day, N., Dooling, E., Kayne, H., Morelock, S., Oppenheimer, E., & Zuckerman, B. Effects of maternal drinking and marijuana use on fetal growth and development. *Pediatrics,* 1982, *70,* 539–546.

Jones, K.L., & Smith, D.W. Recognition of the fetal alcohol syndrome in early infancy. *Lancet,* 1973, *2,* 999–1001.

Lemoine, P., Harousseau, H., Borteyru, J.P., & Menuet, J.C. Les enfants de parents alcooliques. Anomalies observees. A propos de 127 cas [Children of alcoholic parents. Abnormalities observed in 127 cases]. *Ouest Medical [West Medical],* 1968, *21,* 476–482.

Lubchenco, L.O. Assessment of gestational age and development at birth. *Pediatrics Clinics of North America,* 1970, *17,* 125–145.

MacNicholl, T.A. A study of the effects of alcohol on school children. *Quarterly Journal of Inebriety,* 1905, *27,* 113–117.

Ouellette, E.M., Rosett, H.L., Rosman, N.P., & Weiner, L. Adverse effects on offspring of maternal alcohol abuse during pregnancy. *New England Journal of Medicine,* 1977, *297,* 528–530.

Rosett, H.L. A clinical perspective on the fetal alcohol syndrome. *Alcoholism: Clinical and Experimental Research,* 1980, *4,* 119–122.

Ulleland, C., Wennberg, R.P., Igo, R.P., & Smith, N.J. The offspring of alcoholic mothers. *Pediatric Research,* 1970, *4,* 474.

Warner, R.H., & Rosett, H.L. The effects of drinking on offspring: An historical survey of the American and British literature. *Journal of Studies on Alcohol,* 1975, *36,* 1395–1420.

The At-Risk Infant: Psycho/Socio/Medical Aspects
edited by Shaul Harel, M.D., and Nicholas J. Anastasiow, Ph.D.
Copyright © 1985   Paul H. Brookes Publishing Co., Inc.   Baltimore • London

Chapter 14

Smoking and Its Effect
on Pregnancy and the Newborn

LORETTA P. FINNEGAN, M.D.
Jefferson Medical College of the Thomas Jefferson University, Philadelphia, Pennsylvania

NICOTINE IS ONE OF THE MOST POPULAR psychoactive drugs used in the United States today. As a result of its popularity and social acceptability, a large number of babies are chronically exposed to its effects both pre- and postnatally. The effects of smoking on the fetus have been documented by numerous studies. This chapter presents an overview of the current literature on the subject. Included are discussions on the incidence of nicotine use, attitudes toward its use, biochemical and physiological effects on mother and fetus, and the development and behavior of children of smoking mothers.

INCIDENCE

It was reported in *Advance Data,* a publication of the National Center for Health Statistics (NCHS, 1980), that in 1977, 32.1% of all females 20 years of age and over were smokers, with percentages highest in the ages between 20 and 40. Of the current female smokers, 36.2% smoke less than 15 cigarettes daily, 44.2% smoke 15–24, 10.5% smoke 25–34, and 9.1% smoke 35 or more cigarettes daily.

The 1978 Gallup poll on smoking in America (Gallup Opinion Index, 1978) reported that 34% of all females 18 and over were regular smokers, while the National Center for

Health Statistics (1980) reported 29.6% of females 17 and over as smokers. Similar to NCHS data, the Surgeon General's Report on Smoking and Health (United States Department of Health, Education, and Welfare, 1979) reported that peak smoking ages for women coincide with the childbearing years. This is a discouraging report in light of the numerous studies demonstrating definite associations between cigarette smoking and low birth weight, increased mortality and morbidity in the first year of life, intrauterine growth retardation, and impaired scholastic ability among smokers' children through early childhood.

ATTITUDES

A national survey conducted by Fielding (1978) revealed that 62% of women smokers of childbearing age believed that smoking would be harmful to an unborn child, while more than 90% believed that smoking could have detrimental effects on their own health. This is in spite of observations by Simpson (1957) that smoking during pregnancy had an adverse effect on birth weight. While it has been many years since the Surgeon General's Advisory Committee on Smoking and Health first recommended that the United States take action to address the hazardous effects of tobacco smoke, antismoking campaigns directed specifically toward pregnant women were not seriously implemented until the 1970s. A United States Department of Health, Education, and Welfare survey in 1977 showed that about 35% of women smokers in the age range of 18–35 stopped smoking during their pregnancies, and 32% decreased the number of cigarettes per day (Fielding, 1978). In a smaller study done in York, England, in which the percentages were almost identical, the rationales behind the mothers' smoking behavior were probed (Graham, 1976). Pregnant women who had never smoked generally accepted the medical view of fetal growth retardation and, furthermore, viewed pregnant women who continued to smoke as having no regard for the health of their unborn children. Among the expectant mothers who smoked, about one-third accepted the opinion that smoking was detrimental to the fetus. Some of this group gave up smoking during pregnancy; the others felt guilty and inadequate. The majority of smokers did not believe that smoking in general could be harmful to the fetus, or thought that the few cigarettes they were smoking wouldn't do any harm. At the same time, they felt that diet and other personal habits could affect the fetus. These mothers generally put more faith in advice from the first-hand experiences of family and friends than from media sources. They also felt that if they stopped smoking, they would be less able to cope with the problems of daily life, and this would put a burden on their spouses and other children (Graham, 1976). Actually, studies on nicotine addiction have shown that what appears to be a calming effect of nicotine is really the temporary alleviation of adverse effects that can appear with abstinence (Schachter, 1978).

BIOCHEMICAL AND PHYSIOLOGICAL EFFECTS

Cigarette smoke contains or generates over 2,000 compounds in both the gaseous and solid states (United States Department of Health, Education, and Welfare, 1979). The gases of cigarette smoke include: carbon monoxide, carbon dioxide, nitric oxide, ammonia, nitrosamines, hydrogen cyanide, volatile sulphur compounds, volatile nitrites, hydrocarbons, alcohols, aldehydes and ketones, and a number of other toxic nitrogen compounds. In total, there have been 18 major toxic agents identified among the gases of cigarette smoke, many of which are known carcinogens.

The particulates include nicotine and related tobacco alkaloids, nonvolatile N-nitrosamines, aromatic amines (associated with bladder cancer), waxes (alkanes and alkenes), isoprenoids (several hundred), benzenes, naphthalenes, polynuclear aromatic hydrocarbons (17 known tumorigenics and 4 co-carcinogens), phenols, carboxylic acids, radioactive compounds, and metals (primarily calcium, magnesium, potassium, and sodium ions). Table 1 lists 21 classes of tumorigenic agents found in cigarette smoke (United States Department of Health, Education, and Welfare, 1979). The pharmacology of these compounds is diverse although only a minority of them have been specifically studied with respect to their effect on pregnancy and the newborn.

Table 1. Known tumorigenic agents in cigarette smoke particulates

Compound	μg/cig.
Tumor Initiators	
Benzo (a) pyrene	0.01–0.05
Other PAH	0.3–0.4
Dibenz (aj) acridine	0.003–0.01
Other AZA arenes	0.01–0.02
Urethane	0.035
Co-carcinogens	
Pyrene	0.05–0.2
Other PAH	0.5–1.0
1-Methylindoles	0.8
9-Methylcarbazoles	0.14
4,4-Dichlorostilbene	0.5–1.5
Catechol	200–500
Alkylcatechols	10–30
Organ Specific Carcinogens	
N'-Nitrosonornicotine	0.14–3.70
4-(N-methyl-N-nitros-amino)-1-(3-pyridyl)-1-butanone	0.11–0.42
N-Nitrosoanatabine	—[a]
Polonium-210	0.03–0.07 pCi
Nickel compound	0–5.8
Cadmium compounds	0.01–0.07
β-Naphthylamine	0.001–0.022
4-Aminobiphenyl	0.001–0.002
0-Toluidine	0.16

[a]Concentrations unknown.
From the United States Department of Health, Education, and Welfare (1979).

Nicotine

Nicotine in cigarette smoke is efficiently absorbed by the lungs, but less efficiently through the oral mucosa. It has a mean half-life in arterial blood of about 40 minutes (United States Department of Health, Education, and Welfare, 1979). It stimulates both sympathetic and parasympathetic ganglia, causing the release of catecholamines from peripheral nerve endings and chromaffin tissue (adrenal medulla).

Several studies on maternal smoking suggest that the effects of nicotine on the fetus are principally indirect, resulting from maternal responses to nicotine, particularly vasoconstriction. Quigley, Sheehan, and Wilkes (1979) studied eight pregnant women who had smoked 20–40 cigarettes per day at 34 weeks of pregnancy to determine whether neuroendocrine and cardiovascular changes were more evident in the mother or the fetus. Within 2½ minutes of smoking a cigarette, the mother showed elevated levels of norepinephrine and epinephrine. Maternal pulse and blood pressure also increased. Norepinephrine and epinephrine are known not to be transferred to the fetus; nevertheless, within 5 minutes, the fetal heart rate had increased significantly. These results suggest that adrenergic discharges induced by the nicotine caused vasoconstriction in the mother leading to decreased perfusion of the uterus. This, in turn, caused the observed fetal tachycardia. The delayed but prolonged increase in carboxyhemoglobin could result in fetal hypoxia. It should be pointed out that this study was comprised of a small sample of women volunteers who were hospitalized under fasting conditions.

A similar observation was made by Manning, Walker, and Feyerabend (1978) in studies on pregnant ewes. When nicotine was injected into the ewes, the fetal breathing movements decreased, whereas if the nicotine was injected directly into the fetus, rapid breathing was induced. Because reductions in fetal breathing can also be induced by lowering the oxygen concentration in the air the ewe breathes, Manning et al. (1978) concluded that nicotine reduced fetal breathing movements as a consequence of some degree of fetal anoxia, which is produced indirectly by nicotine in the mother's circulation, probably via impairment of uteroplacental perfusion.

Reduction in fetal breathing movements has also been observed in human pregnancies in response to cigarette smoking (Manning & Feyerabend, 1976). The reduction is greatest in fetuses that are small for date or in pregnancies with other clinical evidence of impaired placental function. These observations were made in a study of 64 women in the third trimester of pregnancy who were chronic smokers. Of the 64, only 19 had normal pregnancies, while the other had a variety of complications not necessarily related to smoking. Even among the normal pregnancies, 30 minutes after smoking a cigarette, fetal breathing movements were significantly decreased but returned to close to the precigarette level after 90 minutes. The decrease in fetal breathing was related to the level of nicotine in maternal plasma and was shown to have no relationship to carboxyhemoglobin levels. Thus, it appears that increased nicotine levels in the smoking mother apparently produce transient anoxic effects in the fetus with each cigarette the mother smokes.

Carbon Monoxide

Studies have consistently pointed to carbon monoxide levels as being related to the adequacy of oxygenation in the fetus with the consensus focused on chronic fetal hypoxia associated with increased levels of carboxyhemoglobin. The following results were reported in a study (Hawkins, Cole, & Harris, 1976) that included 200 pregnant women from a prenatal clinic, along with 77 office workers and 97 meat porters, with the purpose of studying carboxyhemoglobin concentrations in an urban population that smokes. The three groups were chosen based upon their different levels of physical exertion and stress. The carbon monoxide content of cigarette smoke is up to 5% by volume. After inhalation, the concentration in alveoli is about 0.04% and retention of carbon monoxide by the body is approximately 80% with an average of 7.5 ml absorbed per cigarette. The net result is that, in a smoking mother and her baby, the levels of carboxyhemoglobin may average 3.5% with levels as high as 8%, whereas normal levels would be less than 1%. In addition to average levels, theoretical plateaus were calculated, resulting in 5.93% of carboxyhemoglobin for both meat porters and pregnant women compared to 16% for office workers. The conclusion reached was that physically active people and pregnant women have lower levels, due to increased pulmonary perfusion (Hawkins et al., 1976). The data from this study were analyzed in a careful and thoroughly statistical fashion that, along with an adequate sample size, provides a base of good information for future use and reference.

An extensive study by the National Institute of Child Health and Human Development (Spira, Philippe, & Spira, 1977) reported the effects of carbon monoxide crossing the placenta by diffusion. Following maternal exposure, 4 or 5 hours are required for fetal carbon monoxide levels to equal those in the mother's circulation. Fetal levels ultimately rise to somewhat higher concentrations than those found in the mother. Carbon monoxide combines with hemoglobin to form carboxyhemoglobin that has an increased affinity for oxygen. Since the fetus normally has a low oxygen tension relative to the mother, blood flow must be increased or oxygen tension must be reduced to a very low level in order to deliver the same amount of oxygen. Because fetal blood flow is unlikely to increase dramatically to compensate for the elevated carbon monoxide levels, adequate oxygenation becomes dependent upon a sharply decreased P_{O_2} in the umbilical artery and vein (Spira et al., 1977).

DeMarisico (1978) reported on the calculations that demonstrate that a level of 9% carboxyhemoglobin in the fetus is equivalent to approximately a 40% reduction of the blood flow. DeMarisico also pointed out that in addition to the competition for hemoglobin between carbon monoxide and oxygen, there may exist competition for enzymes, i.e., cytochrome oxidase and carbonic anhydrase. Davies, Latto, and Jones (1979) investigated whether cessation of smoking for short periods might provide a short-term benefit for pregnant mothers since carboxyhemoglobin levels in the blood are dependent on intake of carbon monoxide. They found that 48 hours without smoking reduced carboxyhemoglobin levels and increased available oxygen in smokers to the same levels as those of controls. On the basis of this evidence, they recommended that smokers be encouraged to stop smoking for a few days before elective deliveries to decrease the chances of fetal anoxia.

Cyanide, Thiocyanate, and Other Substances

Cyanide inhaled in cigarette smoke is detoxified to thiocyanate. Because some foods are also a source of thiocyanate, nonsmokers as well as smokers have thiocyanate in their serum. However, mothers smoking 10 or more cigarettes a day are reported to have significantly higher serum thiocyanate levels at the time of delivery than do nonsmokers (Meberg, Sande, & Foss, 1979). In addition, serum thiocyanate levels were found to correlate highly with low birth weight in a study of 53 women of which 28 were smokers. In the past, thiocyanate has been used as an antihypertensive drug (DeMarisico, 1978). It has been observed that pregnant women who smoke exhibit a lower incidence of hypertension than nonsmokers, which could be a result of the higher thiocyanate levels.

Cyanide ingestion in significant quantities may decrease the availability of vitamin B_{12} as this vitamin is thought to be involved in cyanide detoxification. Serum levels of vitamin B_{12} were found to be lower in pregnant women who smoked than in pregnant nonsmokers (DeMarisico, 1978). The level of vitamin C is also lower in the serum of smokers during pregnancy than in comparable nonsmokers (United States Department of Health, Education, and Welfare, 1979).

The ability of the placenta to hydroxylate zoxazolamine was strikingly increased in mothers who smoked compared with nonsmokers. The ability to metabolize this obscure drug (used several years ago as a muscle relaxant before it was withdrawn due to liver toxicity) may indicate an overall stimulation of metabolic pathways involved in eliminating toxic materials to which smokers expose themselves. This capability in placental secretions may, to some degree, protect the fetus (Kapitulnik, Levin, & Poppers, 1976).

Effects on the Placenta

Smoking has demonstrable effects on both placental metabolism and morphology. This is not surprising in view of the role played by the placenta in adapting to varying levels of oxygen availability. Blood flow in both the umbilical artery and the uterus are generally high; rate of exchange depends upon the resistance of the villous membrane. Based on a study of 12 healthy women between 35 and 40 weeks of pregnancy, Lehtovirta and Forss (1978) showed that smoking cigarettes markedly decreases intervillous placental blood flow.

Diffusing Capacity   The diffusing capacity of the placenta increases directly with the surface area of the villi and fetal capillaries and indirectly with the distance between maternal and fetal blood. These mechanisms are particularly active during the last trimester, when the fetus is growing faster than the placenta. During this period, there is a large increase in the number of terminal villi, concomitant with a decrease in size of each villus (Meyer, 1977). The changes seen in placental tissues due to decreased oxygen supply are similar to those of mothers who live at high altitudes. Intervillous space is reduced in thickness concurrent with increased surface area. There is also a higher incidence of abnormal trophoblast formation and especially of nuclear clumps in the syncytiotrophoblast in placentas of smokers along with the decrease in intervillous space (Spira et al., 1977). Other observations include a broadening of the basement membrane of placental villi, an increased collagen content of the villi, a decrease in vascularization, and edema in the intima of the villous capillaries and arterioles.

Increase in Placental Ratios   With chronic fetal hypoxia, as occurs at high altitudes or in severely anemic women, high ratios of the weight of the placenta to the weight of the fetus are obtained. High placental ratios are

also found in smoking mothers. The high ratios are evident throughout gestation (Wingerd, Christianson, & Lovitt, 1976). However, there is little evidence of placental hypertrophy in the smoking mothers. At all periods of gestation, the size of the placenta is normal. The increase in placental ratios is due almost entirely to the reduced weight of the fetus. In a study of 248 women who smoked at least 5 cigarettes daily during pregnancy and 196 nonsmoking controls, pathological studies of the placenta were performed "blind" for both smokers and controls (Spira et al., 1977). The conclusion was reached that reduced birth weight for infants of smokers, which occurs without an accompanying decrease in placental weight, is suggestive of placental dysfunction. The same increased placental birth weight ratios were reported by Wingerd et al. (1976) in a study of 7,000 pregnancies, and also in a larger study by Naeye (1978) in which the courses of 53,518 pregnancies in 12 hospitals throughout the United States were followed.

Heat Stable Alkaline Phosphatase Concentration

Higher concentrations of heat stable alkaline phosphatase late in gestation or during labor have been reported in smokers (Pirani & MacGillivray, 1978). The function of this enzyme in pregnancy has not been fully determined; however, it is assumed to be associated with growth and development of the fetus. This finding could be symptomatic of abnormal placental function. Human placental lactogen (HPL), often used as an index of placental function, was found by some researchers to be slightly elevated in smokers in the 30th–40th week of pregnancy in a study of pregnant volunteers (Spellacy, Buhi, & Birk, 1977). These findings are inconsistent with those of Boyce (1975) and Moser, Hollingsworth, Carlson, & Lamotte, (1974). In addition, no controls other than smoking/nonsmoking status were instituted. It should also be considered that although HPL levels correlate with placental weight, differentiation between intrauterine growth retardation and prematurity cannot be made (Behrman, 1977).

Vascular Effects

The changes in the aorta and coronary arteries occurring in smokers are indicative of vascular changes throughout the body (National Center for Health Statistics, United States Department of Health, Education, and Welfare, 1979). Umbilical veins from heavy smokers are no exception and were examined in a small study by Asmussen (1978). He reported severe changes in the intima and media such as edema, destruction of intimal elastic membranes, decrease in collagen, and proliferation of myocytes. There was strong indication that smoking is associated with extensive damage to the cord. Possible vascular damage to the fetus is speculative.

BIRTH WEIGHT AND FETAL GROWTH

Numerous studies over the past 24 years have shown that infants born to mothers who smoke are small for gestational age (United States Department of Health, Education, and Welfare, 1979), generally weighing about 200 grams lighter than children of nonsmokers (United States Department of Health and Human Services, 1980). An aggregate of studies has shown that 21%–39% of the incidence of low birth weight could be explained by maternal smoking. The decrease in weight is directly related to the number of cigarettes smoked daily. It has been demonstrated graphically that the distribution of birth weights of infants born to smoking and non-smoking women is of the same shape but with the mean birth weight of smokers' infants displaced at all points by about 200 grams (United States Department of Health and Human Services, 1980). Women who smoked less than a pack a day had 53% more births under 2,500 grams; those who smoked greater than a pack a day had more than twice the number of low birth weight infants compared to nonsmokers (Meyer, Jonas, & Tonascia, 1976). This finding is independent of other variables related to birth weight, including race, prepregnant weight, socioeconomic status, maternal weight gain, maternal age, and alcohol consumption.

In a large, well-controlled study, Naeye (1978) found that women who smoked during one pregnancy but not another had smaller infants in the pregnancy in which they smoked, irrespective of birth order. Heavy smokers gained significantly less weight during pregnancy—an average of 533 grams less than nonsmokers. One-third of this deficit was due to the decreased size of the newborn infant.

There has been considerable controversy about whether the decrease in birth weight of babies born to mothers who smoke is a secondary effect of poor nutrition and decreased appetite induced by smoking. However, some studies, in which birth weights were shown to be reduced by smoking, found no concomitant reduction in maternal weight gain beyond that which could be accounted for by the decreased weight of the baby (Meyer, 1978). The growth pattern of smokers' babies was not the same as that for low birth weight babies born after low maternal weight gain. Babies born to mothers who smoked tended to have shorter body lengths for gestational age, whereas low maternal weight gain babies had, on the average, lower ponderal indices (birth weight in grams multiplied by 100 divided by crown-heel length in cubic centimeters). Attempts to improve the prognosis for the baby by supplementing the smoking mother's diet have been generally unsuccessful. Furthermore, for all classes of maternal weight gain, from less than 5 pounds to more than 40 pounds, the proportion of births under 2,500 grams was directly related to the number of cigarettes smoked (Meyer, 1977).

The lag in birth weight observed in smokers' babies is seen from the 35th week of gestation onward. It reflects an overall depression of fetal growth. Smokers' babies average more than a centimeter shorter than babies of controls and they have decreased head circumference and shoulder circumference. These deficits have been demonstrated from the 28th week onward by ultrasound measurements of the fetal biparietal diameter in a large study of 5,715 pregnancies (Persson, Grennert, & Gennser, 1977).

There was some speculation of self-selection among smokers. That is, mothers who will later become smokers may tend to give birth to infants of low birth weight. However, this is contradicted by the finding that babies of mothers who stop smoking before the third month of pregnancy have no deficit in weight relative to the children of nonsmokers (Kline, Stein, & Susser, 1977). It also appears that the babies of ex-smokers are equal in size to those of mothers who have never smoked. Many of these studies are difficult to interpret because of confounding social factors. There is a tendency for smokers to be younger, unmarried, of low socioeconomic background, and with less education than nonsmokers (United States Department of Health, Education, and Welfare, 1979).

Paradoxically, the incidence of perinatal mortality for the low birth weight infants born to smokers is lower than for low birth weight babies of controls. The rationale for this lowered incidence of perinatal mortality is that the low birth weight of smokers' babies is not due to prematurity, since smoking has been found to decrease average gestation time by only a few days. Therefore, small babies of smokers are more mature by gestational age than are babies of comparable weight born to nonsmokers.

MATERNAL COMPLICATIONS

Smoking appears to increase the risk of a number of conditions that are life-threatening to the mother and the fetus. In the large Ontario study (Meyer, 1977), premature rupture of membranes increased in frequency as the amount of cigarette smoking increased. Smokers had a higher risk of abruptio placenta and of placenta previa at all gestational ages studied. Bleeding early in pregnancy was also a more common complication among smokers than nonsmokers as was the frequency of preterm delivery. All of these complications were strongly associated with increased fetal mortality for smokers' babies. These findings are consistent with the compendium of studies as reported by the Surgeon General (United States Department of Health and Human Services, 1980).

In contrast, there is a decrease in the incidence of preeclampsia among smoking mothers (United States Department of Health and Human Services, 1980). It is postulated that this may be a direct result of the serum concentrations of thiocyanate, which was used in the past as therapy for hypertension.

FETAL AND INFANT MORTALITY

It has been reported in numerous studies from both developed and developing countries that there is a definite increase in the risk of perinatal mortality among infants of mothers who smoked during pregnancy. There are complications, however, in weighing the relative risks, because of intervening socioeconomic factors. However, a number of studies have attempted to control for various factors such as social class, race, age, parity, etc., and have consistently found an increased perinatal mortality risk, especially among heavy smokers, with the ratio of smoker/nonsmoker perinatal mortality ranging from 1.05 to 2.47. The increased perinatal mortality was also linked with tobacco-associated pregnancy complications.

According to a 1973 Public Health Service report of approximately 87,000 infant deaths in the United States, it is estimated that 4,600 were tobacco related. The incidence of spontaneous abortions increased with the number of cigarettes smoked daily. In a study of spontaneous abortions, Kline et al. (1977) found that the proportion of mothers who smoked was 41% as opposed to 28% in a matched sample of term pregnancies. Perinatal deaths are also higher for smokers (Naeye, 1978). Most of these deaths involve infants who die *in utero* without obvious pathology, or who die in the neonatal period after premature delivery. Meyer (1977) has pooled the results of many studies on smoking and infant mortality. She estimated that fetal wastage is increased 33.4% in smokers. As a corollary, smoking has not been associated with congenital abnormalities (Meyer, 1977). In contrast, an increase in the incidence of congenital malformations among infants of smoking mothers has been reported, with the ratio of heavy smokers to controls reported as high as 2.3 to 1 (United States Department of Health and Human Services, 1980).

The increased perinatal mortality ascribed to maternal smoking has been concentrated within a small number of cause-specific categories including: 1) stillbirths with antepartum hemorrhage, abruptio placenta, and "unknown" causes, and 2) neonatal deaths with immaturity, asphyxia, atelectasis, and respiratory distress syndrome (United States Department of Health and Human Services, 1980). Meyer (1978) reported that the largest difference between observed and expected deaths occurred in the "unknown" cause of death category for fetal deaths and the "prematurity alone" category for neonatal deaths. These results are from a large study of 16,549 pregnancies of smoking mothers as compared to 15,420 controls.

The relationship of passive cigarette smoking to sudden infant death syndrome has been evaluated (Bergman & Wiesner, 1976). Smoking habits of 56 families who lost babies to sudden infant death syndrome were compared to those of 86 control families. A higher proportion of sudden infant death syndrome mothers smoked both during pregnancy (61% versus 42%) and after their babies were born (59% versus 37%). The study mothers also smoked a significantly greater number of cigarettes than controls. The investigators also observed that some victims of sudden infant death syndrome were chronically hypoxemic before their death and postulated that this was related to chronic alveolar hypoventilation. Including smoking by any resident family member in future studies may prove to be illuminating.

DEVELOPMENT AND BEHAVIOR

The increased mortality among children of smokers is reported to continue until at least the age of 5. The risk of contracting pneumonia or bronchitis in the first year of life is doubled in babies of pack-a-day smokers as opposed to babies of nonsmoking parents. Until the age of 5, smokers' children were found to be hospitalized more frequently than control children, often with respiratory diseases. They also had a greater predisposition for accidents (Rantakallio, 1978).

It is apparent that the children of mothers who smoke suffer long-lasting and general impairment. A number of studies have indicated that the weight difference observed between children of smokers and nonsmokers persists until at least the age of 7, but this finding has not been reliable. A British study of 11,000 children born during one week in March, 1958, showed a deficit of approximately 1 cm in height of smokers' children at the ages of 7 and 11. Furthermore, the children lagged an average of 3–6 months in scholastic ability. In a battery of psychological tests, children of nonsmoking mothers scored better in 45 out of 48 comparisons; the difference being significant in 14 (United States Department of Health, Education, and Welfare, 1979).

GENERAL CONCLUSIONS AND RECOMMENDATIONS

It is clear that smoking is detrimental to the pregnant smoker as well as to the fetus. Clinical evidence obligates the physician to encourage pregnant patients to stop smoking as soon as possible, preferably in the first trimester. If the woman is of low socioeconomic class and/or has had a poor obstetrical performance, the physician must *strongly* encourage her to break her smoking habit since she is at such a great risk. The physician must show that he or she understands why the patient smokes and then attempt to counteract these reasons and/or influences. Psychological and physiological studies have elucidated some of the motivating factors. A summary of their findings suggests approaches that may be successful.

1. Nicotine is physiologically reinforcing. Studies have shown that increasing excretion of nicotine by acidifying the urine causes an increased desire for cigarettes. When smokers switch to brands of cigarettes containing less nicotine, they compensate by smoking more cigarettes, more of each cigarette, and holding the smoke in their lungs longer so that a desired nicotine level is attained (United States Department of Health, Education, and Welfare,

1979). The patient should be informed that it is less uncomfortable to stop smoking altogether than to gradually decrease. The latter strategy keeps the patient in a lengthy state of withdrawal.

2. Cigarette smoking often separates blocks of time in the day and defines leisure periods. The percentage of housewives who smoke (about 60% in one study) is greater than that for women who work outside the home (about 39% in the same study). Addressing the psychological dependencies is a challenge to behavior modification therapy.

3. Some pregnant women who smoke discount data demonstrating increased risks for their unborn child. The physician must convince the patient that these risks do exist by specifying drugs considered hazardous to pregnant women, including cigarettes. It should be stressed to the patient that smoking adds an especially high risk if there is a history of previous complications of pregnancy. The physician must also express concern about the patient's continued smoking during each subsequent visit, particularly if bleeding occurs. In order to forcefully demonstrate the ill effects of smoking to the patient, carboxyhemoglobin or expired carbon monoxide levels should be obtained from the patient. It might also be discussed that smoking may have a deleterious effect on the physical and mental development of the woman's child.

4. Medical professionals realize that it is not easy to stop smoking. Hospital staffs should be as supportive as possible and smoking should not be permitted in patient areas. Antismoking programs should be available and the patient provided with a list of such clinics. If the patient finds it impossible to quit, but can cut back, she should be informed that this is beneficial. Studies have shown that brief but intensive antismoking counseling by the physician can result in a significant decrease in smoking compared to nonintervention controls (Danaher, Shisslak, & Thompson, 1978). This is an inexpensive form of therapy that can produce a remarkable improvement in perinatal morbidity and mortality.

SUMMARY

Nicotine is one of the most socially acceptable psychoactive drugs in the United States today. The fetus and newborn are chronically exposed to this drug as a result of maternal intake.

Smoking behavior is found in about one-third of the women of childbearing age in the United States. When they become pregnant, one-third quit smoking for the duration of the pregnancy while the others continue or reduce their smoking to varying degrees. Nicotine in the maternal circulation causes vasoconstriction resulting in anoxia along with decreased breathing movements in the fetus. Smoking raises the level of carboxyhemoglobin (response to carbon monoxide) to about 3.5% in the mother and higher in the fetus, thus contributing to anoxia. Some defects in the placenta have been postulated from chronic oxygen deficit.

Infants born to mothers who smoke have been observed to have *in utero* growth retardation. The average 200-gram lag in birth weight cannot be accounted for by decreased maternal weight gain or other factors. Mothers who smoke have increased rates of complications including: premature rupture of membranes, spontaneous abortion, abruptio placenta, placenta previa, and bleeding early in pregnancy. Fetal and infant mortality has been shown to be higher than expected in all studies including those controlling for socioeconomic factors. Some studies also show deficits in health, growth, behavior, and intellectual development for children of smoking parents.

The overwhelming evidence that smoking has a detrimental effect upon the developing fetus and newborn must encourage medical professionals to make every effort to stop pregnant women from smoking as soon as possible, preferably in the first trimester. A critical approach may discourage the mother from seeking prenatal care while compassion and encouragement may help her to protect her developing fetus, newborn, and child.

REFERENCES

Asmussen, I. Ultrastructure of human umbilical veins. *Acta Obstetrica et Gynecologica Scandinavica*, 1978, *57*, 253–255.

Behrman, R.E. (ed.). *Neonatal-perinatal medicine* (2nd ed.). St. Louis: C.V. Mosby Co., 1977.

Bergman, A.B., & Wiesner, L.A. Relationship of passive cigarette-smoking to sudden infant death syndrome. *Pediatrics*, 1976, *58*, 665–668.

Boyce. Smoking, human placental lactogen and birth weight. *British Journal of Obstetrics and Gynaecology*, 1975, *82*, 964–967.

Danaher, B.G., Shisslak, C.M., & Thompson, C.B. A smoking cessation program for pregnant women: An exploratory study. *American Journal of Public Health*, 1978, *68*, 896–897.

Davies, J.M., Latto, I.P., & Jones, J.G. Effects of stopping smoking for 48 hours on oxygen availability from the blood: A study of pregnant women. *British Medical Journal*, 1979, *2*, 355–356.

DeMarisico, R. Smoking and pregnancy. *Journal of the Medical Society of New Jersey*, 1978, *75*, 124–135.

Fielding, J.E. Smoking and pregnancy. *New England Journal of Medicine*, 1978, *298*, 337–338.

Gallop Opinion Index. Smoking in America. Public attitudes and behaviors. *Gallup Opinion Index*, 155, June, 1978.

Graham, H. Smoking in pregnancy: The attitudes of expectant mothers. *Social Science and Medicine*, 1976, *10*, 399–405.

Hawkins, L.H., Cole, P.V., & Harris, J.R.W. Smoking habits and blood carbon monoxide levels. *Environmental Research*, 1976, *11*, 310–318.

Kapitulnik, J., Levin, W., & Poppers, P. Comparison of the hydroxylation of zoxazolamine and benzo(a) pryrene in human placenta. *Clinical Pharmacology and Therapeutics*, 1976, *20*, 557–564.

Kline, J., Stein, Z.A., & Susser, M. Smoking: A risk factor for spontaneous abortion. *New England Journal of Medicine*, 1977, *297*, 793–796.

Lehtovirta, P., & Forss, M. The acute effect of smoking on intervillous blood flow of the placenta. *British Journal of Obstetrics and Gynaecology*, 1978, *85*, 729–731.

Manning, F., & Feyerabend, C. Cigarette smoking and fetal breathing movements. *British Journal of Obstetrics and Gynaecology*, 1976, *83*, 262–270.

Manning, F., Walker, D., & Feyerabend, C. The effect of nicotine on fetal breathing movements in conscious pregnant ewes. *Obstetrics and Gynecology*, 1978, *52*, 563–568.

Meberg, A., Sande, H., & Foss, O.P. Smoking during pregnancy: Effects on the fetus and on thiocyanate levels in mother and baby. *Acta Paediatrica Scandinavica*, 1979, *68*, 547–552.

Meyer, M.B. Effects of maternal smoking and attitude on birth weight and gestation. In: M. Reed & F. Stanley (eds.), *The epidemiology of prematurity*. Baltimore: Urban and Schwarzenberg, 1977.

Meyer, M.B. How does maternal smoking affect birth weight and maternal weight gain? Evidence from the Ontario Perinatal Mortality Study. *American Journal of Obstetrics and Gynecology*, 1978, *131*, 888–893.

Meyer, M.B., Jonas, B.S., & Tonascia, J.A. Perinatal events associated with maternal smoking during pregnancy. *American Journal of Epidemiology*, 1976, *103*, 464–476.

Moser, R.J., Hollingsworth, D.R., Carlson, J.W., & Lamotte, L. Human chorionic sometomammotropin in normal adolescent primiparous pregnancy. I Effect of smoking. *American Journal of Gynecology*, 1974, *120*, 1080–1086.

Naeye, R.L. Effects of maternal cigarette smoking on the fetus and placenta. *British Journal of Obstetrics and Gynaecology*, 1978, *85*, 732–737.

National Center for Health Statistics. *Advance data: Health practices among adults: United States, 1977.* Washington, DC: National Center for Health Statistics, United States Department of Health and Human Services, 1980.

Persson, P.H., Grennert, L., & Gennser, G. A study of smoking and pregnancy with special reference to fetal growth. *Acta Obstetrica et Gynecologica Scandanavica*, 1977, *78*, 33–39.

Pirani, B.K., & MacGillivray, I. Smoking during pregnancy: Its effect on maternal metabolism and fetoplacental function. *Journal of Obstetrics and Gynecology*, 1978, *52*, 257–263.

Quigley, M.E., Sheehan, K.L., & Wilkes, M.M. Effects of maternal smoking on circulating catecholamine levels and fetal heart rates. *American Journal of Obstetrics and Gynecology*, 1979, *133*, 685–690.

Rantakallio, P. The effect of maternal smoking on birthweight and the subsequent health of the child. *Early Human Development*, 1978, *2*, 371–382.

Schachter, S. Pharmacological and psychological determinants of smoking. *Annals of Internal Medicine*, 1978, *88*, 104–114.

Simpson, W.J. A preliminary report on cigarette smoking and the incidence of prematurity. *American Journal of Obstetrics and Gynecology*, 1957, *73*, 808–815.

Spellacy, W.N., Buhi, M.S., & Birk, R.N. The effect of smoking on serum human placental lactogen levels. *American Journal of Obstetrics and Gynecology*, 1977, *27*, 232–234.

Spira, A., Philippe, E., & Spira, N. Smoking during pregnancy and placental pathology. *Biomedicine*, 1977, *27*, 266–270.

United States Department of Health, Education, and Welfare. *Smoking and health: A report of the surgeon general*. Washington, DC: United States Department of Health, Education, and Welfare (Publication Number PHS 79-50066), 1979.

United States Department of Health and Human Services. *The health consequences of smoking for women, a report of the surgeon general*. Washington, DC: United States Department of Health and Human Services, 1980.

Wingerd, J., Christianson, R., & Lovitt, W.V. Placental ratio in white and black women: Relation to smoking and anemia. *American Journal of Obstetrics and Gynecology*, 1976, *124*, 671–675.

Chapter 15

Anticonvulsants during Pregnancy

JANNA G. KOPPE, M.D.
University of Amsterdam, The Netherlands

ANTICONVULSANT AGENTS HAVE BEEN USED in the pharmacotherapy of epilepsy since 1857. Bromium, the first drug used, was not very effective and induced drowsiness as a side effect. In 1912, phenobarbital was introduced and achieved great success in Europe. In 1938, phenytoin became available on the market. The combination of phenobarbital and phenytoin was widely used in the treatment of epilepsy. After the tragedy with Softenon (Thalidomide) in Germany, people became aware of the potential dangers of medications for the embryo and fetus, and the effect of anticonvulsant agents on the unborn was studied by many groups. In this chapter, a brief description is given of the disorders resulting in the offspring from the use of anticonvulsants at various times during pregnancy and the nursing period.

Congenital malformations, fetal hydantoin syndrome, transplacental carcinogenesis, coagulopathy due to a decrease in vitamin K–dependent clotting factors, intrauterine growth retardation, problems with breast-feeding, and long-term follow-up are discussed with special attention to later reproductive function in the offspring.

CONGENITAL MALFORMATIONS

In epileptic women on anticonvulsants, fertility seems to be normal in contrast to male epileptic patients in whom impairment of potency and infertility have been reported. A higher incidence of abortion in epileptic mothers on anticonvulsant drugs has not been proved.

After the first reports of Janz and Fuchs (1964) and Meadow (1968), a number of retrospective studies were done to determine the incidence of malformations in the offspring of epileptic mothers. Elshove and van Eck (1971) found malformations eight times more frequently in the epileptic group taking anticonvulsants than in nonepileptic mothers, with cleft lip and/or palate occurring 29 times more frequently than in controls. Speidel and Meadow (1972) reported 5.1% of infants whose mothers were taking anticonvulsants had malformations (16 babies had congenital heart disease, three had a cleft lip and/or palate, and two had microcephaly).

Other retrospective studies showed similar patterns. There was an incidence of malformations of 8.8% (especially congenital heart disease) in 125 infants of epileptic mothers taking anticonvulsants versus 3% in the total hospital population (Koppe, Bosman, Oppers, Spaans, & Kloosterman, 1973). Among 297 live-born babies of epileptic mothers receiving therapy, 7.4% were referred to a special epilepsy center (Starreveld-Zimmerman, van der Klok, Meinardi, & Elshove, 1973). Nine of the malformed babies in the last study had cleft lip and/or palate, and seven had congenital heart disease.

Annegers, Elveback, Hauser, and Kurland (1974) reported the outcome of a Mayo Clinic study of 141 mothers on anticonvulsants (mainly phenobarbital and phenytoin). There was an incidence of malformations of 7.1%. The increase in malformation rate was borderline statistically significant in epileptic mothers on anticonvulsant therapy compared to those not using drugs. In all these retrospective studies, the same pattern justifies the conclusion that anticonvulsant drugs have a teratogenic effect.

Two prospective studies have confirmed the suspicion that phenytoin is a teratogenic agent. Mirkin (1971) observed the progress of seven pregnancies during which phenytoin was the primary drug taken. Passage of this medication across the placenta was demonstrated in all seven. There were two babies with cleft lip and/or palate, and one with microcephaly. Hill (1973), studying 28 pregnancies during which anticonvulsant agents were taken, found one baby with cleft lip and four with cardiac defects.

FETAL HYDANTOIN SYNDROME

The effect of hydantoin (phenytoin) is probably not restricted to the first trimester, but may influence development in the second and third trimester, resulting in "odd-looking" babies. As aptly described by Speidel and Meadow (1972):

> There does appear to be a group of children with a recognizable pattern of major and minor anomalies. In its full expression the syndrome takes the form of congenital heart disease, cleft lip and/or palate, trigonocephaly or microcephaly and various minor anomalies which include hypertelorism, low-set abnormal ears, short neck with low posterior hair-line, bilateral single transverse palmar creases, and minor peripheral skeletal abnormalities. Mental subnormality is sometimes a feature. This condition is variable in its expression and in its milder forms the minor craniofacial and peripheral abnormalities may be the only ones found (p. 839).

This description agrees with the one published later as the "fetal hydantoin syndrome" (Hanson & Smith, 1975). Phenobarbital also gives rise to similar clinical phenotypes that have been called "fetal barbiturate syndrome" (Feldman, Weaver, & Lovrien, 1977).

In the studies of malformations and the fetal hydantoin or barbiturate syndrome, phenytoin and phenobarbital are the drugs primarily involved. However, carbamazepine and primidone have also produced a significant incidence of defects, although less than those resulting from phenytoin and phenobarbital. A potent teratogenic action has been reported for trimethadione, a drug less frequently used in epilepsy causing either abortion or malformation in 80% of cases.

TRANSPLACENTAL CARCINOGENICITY OF ANTICONVULSANT AGENTS

Carcinogenic substances require certain enzymes that for the most part are missing from fetal tissue in order to assert their effect. Thus, many carcinogenic substances can be found in the cord blood but are not toxic in the fetus. A long-term follow-up of at least 25 years is necessary to determine whether or not drugs or environmental factors can be carcinogenic transplacentally.

Anticonvulsant agents have been suspected of producing cancer transplacentally as described in case reports: a neuroblastoma in a 3-year-old girl (Pendergrass & Hanson, 1976), another neuroblastoma in a 7-day-old boy (Sherman & Roizen, 1976), a malignant mesenchymoma in an 18-year-old boy (Blatner, Henson, Young, & Fraumeni, 1977), and a ganglioneuroblastoma in a 3-year-old boy with signs of fetal hydantoin syndrome and a ventricular septal defect (Seeler, Israel, Royal, Kaye, Rao, & Abulaban, 1979). Phenobarbital, phenytoin, and carbamazepine were the anticonvulsant agents taken during the various pregnancies.

In a long-term follow-up study of 251 liveborn children of 177 epileptic mothers (the malformation rate in this group was 8%) Dukkers van Emden, Koppe, and Peters (1981) discovered one case of Hodgkin's disease. The mother of this boy used phenobarbital, phenytoin, and primidone. On the second day after birth the child had severe intraperitoneal bleeding due to coagulopathy caused by the drugs. Based on the above mentioned reports of neuroblastoma, Miller (1980a, 1980b) concluded that phenytoin is the second transplacental chemical after diethylstilbestrol (DES) that induces cancer in human beings. Certainly, the carcinogenic effects are not common.

COAGULOPATHIES

One life-threatening problem in the newborn of an epileptic mother is the coagulopathy caused by a decrease in vitamin K–dependent clotting factors (Creveld, 1957).

Infants born to mothers taking either phenytoin or a barbiturate derivative or both may show clinical signs of bleeding and diminished levels of coagulation factors. In the mother, the clotting studies are normal. While this effect of anticonvulsant agents may be the consequence of liver enzyme induction accelerating the catabolism of coagulation factors, a more likely hypothesis is that the drugs may be competitive inhibitors of vitamin K.

Severe intracranial, intrathoracic, and intraperitoneal bleeding has been reported. In the liver subcapsular bleeding may start and break through into the peritoneum. Phenobarbital has been blamed for this effect (Mountain, Hirsch, & Gallus, 1970), but phenytoin can also cause a prolonged prothrombin time in the newborn.

Since more than half of the babies whose mothers use anticonvulsant agents (especially phenobarbital, phenytoin, and carbamazepine) have this bleeding tendency, it is important to give extra vitamin K tablets to the mothers during the last weeks of pregnancy or intravenously (for instance 10 mg) when the mother arrives in the clinic in labor.

Hill, Verniaud, Horning, McCulley, and Morgan (1974) describe one infant with evidence of bleeding in the neonatal period that occurred in spite of the administration of vitamin K on admission to the nursery, stressing the fact that vitamin K should be administered to the mother before delivery. The infant was delivered by breech extraction, and had an Apgar score of 6 at birth. Within the first two days of life, ecchymotic areas appeared around the neck, elbow, buttocks, knees, back, and rib cage.

To protect the baby, the supply of vitamin K transplacentally is important. Even the birth trauma itself can be fatal. If administration of vitamin K does not take place prior to delivery, it is necessary to immediately give the infant 1–2 mg of vitamin K intramuscularly. Natural vitamin K (Konakion) should always be used rather than a synthethic vitamin K because of the risk of kernicterus.

INTRAUTERINE GROWTH RETARDATION

A number of investigators reported intrauterine growth retardation in malformed infants of epileptic mothers (Feldman et al., 1977; Hanson & Smith, 1975). Failure to grow may be caused by the malformation itself.

Vert, André, and Deblay (1978) reported low birth weights in infants on antiepileptic medication in general and stressed the fact that 28% of the infants had a head circumference 2 standard deviations below normal at birth. At follow-up, Hanson & Smith (1975) and Vert et al. (1978) reported a postnatal linear growth rate approximately 95% that of normal. In animal studies, growth retardation is seen in otherwise normal offspring of phenytoin-treated mother rats. This is not seen in phenobarbital-treated mother rats (Sonawane & Yaffe, 1983).

BREAST-FEEDING

Mothers who have taken large doses of anticonvulsant agents (e.g., >100 mg of phenobarbital a day) should not breast-feed because the drug can be present in the milk in high concentration, depending on the individual drug. The different breast milk/plasma ratios are reported in Table 1. Only na-valproate is relatively safe because of the low ratio.

EFFECTS ON THE SECOND GENERATION

The question is raised if there is an effect on reproductive performance of daughters and sons of mothers using anticonvulsants as there is in DES daughters. Animal studies point in this direction. Sonawane and Yaffe (1983) and Gupta, Shapira, and Yaffe (1980) published

Table 1. Anticonvulsant agents in breast milk

Breast milk/plasma ratio	
Phenobarbital	0.46
Phenytoin	0.39
Carbamazepine	0.65
Ethosuximide	0.80
Primidone	0.90
Na-valproate	0.15
Diazepam	0.20–0.50

data of studies of rats. The male offspring receiving the drug phenobarbital *in utero* had decreased fertility. A same effect was seen with phenytoin. In the female offspring, fertility was also significantly reduced. The authors blame disturbances in the development of the neuroendocrine axis and hypothesize that prenatal administration of phenobarbital may produce a permanent change in the neuroendocrine axis by producing a suppressed level of progesterone.

To test this hypothesis, a study was done in a group of 95 children of epileptic mothers on anticonvulsants during pregnancy. The mothers had used either phenobarbital alone or in combination with phenytoin and/or other anticonvulsant agents. The children were born between 1952 and 1957. (It is perhaps, therefore, too soon to evaluate the effects of the prenatal anticonvulsants on this first generations' childbearing ability.) A control group was composed of the first baby to be born in the clinic to a nonepileptic mother after the birth of each infant in the study group. The control group babies were matched to the study group for age and parity of the mother and birth weight of the baby. The control mothers had their delivery in the clinic partly because of pathology other than epilepsy, and partly because of social circumstances (mostly a housing problem during those years). This means that the control group was not an example of the normal Dutch population but was more pathological.

Responses were received from 77 children of epileptic mothers on anticonvulsant therapy and from 63 children of control mothers. In this study group, 43 responses were from daughters and 34 from sons, while the control group was made up of 36 daughters and 27 sons. The study group of 77 children of epileptic mothers were all under the prenatal influence of anticonvulsants. The different drugs used are given in Table 2.

The most remarkable but preliminary finding is intrauterine growth retardation and premature delivery in the second generation.

Intrauterine Growth Retardation in the Second Generation

In Table 3, the distribution in different classes of percentile for birth weight and gestational age using the Kloosterman-Huidekoper curve (Kloosterman, 1969) is given for the abovementioned daughters and sons of the first generation in total. In both the study group and the control group, there is a majority under the 50th percentile.

Among the 43 daughters and 34 sons of the study group, 26 women and 15 men have had children; among the control group, 20 of 36 daughters have had children and 11 out of 27 sons have had children.

The distribution of percentiles of this first generation who have had children is given in Table 4. At present, the distribution of percentiles of both the study group and the control group are normal, and there is no longer a predominance under the 50th percentile.

In the study group, a total of 63 children was born to the first generation—35 boys and 28 girls; in the control group, 22 boys and 23 girls were born. Table 5 gives the distribution of percentiles for birth weight and gestational age of these second-generation children. Sixty-two

Table 2. Anticonvulsant agents used by 77 epileptic mothers (1952–1957)

	Number	Percentage
Phenobarbital	27	35.0
Phenobarbital + phenytoin	17	22.0
Phenobarbital + phenytoin + other	13	17.0
Phenobarbital + other	10	13.0
Phenytoin	2	2.5
Phenytoin + other	1	1.0
Unknown	5	6.5

Table 3. Percentiles of first generation offspring of epileptic mothers on anticonvulsants

Percentiles	Study group (N = 77)	Control group (N = 63)
<2.3	3	2
2.3–10	6	9
10–25	10	12
25–50	21	12
50–75	21	12
75–90	9	10
90–97.7	2	4
>97.7	1	1
unknown	4	1

Table 5. Distribution of percentiles of the second generation

Percentile	Study group (n = 63)	Control group (n = 45)
<2.3	2	—
2.3–10	7	4
10–25	9	6
25–50	21	12
50–75	14	12
75–90	4	4
90–97.7	—	4
>97.7	5	3
unknown	1	0

percent (39/63) are under the 50th percentile in the study group versus 49% (22/45) in the control group.

There is a trend of more cases with lower percentiles (i.e., intrauterine growth retardation) in the study group. However, statistically this is not significantly different from the control group. The control group itself shows a normal distribution.

Gestational Age

For the study group of 63 children and an immaturely born pair of twins, and the control group of 45 children, the gestational age is given in Table 6. Both daughters and sons of the first generation had premature/immature deliveries.

Daughters Among the 26 daughters in the first-generation study group who have given birth, five have had a premature delivery and three others were treated for threatened premature labor. In the first-generation control group, of the 20 daughters who have given birth, four had a premature delivery. The reasons included one twin pregnancy at 35 weeks, one mother who was a DES daughter, one induction of labor, and one case of diabetes in

pregnancy. This pathology was not found in the women in the epilepsy group who had had children. There was no case of threatened premature labor in the control group of daughters.

Sons Among the 15 sons in the study group who became fathers, one has an immature pair of twins, two have a prematurely born baby, and three sons' wives experienced a threatened premature labor (one mother on two occasions). In the control group, of the 11 sons whose wives have had children, one has a prematurely delivered baby at 36 weeks and one experienced a threatened premature labor.

These preliminary data about gestational age in the second generation point in the direction of a higher incidence of immaturity/prematurity in the study group. Normal for the Dutch population is ±4% immaturity/prematurity from 25 to 37 weeks; exact numbers are not known, however. The same percentage of ±4% is found in the first generation of epileptic women in general (both in England and in Amsterdam) and in the study group (Table 7).

In a group of 41 men and women (26 first-generation daughters and 15 sons), a number of 8 with immature/premature delivery and 6 with threatened premature labor (one woman two times) represents a very high incidence.

Perinatal Mortality in the Second Generation

Perinatal mortality from 25 weeks until 4 weeks after birth was 6.5% (N = 5) in the study group versus 2% (N = 1) in the control group. The mortality in the study group was due to one intrauterine death, two neonatal deaths due to meningitis (1 spina bifida) and a pair of imma-

Table 4. Distribution of percentiles of the first generation who have had children

Percentiles	Study group (n = 41)	Control group (n = 31)
<2.3	2	2
2.3–10	1	4
10–25	6	6
25–50	10	3
50–75	13	6
75–90	7	5
90–97.7	1	3
>97.7	1	1
unknown	0	1

Table 6.   Gestational age of second generation

	Amenorrhea	Study group (N = 65)	Control group (N = 45)
Immature:	±25 weeks	1 (twins)	—
Premature:	30	1	—
	31	—	—
	32	2	—
	33	1	—
	34	2	—
	35	—	1 (twins)
	36	1	3
Full-term:	37	8	5
	38	6	4
	39	1	—
	40	37	23
	41	—	2
	42	4	5
Unknown:		0	1

ture twins. In the control group there was only one intrauterine death.

Fertility and Fecundity

As reported above, in the study group of 77 children, 41 have had children, versus 31 out of 63 in the control group. The number of abortions is comparable between the two groups: 8 in the study group versus 7 in the control group.

The mean age of the 26 women in the first-generation study group who have given birth was 28 years, versus 27.9 in the control group of 20 women. The mean age of the 15 men was 27.9 years in the study group versus 28.8 in the control group of 11 men.

In the women in the study group, the interval between the first and second baby was slightly longer (32.9 months, $N = 12$) versus that for women in the control group (29.9 months, $N = 8$). The same holds true for the men: the interval is respectively 25.0 months ($N = 6$) versus 20.1 months ($N = 4$).

Congenital Malformations

Table 8 lists the malformations that were found in the second-generation children.

DISCUSSION

In this study the numbers were small. Also, the blood levels of the different anticonvulsant agents were not known during the pregnancies of the epileptic women. It is known that a combination of anticonvulsants can be more deleterious because of biochemical processes enhanced by one drug influencing the metabolism of another. Genetic background also plays a role both for mother and baby (Phelan, Pellock, & Nance, 1982; Spielberg, 1983).

The study group turned out to be a relatively favorable one, as could be expected; no congenital malformations or signs of the fetal hydantoin/barbiturate syndrome were found after retrospectively studying the files. One boy out of 77 first-generation children has

Table 7.   Number of offspring of mothers on anticonvulsants

Gestational age (weeks)	Fedrick (1973) (England) (N = 212)	Dukkers van Emden, Koppe, and Peters (1981) (Amsterdam) (N = 257)	Study group First generation (N = 77)	Second generation (N = 65)
≤30	1	0	0	3
31 to 34	1	2	1	5
35 to 36	6	5	2	1
Percentage premature	3.8%	2.7%	3.9%	13.9%

Table 8. Type and number of congenital malformations present in second-generation children

	Epilepsy group (N = 63)	Control group (N = 45)
Vitium cordis	1	—
Pylorospasmus	2	—
Spina bifida	1	—
Athyroidea	1	1
Benign tumor	1	—
Cataract plus shorter leg	—	1
Hip dysplasia	—	1
	6	3

epilepsy himself. He has no children. Moreover, the first-generation children who have had children can represent a further selection to a more favorable group by nature. Their percentiles in comparison to the entire group point in this direction.

Considering these rather favorable characteristics of the study group children who have borne infants, the abnormal findings in their reproductive performance are the more remarkable and unexpected, but in accordance with the animal studies of Sonawane and Yaffe (1983).

CONCLUSION

This study gives preliminary data on reproductive performance of daughters and sons of mothers on anticonvulsant drugs. There is a trend to both intrauterine growth retardation and premature deliveries in the study group.

A weak point of the study is the small number, making statistical analysis difficult, and also the fact that blood levels of the anticonvulsants during pregnancy are not known.

At the moment, the question of whether it is possible to relate duration of medication, type of drug or combinations of drugs, and later reproductive performance in this group is being studied. An extension of the group to include more numbers also seems desirable for purposes of statistical analysis.

REFERENCES

Annegers, J.F., Elveback, L.R., Hauser, W.A., & Kurland, L.T. Do anticonvulsants have a teratogenic effect? *Archives of Neurology*, 1974, *31*, 364–373.

Bjerkedal, T., & Bahna, S.L. The course and outcome of pregnancy in women with epilepsy. *Acta Obstetrica et Gynecologica Scandinavica*, 1973, *52*, 245–248.

Blatner, W.A., Henson, D.E., Young, R.C., & Fraumeni, J.F. Malignant mesenchymoma and birth defects; prenatal exposure to phenytoin. *Journal of the American Medical Association*, 1977, *238*, 334–335.

Creveld, S. van. Morbus hemorrhagicus neonatorum. *Nederlands Tijdschrift voor Geneeskunde [Netherlands Journal of Medicine]*, 1957, *101*, 2109–2112.

Davies, P.P. Coagulation defect due to anticonvulsant drug treatment in pregnancy. *Lancet*, 1970, *i*, 413.

Dukkers van Emden, D.M., Koppe, J.G., & Peters, G.J.M. Prenatale factoren en het risico van kanker bij kinderen, met name het gebruik van anti-epileptica in de zwangerschap [Prenatal exposure to drugs and the risk in cancer in offspring, especially anticonvulsant agents]. Amsterdam: KWF-projekt Nr.18 (1981).

Elshove, J., & van Eck, J.H.M. Aangeboren misvormingen met name gespleten lip met of zonder gespleten verhemelte bij kinderen van moeders met epilepsie [Congenital malformations (cleft lip and/or palate) in children of mothers with epilepsy]. *Nederlands Tijdschrift voor Geneeskunde [Netherlands Journal of Medicine]*, 1971, *115*, 1371–1375.

Fedrick, J. Epilepsy and pregnancy: A report from the Oxford Record Linkage Study. *British Medical Journal*, 1973, *i*, 442–448.

Feldman, G.L., Weaver, D., & Lovrien, E.W. The fetal trimethadione syndrome. *American Journal of Diseases of Children*, 1977, *131*, 1389–1392.

Gupta, C.H., Shapiro, B.H., & Yaffe, S.J. Decreased neonataol testosterone in plasma and brain with subsequent reproductive dysfunction of the offspring exposed to phenobarbital (PB) prenatally. *Pediatric Research*, 1980, *14*, 467.

Hanson, J.W., & Smith, D.W. The fetal hydantoin syndrome. *The Journal of Pediatrics*, 1975, *87*, 285–290.

Hill, R.M. Drugs ingested by pregnant women. *Clinical Pharmacology and Therapeutics*, 1973, *14*, 654–659.

Hill, R.M., Verniaud, W.M., Horning, M.G., McCulley, L.B., & Morgan, N.F. Infants exposed in utero to antiepileptic drugs. *American Journal of Diseases of Children*, 1974, *127*, 645–653.

Janz, D., & Fuchs, U. Sind antiepileptische Medikamente während der Schwangerschaft schädlich? [Are anticonvulsant agents toxic during pregnancy?] *Deutsche Medizinische Wochenschrift [German Medical Weekly]*, 1964, *89*, 241–243.

Kloosterman, G.J. Over intra-uteriene groei en de intra-uteriene groeicurve [On intra-uterine growth and the intra-uterine growth curve]. (Verslag vergadering dd 9-11-1968). *Nederlands Tijdschrift voor Verloskunde [Netherlands Journal for Obetetrics]*, 1969, *69*, 349–365.

Koppe, J.G., Bosman, W., Oppers, V.M., Spaans, F., & Kloosterman, G.J. Epilepsie en aangeboren afwijkingen [Epilepsy and congenital malformations]. *Nederlands Tijdschrift voor Geneeskunde [Netherlands Journal of Medicine]*, 1973, *117*, 220–224.

Meadow, S.R. Anticonvulsant drugs and congenital abnormalities. *Lancet*, 1968, *ii*, 1296.

Miller, R.W. Clinical clues to interactions in carcinogenesis. In: Gelboin et al. (eds.), *Genetic and environmental factors in experimental and human cancer*. Tokyo: Japan Sci. Soc. Press, 1980. (a)

Miller, R.W. Prevention - The ultimate solution. In: Van Eys & Sullivan (eds.), *Status of the curability of childhood cancers*. New York: Raven Press, 1980. (b)

Mirkin, B.L. Diphenylhydantoin: Placental transport, fetal localization, neonatal metabolism and possible teratogenic effects. *The Journal of Pediatrics*, 1971, *78*, 329–337.

Mountain, K.R., Hirsch, J., & Gallus, A.S. Neonatal coagulation defect due to anticonvulsant drug treatment in pregnancy. *Lancet*, 1970, *i*, 265–268.

Pendergrass, T.W., & Hanson, J.W. Fetal hydantoin syndrome and neuroblastoma. *Lancet*, 1976, *ii*, 150.

Phelan, M.G., Pellock, J.M., & Nance, W.E. Discordant expression of fetal hydantoin syndrome in heteropaternal dizygotic twins. *New England Journal of Medicine*, 1982, *307*, 99–101.

Seeler, R.A., Israel, J.N., Royal, J.E., Kaye, C.I., Rao, S., & Abulaban, M. Ganglioneuroblastoma and fetal hydantoin-alcohol syndromes. *Pediatrics*, 1979, *63*, 524–527.

Sherman, & Roizen, N. Fetal hydantoin syndrome and neuroblastoma. *Lancet*, 1976, *ii*, 517.

Sonawane, B.R., & Yaffe, S.J. Delayed effects of drug exposure during pregnancy: Reproductive function. *Biological Research in Pregnancy*, 1983, *4*, 48–55.

Speidel, B.D., & Meadow, S.R. Maternal epilepsy and abnormalities of the fetus and newborn. *Lancet*, 1972, *ii*, 839–843.

Spielberg, S.P. Pharmacogenesis and the fetus. *New England Journal of Medicine*, 1982, *307*, 115–116.

Starreveld-Zimmerman, A.A.E., van der Klok, W.J., Meinardi, H., & Elshove, J. Are anticonvulsants teratogenic? *Lancet*, 1973, *ii*, 48–49.

Vert, P., André, M., & Deblay, M.E. Infants of epileptic mothers. In: L. Stern (ed.) *Intensive care in the newborn*, Vol. II. New York: Masson Publishing, USA, Inc., 1978.

The At-Risk Infant: Psycho/Socio/Medical Aspects
edited by Shaul Harel, M.D., and Nicholas J. Anastasiow, Ph.D.
Copyright © 1985   Paul H. Brookes Publishing Co., Inc.   Baltimore • London

Chapter 16

Fetal Brain Damage
of Circulatory Origin

JEANNE-CLAUDIE LARROCHE, M.D.
Port-Royal Hospital, Paris, France

U NDER THE GENERAL HEADING OF FETAL brain damage can be grouped a variety of lesions that occur *in utero* and are related either to fetal or maternal conditions and/or to anomalies of the placenta and cord. The morphological aspects of the lesions depend on the time of occurrence of the insult *in utero,* that is, the state of maturation of the fetal brain, and on the time elapsed between the insult and the examination of the brain. Now, with ultrasound (US) examinations of the fetus and US or CT scan of the neonate done within the first hours of life, these lesions can easily be detected and even dated. Therefore, lesions should no longer be attributed automatically to difficult labor and birth, but instead could be linked to conditions that arise earlier in the course of development.

A classification of these lesions can now be based on morphological criteria and on circumstances in which they arise. The classifications are presented below. The first group includes those damages that are related to abnormal fetal conditions.

ABNORMAL FETAL CONDITIONS

Multiple Pregnancies

Until recently, the relationship between brain damage and multiple pregnancy has been poorly appreciated (Aicardi, Goutieres, & Hodeborg de Verbois, 1972; Manterola, Towbin, & Yakovlev, 1966; Smith & Rodeck, 1975). One condition that should be examined is the monochorionic placenta. In monochorionic placentas, large anastomoses between the two circulations are frequent, leading to the so-called transfusion syndrome. The author and her colleagues have observed various situations upon delivery, three of which are described below.

In the first situation, neither twin survived. At delivery, one fetus was macerated; the other, born alive, presented respiratory distress, convulsions, and inactive EEG. Echography showed enlarged ventricles. Multiple areas were poorly echogenic. Death occurred within a few hours. At autopsy, the brain was small for the age of the infant, the hemispheres were soft and collapsed. Parts of frontal and temporal lobes were relatively preserved as well as the brain stem and cerebellum. Horizontal serial celloidin sections disclosed hydranencephaly. The hemispheres were nearly "empty," maintained only by the meninges and the molecular layer. Temporal lobes, basal ganglia, brain stem, and cerebellum were recognizable as can be seen in Figure 1.

In a second situation deserving of attention, both twins were born alive. One infant died soon after birth. At autopsy, there was a severe

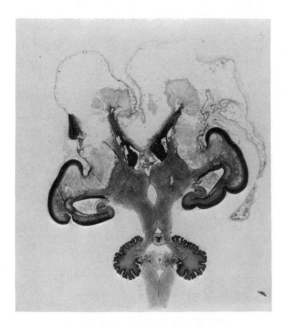

Figure 1. Hydranencephaly in a twin. Thalamus and brain stem are relatively preserved (serial celloidin sections).

softening in the territory of the middle cerebral artery on one side. The surviving twin was normal. In another similar case, there were old cystic lesions in the white matter of both hemispheres of a twin who died. The surviving twin was also normal.

In a third situation, both twins were born alive and survived. One was normal, the other showed signs of abnormal neurological status. A CT scan done at 2 days showed characteristic features of hydranencephaly.

The cause of these cerebral lesions is not clear. Their distribution is not consistent with venous infarction; in a few cases the lesions were located in a particular arterial territory, but they may also predominate in the white matter. Circulatory impairment in twins can arise in several ways. In monochorionic placentas, anastomoses between the two fetal placental circulations frequently exist and differences in blood pressure between the two circulations often lead to disparate growth of the fetuses. If blood flow is severely impaired in one circulation, the corresponding fetus may die and become macerated. Subsequently, necrotic or thrombotic material may pass from the macerated placenta to the surviving fetus, causing single or multiple emboli or dissemi-

nated intravascular coagulation. Occlusions of large arteries have been demonstrated on angiography, but the mechanism is poorly understood (Yoshioka, Kadomoto, Mino, Morikawa, Kasubuchi, & Kusumoki, 1979). Alternatively, an episode of severe maternal arterial hypotension can lead to death of one fetus and to brain damage in the survivor. Or, depending on the severity of the vascular impairment, both infants may be born alive and brain lesions can be apparent in one or both twins.

Neurological signs may be obvious at birth, but they are not specific and are often overshadowed by respiratory distress. Cases with an interval between birth and the onset of abnormalities have been reported with no satisfactory explanation. A CT scan (Choulot, LeClerc, & Saint Martin, 1982) or US examination, as mentioned earlier, permits early diagnosis and evaluation of both localization and extent of the damage. In infants who survive, a wide range of neurological disabilities has been described. Microcephaly is the rule, but normal or even increased head circumference with intracranial hypertension may develop.

In multiple pregnancies, growth and vitality of the fetuses can be closely followed by frequent US examinations. Unfortunately, ultrasound is not helpful in detecting a possible compromised fetal circulation, and brain damage is likely to occur before appropriate obstetrical action can be taken.

Arterial Occlusions

Softening in a particular cerebral arterial territory has been observed at autopsy of stillborn infants and in those who died soon after birth (Clark & Linell, 1954; Larroche, 1977; Larroche & Amiel, 1966). The lesions may be recent or old. The pathogenesis is poorly understood. It has been suggested that emboli arising from the fetal veins or placenta might reach cerebral arteries because of the large right-left shunt during fetal life.

At autopsy, the lesions are very similar to those observed later in life. In one such case (Figure 2), one hemisphere was smaller than the other and was the site of palpable softening

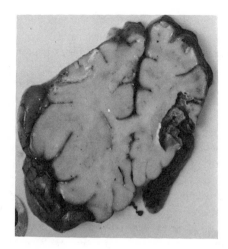

Figure 2. Occlusion of the left middle cerebral artery in a stillborn infant.

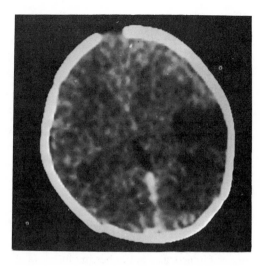

Figure 3. Occlusion of the right middle cerebral artery as detected by CT scan at 2 days. (Courtesy of Dr. Amiel.)

consisting of cavitations of various sizes crossed by trabeculae in the territory of the occluded middle cerebral artery. On histological examination, the cortex was found to be a ribbonlike structure devoid of neurons. The underlying tissue showed multiple cavitations, and the walls of the pseudocysts contained glial cells, macrophages, and encrusted neurons. In another case, cerebral peduncles, pons, and medulla oblongata were asymmetrical with marked atrophy of the pyramidal tract; these features suggested that the vascular accident had occurred long before birth. The middle cerebral artery was dissected and cut in serial sections that disclosed an old parietal thrombus and disrupted lamina elastica interna; there was no inflammatory reaction. On the basis of morphological criteria, however, it was not possible to differentiate this thrombus from an old embolus. When occlusion occurs early in fetal life, anomalies of morphogenesis and cytoarchitecture (Larroche, 1977; Norman, 1980) can be observed. Now, when CT scan and US are performed within the first hours of life, such softenings as seen in Figure 3 can easily be detected and dated. In survivors, the diagnosis of hemiplegia is usually confirmed within a few months.

Blood Dyscrasia

Intracerebral hemorrhage occurring *in utero* has been described in cases of throm-

bocytopenia (Zalneraitis, Young, & Krishnamoorthy, 1979) and in a case of hydrops fetalis due to hemolytic disease (Bose, 1978). In a case of thromboembolic disease of unknown origin that developed in fetal life, the brain abnormalities were diagnosed by US in a 2-day-old infant. On coronal view, the ventricles were enlarged with irregular, crenated borders. In addition, the infant presented diffuse hemorrhagic necrosis of the skin and various viscera. At autopsy, the ventricular cavities were ill defined with multiple disruptions in a necrotico-hemorrhagic parenchyma (Figure 4). Histological examination showed disseminated thrombi and diffuse, massive calcifications. These features, observed in an

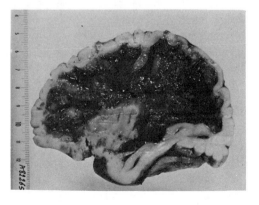

Figure 4. Fetal thromboembolic disease. Severe necrotico-hemorrhagic lesions.

infant who died at 3 days of age, suggested that the insult had occurred at least 1 week before birth.

MATERNAL PATHOLOGICAL CONDITIONS

The second group of lesions may be related to various maternal pathological conditions.

Hypertension

Hypertension has long been incriminated in the pathogenesis of fetal cerebral damage, mainly in the 1950s and 1960s (Rizzuto & Martin, 1967). However, the lesions were rarely described in neonates but rather in older infants. Because of apparently normal labor and delivery, there was no doubt, for Rizzuto and Martin, that the lesions had occurred *in utero*.

Maternal Bee Sting Anaphylaxis

Erasmus, Blackwood, and Wilson (1982) have reported that maternal bee sting anaphylaxis during pregnancy leads to severe fetal brain damage. The lesions were diagnosed *in utero* by US; they were confirmed in the neonate by CT scan and finally described at autopsy.

Maternal Trauma during Pregnancy

Maternal trauma during pregnancy and its potential deleterious effects on the fetal circulation have been mentioned several times in the recent literature (Coignet, Palix, Tommasi, & Raybaud, 1979; Ferrer & Navarro, 1978). Direct trauma to the abdominal wall of the mother with cephalhematoma of the fetus has been reported. Diagnosis of the cephalhematoma was made *in utero* by US. The infant was delivered by cesarean section and the cephalhematoma resolved completely within 3 weeks (Grylack, 1982).

Car Accident without Direct Trauma

In several cases, car accident without direct trauma was incriminated in the origin of fetal brain damage, posing difficult legal problems. In the first case, the mother had three normal US studies during early and mid-pregnancy. At 34 weeks, she had a car accident. She was not hurt but only deeply stressed and also noticed that the baby stopped moving. At 37 weeks,

US showed dilated ventricles in an otherwise normal fetus. She gave birth soon after to a baby who died at 7 minutes of life. At autopsy, the brain was normally convoluted for the gestional age; the meninges over the brain stem and cerebellum showed a brownish discoloration; the ventricles were enlarged, the ependyma was covered with a fine, granular, rusty deposit, suggesting posthemorrhagic hydrocephaly. In addition, the left hemisphere was the site of multicystic malacia. Both macroscopic and microscopic aspects were consistent with lesions several weeks old. In two other cases, the babies were delivered at term, several weeks after the mothers' car accidents. At autopsy, the brains were atrophic and showed bilateral multicystic encephalomalacia and dilated ventricles (Figure 5). The diffuse ischemic lesions might have resulted from temporary impairment of placental blood flow due to maternal stress during the accident. It has been demonstrated in the pregnant rhesus monkey (Myers, 1975) that maternal psychological stress may produce episodes of fetal asphyxia and ischemia with brain damage similar to that just described in neonates. Catecholamine discharge might have

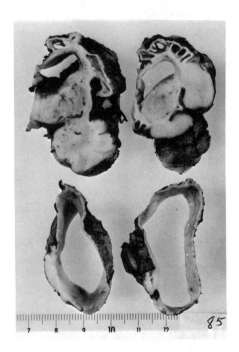

Figure 5. Multicystic encephalopathy following maternal car accident. (Courtesy of Dr. Hanau.)

led to uterine vasoconstriction and impaired intervillous space perfusion.

Inhalation of Carbon Monoxide

Another maternal pathological condition that may be related to fetal cerebral damage is inhalation of carbon monoxide. Microgyria was reported after an accident early in fetal life, and softening of white matter and basal ganglia was observed when the accident occurred later in fetal life.

Inhalation of Butane Gas

A case of attempted suicide by inhalation of butane gas at 30 weeks gestation illustrates the effects of pure total anoxia, probably followed by prolonged cardiovascular collapse (Gosseye, Golaire, & Larroche, 1982). The pregnant woman was found comatose and needed resuscitation. Four weeks later, labor began spontaneously and she gave birth to an infant who died soon after. The external surface of the hemispheres corresponded to 30 weeks gestation. Sections of the brain disclosed severe, diffuse, multicystic encephalomalacia and enlarged ventricles as seen in Figure 6. Histological examination showed old infarcts with loss of neurons, glial and macrophagic reaction, and abundant calcium deposits. Brain stem and cerebellum were also severely damaged.

ANOMALIES OF THE PLACENTA AND CORD

The third group of lesions may be related to anomalies of the placenta and cord. A case of severe placental calcification without intrauterine growth retardation has been observed. The infant was born at term, suffering from asphyxia and in a coma. A CT scan at 2 days showed a diffuse hypodensity interpreted at first as hydranencephaly (Figure 7). The infant died a few hours later. The brain at autopsy was edematous but grossly preserved. Histological

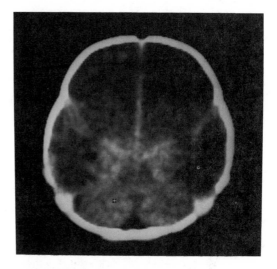

Figure 7. CT scan at 2 days. Hydranencephaly.

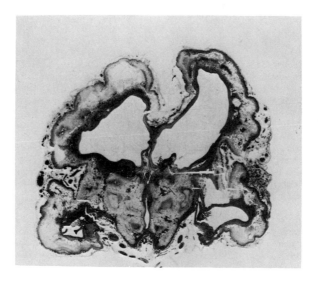

Figure 6. Hydranencephaly following maternal butane gas inhalation (serial celloidin sections).

examination as shown in Figure 8 revealed total loss of neurons in the hemispheres with diffuse glial and macrophagic proliferation and prominent capillary endothelial cells, features that suggested that the lesions had developed at least a week before birth.

The marked and diffuse hypodensity observed on CT corresponded to a near total loss of cells without macroscopic loss of tissue; with longer survival these lesions might have evolved to true hydranencephaly.

CONCLUSION

Fetal brain damage may be due to a variety of pathological conditions resulting in circulatory impairments. These lesions have long been described by pathologists and have recently received the renewed interest of obstetricians and pediatricians. The widespread utilization of ultrasound has made it possible to visualize the lesions in fetuses or soon after birth, and to

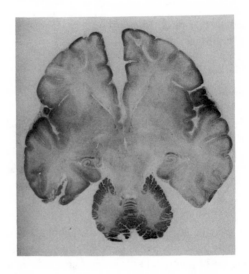

Figure 8. Brain of Figure 7, grossly normal. Near total loss of neurons on serial celloidin sections.

approximately date them. Although the pathogenesis is not fully understood, birth trauma, as a cause, can be discarded in most cases.

REFERENCES

Aicardi, J., Goutieres, F.F., & Hodeborg de Verbois, A. Multicystic encephalomalacia of infants and its relation to abnormal gestation and hydranencephaly. *Journal of Neurological Sciences*, 1972, *15*, 357–373.

Bose, C. Hydrops fetalis and *in utero* intracranial haemorrhage. *The Journal of Pediatrics*. 1978, *93*, 1023.

Choulot, J.J., LeClerc, M.A., & Saint Martin, J. Malformation Cérébrale et jumeau survivant [Cerebral malformation and surviving twins]. *Archives Francaises de Pediatrie [Archives of French Pediatrics]*, 1982, *39*, 105–107.

Clark, R.M., & Linell, E.A. Case report: Premature occlusion of the internal carotid artery. *Journal of Neurology, Neurosurgery and Psychiatry*, 1954, 295–297.

Coignet, J., Palix, C., Tommasi, C., & Raybaud, Ch. Apport de la scanographie dans la souffrance cérébrale du nouveau-né [Contribution of the scan in cerebral distress of the newborn child]. *Pediatrie [Pediatrics]*, 1979, *XXXIV*, 787–797.

Erasmus, C., Blackwood, W., & Wilson, J. Infantile multicystic encephalomalacia after maternal bee sting anaphylaxis during pregnancy. *Archives of Disease in Childhood*, 1982, *57*, 785–787.

Ferrer, I., & Navarro, C. Multicystic encephalomalacia of infancy. *Journal Neurological Sciences*, 1978, *38*, 179–189.

Gosseye, S., Golaire, M.C., & Larroche, J. Cl. Cerebral, renal and splenic lesions due to fetal anoxia and their relationship to malformations. *Developmental Medicine and Child Neurology*, 1982, *24*, 510–518.

Grylack, L. Prenatal sonographic diagnosis of cephalohematoma due to pre-labor trauma. *Pediatric Radiology*, 1982, *12*, 145–147.

Larroche, J. Cl. *Developmental pathology of the neonate*. Amsterdam: Excerpta Medica, 1977.

Larroche, J. Cl., & Amiel, Cl. Thrombose de l'artère sylvienne á la période neonatale. Etude anatomique et discussion pathogénique des hémiplégies dites congénitales [Thrombus of the middle cerebral artery in the neonatal period. Anatomical study and pathogenic discussion of congenital hemiplegias]. *Archives Francaise de Pédiatrie [Archives of French Pediatrics]*, 1966, *XXIII*, 257–274.

Manterola, A., Towbin, A., & Yakovlev, P.I. Cerebral infarction in the human fetus near term. *Journal Neuropathology and Experimental Neurology*, 1966, *25*, 479–488.

Myers, R.E. Maternal psychological stress and fetal asphyxia: A study in the monkey. *American Journal of Obstetrics and Gynecology*, 1975, *122*, 47–59.

Norman, M.G. Bilateral encephaloclastic lesions in a 26 week gestation fetus: Effect on neuroblast migration. *Journal Canadien des Sciences Neurologiques [Canadian Journal of Neurological Sciences]*, 1980, *7*, 191–194.

Rizzuto, N., & Martin, L. Le problème de l'encéphalopathie foetale kystique survenant au cours du deuxième tiers de la grossesse [The problem of the fetal cystic encephalopathy occurring during the mid trimester]. *Biology of the Neonate*, 1967, *11*, 115–127.

Smith, J.F., Rodeck, C. Multiple cystic and focal encephalomalacia in infancy and childhood with brainstem
damage. *Journal Neurological Sciences,* 1975, *25,*
377–388.

Yoshioka, H., Kadomoto, Y., Mino, M., Morikawa, Y.,
Kasubuchi, Y., & Kusumoki, T. Multicystic en-
cephalomacia in liveborn twin with a stillborn macerated
co-twin. *The Journal of Pediatrics,* 1979, *95,* 798–800.

Zalneraitis, E.L., Young, R.S.K., & Krishnamoorthy,
K.S. Intracranial hemorrhage *in utero* as a complication
of isoimmune thrombocytopenia. *The Journal of Pediatrics,* 1979, *95,* 611–614.

Chapter 17

Perinatal Hypoxic-Ischemic Brain Damage and Periventricular Hemorrhage
The Pathogenetic Significance of Arterial Pressure Changes

HANS C. LOU, M.D.
The John F. Kennedy Institute, Glostrup, Denmark

ABNORMAL NEUROLOGICAL AND INTELLEC-tual development affects the lives of an estimated 10% of children in modern society. Among the causes of impairment, perinatal hypoxia, ischemia, and periventricular hemorrhage (PVH) rank high.

Hypoxic-ischemic lesions and severe PVH often occur in the same patient. They are related to perinatal asphyxia and consequent hypoxia and hypercarbia (De Reuck, Chatta, & Richardson, 1972; Fujimura, Salisbury, Robinson, et al., 1979). Recent data permit establishment of a comprehensive model of the pathogenesis of both of these disorders.

FACTORS THAT PREDISPOSE TO PERINATAL ASPHYXIA

Conditions leading to perinatal asphyxia are insufficient gas exchange or transport, either via the placenta or, postnatally, via the lungs. They may be prenatal, intrapartum, or postnatal.

DEFICIENT AUTOREGULATION IN PERINATAL DISTRESS

Crucial to the understanding of the pathogenesis of perinatal hypoxic ischemia and of PVH is the recent finding of deficient autoregulation of cerebral blood flow (CBF) in the distressed fetus (Lou, Lassen, Tweed et al., 1979) and neonate (Lou, Lassen, & Friis-Hansen, 1979a). Cerebral blood flow was studied *in utero* in fetal sheep by the radioactive microsphere technique. In slightly hypertensive asphyxia, CBF was increasesd fivefold, but it decreased proportionally in hypotension induced by bleeding, indicating arteriolar dilation and pressure-passive CBF.

In 19 distressed newborns, a proportional relationship was found between arterial blood pressure (aBP) and CBF several hours after birth. This relationship was also seen in subgroups defined by birth weight (<2,000 grams or >2,000 grams) and by the degree of asphyxia at birth (Apgar score <7 at 1 minute and Apgar score >7), indicating pressure-passive CBF in neonatal distress. In these infants, CBF was studied by the Xe clearance technique. CBF is normally independent of variations in aBP within a wide range, and cerebral circulation is not greatly decreased even at low pressures due to decreased vascular resistance (arteriolar dilation) (Lassen & Paulson, 1969). Hence, the energy state of the brain is preserved (Siesjö & Nilsson, 1971), a prerequisite for normal functional activity and morphological integrity (Astrup, Symon, & Branston, 1977). Conversely, higher aBP induces arteriolar constriction, and CBF and the transmural pressure gradient in capillaries remain fairly constant (Lassen & Paulson, 1969). Since normal autoregulation is absent in the distressed newborn, even moderate hypotension leads to a proportionate decrease in CBF, and hence, ischemia. The effect of ischemia is further aggravated by hypoxemia. In hypertension, the high pressure is transmitted unhampered to the capillary wall with the risk of rupture, as protective arteriolar constriction does not occur. Thus, pressure changes become of prime pathological relevance.

ARTERIAL PRESSURE CHANGES IN ASPHYXIA

There are no data on blood pressure in the human fetus so that deductions must be made from observations in animals. In the preterm sheep fetus, the difference in pressure between the umbilical artery and vein is about 20 mm Hg, and this difference increases toward term to 35 mm Hg (Purves & James, 1969). The deduction that low arterial pressures occur in the human preterm fetus is supported by the finding by many pathologists that the smooth cell layer of the arteries and arterioles is very thin. There are reasons to suspect that aBP increases during birth as even slight or moderate asphyxia initially leads to hypertension, and the birth process itself is a hypoxic insult (Vanucci & Plum, 1975). This is also the case, although to a lesser degree, in cesarean sections. Furthermore, during delivery of the head, cardiac decelerations are produced with each uterine contraction. Deformation of the head probably raises intracranial pressure and elicits a Cushing's response: arterial hypertension and bradycardia (Lou et al., 1979). The mean arterial pressure in normal full-term infants is about 45 mm Hg, and about 40 mm Hg in infants with birth weights of 1,500 grams. These pressures are probably higher than those of a fetus of corresponding gestational age or size and reflect the well-established pattern of a rise in systemic arterial pressure and a fall in

pulmonary arterial pressure as the ductus arteriosus closes.

If asphyxia is prolonged, arterial hypotension will supervene, possibly due to exhaustion of myocardial carbohydrate stores. Actually, hypotension is the rule during the first few hours after birth in moderately or severely distressed infants (Fujimura et al., 1979). As the infant recovers, arterial pressure returns to normal. However, longitudinal studies of aortic blood pressure during the first days of life have shown that further considerable rises occur with a number of events: motor activity, handling procedures such as sucking or physiotherapy, or during apnea or convulsions (Lou & Friis-Hansen, 1979). These events may raise the mean aBP from 80 to 100 mm Hg, even in the small premature infants, probably due to increased sympathetic activity.

Pathological Effects of Pressure Changes

It would seem from the above that in the distressed infant, periods of hypertension and hypotension alternate. As CBF is pressure passive, lesions due to both can be expected, and new data have confirmed this.

PERIVENTRICULAR HEMORRHAGE

As mentioned at the beginning of this chapter, PVH is a frequent event in small premature infants. Labeled RBCs injected soon after birth and ultrasound studies have shown that PVH usually occurs 12–72 hours after birth. In a few cases, however, there is clinical and pathological evidence that the hemorrhages were present at birth. The hemorrhages usually arise from the capillaries of the subependymal germinal matrix which is still present in the premature infant (Hambleton & Wigglesworth, 1976). It is easy to understand why this region is particularly vulnerable: it is the most richly perfused region in the brain and is very loosely organized with poor mechanical support of the vessels. As autoregulation is deficient and dramatic increases in arterial pressure are frequent during recovery from asphyxia or even normal birth, it has been hypothesized that the hemorrhages are due to elevations in arterial pressure (Hambleton & Wigglesworth, 1976; Lou, Lassen, & Friis-Hansen, 1979b). This hypothesis has received support from experimental studies: it is possible to induce intraventricular hemorrhage (IVH) in newborn puppies by raising the mean aBP from 50 to 80 mm Hg (Goddard, Lewis, Armstrong et al., 1979), and clinical data are consistent with this hypothesis (Lou & Friis-Hansen, 1979).

ISCHEMIA

Edema (due to lactic acid accumulation and damage to the blood brain barrier [BBB]) and PVH raise cranial pressure and decrease perfusion pressure (arterial pressure minus intracranial pressure) with ischemia as a result, as autoregulation is lacking. The PVH in itself induces vasospasm and hence, ischemia, as demonstrated by Doppler ultrasound detection of pulsations in the anterior cerebral artery. Infusion of bicarbonate in asphyxiated neonates also seems to aggravate cerebral ischemia. This effect is to be expected if the blood brain barrier is damaged and permits passage of bicarbonate into the perivascular tissues, since increased pH will induce vasoconstriction. Finally, cerebral ischemia can be the direct result of circulatory depression and hypotension often seen in distressed neonates.

IMPACT OF NEONATAL ISCHEMIA ON NEUROLOGICAL DEVELOPMENT

The above study of neonatal CBF (Skov, Lou, & Pedersen, 1984) involved 19 newborns with varying degrees of respiratory distress. Ten of these neonates had had proven episodes of ischemia with CBF values of <20 ml/100 g/min within the first few hours after birth.

Death with clinical signs of severe periventricular hemorrhage (circulatory collapse and a sudden drop in hematocrit) occurred on days 2, 9, and 37 in three of these patients, and in a fourth who had an initial CBF of 26 ml/100 g/min on day 4.

These data suggest that initial ischemia precedes severe PVH and may be a significant pathogenetic factor. Further support for this interpretation is provided by the work of Fu-

jimura et al. showing that lethal PVH is preceded by hypotension (Fujimura et al., 1979). A close association of cerebral ischemia and PVH is also supported by recent data obtained by positron emission tomography, where it has been demonstrated that a large ischemic zone surrounds the hemorrhage (Volpe, Perlman, Herscovitch, & Raichle, 1982).

In 6 of the 10 infants with initial ischemia, atrophic encephalopathy was demonstrated, either at autopsy, or by CT at 1 year of age. None of the other children had developed detectable atrophic lesions. Clinical neurological symptoms such as truncal instability, discoordination, and abnormalities of muscle tone, as well as low scores on The Cattell Infant Intelligence Scale, were also found predominantly in the group with proven neonatal ischemia (Lou, Skov, & Pedersen, 1979).

At reexamination at the age of 4 years, poor articulation, dysphasia, attention deficit, and low IQ (Stanford-Binet) were found significantly more often in the group with low neonatal CBF ($p < .05$, chi-square test, Yates' correction). Dyspraxia, dyssynergia, spasticity, and short-term memory dysfunction were also seen more frequently in this group, although the differences were not statistically significant. By summarizing the abnormal findings in each of the two groups, the severe impact of neonatal ischemia on neurological development became particularly striking: the difference between the groups was significant at the $p < .001$ level (Skov et al., 1984).

All of these infants had been vigorously treated with oxygen, and, where necessary, with ventilation with continuous positive airway pressure, so that Pa_{O_2} values that could be critically low per se (<60 mm Hg) were avoided, except in two infants who had isolated episodes of Pa_{O_2} of 40 and 21 mm Hg, respectively.

It may therefore be concluded that neonatal ischemia is a critical determinant for later neurological and intellectual development, probably the most important single factor at the present state of the art. In accordance with this hypothesis is the consistent finding of hypoperfusion, low metabolic activity, and possible minor structural changes in the white matter border zones between major arterial territories in children with severe learning disorders who were examined with the 133 Xe inhalation computerized emission tomography technique (Lou, Henriksen, & Bruhn, in press).

PREVENTION

It seems from the present discussion that the principal lesions of perinatal cerebral hypoxia-ischemia and PVH in the premature infant are pathogenetically interrelated, a concept that has long been suspected by pathologists.

There are several points in the chain of events leading to such lesions that can be interfered with in an attempt at prevention.

1. The hypoxic insult of birth could be minimized. In fact, an increasing number of clinical studies indicate that PVH is less frequent after cesarean section than after normal birth.

2. Measures such as immediate ventilatory support and adequate monitoring of blood gases and blood pressure could be taken. This means immediate naso-tracheal intubation and cauterization of the umbilical artery in small prematures. It is probably wiser to allow the infant to prove that it can be safely extubated than to wait for respiratory insufficiency to develop

It seems that hyperventilation at birth protects against the development of early PVH. Retrospective analysis of 63 premature infants with birth weights of <1,350 grams at the University of California in San Francisco have shown that among the 26 accidentally hyperventilated babies, none developed early PVH, a fact that could not be explained by differences in pulmonary function (Lou, Phibbs, Wilson, & Gregory, 1982). Removal of hydrogen ions by decreasing Pa_{CO_2} from the perivascular tissue of the brain could possibly enhance restoration of a normal autoregulation. Further studies will be needed before the safety and efficacy of hyperventilation can be ascertained.

3. Circulatory support to prevent hypotension is important in the absence of normal autoregulation in order to prevent ischemia. Prudent administration of repeated, small transfusions aimed at correcting hypotension may be used.

4. Means to avoid excessive arterial pressure peaks in the early neonatal period should be sought. The possible effect of barbiturates in the prevention of PVH may be related to sedation, with stabilization of blood pressure. Another possibility is to use muscle relaxants that effectively seem to stabilize blood pressure in infants on a ventilator (Perlman, McMenamin, & Volpe, 1983).

5. Finally, attempts have been made to stabilize the capillary membranes with ethamsylate.

In summary, the "lost autoregulation hypothesis" points to a number of possible methods of prevention of PVH in premature infants. The ideal solution to the problem would, however, be elimination of premature birth. Sadly, this possibility is not yet in sight.

REFERENCES

Astrup, J., Symon, L., & Branston, N.M. Cortical evoked potentials and extracellular K and H at critical levels of brain ischemia. *Stroke, 1977, 8,* 51–57.

De Reuck, J., & Chatta, A.S., & Richardson, E.P. Pathogenesis and evolution of periventricular leukomalacia. *Archives of Neurology, 1972, 27,* 299–336.

Fujimura, M., Salisbury, D.N., Robinson, R.O., et al. Clinical events relating to intraventricular haemorrhage in the newborn. *Archives of Diseases in Childhood,* 1979, 409–414.

Goddard, H., Lewis, R.M., Armstrong, D.L., et al. *Intraventricular hemorrhage—an animal model: Initial hypertension studies.* Paper presented at the annual meeting of the Child Neurology Society, Hanover, NH, September, 1979.

Hambleton, G., & Wigglesworth, J.S. Origin of intraventricular haemorrhage in the preterm infant. *Archives of Diseases in Childhood, 1976, 51,* 651–659.

Lassen, N.A., Paulson, O.B. Partial cerebral vasoparalysis in patients with apoplexy: Dissociation between carbon dioxide responsiveness and autoregulation. In: M. Brock, C. Fieschi, D.H. Ingvar, et al. (eds.), *Cerebral blood flow.* Berlin: Springer Verlag, 1969.

Lou, H.C., & Friis-Hansen, B. Elevations in arterial blood pressure during motor activity and epileptic seizures in the newborn. *Acta Pediatrica Scandinavica*, 1979, *68*, 803–806.

Lou, H.C., Henriksen, L., & Bruhn, P. Is childhood attention deficit disorder (ADD) a frontal cortex dysconnection syndrome? Focal cerebral hypoperfusion in children with dysphasia and/or ADD. *Archives of Neurology*, in press.

Lou, H.C., Lassen, N.A., & Friis-Hansen, B. Impaired autoregulation of cerebral blood flow in the distressed newborn infant. *The Journal of Pediatrics*, 1979, *94*, 118–212.(a)

Lou, H.C., Lassen, N.A., & Friis-Hansen, B. Is arterial hypertension crucial for the development of intraventricular haemorrhage in the neonatale? *Lancet*, 1979, *1*, 1215–1217.(b)

Lou, H.C., Lassen, N.A., Tweed, W.A., et al. Pressure passive cerebral blood flow and breakdown of the blood-brain barrier in experimental fetal asphyxia. *Acta Pediatrica Scandinavica*, 1979, *68*, 57–63.

Lou, H.C., Phibbs, R., Wilson, S., & Gregory, G. Hyperventilation at birth may prevent early periventricular hemorrhage. *Lancet*, 1982, *1*, 1407.

Lou, H.C., Skov, H., & Pederson, H. Low cerebral blood flow: A risk factor in the neonatale. *The Journal of Pediatrics*, 1979, *95*, 606–609.

Perlman, J.M., McMenamin, J.B., Volpe, J.J. Fluctu-

ating cerebral blood flow velocity in respiratory-distress syndrome. Relation to the development of intraventricular hemorrhage. *New England Journal of Medicien*, 1983, *309*, 204–209.

Purves, J.M., & James, I.M. Observations of the control of cerebral blood flow in the sheep fetus and newborn lamb. *Circulation Research*, 1969, *25*, 651–667.

Siesjö, B.K., & Nilsson, L. The influence of arterial hypoxemia upon labile phosphates and upon extracellular and intracellular lactate and pyruvate concentrations in the rat brain. *Scandinavian Journal of Clinical and Laboratory Investigations*, 1971, *27*, 83–96.

Skov, H., Lou, H.C., & Pedersen, H. Neonatal ischemia-impact on the four-year-old child. *Journal of Developmental Medicine and Child Neurology*, 1984, *26*, 353–357.

Vanucci, R.C.M., & Plum, F. Pathophysiology of perinatal hypoxic-ischemic brain damage. In: G. Garell (ed.), *Biology of brain dysfunction*. New York: Plenum Publishing Corp., 1975.

Volpe, J., Perlman, J.M., Herscovitch, P., & Raichle, M.E. Positron emission tomography in the assessment of regional cerebral blood flow in the newborn. *Annals of Neurology*, 1982, *12*, 225–226.

Chapter 18

Neonatal Hypoxic-Ischemic Encephalopathy

ALFRED W. BRANN, JR., M.D.

Emory University School of Medicine, Atlanta, Georgia

O VER THE PAST CENTURY, NUMEROUS ETI- ologies for perinatally related central nervous system pathology and neurological dysfunction seen in children have been defined. They include the following:

1. Chromosomal abnormalities
2. Dysmorphic syndromes
3. Infections
4. Inherited metabolic diseases
5. Trauma
6. Intracranial hemorrhage
7. Metabolic disorders
   a. *Hypoxic ischemia*
   b. Hypoglycemia
   c. Hyperbilirubinemia
   d. Hypernatremia

This chapter concentrates on the effects of hypoxic ischemia on the brain of the full-term fetus/neonate. Much has been and continues to be written about this area. In a landmark treatise written in 1862, a causal link between suboptimal perinatal events and subsequent neurological dysfunction and brain damage in both preterm and full-term infants was first made. This article, by W. J. Little, was entitled "On the Influence of Abnormal Parturition, Difficult Labours, Premature Birth, and Asphyxia Neonatorum on the Mental and Physical Condition of the Child, Especially in Re-

lation to Deformities'' (Little, 1861). From this article and other classical retrospective clinical and neuropathological studies using human autopsy material, the term "birth injury" was coined. Since its inception, this term has been used in a broad, nonselective manner to include both physical injury ("birth trauma") and asphyxial insult to the neonate's brain during the actual birthing process ("birth asphyxia")(Courville, 1971).

Prior to the 1940s, "birth trauma" was felt to be the overriding etiological and pathogenetic mechanism leading to the bulk of perinatally related brain damage. With improvement both in the management of dysfunctional labor and in the management of fetuses of abnormal size and position, actual birth trauma to the nervous system has been almost totally reduced to brachial plexus and facial nerve injury.

Information concerning the specific effect of "birth asphyxia" on the fetus/neonate has been possible only since the development of techniques for determining the value of blood pH and blood gases. Articles began to appear in the 1940s that strongly suggested a link between neonatal brain damage and perinatal asphyxia. In a second landmark article, Stewart Clifford described a group of neonates who died following delivery by cesarean birth for premature separation of the placenta (Clifford,

1941). At the time of death, these infants were found to have brain swelling and cerebral necrosis. During the infants' clinical course, devoid of evidence for birth trauma, an asphyxial etiology was suggested from acid base and blood gas studies. There was also a strong suggestion that asphyxia during the perinatal period was the etiology that led to the development of ulegyria in children who as neonates survived a perinatal insult (Courville, 1971; Friedman & Courville, 1941). Recent human and animal studies have permitted a clearer distinction between the effects of asphyxia and trauma on the fetal/neonatal nervous system.

Classical clinical neuropathological studies of brains from neonates who have experienced an episode of "perinatal distress" have identified three distinct sites of damage to the neonatal brain (Banker, 1967; Terplan, 1967; Towbin, 1970). These sites are: 1) the region of the subependymal germinal matrix, 2) the periventricular white matter, and 3) the cortical and subcortical gray matter. When babies with these three loci of brain lesions are classified by gestational age, it becomes apparent that there are differences in the loci of lesions seen in the preterm infant as compared to lesions seen in the full-term neonate. The principal lesion seen in the preterm infant is located at the center of the hemisphere in the germinal matrix along the periventricular region, with sparing of the cortical mantle. This was a hemorrhagic lesion giving rise to the term *subependymal germinal matrix hemorrhage/intraventricular hemorrhage* (SE/IVH). The second lesion, noted in the white matter of the periventricular region at the angles of the ventricle, superior to the germinal matrix, is cystic in nature and has been called *periventricular leucomalacia* (PVL). Although it is seen predominantly in preterm infants, it has been described in full-term infants. The third lesion seen in the full-term infant is located principally in the peripheral and dorsal areas of the cerebral cortex gyri at the depths of sulci and the neuronal nuclei of the basal ganglia. The term used to designate intrapartumally asphyxiated full-term infants with this third type of lesion and a particular type of neonatal neurological dysfunction is *neonatal hypoxic-ischemic encephalopathy* (HIE).

The magnitude of the problem of neonatal hypoxic-ischemic encephalopathy is not fully appreciated. Three important factors contribute to the magnitude of this problem. First, more children with cerebral palsy were full-term infants than preterm infants. The reason for this discrepancy is that even though the incidence of cerebral palsy (Nelson & Ellenberg, 1979) is lower in the full-term infant (3.38/1,000 lb.) than in the preterm infant (90/1,000 lb.), the denominator to which this lower incidence is applied is 92% of the births in the United States. Second, more full-term infants who have been asphyxiated survive than do preterm infants (Mulligan, Painter, O'Donoghue, MacDonald, Allen, & Taylor, 1980). Third, the problem of HIE is accentuated because there does not appear to have been a significant reduction in the types of cerebral palsy seen in children who were full-term neonates. A comprehensive population-based Swedish study showed that a decrease in the total incidence of cerebral palsy from 1954 to 1974 was due to a reduction of spastic diplegia in neonates weighing less than 2,500 grams (Hagberg, 1971). Data from hospital-based studies in the United States show a similar reduction in the incidence of CNS sequelae in infants weighing less than 2,500 grams (Koops & Harmon, 1980). Data from the Swedish study do not show any reduction in the incidence of the types of cerebral palsy seen in full-term infants. Thus, in the absence of U.S. data to the contrary, there is no reason to believe that the problem of the full-term asphyxiated neonate is different from that in Sweden.

The current status of knowledge concerning neonatal hypoxic-ischemic encephalopathy is described in the following sections.

CLINICAL FEATURES

The full-term infant, following a period of intrapartum asphyxia from whatever cause, was thought in the past to have a clinical course that reflected primarily an altered state of the brain. However, it is now known that such an infant can have a varied clinical course because of the involvement of different organ systems to varying degrees. The variation in the clinical course of asphyxia in full-term infants probably arises from factors such as the ability of the fetus to redistribute blood flow in protecting vital organs (Meschia & Giacomo, 1979; Peeters, Sheldon, Jones, Makowski, & Meschia, 1979); the current inability to accurately estimate the length, severity, and acuteness of onset of the asphyxial episode; and possibly the existence of components of the asphyxial insult that are as yet unidentified.

To appropriately manage a full-term neonate who has experienced a period of intrapartum asphyxia, the infant must be identified as early as possible. The preferable time of identification is during the intrapartum period so as to reduce the length of the asphyxial episode by appropriate and timely delivery. However, since not all fetuses experiencing asphyxia can be so identified, all neonates must be appropriately evaluated from birth in a sequential fashion.

In order to accomplish an early identification of the full-term infant who has experienced an asphyxial episode, the spectrum of clinical responses is described with a specific concentration on the neonate with neurological dysfunction. This description has three parts: 1) varied multi-organ response, 2) specific signs and chronology of neonatal neurological dysfunction seen in the syndrome of HIE, and, 3) the value of the neonatal neurological exam in the prediction of later outcome following this particular neonatal syndrome.

Varied Multi-Organ Response

The varied clinical course was documented in a retrospective study involving 6,045 consecutive deliveries (Sexson, Sexson, Rawson, & Brann, 1976). Fifty-three full-term infants were found to have had an Apgar score of 5 or less at 1 and 5 minutes, which was thought to be secondary to intrapartum asphyxia. Eighteen of the 53 infants had no clinically apparent disease throughout their hospitalization. However, 35 of the 53 infants had at least one, or as many as five abnormal organ systems. Nineteen of the 35 infants had more than one system

involved. The organ systems involved in the 35 affected infants with low Apgar scores, in order of their decreasing fequency, were the pulmonary system, the cardiovascular system, the central nervous system, the gastrointestinal system, and the renal system. No infants demonstrated problems with the coagulation system although this has been described. Nine of these 35 died during the neonatal period. The common cause of death was persistent pulmonary hypertension that occurred in four infants. No one system or group of systems appeared to be the primary target of the intrapartum asphyxial episode. Only one-third of the infants had clinical signs that suggested central nervous system involvement. Only two of the nine infants who expired died from central nervous system disturbances. These two infants had massive brain swelling with cortical necrosis. It was impossible to clinically predict the CNS or any other organ system as being the affected organ from either the intrapartum course and/or the status of the neonate in the delivery room.

Specific Signs and Chronology

The functional state of the nervous system in an asphyxiated full-term neonate during the first 2 weeks of life is felt to be characteristic enough to be labeled as a specific entity, neonatal hypoxic-ischemic encephalopathy. Data presently indicates that full-term neonates at risk of developing long-term neurological sequelae secondary to intrapartum asphyxia will demonstrate signs of neurological dysfunction within the first few hours after birth. These infants may or may not have a low Apgar score. The major signs of CNS dysfunction include seizures, abnormalities in state of consciousness, tone, posture, reflexes, respiratory pattern, oculovestibular response, autonomic function, and anterior fontanel (Clark, 1964; Finer, Robertson, Richards, Pinnell, & Peters, 1981; Sarnat & Sarnat, 1976; Ziegler, Calame, Marchand, Passera, Reymond-Goni & Prod'hom, 1976).

As the physician assesses the relative risk of an individual neonate developing cerebral palsy, obstetrical complications must be considered as possible risk factors. Numerous prenatal and intrapartum complications have been described as placing the fetus at an increased risk for experiencing intrapartum asphyxia. In a prospective study, the relative risk of cerebral palsy in infants weighing 2,500 grams or more following certain obstetric complications was described in association with the Apgar score (Nelson & Ellenberg, 1983). It was noted that infants born in association with "anoxigenic" obstetrical complications were at no greater risk for developing cerebral palsy when their 5 minute Apgar scores were 6 or higher than in infants whose births were uncomplicated. This group comprised about 62% of the study group and accounted for less than its proportional share of cerebral palsy. There was an increased risk for cerebral palsy when the infant born with an obstetrical complication had an Apgar score less than or equal to 3. This group of patients accounted for only 1.5% of the population, but it accounted for 17% of infant deaths and 13% of cerebral palsy in the study population. These data indicate that an obstetrical complication per se does not place the infant at increased risk for cerebral palsy unless there is an associated significantly low Apgar score.

The Apgar score, when low, is indicative of an abnormal condition but does not imply any specific etiology. It can be due to any one of the following six major causes: asphyxia, drugs, trauma, hypovolemia, infection, and/or anomalies. In ascribing a low Apgar score to asphyxia, one should have positive signs of intrapartum asphyxia, while also ruling out the other five causes of a low score.

Data now show that a significantly low Apgar score is a score of 0–3 (Nelson & Ellenberg, 1979). The level of 0–3 is a "significantly low score" because of the higher mortality and CNS morbidity in infants with this score than with either a 4–6 or a 7–10 score. The longer the score is low, the greater is its significance (Nelson & Ellenberg, 1981). An infant with a 0–3 Apgar score at 1 minute has a mortality of some 5%–10% which rises to approximately 53% if that Apgar score is maintained for 20 minutes. In surviving full-term neonates with an Apgar score of 0–3 at 5 minutes, the incidence of cerebral palsy is approximately 1%. If this Apgar score is sus-

tained for 15 minutes, the percentage of survivors having cerebral palsy rises to 9%, with a dramatic increase to 57% for infants with a sustained Apgar of 0–3 for 20 minutes (Nelson & Ellenberg, 1981).

The following clinical observations are felt to be helpful in estimating the length of an asphyxial episode. Five areas are assessed in assigning the Apgar score. When a low score occurs, the order of their disappearance tends to be: color, respirations, tone, reflexes, and heart rate. Following effective resuscitation, these functions tend to reappear in the following order: heart rate, reflexes, color, respirations, and tone. The length of time it takes for the return of tone and respirations is felt to be an indicator of the severity of the insult to the central nervous system. A delay in return of tone, if greater than 2 hours, is associated with an increased incidence of HIE as well as significant neurological sequelae in surviving neonates (Brown, Parvis, Forfar, Cochburn, 1974). The mean age at onset of respirations in an intrapartumally asphyxiated neonate is significantly greater in those neonates who developed seizures (Mulligan et al., 1980). Three other delivery room observations that may also give some estimate of the length and/or severity of the asphyxial episode are: 1) delay in return of heart rate if resuscitative efforts are considered adequate, 2) meconium in the trachea, and 3) meconium staining of the neonate's umbilical cord, skin, or nails. The last observation indicates previous exposure to meconium for at least 3–6 hours (Fiyikura & Klionsky, 1975).

Seizures have been reported in from 8% to 22% of infants with low Apgar scores and in up to 68% of infants presenting with abnormal neurological examinations following an intrauterine asphyxial episode. Classically, the onset of seizures has been reported to occur at 12–24 hours after delivery. However, if signs other than just tonic clonic movements are used to identify a seizure, the onset of seizures may be as early as 2–6 hours. Seizures, per se, are not invariably associated with late neurological sequelae. However, the occurrence of seizures within the first 12 hours, the appearance of status or serial seizures, or a persistently abnormal electroencephalogram (electrical silence, burst suppression, or low voltage background) are signs of significant neonatal neurological dysfunction (Finer et al., 1981; MacDonald, Mulligan, Allen, & Taylor, 1980; Sarnat & Sarnat, 1976; Volpe, 1977). The presence of seizures especially in infants with HIE increases the likelihood of long-term neurological sequelae (Mulligan et al., 1980; Nelson & Ellenberg, 1979; Volpe, 1977).

Abnormalities in the level of consciousness are very helpful in delineating the severity of an asphyxial insult and in predicting which infants may have neurological sequelae if they survive. In a recent study, full-term infants who were thought to have hypoxic-ischemic encephalopathy were categorized into three clinical states (Sarnat & Sarnat, 1976). The distinguishing features of the three states were: level of consciousness, neuromuscular control, complex reflexes, autonomic function, seizures, EEG findings, and duration of abnormality. Although the last six categories were important in delineating the states of encephalopathy, the level of consciousness seemed to be the primary determinant. The level of consciousness in each state is: state 1—hyperalertness; state 2—lethargy or obtundation; and state 3—stupor. The delineating feature regarding the severity of HIE and predictability of status of long-term outcome was the duration of time the infant stayed in a given state. It was concluded that infants who did not enter state 3 and had signs of state 2 for fewer than 5 days appeared to be normal later in infancy. It was also demonstrated that infants who entered state 3 or who had signs of state 2 for more than 7 days, or whose EEG failed to revert to normal, either expired or developed significant neurological sequelae. These results have been confirmed using this same scoring system, even without using EEG criteria (Finer et al., 1981).

Prediction of Later Outcome

The value of signs as seen in hypoxic-ischemic encephalopathy has been confirmed in identifying neonates at increased risk for later neurological dysfunction. From the National Collaborative Perinatal Project (Nelson & Ellenberg, 1979), approximately 11% of surviving children were considered to demonstrate a specific abnormality of brain during the nursery course. Of this group, 1% later had cerebral palsy, a sixfold increased risk. Of neonates with even suspect neurological status during the nursery course, 6% died. When the infant was said to have a definite neurological abnormality at time of discharge (occurring in only 0.5% of surviving infants), the incidence of cerebral palsy in survivors was 15.8%, a 99-fold increased incidence of cerebral palsy. Fifty-three percent of these children died in the first year.

Among a group of full-term neonates with a history of an asphyxial episode and an abnormal neurological exam, during the first week of life the incidence of early death was 7% and the incidence of neurological handicaps was 28%. When abnormalities of tone were isolated as a predictor of severe handicap in full-term neonates with a history and a clinical course compatible with asphyxia, the risk for cerebral palsy in children surviving the neonatal period was 25%. Combination of abnormal signs with regard to chronology of these signs is more helful than using a single sign (Sarnat & Sarnat, 1976; Ziegler et al., 1976). From existing literature, the most helpful signs to be used in clusters include: an Apgar score of 3 or less at 5 minutes; an Apgar score that stays below 3 for 10, 15, 20 minutes or longer; reduced levels of activity, tone, and consciousness lasting for more than a day; need for gavage feeding; hypotonia, or single or multiple episodes of apnea during the first week; Sarnat state 2 or 3 lasting longer than 7 days; asymmetrical neurological signs; seizures with onset during the first day of life; and an overall impression of abnormality of brain function during the time the infant was in the nursery.

More work is needed to define the predictive powers of the neonatal neurological examination. However, an abnormal neurological examination in a full-term infant, interpreted in light of a history compatible with intrapartum asphyxia, is an extremely powerful tool in identifying neonates with HIE, in predicting early death, and/or in identifying neonates who should be especially followed for the increased risk of the later development of neurological sequelae. As treatment for HIE is improving and as potential treatments for children with early developmental delays are appearing, it becomes extremely important to categorize, *as early as possible,* newborns who are at risk for any of these conditions.

PATHOLOGICAL FEATURES

The pathological changes in the brain of a full-term infant who has experienced an episode of asphyxia during the intrapartum period depend on the length of survival of the patient and the length and severity of the asphyxial episode. In those patients dying in the first few hours after birth, there may be no gross or microscopic changes. Animal studies, however, suggest that there may be light and electron microscopic changes in both neurons and astrocytes shortly after an asphyxial insult. Full-term neonates dying after the first 24 hours of age frequently have brain swelling and cerebral necrosis (Terplan, 1967; Towbin, 1970). Brain swelling was found as an isolated lesion in as many as 39% of the cases. The cerebral necrosis involves the cortical gray matter (especially at depths of sulci), underlying white matter, and the gray matter of the basal ganglia. In some patients, cerebral necrosis involves the region of the postcentral gyrus and posterior parietal-anterior occipital regions as was seen in the full-term newborn monkey following experimentally produced intrapartum asphyxia (Brann, Myers, & DiGiacomo, 1971; Brann & Myers, 1975; Myers, 1977). Areas of petechial periventricular hemorrhage and leucomalacia can also be seen. SE/IVH as pointed out previously is not usually a part of the pattern of cerebral damage seen in the full-term infant.

Those full-term infants who survive the perinatal asphyxial episode and neonatal period will have two primary neuropathological conditions: ulegyria and status marmoratus of the basal ganglia. The reader is referred to other sources for a more thorough discussion of these late sequelae, since the present discussion deals primarily with the nervous system findings in the neonatal period (Norman, 1969).

EXPERIMENTAL OBSERVATIONS

Data from two primate animal models using the rhesus monkey have given insights into the pathogenesis of damage seen in the normally formed brain of an asphyxiated full-term fetus/neonate and the surviving child who as a neonate experienced intrapartum asphyxia. These two models, termed *acute total asphyxia,* and *prolonged partial asphyxia,* are summarized in Table 1.

The experimental design using these two different animal models replicates as closely as possible the two different types of perinatal asphyxial events that most frequently occur in the human fetus/neonate—an acute asphyxial episode such as occurs with cord prolapse, and a prolonged partial asphyxial episode such as occurs with a placental abruption. When combined, the identified clinical spectrum and neuropathological findings seen in monkeys from these two animal models very closely replicate short- and long-term clinical and neuropathological findings that usually occur in the human following perinatal asphyxia. In most cases, the perinatal insult in the human setting is a combined partial prolonged asphyxial episode with a terminal acute asphyxial episode.

The description of the separate findings in the two animal models is as follows:

1. *Acute total asphyxia* produces in the monkey a long-term neurological dysfunction similar to that seen in patients with cerebral palsy (Ranck & Windle, 1959). In the neonatal period, neither seizures nor brain swelling are seen. The neuropathological findings occur primarily in the nuclei located in the brain stem, thalamus, and basal ganglia with sparing of the cerebral cortex. This particular animal model of asphyxia most closely duplicates the findings in the human brain following an acute deprivation of oxygen such as with cord prolapse (Leech & Alvord, 1977).

2. *Prolonged partial asphyxia* in the monkey fetus produces a clinical course in the neonatal period that is similar to that seen in the depressed human neonate following

Table 1. Partial and total asphyxia in the full-term newborn rhesus monkey

		Prolonged partial asphyxia	Acute total asphyxia
Insult	Length	3–4 hours	13 minutes
	pH	6.9	6.9
	P_{O_2}	15 mm Hg	3 mm Hg
	P_{CO_2}	90 mm Hg	120 mm Hg
	Blood pressure	40 mm Hg	5 mm Hg
Clinical course	Resuscitation	Yes	Yes
	Seizures	Yes	No
	Retinal hemorrhage		
	Survival	Variable	Variable
	Sequelae	No detected dysfunction	Spasticity; sensory loss
Pathological aspects	Brain swelling	Yes	No
	Site of edema	Intracellular	
	Brain necrosis	Yes	Yes
	Locus of necrosis	Cerebral cortex; basal ganglia; thalamus	Brain stem; thalamus, basal ganglia, spinal cord
	Cerebral blood flow	Abnormal at birth Cortex	Abnormal at birth Brain stem

a placental abruption (Brann et al., 1971; Brann & Myers, 1975; Myers, 1977). Seizures occur in approximately 50% of the monkeys within the first 24 hours of life. The spectrum of brain lesions in the cortex is similar to that seen in neonates who die following intrapartum asphyxia as well as in children or adults said to have cerebral palsy secondary to a perinatal insult. The surviving monkey, unlike the human, has no motor deficit in spite of significant brain lesions in the association areas of the cortex. The brain edema seen in the neonatal period is of the cytotoxic variety (Bondareff, Myers, & Brann, 1970). Cerebral blood flow studies in the monkey show that the brain is abnormal at birth as demonstrated by focal areas of ischemia (Reivich, Brann, Shapiro, & Myers, 1972). These three studies from the animal model strongly suggest that prolonged partial asphyxia of the fetus from any cause in the absence of fetal circulatory collapse or fetal head compression is the primary event that sets in motion a downward spiral of cytotoxic edema with impaired cerebral blood flow leading to cerebral necrosis and/or ulegyria.

PATHOGENESIS

Based on currently available human and animal data, a proposed pathogenesis for hypoxic-

ischemic encephalopathy in the full-term infant, and its sequelae in the neonate who survives, is outlined in Figure 1. The extent of the changes seen in the brain can vary depending on the acuteness of onset and on the length and severity of the asphyxial episode. The entire sequence of events leading to the various types of neuropathological outcomes is not totally clear from the data currently available, although the points represented in each of the rectangles in Figure 1 have been demonstrated in either animal or human material. The figure is drawn as though there was a continuum of the intrapartum asphyxial episode from top to bottom with the outcomes seen on the right side of the figure.

Numerous infants born following intrapartum asphyxial episodes with low Apgar scores have no evidence of hypoxic-ischemic encephalopathy. This has been seen in asphyxiated infants who succumb because of other dysfunctions such as persistent fetal circulation (Sexson et al., 1976). The lack of findings in the central nervous system could be explained by the fact that the brain received an increased percentage of cardiac output, thus maintaining adequate tissue oxygenation, and preventing the development of tissue ischemia (Meschia & Giacomo, 1979; Peeters et al., 1979) (Figure 1, Step 1).

If the intrauterine asphyxial episode continues and homeostatic mechanisms to maintain oxygenation to the brain begin to fail (e.g.,

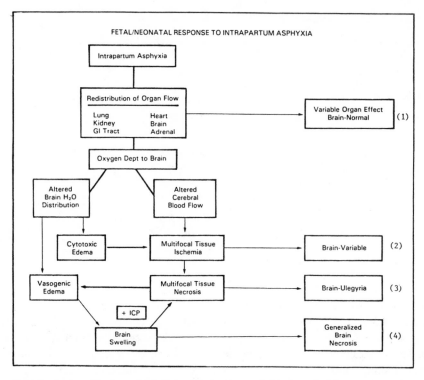

Figure 1. A proposed pathogenesis for hypoxic-ischemic encephalopathy in the full-term infant, and its sequelae in the neonate who survives.

when the oxygen content in the ascending aorta falls below the $1mM(O_2)a$ in the sheep fetus) (Peeters et al., 1979), two major alterations in the brain begin to occur: an alteration of brain water distribution and an alteration of cerebral blood flow. Both of these alterations in the brain are thought to act synergistically and contribute to the key finding (i.e., multifocal tissue ischemia as described in the fetal monkey). There is a general reduction of blood flow with focal areas of total ischemia. The brains of monkey fetuses subjected to greater intensities and length of asphyxia showed greater degrees of ischemia (Reivich et al., 1972). An understanding of the multiple factors that lead to this multifocal tissue ischemia is of central importance in the overall pathogenetic mechanism leading to the brain damage seen in neonatal hypoxic-ischemic encephalopathy.

It is unclear from the literature what length of time is required for tissue ischemia to be present before actual death of tissue occurs in the cerebral cortex. It is conceivable that if the intrauterine asphyxial episode is relieved and

appropriately treated after the development of only mild multifocal tissue ischemia, the brain in the surviving infant could escape evidence of tissue necrosis (Figure 1, Step 2).

If the intrapartum insult is not extremely severe and/or is terminated, smaller areas of multifocal tissue necrosis do occur but not to an extent that would lead to significant areas of vasogenic edema with the development of increased intracranial pressure. Through the reparative process of the brain, these areas of multifocal tissue necrosis are converted into areas of ulegyria as described in the monkey brain. The extent and pattern of ulegyria are dependent on the degree and location of cerebral necrosis (Figure 1, Step 3).

If the intrapartum episode is severe and persists for a prolonged period of time, multifocal areas of tissue ischemia initially located at the depths of sulci and within neuronal nuclei spread to involve the entire cerebral hemisphere (Reivich et al., 1972). The existing tissue ischemia, if not relieved, will lead to tissue necrosis. At the same time that multifocal tissue necrosis is developing, vasogenic edema is also developing (Goldstein, 1979; Katzman, Clasen, Klatzo, Meyer, Pappius, & Waltz, 1977). This type of edema develops following disruption of the tight junctions of the capillary endothelium with leakage of osmotic materials into the interstitial tissues of the brain, which pulls water from the intravascular space. As the multifocal areas of necrotic brain begin to coalesce, and significant increases in intracranial pressure begin to occur in association with vasogenic edema, progressive brain swelling occurs. This would produce clinically measurable increases in intracranial pressure. From animal data it is known that when intracranial pressure reaches one-half to two-thirds of the mean arterial pressure, tissue ischemia from a reduction of cerebral blood flow begins to occur, especially in areas of cortex at depths of sulci (Baldy-Mouliner & Frerebeau, 1968). As can be seen in Figure 1, the triad of multifocal tissue necrosis, vasogenic edema, and brain swelling with increasing intracranial pressure leads to a vicious downward spiral with an ever-increasing oxygen debt to the brain leading to almost total tissue necrosis and death (Figure 1, Step 4).

At autopsy in some neonates, lack of clinically apparent increased intracranial pressure, or findings of brain edema following intrapartum asphyxia, are known to occur. This may be related to the ability of the fetus to compensate with redistribution of flow to protect the brain, but with inadequate oxygen to the lung, kidney, or gastrointestinal tract, which may lead to a fatal outcome secondary to dysfunction of these organs. The absence of edema may also be related to the type and length of the asphyxial episode. There is consistently an absence of brain swelling in the monkey experiencing acute total asphyxia. However, there can be enough neuronal necrosis principally confined to the brain stem and basal ganglia to lead to death through impaired respiratory control. It is important to recognize that unkown and as yet unidentified or poorly quantified factors leading to cerebral infarction may play a role in the pathogenesis of ulegyria without a phase of brain swelling during the neonatal period.

TREATMENT

Except for the use of glucose, there is general agreement regarding the symptomatic management of an infant with hypoxic-ischemic encephalopathy. At the present time, clinical studies have not reached a point where any specific therapy can be recommended for prospective management, from birth, of an infant at high risk for developing hypoxic-ischemic encephalopathy.

There are at least three unanswered questions regarding the appropriate prospective therapeutic management of a neonate at risk of developing hypoxic-ischemic encephalopathy:

1. Can the asphyxiated neonate, whose central nervous system is altered enough to develop HIE, be identified within the first 2–6 hours after birth?
2. Is there a critical time after which treatment is ineffective in eliminating or significantly reducing permanent brain damage in this infant?
3. What is the appropriate prospective intervention for this asphyxiated neonate?

The first question is the most important. If a patient cannot be recognized as abnormal, therapy cannot be initiated to alleviate the condition. Current data support the position that the full-term neonate who has had a history of fetal distress, with either an Apgar score of less than or equal to 3 at 5 or 10 minutes, failure to have spontaneous and sustained respiration by 5 minutes, and/or altered tone or level of consciousness during the first 2–6 hours of life is at great risk for having HIE. This neonate, who probably has focal areas of brain ischemia at birth, similar to those seen in the fetal monkey following prolonged partial asphyxiation (Reivich et al., 1972), has a 50% chance of having seizures (Finer et al., 1981; Mulligan et al., 1980) and at least a 20% chance of having long-term neurological sequelae (Nelson & Ellenberg, 1979, 1981).

Certainly, some neonates who have subsequently developed neurological findings and a clinical course of HIE have presented with an Apgar score of 7–10. However, they usually have had an intrapartum course suggestive of asphyxia. It is extremely important in such cases to be sure that the neurological dysfunction seen in the first 2–6 hours after birth is not secondary to an etiology other than intrapartum asphyxia. Data indicate at the present time that a neonate experiencing intrapartum asphyxia significant enough to lead to long-term neurological sequelae will have clinically recognizable neurological dysfunction during the first 24 hours of life, if followed closely.

The second question relates to the stage of the asphyxial process in which the neonate presents. If the infant is born after a prolonged intrapartum asphyxial episode following which the processes of vasogenic edema and increased intracranial pressure are far advanced, there will, more than likely, be no therapeutic intervention that is effective. However, with earlier detection of intrapartum asphyxia leading to delivery of a baby without any clinically apparent disease or very early stages of hypoxic-ischemic encephalopathy, therapeutic intervention certainly seems justified on theoretical grounds from animal and human data.

The third question relates to the appropriate prospective intervention for the asphyxiated neonate. In order to alleviate or reduce brain damage secondary to HIE, the therapeutic management should be directed first at eliminating the hypoxic environment and then at reducing brain ischemia/edema and/or reducing the metabolic requirements of the brain. A number of therapeutic modalities, including steroids (Anderson & Cranford, 1979), diuretics (Wilkenson, Wepsic, & Austin, 1971), mannitol (Marchal, Leveau, Genet, & Andree, 1972), and barbiturates (Katzman et al., 1977; Marsh, Marshall, & Shapiro, 1977) have been suggested. At the present time, barbiturates appear to hold the theoretical edge as the first agent to be used in a randomized clinical trial because of their "protective effect." This relates to the ability of barbiturates to reduce seizures (Todd, Chadwich, Shapiro, Dunlop, Marshall, & Dueck, 1982), catecholamine secretion (Smith, Rehncuoma, Siesjo, 1980; Steen & Michenfelder, 1980), toxic free radicals (Steen & Michenfelder, 1980), cerebral edema (Marsh et al., 1977; Nordstrom, Rehncuoma & Siesjo, 1978), and general metabolic activity (Marsh et al., 1977; Nordstrom et al., 1978).

Because of the relatively small numbers of neonates with HIE cared for in any given center, progress has been slow in resolving the question of appropriate therapy for them. A collaborative, randomized clinical trial involving a specific therapeutic modality is needed.

REFERENCES

Anderson, D.C., & Cranford, R.E. Corticosteroids in ischemic stroke. *Current Concepts of Cerebrovascular Disease-Stroke*, 1979, *10*(1), 68–71.

Baldy-Mouliner, M., & Frerebeau, P. Blood flow of the cerebral cortex in intracranial hypertension. *Scandinavian Journal of Clinical Laboratory Investigations*, 1968, Suppl. 102.

Banker, B.Q. The neuropathological effects of anoxia and hypoglycemia in the newborn. *Developmental Medicine and Child Neurology*, 1967, *9*, 544–550.

Bondareff, W., Myers, R.D., & Brann, A.W. Brain extracellular space in monkey fetuses subjected to prolonged partial asphyxia. *Experimental Neurology*, 1970, *28*, 167–168.

Brann, A.W., & Myers, R.E. Central nervous system findings in the newborn monkey following severe in utero partial asphyxia. *Neurology*, 1975, *25*, 327–338.

Brann, A.W., Myers, R.E., & DiGiacomo, R. The effect of halothane-induced maternal hypotension on the fetus. In: *Medical Primator 1970*. Proceedings of the Second Conference of Experimental Medicine and Surgery in Primates. Basel, Switzerland: S. Karger Publishing Co., 1971.

Brown, J.K., Parvis, R.J., Forfar, J.D., Cochburn, F. Neurological aspects of perinatal asphyxia. *Developmental Medicine and Neurology*, 1974, *16*, 567–580.

Clark, D.B. Abnormal neurologic signs in the neonate. In: J. Kay (ed.), *Physical diagnosis of the newly born*. Report of the 46th Ross Conference on Pediatric Research. Columbis, OH: Ross Laboratories, 1964.

Clifford, S.H. The effects of asphyxia on the newborn infant. *The Journal of Pediatrics*, 1941, *18*, 567–578.

Courville, C.B. *Birth and brain damage*. Unpublished doctoral dissortation, Pasadena, 1971, Courville MF.

Finer, N.N., Robertson, C.M., Richards, R.T., Pinnell, L.E., & Peters, K.L. Hypoxic-ischemic encephalopathy in term neonates: Perinatal factors and outcome. *The Journal of Pediatrics*, 1981, *98(1)*, 112–117.

Fiyikura, T., & Klionsky, B. The significance of meconium staining. *American Journal of Obstetrics and Gynecology*, 1975, *121*, 45–50.

Friedman, S.P., & Courville, C.B. Atrophic lobar sclerosis of early childhood (Ulegyria). Report of two verified cases with particular reference to their asphyxial etiology. *Bulletin of the Los Angeles Neurological Society*, 1941, *6*, 32–45.

Goldstein, G.W. Pathogenesis of brain edema and hemorrhage: Role of the brain capillary. *Pediatrics, 1979, 64,* 357–360.

Hagberg, B. Epidemiological and preventive aspects of cerebral palsy and severe mental retardation in Sweden. *European Journal of Pediatric Research,* 1971, *7,* 691.

Katzman, R., Clasen, R., Klatzo, I., Meyer, J.S., Pappius, H.M., & Waltz, A.G. Brain edema in stroke. Report of joint committee for stroke resources. *Stroke,* 1977, *8,* 512–540.

Koops, B.L., & Harmon, R.J. Studies on long-term outcome in newborns with birth weights under 1500 grams. *Advances in Behavioral Pediatrics,* 1980, *1,* 1–28.

Leech, R.W., & Alvord, E.C. Anoxic ischemic encephalopathy in the human neonatal period: The significance of brain stem involvement. *Archives of Neurology,* 1977, *34,* 109–113.

Little, W.J. On the influence of abnormal parturition, difficult labours, premature birth, and asphyxia neonatorum on the mental and physical condition of the child, especially in relation to deformities. *Transactions of the Obstetrical Society of London,* 1861, *3,* 293–346.

MacDonald, H.M., Mulligan, J.C., Allen, A.C., & Taylor, P.M. Neonatal asphyxia. I. Relationship of obstetric and neonatal complications to neonatal mortality in 38,405 consecutive deliveries. *The Journal of Pediatrics,* 1980, *96,* 898–909.

Marchal, C., Leveau, P., Genet, Y., & Andree, M. Traetment des souffrances cerebrales neonatales. *Pediatrie [Pediatrics],* 1972, *27,* 709.

Marsh, M.L., Marshall, L.F., & Shapiro, H.M. Neurosurgical intensive care. *Anesthesiology,* 1977, *47,* 149–163.

Meschia & Giacomo. Supply of oxygen to the fetus. *Journal of Reproductive Medicine,* 1979, *23,* 160–165.

Mulligan, J.C., Painter, M.J., O'Donoghue, P.A., MacDonald, H.M., Allen, A.C., & Taylor, P.M. Neonatal asphyxia. II. Neonatal mortality and long-term sequelae. *The Journal of Pediatrics,* 1980, *96,* 903–907.

Myers, R.E. *Experimental models of perinatal brain damage: Revelance to human pathology. Intrauterine asphyxia and the developing fetal brain.* Chicago: Year Book Medical Publishers, 1977.

Nelson, K.B., & Ellenberg, J.H. Neonatal signs as predictors of cerebral palsy. *Pediatrics,* 1979, *64,* 225–232.

Nelson, K.B., & Ellenberg, J.H. Apgar scores as predictors of cerebral palsy. *Pediatrics,* 1981, *68,* 36–44.

Nelson, K.B., & Ellenberg, J.H. Obstetric complications as risk factors for cerebral palsy or seizure disorder. *The Journal of the American Medical Association,* 1983.

Nordstrom, C.H., Rehncuoma, S., Siesjo, B.K. Effects of phenobarbital on cerebral ischemia, Part II: Restriction of cerebral energy state as well as glycolytic metabolites, citric acid cycle intermediates and associated amino acids after pronounced incomplete ischemia. *Stroke,* 1978, *9,* 335–343.

Norman, R.M. Late neuropathological sequelae of birth injury. In: *Greenfield's neuropathology.* London: Edward Arnold Publishers, Ltd., 1969.

Peeters, L.H., Sheldon, R.E., Jones, M.D., Makowski, E.L., & Meschia, G. Blood flow to fetal organs as a function of arterial oxygen content. *American Journal of Obstetrics and Gynecology,* 1979, *135,* 1071–1078.

Ranck, J.B., & Windle, W.F. Brain damage in the monkey, macaca malatta, by asphyxia neonatorum. *Experimental Neurology,* 1959, *1,* 130–154.

Reivich, M., Brann, A.W., Shapiro, H., & Myers, R.E. Regional cerebral blood flow during intrauterine prolonged partial asphyxia. Research on the Cerebral Circulation. In: S.S. Meyer, M. Reivich, & O. Elckhorn (eds.), *Fifth international Salzburg conference.* Springfield, IL: Charles C Thomas, 1972.

Sarnat, H.B., & Sarnat, M.S. Neonatal encephalopathy following fetal distress. A clinical and electroencephalographic study. *Archives of Neurology,* 1976, *33,* 696–705.

Sexson, W.R., Sexson, S.B., Rawson, J.E., & Brann, A.W. The multisystem involvement of the asphyxiated newborn. *Pediatric Research,* 1976, *10,* 432–439.

Smith, D.S., Rehncuoma, S., & Siesjo, B.K. Barbiturates as protective agents in brain ischemia and as free-radical scavengers in vitro. *Acta Physiologica Scandinavia,* 1980, *492,* 129.

Steen, P.A., & Michenfelder, J.D. Mechanism of barbiturate protection. *Anesthesiology,* 1980, *53,* 183–185.

Terplan, K.L. Histopathologic brain changes in 1152 cases of the perinatal and early infancy period. *Biology of the Neonate,* 1967, *11,* 348–353.

Todd, M.M., Chadwich, H.S., Shapiro, H.M., Dunlop, B.J., Marshall, L.F., & Dueck, R. The neurologic effects of thiopental therapy following experimental cardiac arrest in cats. *Anesthesiology,* 1982, *57,* 76–86.

Towbin, A. Central nervous system damage in the human fetus and newborn infant: Mechanical and hypoxic injury incurred in the fetal-neonatal period. *American Journal of Diseases of Children,* 1970, *119,* 259.

Volpe, J.J. Neonatal seizures. *Clinics in Perinatology,* 1977, *4,* 43–63.

Wilkenson, H.A., Wepsic, J.J., & Austin, B.S. Diuretic synergy in the treatment of acute experimental cerebral edema. *Journal of Neurosurgery,* 1971, *34,* 203–208.

Ziegler, A.L., Calame, A., Marchand, C., Passera, M., Reymond-Goni, I., & Prod'hom, L.S. Cerebral distress in full term newborns and its prognostic value. A follow-up study of 90 infants. *Helvetica Paediatrica Acta,* 1976, *31,* 299–317.

Chapter 19

Postnatal Screening for Hereditary and Metabolic Disorders

JOSEPH H. FRENCH, M.D.
*New York State Office of Mental Retardation and Developmental Disabilities,
Institute for Basic Research in Developmental Disabilities, Staten Island, New York*

MAN'S EXTRAORDINARY COGNITIVE FUNC-tioning capabilities are biologically unmatched. This information-processing potential and its creative products—scientific knowledge, culture, technology—are based in part on human central nervous system structure and function. Human nervous system developmental maturation, however, is associated with an ontogenetic loss of nerve cell replicative capability; human postencephaloclastic functional recovery is often limited. Thus, it is essential to, preclinically, detect and treat those familial neurometabolic and endocrine diseases that diminish normal human nervous system development in order to ensure our progeny's continuing uniqueness.

The public health technique of neonatal mass screening has enabled health professionals to advance toward the goal of secondary prevention of mental retardation and other developmental disabilities. Neonatal mass screening is now used regularly to detect phenylketonuria (PKU) and the other hyperphenylalaninemias, as well as diseases such as congenital hypothyroidism, galactosemia, and maple syrup urine disease. A relatively simple bacterial-growth inhibition blood test (Guthrie, 1961; Guthrie & Susi, 1962) is used to detect these and other diseases. Table 1 lists some of the disorders that can be screening test–assessed

using a dried PKU blood spot sample for testing. These and other screening tests have also used chromatographic (Levy, Coulombe, & Shih, 1980; Shapcott, Lemieux, & Shapoglu, 1972), radioimmunoassay (Dussault & Laberge, 1973; Irie, Enomato, & Naruse, 1975), and electrophoretic (Garrick, Dewbure, & Guthrie, 1973) measurement methods. Some of these methods can also be applied to urine specimens.

Table 1 also shows the estimated frequency of occurrence of these diseases. Congenital hypothyroidism and the hyperphenylalaninemias, among the treatable genetic neurometabolic-endocrine diseases, have a relatively high incidence. Galactosemia, homocystinuria, and maple syrup urine disease occur less frequently.

HISTORY OF POSTNATAL SCREENING

Mass screening for inherited neurometabolic and endocrine diseases is based on Gregor Mendel's 19th century investigations of eukaryote heredity. Garrod (1908) subsequently developed the concept of ''inborn error of metabolism'' by noting the familial occurrence of, as well as the increased consanguinity rate in, albinism, alcaptonuria, cystinuria, and pentosuria. Beadle (1945), as a consequence of his

Table 1. Estimated North American frequency of newborn mass screening–detected metabolic and endocrine diseases[a]

Disease	Estimated frequency
Hypothyroidism	1: 3,500–5,000
Iminoglycinuria	1: 11,000[c]
Cystinuria[b]	1: 13,000
Classical PKU	1: 10,000–16,000
Atypical PKU[b]	1: 16,000
Hartnup disease[b]	1: 18,000
Histidinemia	1: 20,000
PKU and maternal PKU[b]	1: 30,000
Cystathionemia	1: 65,000
Argininocussinic acidemia (ASA)	1: 70,000
Galactosemia	1: 75,000
Methylmalonic acidemia	1: 75,000
Maternal histidinemia	1: 75,000
Nonketotic hyperglycinemia	1:190,000
Sarcosinemia	1:275,000
Homocystinuria	1:290,000
Hyperlysinemia[b]	1:290,000
Hyperprolinemia[b]	1:290,000
Maple syrup urine disease	1:290,000
Atypical ASA	<1:500,000
Proprionic acidemia	<1:500,000
Hyperornithenemia[b]	<1:500,000
Carnosinemia	<1:500,000
Urocanicaciduria	<1:500,000
Hyperglutamicaciduria	<1:500,000
Fanconi syndrome	<1:500,000
Vitamin D dependent rickets	<1:500,000

Italics represent diseases with well-established symptoms.

[a]Modified from Acosta, 1982; Eaton, Doody, Zipf, Ackerman, Croft, & Porter, 1982; Fernhoff, Fitzmaurice, Milner, McEwen, Dembure, Brown, Wright, Acosta, & Elsas, 1982; Haibach & Woodruff, 1982; Moser, 1982; Reddy, 1982; Somers & Favreau, 1982; and United States General Accounting Office, 1977.

[b]Diseases that may or may not be associated with clinical symptoms.

[c]Carriers may have iminoglycine excretion during the neonatal period and falsely increase the homozygotic incidence rate.

studies of *Drosophila* eye color, formulated the concept of "one gene—one enzyme"; the applicability of this concept in a genetically determined human disease was promptly confirmed by the Coris' (1952) investigations of the glycogenoses.

Soon after the Coris' work, Jervis (1953) delineated the enzyme deficiency in phenylketonuria. Bickel, Gerrard, and Hickmans (1953) promptly reported a treatment strategy: phenylalanine dietary restriction. Next, Centerwall (1957) applied Folling's acidified FeCl₃ PKU urine test (1934) on wet diapers as a neonatal screening procedure. A more sensitive and specific bacterial-growth inhibition blood test for phenylalanine concentration was subsequently introduced by Guthrie (1961; Guthrie & Sussi, 1962). A spectrophotofluorimetric measurement of serum phenyl-alanine content (McCamman & Robins, 1962) has a similar efficiency (Table 2). Table 3 provides a conceptual and technological history of neonatal mass screening.

CURRENT STATUS OF NEWBORN MASS SCREENING FOR SELECTED DISEASES

Table 4 lists some of the conditions that must exist in order to justify instituting a mass screening program for an inherited neurometabolic or endocrine disease (Research Group on Ethical, Social and Legal Issues in Genetic Counselling and Genetic Engineering of the Institute of Society, Ethics and the Life Sciences, 1972). PKU and congenital hypothyroidism have been found to adequately meet most of these criteria.

Table 2. Screening test efficacy measures

Sensitivity = S_n	$S_n = \dfrac{TP}{TP + FN} \times 100$
Specificity = S_p	$S_p = \dfrac{TN}{TN + FP} \times 100$
Efficiency = E_f	$E_f = \dfrac{TP + TN}{\Sigma\ tests} \times 100$

FN = number of false negative results; TN = number of true negative results; FP = number of false positive results; TP = number of true positive results; Σ tests = total number of results.

Phenylketonuria

Detection The technological foundation of neonatal mass screening for PKU and the other hyperphenylalaninemias (Tourian & Sidbury, 1978) is the use of a dried blood spot analytical sample. A special filter paper is impregnated with a few drops of capillary blood drawn from a "heel stick." The blood content per unit area on the filter paper is exceptionally constant (Manning, 1982), and the dried blood–containing filter paper is stable at common environmental temperatures. It can be mailed to a central reference laboratory without being refrigerated. There, the blood sample is placed on an inoculated culture medium that requires large amounts of phenylalanine for growth. If an excessive amount of the amino acid is present, bacterial growth will be readily evident. Blood phenylalanine concentration is a more specific (Table 2) indicator of the presence of PKU than urinary phenylpyruvic acid excretion because of a transient neonatal developmental deficiency of phenylalanine transamination (Auerbach, DiGeorge, & Carpenter, 1967).

False negative results are obtained at a frequency of 1:217,000 in U.S. screening programs for PKU (Erbe, 1981). This rate may be decreased by follow-up screening; however, the case detection cost is increased 30-fold ($263,000 versus $8,700) when compared to newborn screening costs. As implied above, the serum phenylalanine concentration population distribution curve is skewed in the early hours after birth. Thus, the American Academy of Pediatrics Committee on Genetics (1982) has recommended that infants who are discharged before 24 hours of life should be screened for hyperphenylalaninemia at the time of discharge and rescreened at a later time before the age of 3 weeks. This group also states that "heel stick" capillary blood is the only adequate sample for hyperphenylalaninemia screening; premature infants, sick infants, and infants who receive parenteral alimentation should be screened on day 7.

Treatment Limitation, early in the affected infant's life, of the intake of phenylalanine, which undergoes toxic and alternate metabolic products accumulation, effectively prevents the mental retardation that is an almost inevitable clinical finding in classical PKU (Wrona, 1979). This is accomplished by placing the child, within the first months of life, on a diet restricting the intake of phenylalanine. Galactosemia, maple syrup urine disease, and some disorders of fatty acid metabolism are similarly responsive to dietary restrictions that prevent accumulation of harmful metabolic products.

Parents usually accept the necessity of a low phenylalanine diet for PKU-affected offspring when it is prescribed and monitored by an experienced metabolic disease health care team. A relaxed attitude usually permits the maintenance of a low phenylalanine diet for a longer period than the prudent minimum of 4–5 years of age (Scriver & Clow, 1980).

Table 3. Conceptual and technological history of neonatal mass screening

Contribution	Contributor	Year
Heredity	Mendel	mid 1800s
Inborn error of metabolism	Garrod	1908
FeCl$_3$ test	Følling	1934
One gene—one enzyme	Beadle	1945
Enzyme deficiency cause of disease	Cori & Cori	1952
PKU enzyme deficiency	Jervis	1953
PKU treatment	Bickel et al.	1953
Effective blood screening test for PKU	Guthrie	1961

Table 4. Disease-selection criteria for appropriate mass screening

Category	Necessary characteristics
Available treatment	Public acceptance; Health care deliverer acceptance
Early treatment response	Significant amelioration of mortality and morbidity, i.e., favorably alters natural history of the disease
Available screening test	Acceptance by test performer Specificity Sensitivity Efficiency Low cost
Frequency of selected disease	Relative incidence that is of sufficient magnitude to make cost/test "reasonable"
Available health care facilities	Sufficient number, quality, and organization to diagnose as well as treat individuals with positive screening tests
Demonstrated screening test cost-effectiveness	Human suffering, lost productivity, and late diagnosis clinical care costs are less than neonatal screening, early diagnosis, and early onset treatment costs

Congenital Hypothyroidism

Detection Heel cord blood, as drawn for PKU testing, is an adequate sample for congenital hypothyroidism mass screening. The cost per screening test in North America is $.70 to $1.60 (Fisher, Dussault, Foley, LeFranchi, Larsen, Mitchell, Murphey, & Walfish, 1979). Most of the detected infants have primary hypothyroidism; secondary-tertiary hypothyroidism occurs at a rate that is approximately 10 times less than the incidence of primary hypothyroidism. Thus, a T_4 assay is an "adequate" initial screening procedure; positive results are confirmed by T_4 reassay and a thyroid stimulating hormone determination.

The false negative rate (Table 2) in congenital hypothyroidism mass screening is estimated to be approximately 10% (Holtzman, Leonard, & Farfel, 1981; LeFranchi, Murphey, Foley, Larsen, & Buist, 1979; Report of the New England Regional Screening Program and the New England Congenital Hypothyroidism Collaborative, 1982). Failure of sample submission, laboratory processing errors, and a lack of T_4 test measurement specificity (Table 2) are felt to cause this false negative rate. Radioimmunoassay measurements of neonatal blood T_4 are less precise and accurate than adult blood measurements (Walfish, Gera, & Wood, 1981).

Treatment Thyroid hormone replacement therapy (Stanbury, 1978) is an effective treatment for congenital hypothyroidism (Klein, Meltzer, & Kenny, 1972) when admin-

istered early in life. Preliminary results indicate that there is improved mental development of hypothyroid infants who were treated from birth in the Quebec Screening Program (Glorieux, Dussault, Letarte, Guyda, & Morrissette, 1983), in comparison to later-age diagnosis and treatment results (Mäenpää, 1972; Raiti & Newns, 1971). However, early postnatal treatment expectations will probably require a "hypothyroidism age of onset" correction (Wolter, Nöel, DeCock, Craen, Ernould, Malvaux, Verstraeten, Simons, Mertens, Van Broeck, & Vanderschueren-Lodeweyckx, 1979). Thyroid supplementation has not posed any problems of parent or physician acceptance.

COST-EFFECTIVENESS OF SCREENING

The cost of PKU screening for each productive year of life gained compares favorably to other accepted health programs (Bush, Chen, & Patrick, 1973). A cost-benefit analysis of PKU newborn screening indicates that long-term savings are achieved (Massachusetts Department of Health, 1973). This finding is corroborated by a marked reduction in U.S. institutional admissions of mentally retarded persons with PKU since near universal screening was instituted (MacCready, 1974). Cost-benefit analysis of congenital hypothyroidism screening is also positive (Layde, von Allmen, & Oakley, 1979).

Although there are effective treatments for maple syrup urine disease and galactosemia, prompt diagnosis of these diseases is not always achieved. Neonatal symptoms may develop before a positive screening-test result is communicated to an infant's physician (Holtzman et al., 1981).

Neonatal mass screening for sickle cell disease and related hemoglobinopathies can reduce early deaths (Warren, Carter, Humbert, & Rowley, 1982) if specialized outreach services are available to detected cases (Grover, Sahidi, Fisher, Goldberg & Wethers, 1983). However, there is presently no case control substantiation of this finding.

EFFICACY OF MASS SCREENING

The United States health care delivery system has several independent components, i.e., solo and private group practices, as well as institutional practices and their numerous permutations. Patients are free to obtain services from any of these components at any moment in time. Thus, it is difficult to achieve efficient communication between a neonatal mass screening laboratory and the responsible health caregiver. Frequent changes of patients' addresses in large urban areas compound this problem. An effective response to such difficulties has been the establishment of outreach and regional services for the parents of infants who have positive mass screening test results (Grover et al., 1983; Harris & Dreyfus, 1982). However, this method runs the risk of an accurate accusation that it threatens the "private practice of medicine." Yet, the failure to use specialized services for the preclinical diagnosis and treatment of a metabolic or endocrine disease obviously cannot prevent disease sequelae (Warren et al., 1982).

Contemporary society perceives that disease is externally caused. Genetic variability and an individual, genetically determined intrinsic susceptibility to environmental experience are not widely appreciated. Individual health is not viewed as an equilibrium between genetically determined adaptability and multiple environmental factors; disease represents a disequilibrium of these factors. Ethical traditions have not yet incorporated this reality. Thus, ethical questions concerning neonatal mass screening may be anticipated.

"Ideal" clinical genetics presumably would permit informed citizens to assess the potential risks to individual health that a variety of environmental exposures pose, as well as the risks for inherited metabolic disease in future offspring. Following this, they would make informed health-related decisions. Mandatory neonatal mass screening programs, however, may subvert this personal right.

One of the rationales for mandatory neonatal mass screening programs is that the state may restrict parental liberty if the parents' action could result in harm to their offspring. However, this fear of harm to infants, by their parents refusing neonatal screening services, appears to be unfounded. The neonatal mass screening program in the state of Maryland is voluntary and requires informed parental consent. The screening rate in Maryland is equal to that of mandated state programs in the United States (Holtzman et al., 1981). A questionnaire survey of test performers and parents in Maryland (Faden, Chwalow, Holtzman, & Horn, 1982) documents preference for a voluntary program and an educational benefit that occurs during the process of obtaining parental informed consent.

SUMMARY

The benefits of PKU and congenital hypothyroidism neonatal mass screening appear to outweigh the costs, risks, and problems. Improved treatment of other disorders by neonatal mass screening identification has not yet been established.

REFERENCES

Acosta, P.B. Prevention of mental retardation through screening retrieval, diagnosis and management of inherited metabolic disease. *Alabama Journal of Medical Science*, 1982, *19* (4 Suppl. 1), 10–16.

American Academy of Pediatrics Committee on Genetics. New issues in newborn screening for phenylketonuria and congenital hypothyroidism. *Pediatrics*, 1982, *69*, 104–106.

Auerbach, V.H., DiGeorge, A.M., & Carpenter, G.C. Phenylalaninemia: A study of the diversity of disorders which produce elevation of blood concentrations of phenylalanine. In: W.C. Nyhan (ed.), *Amino acids metabolism and genetic variation*. New York: McGraw-Hill Book Co., 1967.

Beadle, G.W. Biochemical genetics. *Chemistry Review*, 1945, *37*, 15–96.

Bickel, H., Gerrard, J.W., & Hickmans, E.M. Influence of phenylalanine intake on phenylketonuria. *Lancet*, 1953, *2*, 812–813.

Bush, J.W., Chen, M.M., & Patrick, D.L. Health status index in cost-effectiveness: analysis of PKU program. In: L. Berg (ed.), *Health status indexes*. Chicago: Hospital Residency Education Trust, 1973.

Centerwall, W.R. Phenylketonuria. *Journal of the American Medical Association*, 1957, *165*, 392.

Cori, G.T. & Cori, C.F. Glucose-6-phosphatase of liver in glycogen storage disease. *Journal of Biological Chemistry*, 1952, *199*, 661–667.

Dussault, J.H. & Laberge, C. Dosage de la thyroxine (T$_4$) par methode radio-immunologique dans l'eluat de sang seche: nouvelle methode de depistage de l'hypothyroidie neonatale. [Radioimmunoassay of thyroxine (T$_4$) via elution of dried blood: A new method for neonatal hypothyroidism screening.] *Union Medicale du Canada*, 1973, *102*, 2062–2064.

Eaton, A.P., Doody, D.M., Zipf, W.B., Ackerman, J.H., Croft, C., & Porter, L. Neonatal hypothyroid screening in Ohio. *Ohio State Medical Journal*, 1982, *78*, 360–361, 365, 368.

Erbe, R.W. Issues in newborn genetic screening. *Birth Defects*, 1981, *17*, 167–179.

Faden, R., Chwalow, A.J., Holtzman, N.A., & Horn, S.D. A survey to evaluate parental consent as public policy for neonatal screening. *American Journal of Public Health*, 1982, *72*, 1347–1352.

Fernhoff, P.M., Fitzmaurice, N., Milner, J., McEwen, C.T., Dembure, P.P., Brown, A.L., Wright, L., Acosta, P.B., & Elsas, L.J. 2d. Coordinated system for comprehensive newborn metabolic screening. *Southern Medical Journal*, 1982, *75*, 529–532.

Fisher, D.A., Dussault, J.H., Foley, T.P., Jr., LeFranchi, S., Larsen, P.R., Mitchell, M.L., Murphey, W.H., & Walfish, P.G. Screening for congenital hypothyroidism: Results of screening one million North American infants. *The Journal of Pediatrics*, 1979, *94*, 700–705.

Følling, A. Uber Aussscheidung von Phenylbenztraubensaure in den Harn als Stoffwechsanomalie in Verbindung mit Imbezillitat. [Phenylpyruvic acid urinary excretion in association with mental retardation: A metabolic anomaly.] *Hoppe-Seylers Zeitschrift fuer Physiologische Chemie*, 1934, *227*, 169–176.

Garrick, M.D., Dewbure, P., & Guthrie, R. Sickle cell anemia and other hemoglobinopathies. *New England Journal of Medicine*, 1973, *288*, 1265–1268.

Garrod, A.E. Croonian lectures: Inborn errors of metabolism. *Lancet*, 1908, *2*, 1–7, 73–79, 142–148, and 214–220.

Glorieux, J., Dussault, J.H., Letarte, J., Guyda, H., & Morrissette, J. Preliminary results on the mental development of hypothyroid infants detected by the Quebec Screening Program. *The Journal of Pediatrics*, 1983, *102*, 19–22.

Grover, R., Sahidi, S., Fisher, B., Goldberg, D., &

Wethers, D. Current sickle cell screening program for newborns in New York City, 1979–80. *American Journal of Public Health*, 1983, *73*, 249–252.

Guthrie, R. Blood screening for phenylketonuria. *Journal of the American Medical Association*, 1961, *178*, 863 (Letter).

Guthrie, R., & Susi, A. A simple phenylalanine method for detecting phenylketonuria in large populations of newborn infants. *Pediatrics*, 1962, *32*, 338–343.

Haibach, H., & Woodruff, C.W. Neonatal screening for metabolic diseases in Missouri. *Missouri Medicine*, 1982, *79*, 615–620.

Harris, P., & Dreyfus, N.G. Newborn thyroid screening in municipal hospitals. *American Journal of Diseases in Children*, 1982, *136*, 248–250.

Holtzman, N.A., Leonard, C.O., & Farfel, M.R. Issues in antenatal and neonatal screening and surveillance for hereditary and congenital disorders. *Annual Review of Public Health*, 1981, *2*, 219–251.

Irie, M., Enomato, K., & Naruse, H. Measurement of thyroid stimulating hormone in dried blood spot. *Lancet*, 1975, *2*, 1233–1234.

Jervis, G.A. Phenylpyruvic oligophrenia deficiency of phenylalanine-oxidizing system. *Proceedings of the Society for Experimental Biology and Medicine*, 1953, *82*, 514–515.

Klein, A.H., Meltzer, S., & Kenny, F.M. Improved prognosis of congenital hypothyroidism treated before 3 months. *The Journal of Pediatrics*, 1972, *81*, 912–915.

Layde, P.M., von Allmen, S.D., & Oakley, G.P., Jr. Congenital hypothyroidism control programs: A cost benefit analysis. *Journal of the American Medical Association*, 1979, *241*, 2290–2292.

LeFranchi, S.H., Murphey, W.H., Foley, T.P., Jr., Larsen, P.R., & Buist, N.R.M. Neonatal hypothyroidism detected by the Northwest Regional Screening Program. *Pediatrics*, 1979, *63*, 180–191.

Levy, H.L., Coulombe, J.T., & Shih, V.E. Newborn urine screening in maple syrup disease. In: H. Bickel, R. Guthrie, and G. Hemmersen (eds.), *Neonatal screening for inborn errors of metabolism*. Heidelberg: Springer-Verlag, 1980.

McCamman, M., & Robins, E. Fluorometric method for the determination of phenylalanine in the serum. *Journal of Laboratory and Clinical Medicine*, 1962, *59*, 885–890.

MacCready, R.A. Admissions of phenylketonuric patients to the residential institutions before and after screening programs of the newborn infant. *The Journal of Pediatrics*, 1974, *85*, 383–385.

Mäenpää, J. Congenital hypothyroidism: Aetiological and clinical aspects. *Archives of Disease in Childhood*, 1972, *47*, 914–923.

Manning, D.N. Dried blood spots: A convenient technique for neonatal hormone screening. *Medical Laboratory Science*, 1982, *39*, 257–260.

Massachusetts Department of Public Health. Newborn screening for metabolic disorders. *New England Journal of Medicine*, 1973, *288*, 1299–1300.

Moser, H.W. Mental retardation due to genetically determined metabolic and endocrine disorders. In: I. Jakab (ed.), *Mental retardation*. Basel: S. Karger AG, 1982.

Raiti, S., & Newns, G.H. Cretinism: Early diagnosis and its relation to mental prognosis. *Archives of Disease in Children*, 1971, *46*, 692–694.

Reddy, U.B. Delaware's hereditary metabolic disorders infant screening program. *Delaware Medical Journal,* 1982, *54,* 555–557.

Report of the New England Regional Screening Program and the New England Congenital Hypothyroidism Collaborative. Pitfalls in screening for neonatal hypothyroidism. *Pediatrics,* 1982, *70,* 16–20.

Research Group on Ethical, Social and Legal Issues in Genetic Counselling and Genetic Engineering. Ethical and social issues in screening for genetic disease. *New England Journal of Medicine,* 1972, *286,* 1129–1132.

Scriver, C.R., & Clow, C.L. Phenylketonuria: Epitome of human biochemical genetics. *New England Journal of Medicine,* 1980, *303,* 1336–1342.

Shapcott, D., Lemieux, B., & Shapoglu, A. A semiautomated device for multiple sample application to thin-layer chromatography plates. *Journal of Chromatography,* 1972, *70,* 174–178.

Somers, D.G., & Favreau, L. Newborn screening for phenylketonuria: Incidence and screening procedures in North America. *Canadian Journal of Public Health,* 1982, *73,* 206–207.

Stanbury, J.B. Familial goiter. In: J.B. Stanbury, J.B. Wyngaarden, & D.S. Frederickson (eds.), *The metabolic basis of inherited disease (4th ed.).* New York: McGraw-Hill Book Co., 1978.

Tourian, A.Y., & Sidbury, J.B. Phenylketonuria. In: J.B. Stanbury, J.B. Wyngaarden, & D.S. Frederickson (eds.), *The metabolic basis of inherited disease (4th ed.).* New York: McGraw-Hill Book Co., 1978.

United States General Accounting Office. *Preventing mental retardation—More can be done.* Washington, DC: Government Printing Office, 1977.

Walfish, P.G., Gera, E., & Wood, M.M. Problems in screening for congenital hypothyroidism using thyroxine assays from small dried blood discs. *Journal of Nuclear Medicine,* 1981, *22,* 818–823.

Warren, N.S., Carter, T.P., Humbert, J.R., & Rowley, P.T. Newborn screening for hemoglobinopathies in New York State: Experience of physicians and parents of affected children. *The Journal of Pediatrics,* 1982, *100,* 373–377.

Wolter, R., Nöel, P., DeCock, P., Craen, M., Ernould, C.H., Malvaux, P., Verstraeten, F., Simons, J., Mertens, S., Van Broeck, N., & Vanderschueren-Lodeweyckx, M. Neuropsychological study in treated thyroid dysgenesis. *Acta Paediatrica Scandinavica,* 1979 (Supp. 277), 41–46.

Wrona, R.M. A clinical epidemiological study of hyperphenylalainemia. *American Journal of Public Health,* 1979, *69,* 673–679.

The At-Risk Infant: Psycho/Socio/Medical Aspects
edited by Shaul Harel, M.D., and Nicholas J. Anastasiow, Ph.D.

Chapter 20

Neonatal Apnea

MICHAEL KAPPLUS, M.D.
Soroka Medical Center, Beer-Sheba, Israel

A PNEA IS A FREQUENT EVENT DURING THE early postnatal period of the preterm infant and is due to the failure of an unstable respiratory control system. Failure of the respiratory control system is likely to occur when a premature infant with structural and functional neuronal immaturity goes into active sleep. In this state, it becomes difficult for the small premature infant to maintain a strong excitation of the respiratory neurons over a long period of time and with a regular recurrence rate. It is under these conditions that periodic breathing and apnea are most likely to occur. Figure 1 shows the typical sequence of events preceding an apneic episode.

APNEA AND THE IMMATURE BRAIN

Neurohistological research on the developing brain has shown that the premature infant is disadvantaged by certain morphological features of neuronal immaturity. Using Golgi staining techniques, Purpura has found poorly developed neuronal dendrites and an absence of dendritic spines in infants of 25 and 27 weeks gestation. As the fetus matures during the third trimester, there is a considerable increase of dendritic surface area. This provides the structural base for the progressive improvement of synaptic linkages (Purpura, 1977).

Recent studies of brain stem function in small preterm infants by Dubowitz and Henderson-Smart suggest that brain stem conduction time of the auditory response is significantly prolonged when compared with brain stem conduction time of term infants (Fawer & Dubowitz, 1982; Henderson-Smart, Pettigrew, & Campbell, 1983).

Henderson-Smart et al. (1983) also noticed a positive correlation between apneic spells and increased brain stem conduction time. The prolonged brain stem conduction time present in small preterm infants may not entirely be due to the structural immaturity described by Purpura. Although not proved, it is likely that low levels of neurotransmitters in the immature brain may have a synergistic effect.

BREATHING AND SLEEP

Sleep is an important factor in the generation of the apneic episode. The newborn infant fluctuates constantly through different, brief states of sleep and wakefulness. It is well known that the small preterm infant spends most of his or her time in active sleep. This particular sleep state is considered an ontogenetically primitive sleep state.

Active sleep is controlled by lower brain stem mechanisms located in the pontine reticular formation, and precedes maturation of

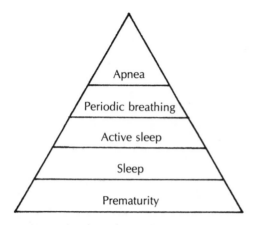

Figure 1. The apneic episode—predisposing factors.

many neuronal elements of the forebrain. It is characterized by the simultaneous presence of nervous system excitation and inhibition. It can be recognized by typical bursts of rapid eye movements, jerky face, limb and body movements, and large variations in respiratory rate and amplitude (Cohen, Gutnik, Zmora, & Karplus, 1982).

Active sleep decreases with maturation of the central nervous system. According to Parmelee, it decreases from about 85% of total sleep time at 29 weeks gestation to 40% at 3 months postterm and 20% in the adult (Parmelee, Stern, & Harris, 1972; Parmelee, Wenner, Akiyama, Schultz, & Stern, 1967).

Quiet sleep presents a high degree of central nervous organization control and regulation. Rapid eye movements are absent and body movements are reduced. There is little variation in heart rate, respiration is more regular, and respiratory muscle activity is well synchronized.

Breathing is controlled by a number of anatomically separate but functionally integrated systems: the metabolic control system with its center located in the brain stem reticular substance, and the behaviorial or voluntary control system which arises in the cortex and centers in the hypothalamus.

There is now good evidence that breathing is regulated by different control systems during sleep and wakefulness. During quiet sleep, breathing is regulated solely by the metabolic control system. In this state, breathing is reg-

ular with little variations in rate and amplitude. During active sleep, the influence of the metabolic control system on breathing is reduced. Respiration is affected by the simultaneous presence of nervous system excitation and inhibition and is therefore irregular or periodic in nature (Phillipson, 1978).

APNEA AND ACTIVE SLEEP

Schulte and Parmelee were among the first to document a significantly high incidence of apneic episodes during active sleep in small preterm infants. Mild apneic episodes were found to be 10 times more common during active sleep, and longer apneic spells were 20 times more frequent (Gabriel, Albani, & Schulte, 1976). A relevant feature of active sleep is the fluctuating inhibition of brain stem and spinal motor neurons described by Schulte, Busse, and Eichhorn (1977). This inhibition plays a major role in the formation of the typical pattern of irregular breathing with frequent apneic intervals of variable duration.

The fluctuating inhibition of brain stem and spinal motor neurons also causes recurrent loss of tonic muscle activity in the upper airways and intercostal muscles. The loss of muscle tone is primarily due to supraspinal inhibition of motor neurons. The diaphragm, which is almost exclusively driven by motor neurons, escapes this inhibition of tone. The inhibition of intercostal muscle activity while diaphragmatic contractions continue causes asynchronous paradoxical respiration. Davi, Koravangattu, MacCallum, Gates, and Rigatto (1979), and Martin, Okken, and Rubin (1979) have shown that the asynchronous chest wall movements present during active sleep are accompanied by a drop in arterial oxygen tension.

Even the diaphragm of the premature infant is likely to fail. The resistance of a muscle to fatigue depends largely on the presence of type 1 high oxidative fibers in it. The adult diaphragm has about 50% of type 1 fibers, the premature infant's diaphragm has only 10%. The high work load of the diaphragm during active sleep is thus likely to cause fatigue patterns characterized by slow respiration, decrease of tidal volume, and frequent apneic episodes.

Not all apneic episodes during active sleep are due to inhibition of respiratory muscle activity. Some of them may be due to upper airway obstruction. The mechanism involved is loss of postural tone in the upper airways which causes obstructive apnea by pharyngeal collapse, laryngeal narrowing, and relapse of the tongue.

Small premature infants spend 16–18 hours each day in the state of active sleep. With maturation of the brain stem reticular system, the development of more neuronal synapses, and the reduction of active sleep time, respiratory neuron activity becomes more stable and the size and incidence of apneic spells are reduced.

THE APNEIC EPISODE

Time is the most crucial factor in determining the sequence of pathophysiological events as-sociated with apnea. The longer the apneic episode lasts, the more serious are the metabolic, circulatory, and cerebral effects.

Until today, there was no universal agreement as to the definition of apnea. Some definitions included all apneic intervals of over 10 seconds duration, others counted only those longer than 20 seconds, or those associated with bradycardia. The initial 10–15 seconds of apnea usually have little effect on the infant except for some variations in heart rate. These early variations are not due to hypoxemia and most probably reflect fluctuations of sympathetic output during active sleep. The apneic episode becomes clinically significant when followed by serious slowing of the heart rate or hypoxemia. This occurs inevitably if breathing does not resume (Lucey, Shannon, & Soyka, 1977).

Figure 2 shows the hemodynamic and metabolic effects of a severe apneic episode, and the impact of these events on the causation of hypoxic metabolic and ischemic brain damage. The main metabolic effects of a severe apneic

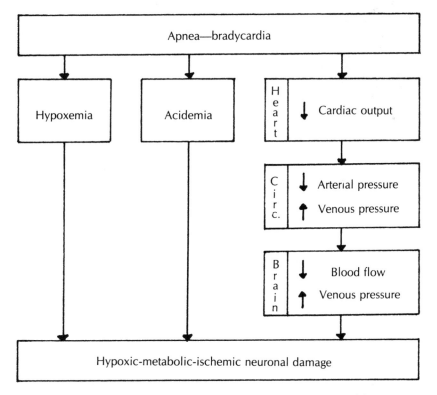

Figure 2. The apneic episode—metabolic and hemodynamic effects causing neuronal damage.

episode are hypoxemia and acidemia. The cardiocirculatory consequences are reduced cardiac output, fall in arterial blood pressure, and increase in central venous pressure. Most important, however, are the effects on the cerebral blood flow. In Chapter 17, Hans Lou has shown that cerebral blood flow is pressure passive in the distressed newborn infant. Hypotension will thus inevitably cause reduction of cerebral blood flow and cerebral ischemia. On the other hand, reduced venous return and increased central venous pressure may increase cerebral venous pressure and cause periventricular hemorrhage.

The hypoxic-ischemic insult may cause serious damage to a number of other organs. Among the most critical complications are necrotizing enterocolitis, reopening of the ductus arteriosus, and renal ischemia.

APNEA AND
METHYLATED XANTHINES

Five years ago at the First International Workshop on the "At Risk" Infant data were presented on the effect of caffeine on apnea. Caffeine and theophylline have since become well-established drugs in neonatal intensive care units all over the world. In fact, they are so well established that it has become difficult to perform any prospective controlled study. Murat, Bun, Couchard, Flouvat, DeGamarra, Relier, and Dreyfus-Brisal (1981) began such a study, but six out of nine infants in the control group had such severe and frequent apneic episodes that withholding the use of caffeine seemed ethically impossible. They, therefore, were also treated with caffeine.

Knowledge concerning the effects of methylated xanthines is constantly growing. These drugs increase the sensitivity of the respiratory center to carbon dioxide and also increase the output of neuronal activity of the respiratory center (Gerhardt, McCarthy, & Bancalari, 1983). Opinions differ concerning the effects of xanthines on sleep states and there is as yet no information about their effects on brain stem conduction time.

Methylxanthines have dramatic effects on the respiration of the small preterm infant. They not only reduce the number and severity of the apneic episodes with respiration becoming less periodic and more regular, but also increase alveolar ventilation causing a reduction in arterial P_{CO_2}.

One should, however, remember that xanthines are not innocent drugs and that they have a wide range of action. Among the possible harmful effects produced by high doses in rats are reduction of cerebral blood flow, inhibition of neuronal division in tissue culture, reduced synthesis of cholesterol in glial cells, chromosomal breakage, and inhibition of thyroid stimulating hormone (TSH) and growth hormone secretion.

Research at the moment is focused on the effects of xanthines on neuronal metabolism and on neurotransmitter synthesis. Initially, the mechanism of action of these drugs was thought to be through the inhibition of cyclic nucleotide phosphodiesterase and a subsequent increase in levels of cyclic adenosine monophosphate (AMP). It is known that cyclic nucleotides play an important role in the production of a variety of neurotransmitters. More recent study does not support this assumption since the concentration of methylated xanthines necessary to obtain such an effect would be extremely high. On the other hand, there is now some evidence that xanthines in therapeutic doses act by competitive antagonism by blocking adenosine receptors. Adenosine is known to inhibit the release of excitatory neurotransmitters in the central nervous system (Goodman & Gilman, 1980).

At present, no serious effects that should prevent the use of xanthines in the treatment of apnea have been identified. Not many follow-up studies are available, however. The study of Gunn, Metrakos, Riley, Willis, and Aranda (1979) could not find any difference in growth and development between control and caffeine-treated infants at 2 years age. Such studies will become more difficult to perform in the future as an increasing number of preterm infants with apneic spells are now treated with methylxanthines. The difficulty of performing clinically controlled studies should not lessen the alertness to possible long-term harmful effects of these potent drugs. More time and energy should be invested in experimental and clinical research aimed at increasing the understanding of the effects of these drugs on the premature infant.

REFERENCES

Cohen, A., Gutnick, M., Zmora, E., & Karplus, M. On quantitative analysis of periodicity in neonatal respiratory signals. *IEEE Transactions of Biomedical Engineering BME*, 1982, *29*, 469.

Davi, M., Koravangattu, S., MacCallum, M., Gates, D., & Rigatto, H. Effects of sleep state on chest distortion and on the ventilatory response to CO_2 in neonates. *Pediatric Research*, 1979, *13*, 982.

Davi, M., Sankaran, K., Simons, J.K., Simons, F.E.R., Seshia, M.M., & Rigatto, H. Physiologic changes induced by theophylline in the treatment of apnea in preterm infants. *The Journal of Pediatrics*, 1978, *92*, 91.

Fawer, C.L., & Dubowitz, L.M.S. Auditory brainstem response in neurologically normal preterm and full term newborn infants. *Neuropediatrics*, 1982, *13*, 200.

Gabriel, M., Albani, M., & Schulte, F.J. Apneic spells and sleep states in preterm infants. *Pediatrics*, 1976, *57*, 142.

Gerhardt, T., McCarthy, J., & Bancalari, E. Effects of aminophylline on respiratory center and reflex activity in premature infants with apnea. *Pediatric Research*, 1983, *17*, 188.

Goodman, L.S., & Gilman, A. *The pharmacological basis of therapeutics* (6th ed.). 1980.

Gunn, T.R., Metrakos, K., Riley, P., Willis, D., & Aranda, J.V. Sequelae of caffeine treatment in preterm infants with apnea. *The Journal of Pediatrics*, 1979, *94*, 106.

Henderson-Smart, D.J., Pettigrew, A.G., & Campbell, D.J. Clinical apnea and brainstem neural function in preterm infants. *New England Journal of Medicine*, 1983, *308*, 353.

Lucey, J.F., Shannon, D.C., & Soyka, L.F. (eds.). *Apnea of prematurity*. Report of the 71st Ross Conference on Pediatric Research. Columbus, OH: Ross Laboratories, 1977.

Martin, R.J., Herrell, N., Rubin, D., & Fanaroff, A. Effects of supine and prone positions on arterial oxygen tension in the preterm infant. *Pediatrics*, 1979, *63*, 528.

Martin, R.J., Okken, A., & Rubin, D. Arterial oxygen tension during active and quiet sleep in the normal neonate. *The Journal of Pediatrics*, 1979, *94*, 271.

Murat, I.M., Bun, M.C., Couchard, M., Flouvat, B., DeGamarra, E., Relier, J.P., & Dreyfus-Brisal, C. The efficacy of caffeine in the treatment of recurrent idiopathic apnea in premature infants. *The Journal of Pediatrics*, 1981, *99*, 984.

Parmelee, A., Stern, E., & Harris, B.A. Maturation of respiration in premature and young infants. *Neuropediatrics*, 1972, *3*, 294.

Parmelee, A., Wenner, W.H., Akiyama, Y., Schultz, M., & Stern, E. Sleep states in premature infants. *Developmental Medicine and Child Neurology*, 1967, *9*, 70.

Phillipson, E.A. Control of breathing during sleep. *American Review of Respiratory Diseases*, 1978, *118*, 909.

Purpura, D.P. *Developmental pathobiology of cortical neurons in immature human brain. Intrauterine asphyxia and the developing fetal brain*. Chicago: Year Book Medical Publishers, 1977.

Schulte, F., Busse, C., & Eichhorn, W. Rapid eye movement sleep, motorneurone inhibition and apneic spells in preterm infants. *Pediatric Research*, 1977, *11*, 709.

Chapter 21

Neurological Assessment of the Full-Term and Preterm Newborn Infant

LILLY M. S. DUBOWITZ, M.D.
Hammersmith Hospital, London, England

THE MAIN AIM OF NEONATAL INTENSIVE CARE is to maintain the integrity of the nervous system. However, until fairly recently, there have been no adequate tools for assessment of the nervous system. The impetus for a standardized neurological examination of the newborn infant came originally from Saint-Anne Dargassies and her associates in Paris (Amiel-Tison, 1968; Andre-Thomas & Saint-Anne Dargassies, 1960; Saint-Anne Dargassies, 1955, 1977), who mapped out the maturation process of tone and primitive reflexes in the preterm infant, and from Prechtl in Holland (Prechtl, 1977), who carefully defined the neurophysiological behavior of the normal full-term infant. Parmelee and his co-workers attempted to develop a simplified quantitative system based mainly on the French work and Prechtl's criteria (Parmelee & Michaelis, 1971). Brazelton developed a neurobehavioral examination (Brazelton, 1973) intended as a behavioral rather than a neurological examination but it has been used for the latter purpose as well. Its main importance has been that it has drawn attention 1) to the fact that the newborn has a complex behavioral pattern, some of which can be objectively assessed,

particularly the ability to hear and see, and 2) to how quickly an infant will become irritable and will quiet with intervention.

All of these newborn neurological examinations have various shortcomings. The French examination was mainly based on tone and reflexes, and though it was standardized for premature infants, it was not advocated for use in the first few days of life and, thus, no normative data are available for this period. The original recording was expressed in terms of maturity reached, which required considerable experience of the recorder for proper administration. Prechtl was the first to draw attention to the "state" of the infant as being an important variable affecting neurological signs. This examination, however, has only been geared to the term infant; thus, preterm infants can only be examined on reaching 40 weeks postmenstrual age.

Parmelee tried to combine some elements from the French school with those of Prechtl and use an objective scoring system with the aid of diagrams. The examination was also geared for 40 weeks postmenstrual age, but could have been adapted to earlier gestation. Its greatest shortcoming was that it aimed for a

The author is grateful to Val Chalk and Doig Simmonds for their help with the preparation of the charts, and to various research associates who have helped to validate stages of this study.

total score. Unfortunately, in neurologically abnormal infants, some neurological signs might be increased while others are decreased; thus, a total score might result in a neurologically normal infant.

Brazelton's examination is also only geared to the full-term infant. It is complex, with 26 individual criteria scored on a nine-point scale. According to Brazelton himself, two examiners are needed to perform two examinations in half a day. The assessment scale is thus better suited as a research tool of infant behavior than as a routine means of assessing neurological normality by a neonatologist.

All of these drawbacks led to a rather negative attitude on the part of neonatal staff toward the neurological examination of newborn infants. This in turn led to poor documentation of the state of the nervous system—the very function whose integrity intensive care aims to maintain. Thus, there has been an increasing need for a neurological examination that would meet the following basic requirements:

1. It can be carried out by staff with no particular experience in neonatal neurology and therefore should have a recording system that is simple and objective.
2. It should be applicable to preterm as well as full-term infants and reliable as soon after birth as possible in order to show the pattern of changes due to drugs, anoxia, difficult delivery, and other environmental influences in the perinatal period.
3. The same examination should be reliable for sequential examination of preterm infants after birth in order to compare their neurological behavior with that of newborn infants of corresponding postconceptional age and also to assess the resolution or development of abnormalities.
4. The full examination and its recording should not take longer than 10–15 minutes at most.

METHOD

Choice of Items

To achieve the above aims, the items selected had to meet the following requirements:

1. Applicable to full-term infants within the first 3 days of life
2. Applicable to preterm infants in an incubator in the first few days of life and also suitable for sequential assessment of the preterm infant
3. Should be easy to define and show good interobserver correlation
4. Should include some items covering aspects of higher neurological function

After all available neurological criteria from the studies of the earlier authors were tested in a series of some 300 infants, the items tabulated in Table 1 were eventually selected.

Method of Recording

From experience with the recording of the assessment of gestation, it was found that by using a flat sheet with the charts printed on it for each infant and recording the appropriate items by circling the item directly on the sheet, recording was vastly improved in both accuracy and speed. In this way, the gestational assessment could be done and recorded within 2 or 3 minutes, and this also provided a permanent objective record for each infant. A similar approach was accordingly adopted in the development of the neurological assessment.

The author and her colleagues decided to record the items on a five-point scale as they found from experience that it provided a reasonable number of gradations to objectively categorize most neurological parameters. Thus, such a scale was used to record items. Because the nine-point scale of the Brazelton technique was somewhat cumbersome and difficult to apply, the Brazelton neurobehavioral criteria were modified to fit the five-point scale as well. Clear instructions for the elicitation of each item were entered on the actual recording sheet, followed by descriptions of the five grades and, wherever possible, illustrative diagrams (see Figure 1). Items such as posture and type of mobility are not static but are constantly changing; therefore, the predominant status during the examination is recorded. Because the newborn infant is not obliging enough to always adhere strictly to the individual dia-

Table 1. Neurological signs used for assessment

Response decrement (Habituation)	Movement and tone	Reflexes	Neurobehavior
Light (torch)	Posture	Tendon reflexes	Eye appearance
Auditory (rattle)	Arm recoil	Palmar grasp	Auditory orientation
	Arm traction	Rooting	Visual orientation
	Leg recoil	Sucking	Alertness
	Popliteal angle	Moro	Peak of excitement
	Head lag		Irritability
	Ventral suspension		Consolability
	Head control		Cry
	(posterior neck muscle)		
	(anterior neck muscle)		
	Head raising (prone)		
	Arm release		
	Body movement		
	Abnormal movement		
	Tremor		
	Startle		

grams, some latitude is allowed by actually recording the asymmetry or aberration on the nearest corresponding figure instead of merely circling the appropriate figure.

This scheme proved to be immensely practical and easy to handle in spite of the large number of items used. It has undergone a number of modifications and amendments during the past few years of use. Some items have been deleted. These include the auditory orientation to a bell, which seemed to be an unnecessary duplication of a similar response to a rattle; the withdrawal response to pinprick as this was often upsetting to the mother and did not seem to be discriminative under pathological circumstances; and the Galant (spinal incurvation) response, which seemed to be invariably present. Other items such as popliteal angle and head lag have been added because they were noted to be aberrant on some of the assessments of gestation of the premature infant and it was thought that they might thus have additional discriminative value in relation to the neurological assessment of the infant, apart from their reflection of the process of maturation of the infant with increasing gestation. The tendon reflexes were initially removed as they seemed of little discriminative value in premature infants or in the first 48 hours of life, but were subsequently included again when it was noted that residents were no longer doing tendon jerks on any infants, even in overtly pathological circumstances such as floppy or paralyzed infants.

Timing and Sequence of Recording

Because many of the neurological items are influenced by the state of the baby, it is important to elicit the individual items with the infant in an optimal state for that item and also to record the state at the time. Accordingly, the examination was done about two-thirds of the way between one feeding and the next (irrespective of the frequency of feeding) in order to try to standardize the state of the infant as much as possible. Preterm infants on continuous feeding (intravenous or alimentary) were examined at any time.

The sequence of examinations was intentionally selected so that those assessments requiring the baby to be in a relatively quiet or sleep state (state 1 or 2) were done first, followed by those not particularly influenced by the state, and subsequently completing the examination with the Brazelton criteria for which the baby needed to be fully awake. The six gradings of state as defined by Brazelton were used rather than the five grades of Prechtl (although the latter might be neurophysiologically more precise), as Brazelton's Grade 3, although a transitional state, was commonly present in preterm as well as full-term infants.

Assessment of Gestation

During their initial examination, all infants had an assessment of gestation done in the course of their neurological examination (Dubowitz, Dubowitz, & Goldberg, 1970).

Name						STATES 1. Deep sleep, no movement, regular breathing. 2. Light sleep, eyes shut, some movement. 3. Dozing, eyes opening and closing. 4. Awake, eyes open, minimal movement. 5. Wide awake, vigorous movement. 6. Crying.	State	Comment	Asymmetry
HOSP. NO.	D.O.B./TIME DATE OF EXAM	WEIGHT HEIGHT	E.D.D. L.N.M.P.	E.D.D. ·U/snd.				
RACE SEX	AGE	HEAD CIRC.	GESTATIONAL SCORE WEEKS ASSESSMENT					

Habituation (≤ state 3)

| Light
Repetitive flashlight stimuli (10) with 5 sec. gap. Shutdown = 2 consecutive negative responses | No response | A. Blink response to first stimulus.
B. Tonic blink response.
C. Variable response. | A. Shutdown of movement but blink persists 2-5 stimuli.
B. Complete shutdown 2-5 stimuli. | A. Shutdown of movement but blink persists 6-10 stimuli.
B. Complete shutdown 6-10 stimuli. | A. Equal response to 10 stimuli.
B. Infant comes to fully alert state.
C. Startles + major responses throughout. | | | |
| Rattle
Repetitive stimuli (10) with 5 sec. gap. | No response | A. Slight movement to first stimulus.
B. Variable response. | Startle or movement 2-5 stimuli, then shutdown. | Startle or movement 6-10 stimuli, then shutdown | A.
B. Grading as above
C. | | | |

Movement & tone — Undress infant

Posture (At rest - predominant)	*			(hips abducted)	(hips adducted)	Abnormal postures: A. Opisthotonus. B. Unusual leg extension. C. Asymm. tonic neck reflex			
Arm recoil Infant supine. Take both hands, extend parallel to the body; hold approx. 2 secs. and release.	No flexion within 5 sec.	Partial flexion at elbow >100° within 4-5 sec.	Arms flex at elbow to <100° within 2-3 sec.	Sudden jerky flexion at elbow immediately after release to <60°	Difficult to extend; arm snaps back forcefully			
Arm traction Infant supine; head midline; grasp wrist, slowly pull arm to vertical. Angle of arm scored and resistance noted at moment infant is initially lifted off and watched until shoulder off mattress. Do other arm.	Arm remains fully extended	Weak flexion maintained only momentarily	Arm flexed at elbow to 140° and maintained 5 sec.	Arm flexed at approx. 100° and maintained	Strong flexion of arm <100° and maintained			
Leg recoil First flex hips for 5 secs, then extend both legs of infant by traction on ankles; hold down on the bed for 2 secs and release.	No flexion within 5 sec.	Incomplete flexion of hips within 5 sec.	Complete flexion within 5 sec.	Instantaneous complete flexion	Legs cannot be extended; snap back forcefully			
Leg traction Infant supine. Grasp leg near ankle and slowly pull toward vertical until buttocks 1-2" off. Note resistance at knee and score angle. Do other leg.	No flexion	Partial flexion, rapidly lost	Knee flexion 140-160° and maintained	Knee flexion 100-140° and maintained	Strong resistance; flexion <100°			
Popliteal angle Infant supine. Approximate knee and thigh to abdomen; extend leg by gentle pressure with index finger behind ankle.	180-166	150-140°	130-120°	110-90°	<90°			
Head control, post. neck m. Grasp infant by shoulders and raise to sitting position; allow head to fall forward; wait 30 sec.	No attempt to raise head	Unsuccessful attempt to raise head; upright	Head raised smoothly to upright in 30 sec. but not maintained.	Head raised smoothly to upright in 30 sec. and maintained	Head cannot be flexed forward			
Head control, ant. neck m. Allow head to fall backward as you hold shoulders; wait 30 sec.	Grading as above	Grading as above	Grading as above	Grading as above				
Head lag Pull infant toward sitting posture by traction on both wrists. Also note arm flexion.	*							
Ventral suspension Hold infant in ventral suspension; observe curvature of back, flexion of limbs and relation of head to trunk.	*							
Head raising, prone Infant in prone position with head in midline.	No response	Rolls head to one side	Weak effort to raise head and turns raised head to one side	Infant lifts head, nose and chin off	Strong prolonged head lifting			
Arm release, prone Head in midline. Infant in prone position; arms extended alongside body with palms up.	No effort	Some effort and wriggling	Flexion effort but neither wrist brought to nipple level	One or both wrists brought at least to nipple level without excessive body movement	Strong body movement with both wrists brought to face or 'press-ups'			
Spont. body movement If no spont. movement try to elicit by cutaneous stim.	None or minimal	A. Sluggish. B. Random, incoordinated. C. Mainly stretching.	Smooth movements alternating with random, stretching, athetoid or jerky	Smooth alternating movement of arms and legs with medium speed and intensity	Mainly: A. Jerky movement. B. Athetold movement. C. Other abnormal movement.	1 2		
Tremors Fast (>6/sec) Mark: or Slow (<6/sec)	No tremor	Tremors only in state 5-6	Tremors only in sleep or after Moro and startles	Some tremors in state 4	Tremulousness in all states			
Startles	No startles	Startles to sudden noise, Moro, bang on table only	Occasional spontaneous startle	2-5 spontaneous startles	6 + spontaneous startles			
Abnormal movement or posture	No abnormal movement	A. Hands clenched but open intermittently. B. Hands do not open with Moro.	A. Some mouthing movement. B. Intermittent adducted thumb	A. Persistently adducted thumb. B. Hands clenched all the time.	A. Continuous mouthing movement. B. Convulsive movements.			

Figure 1. Protocol of neurological examination of the newborn infant.

Scoring of Items

Items were intentionally not rated to result in a single total score as this might mask variations in individual items, and significant changes in opposite directions might merely cancel each other out. The preferred method was to document individual items on a *pro forma* sheet so that patterns of responses could be readily seen. This approach also allows one to use part of the *pro forma* when the infant may be too ill to elicit all the responses. It will also allow flexibility and ready modifications if one wants

Reflexes

						State	Comment	Asymmetry
Tendon reflexes Biceps jerk / Knee jerk / Ankle jerk	Absent	Present	Exaggerated	Clonus				
Palmar grasp Head in midline. Put index finger from ulnar side into hand and gently press palmar surface. Never touch dorsal side of hand.	Absent	Short, weak flexion	Medium strength and sustained flexion for several secs.	Strong flexion; contraction spreads to forearm.	Very strong; infant easily lifts off couch			
Rooting Infant supine, head midline. Touch each corner of the mouth in turn (stroke laterally).	No response	A. Partial weak head turn but no mouth opening. B. Mouth opening, no head turn.	Mouth opening on stimulated side with partial head turning.	Full head turning, with or without mouth opening.	Mouth opening with very jerky head turning			
Sucking Infant supine; place index finger (pad towards palate) in infant's mouth; judge power of sucking movement after 5 sec.	No attempt	Weak sucking movement; A. Regular. B. Irregular.	Strong sucking movement, poor stripping: A. Regular. B. Irregular.	Strong regular sucking movement with continuing sequence of 5 movements. Good stripping.	Clenching but no regular sucking.			
Walking Hold infant upright, feet touching bed, neck held straight with fingers.	Absent		Some effort but not continuous with both legs.	At least 2 steps with both legs.	A. Stork posture; no movement B. Automatic walking.			
Moro One hand supports infant's head in midline, the other the back. Raise infant to 45° and when infant is relaxed let his head fall through 10°. Note if jerky. Repeat 3 times.	No response, or opening of hands only	Full abduction at the shoulder and extension of the arm.	Full abduction but only delayed or partial adduction	Partial abduction at shoulder and extension of arms followed by smooth adduction. A. Abd>Add B. Abd=Add C. Abd<Add	A. No abduction or adduction; extension only. B. Marked adduction only.	J / S		

Neurobehavioural items

						State	Comment	Asymmetry
Eye appearances	Sunset sign / Nerve palsy	Transient nystagmus. Strabismus. Some roving eye movement.	Does not open eyes	Normal conjugate eye movement.	A. Persistent nystagmus. B. Frequent roving movement. C. Frequent rapid blinks.			
Auditory orientation To rattle. (Note presence of startle.)	A. No reaction. B. Auditory startle but no true orientation.	Brightens and stills; may turn toward stimuli with eyes closed.	Alerting and shifting of eyes; head may or may not turn to source.	Alerting; prolonged head turns to stimulus; search with eyes	Turning and alerting to stimulus each time on both sides			S
Visual orientation To red woollen ball	Does not focus or follow stimulus	Stills; focuses on stimulus; may follow 30° jerkily; does not find stimulus again spontaneously.	Follows 30-60° horizontally; may lose stimulus but finds it again. Brief vertical glance.	Follows with eyes and head horizontally and to some extent vertically, with frowning	Sustained fixation; follows vertically, horizontally, and in circle.			
Alertness	Inattentive; rarely or never responds to direct stimulation	When alert, periods rather brief; rather variable response to orientation	When alert, alertness moderately sustained; may use stimulus to come to alert state.	Sustained alertness; orientation frequent, reliable to visual but not auditory stimuli	Continuous alertness, which does not seem to tire, to both auditory and visual stimuli			
Defensive reaction A cloth or hand is placed over the infant's face to partially occlude the nasal airway.	No response.	A. General quietening. B. Non-specific activity with long latency.	Rooting; lateral neck turning; possibly neck stretching.	Swipes with arm	Swipes with arm with rather violent body movement			
Peak of excitement	Low level arousal to all stimuli; never > state 3	Infant reaches state 4-5 briefly but predominantly in lower states	Infant predominantly state 4 or 5; may reach state 6 after stimulation but returns spontaneously to lower state.	Infant reaches state 6 but can be consoled relatively easily	A. Mainly state 6. Difficult to console, if at all. B. Mainly state 4-5 but if reaches state 6 cannot be consoled.			
Irritability Aversive stimuli: Uncover / Ventral susp. Undress / Moro Pull to sit / Walking reflex Prone	No irritable crying to any of the stimuli	Cries to 1-2 stimuli	Cries to 3-4 stimuli	Cries to 5-6 stimuli	Cries to all stimuli			
Consolability	Never above state 5 during examination, therefore not needed.	Consoling not needed. Consoles spontaneously.	Consoled by talking, hand on belly or wrapping up.	Consoled by picking up and holding; may need finger in mouth.	Not consolable.			
Cry	No cry at all	Only whimpering cry.	Cries to stimuli but normal pitch.	Lusty cry to offensive stimuli; normal pitch	High-pitched cry, often continuous			

Notes *If asymmetrical or atypical, draw in on nearest figure. Record any abnormal signs (e.g. facial palsy, contractures, etc.). Draw if possible.

Record time after feed:

Examiner:

Figure 1. (continued)

RESULTS

The format of the final *pro forma* (Dubowitz & Dubowitz, 1981) is shown in Figure 1. The examination could be recorded on a single flat sheet. Since the instructions are included on the sheet itself and the recording is directly on the sheet (Figure 2), it can be done quickly and accurately. The average time for examination and recording done by one examiner is under 15 minutes; if a second person is available for recording, it can be completed on a premature

to add or remove items in one particular area, for example neurobehavioral, in relation to particular studies.

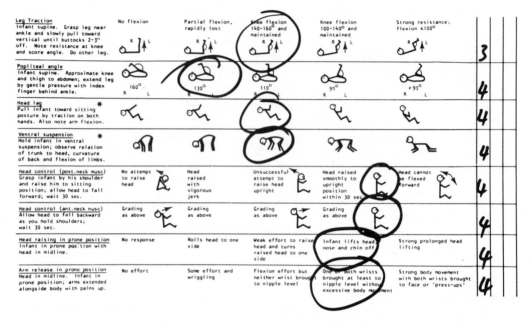

Figure 2. Part of protocol to show the method of scoring/documentation.

infant within 5–10 minutes. The entire procedure was well tolerated by preterm infants as young as 28 weeks gestation and within 24 hours of birth.

Members of the junior medical staff with no prior expertise in neonatal neurology could readily be trained in administration, and they showed good interobserver recording on the same infant. Quality of interobserver recording was determined by either one examiner doing the examination while the other was watching and both recording the data independently, or by two examiners performing the same examination independently of each other on the same day and in the same time-relationship to the infant's last feed.

In a comparative assessment of 352 individual criteria in 11 infants by two observers at the same time (one examining and both recording independently), there was a difference of three grades on only one occasion, of two grades on two occasions, and of one grade on 24 occasions, and the remainder did not differ at all. In a separate study of 12 infants with recording of 340 individual items by two observers separately, there were 10 items differing by three grades (all habituation or startle items), 19 differing by two grades, 82 by one grade, and the remaining 229 were identical.

Observations to Date

This objective type of recording (instead of the customary abnormal/normal) has been invaluable in longitudinal studies and has also drawn attention to a number of things hitherto unrecognized such as changes associated with periventricular hemorrhage.

Normal Infants Full-term infants born after normal pregnancy with minimal medication during delivery and no complications showed a fairly consistent pattern on the *pro forma.*

Preterm Infants Some of the most interesting observations to date have been on the process of maturation in preterm infants. The method has made it possible to study the development of some of the functions not previously studied in newborn preterm infants, such as auditory and visual responses. It has also enabled longitudinal following of the evolution of some of the neurological signs previously only compared in preterm infants at term with full-term newborn infants. Results of these studies show that visual fixation and orientation can be consistently documented in preterm infants from 30 weeks gestation onward and that by 36 weeks postconceptional age, the pattern is fully mature and comparable to full-term infants. Longitudinal studies in preterm infants born at 28–34 weeks gestation have shown a very different pattern of changes in a number of neurological parameters as they approach term (40 weeks postmenstrual age) in comparison with full-term newborn infants. For instance, in the supine posture, premature infants reaching 40 weeks postmenstrual age (PMA) tended to be less flexed than newborn full-term infants, thus appearing "less mature," while in ventral suspension preterm infants reaching 40 weeks PMA had more extensor tone and thus showed better head control and more leg extension (Figure 3). Other neurological criteria have also shown different development in premature infants reaching 40 weeks PMA (Palmer, Dubowitz, Verghote, & Dubowitz, 1982).

Abnormal Infants: Intraventricular Hemorrhage (IVH) Sequential examinations helped identify infants with IVH. Figure 4 shows the examinations on a 30-week-old

infant at 24 hours and on the 5th day of life. The infant shows no habituation to light. Auditory response was present. There was good tone of the limbs on traction and a good flexed posture and popliteal angle, which was commensurate with the gestation. (The flexor tone in the arm would now be regarded as excessive for the gestation.) Some head control was present in the sitting posture and also when the infant was pulled to sit. There was quite good mobility. Excessive tremors and startles were present. Four days later, the posture was extended, limb tone was less, but the popliteal angle (PA) was tighter. Head control was poor, mobility was less, startles and tremors were absent. When these findings were later compared with the ultrasound examinations, it was discovered that this infant sustained a germinal layer hemorrhage on the third day of life. Neurological examinations and ultrasound findings were compared in 100 consecutive infants, and correlations were found with IVH in the following

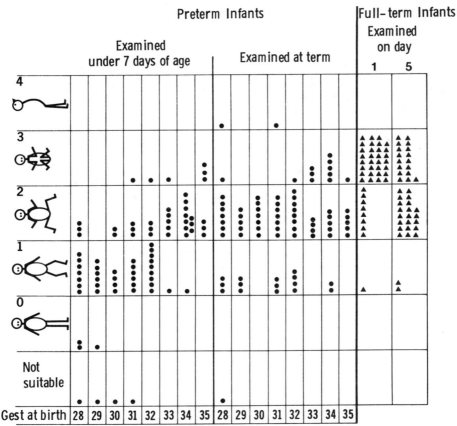

Figure 3. Evolution of posture in preterm infants of varying gestational age examined in the first week and at term. Comparative study of full-term normal infants examined on day 1 and day 5.

Name Ta.	D.O.B./TIME	WEIGHT 1360	E.D.D.	E.D.D.	STATES	State	Comment	Asymmetry
HOSP. NO.	DATE OF EXAM	HEIGHT	L.N.M.P.	U/snd.	1. Deep sleep, no movement, regular breathing. 2. Light sleep, eyes shut, some movement. 3. Dozing, eyes opening and closing. 4. Awake, eyes open, minimal movement. 5. Wide awake, vigorous movement. 6. Crying.			
RACE SEX	AGE 24hrs	HEAD CIRC.	GESTATIONAL ASSESSMENT	SCORE WEEKS				

Habituation (≤ state 3)

Light. Repetitive flashlight stimuli (10) with 5 sec. gap. Shutdown = 2 consecutive negative responses	No response	A. Blink response to first stimulus. B. Tonic blink response. C. Variable response.	A. Shutdown of movement but blink persists 2-5 stimuli. B. Complete shutdown 2-5 stimuli.	A. Shutdown of movement but blink persists 6-10 stimuli. B. Complete shutdown 6-10 stimuli.	A. Equal response to 10 stimuli. B. Infant comes to fully alert state. C. Startles + major responses throughout.	
Rattle. Repetitive stimuli (10) with 5 sec. gap.	No response.	A. Slight movement to first stimulus. B. Variable response	Startle or movement 2-5 stimuli, then shutdown	Startle or movement 6-10 stimuli, then shutdown	A. B. Grading as above C.	

Movement & tone

Posture * (At rest - predominant)	Undress infant			(hips abducted)	(hip adducted)	Abnormal postures. A. Opisthotonus. B. Unusual leg extension C. Asymm. tonic neck reflex	3
Arm recoil. Infant supine. Take both hands, extend parallel to the body; hold approx. 2 secs. and release.	No flexion within 5 sec.	Partial flexion at elbow >100° within 4-5 sec.	Arms flex at elbow to <100° within 2-3 sec.	Sudden jerky flexion at elbow immediately after release to <60°	Difficult to extend; arm snaps back forcefully	3
Arm traction. Infant supine; head midline; grasp wrist, slowly pull arm to vertical. Angle of arm scored and resistance noted at moment infant is initially lifted off and watched until shoulder off mattress. Do other arm.	Arm remains fully extended	Weak flexion maintained only momentarily	Arm flexed at elbow to 140° and maintained 5 sec.	Arm flexed at approx. 100° and maintained	Strong flexion of arm <100° and maintained	3
Leg recoil. First flex hips for 5 secs. then extend both legs of infant by traction on ankles; hold down on the bed for 2 secs and release.	No flexion within 5 sec.	Incomplete flexion of hips within 5 sec.	Complete flexion within 5 sec.	Instantaneous complete flexion	Legs cannot be extended; snap back forcefully	
Leg traction. Infant supine. Grasp leg near ankle and slowly pull toward vertical until buttocks 1-2" off. Note resistance at knee and score leg. Do other leg.	No flexion	Partial flexion, rapidly lost	Knee flexion 140-160° and maintained	Knee flexion 100-140° and maintained	Strong resistance; flexion <100°	3
Popliteal angle. Infant supine. Approximate knee and thigh to abdomen; extend leg by gentle pressure with index finger behind ankle.	180-160°	150-140°	130-120°	110-90°	<90°	
Head control, post. neck m. Grasp infant by shoulders and raise to sitting position; allow head to fall forward; wait 30 sec.	No attempt to raise head	Unsuccessful attempt to raise head upright	Head raised smoothly to upright in 30 sec. but not maintained	Head raised smoothly to upright in 30 sec. and maintained	Head cannot be flexed forward	3
Head control, ant. neck m. Allow head to fall backward as you hold shoulders; wait 30 sec.	Grading as above	Grading as above	Grading as above	Grading as above		
Head lag * Pull infant toward sitting posture by traction on both wrists. Also note arm flexion.						3
Ventral suspension * Hold infant in ventral suspension; observe curvature of back, flexion of limbs and relation of head to trunk.						
Head raising, prone. Infant in prone position with head in midline.	No response	Rolls head to one side	Weak effort to raise head and turns raised head to one side	Infant lifts head, nose and chin off	Strong prolonged head lifting	4
Arm release, prone. Head in midline. Infant in prone position; arms extended alongside body with palms up.	No effort	Some effort and wriggling	Flexion effort but neither wrist brought to nipple level	One or both wrists brought at least to nipple level without excessive body movement	Strong body movement with both wrists brought to face or 'press-ups'	
Spont. body move, supine. If no spont. movement try to elicit by cutaneous stim.	None or minimal	A. Sluggish. B. Random, incoordinated. C. Mainly stretching.	Smooth movements alternating with random stretching, athetoid or jerky.	Smooth alternating movements of arms and legs with medium speed and intensity	Mainly: A. Jerky movement. B. Athetoid movement. C. Other abnormal movement.	1, 2
Tremors. Fast (>6/sec) Mark: or Slow (<6/sec)	No tremor	Tremors only in state 5-6	Tremors only in sleep or after Moro and startles	Some tremors in state 4	Tremulousness in all states	
Startles	No startles	Startles to sudden noise, Moro bang on table only	Occasional spontaneous startle	2-5 spontaneous startles	6+ spontaneous startles	
Abnormal move. or post.	No abnormal movement	A. Hands clenched but open intermittently. B. Hands do not open with Moro	A. Some mouthing movement. B. Intermittent adducted thumb.	A. Persistently adducted thumb. B. Hands clenched all the time.	A. Continuous mouthing movement. B. Convulsive movements.	

Figure 4. Infant with intraventricular hemorrhage on day 4. Part of neurological examination shows a *pro forma* on day 1 and day 5 (before and after IVH).

items: reduction in tone, tight PA, poor mobility, poor visual orientation, roving eye movement. Comparisons under 34 weeks gestation showed that 80% of infants with IVH had more than three positive signs.

The examination also helped to define the evolution of IVH. At the time of the hemorrhage (stage 1), there is usually no auditory response, and arm recoil is greater than leg recoil. There is excessive mobility often ac-

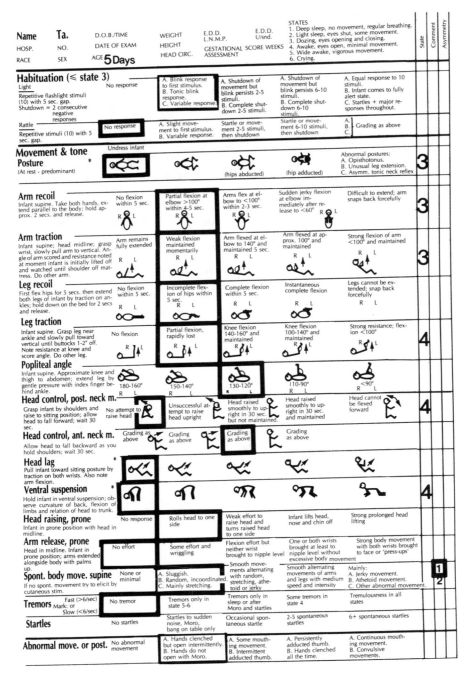

Figure 4. *(continued)*

companied by tremor and startles. Abnormal Moro reflex may be present. Tendon reflexes are often brisk. Visual orientation is absent. Stage 2 is when the hemorrhage is established. Tone and mobility are decreased, and the popliteal angle is relatively tighter. There is generally poor reactivity. Tremors and startles are absent. Visual orientation is absent. Stage 3 is the phase of recovery. Limb tone becomes normal and there is also a decrease in the PA.

Table 2. Neurological signs in various stages of IVH—deviant signs

Stage 1	Stage 2	Stage 3
No auditory response	Tone ↓	Limb tone normal
Arm recoil > leg recoil	Politeal angle ↑	Politeal angle < tone
Excessive mobility	Mobility ↓	Head control ↓
± Abnormal Moro	No tremor or startle	Mobility ↓
Tendon reflexes ↑	No visual orientation	Visual orientation ±
No orientation	Poor reactivity	Roving eye movements ±

Mobility improves next, visual orientation recovers later, and head control appears to be the first to return to normal. During this phase, roving eye movements are often noted (Table 2).

Abnormal Infants: Asphyxiated Infants Asphyxia has been graded in a similar way (Table 3). In mild asphyxia (stage 1), the common findings are poor habituation, flexor hypertonicity, startles and tremors, and hyperalertness. If the asphyxia has been more severe (stage 2), one may find, in addition, neck extension hypertonia. Irritability is often present, which makes the elicitation of orientation difficult. Adducted thumbs are usually present. In even more severe states (stage 3), there is usually marked flexion of the arm with extended legs; often intermittent opisthotonus can be seen. Neck extensor hypertonia can always be elicited. The Moro response is abnormal, and fisting, mouthing, and other abnormal movement may be present; this state is often preconvulsive. Infants with hypoxic encephalopathy may remain in stage 2 or 3 for several days, while infants with a hemorrhage rapidly become hypotonic and unresponsive.

Prediction of Outcome

An attempt was made to compare the predicted outcome of the 129 infants who were followed for 1 year based on an initial ultrasound examination and on a neurological examination at 40 weeks PMA. Fourteen were unable to be traced.

Ninety-one percent of the infants who were classified as being normal at 40 weeks were still normal at 1 year. There was no marked difference between those who had an initial IVH and those who did not. Of the infants who were abnormal at 40 weeks, only 35% were normal at 1 year. Infants who did not have an IVH did slightly better than those where IVH was present: 47% of those without an IVH became normal, compared to 25% of those who did have one. This leads to the conclusion that the clinical course is still probably a more reliable indicator for later outcome than deductions drawn from imaging techniques.

DISCUSSION AND CONCLUSIONS

The neurological scheme that has been evolved has proved to be practical and effective for the assessment of preterm and full-term infants and for the sequential study of the same infant. A combination of neurobehavioral and neurological criteria has proved feasible and, the entire examination can be completed in most infants if the particular sequence of the examination is followed.

At the present time, this scheme has the following to offer:

1. It can be used to record objectively the neurological status of the preterm as well as the full-term infant within 24 hours of birth.

Table 3. Neurological signs in asphyxia—deviant signs

Stage 1	Stage 2	Stage 3	Stage 4
Poor habituation	Poor habituation	No habituation	Convulsions
Hypertonia (flexor)	Hypertonia (flexor)	Extended posture with	
Startles, tremors	Neck extension hypertonia (sit)	flexed arms	
Hyperalertness	Startles, tremors	Differential head control ++	
	Irritability	Startles, tremors	
	± Adducted thumb	Abnormal Moro	
	± Hyperalertness	Fisting, mouthing	
		Poor alertness	

2. It can provide a means to study the preterm infant under normal and abnormal circumstances.
3. It can help to identify and document the effects of perinatal insults, such as drugs in the perinatal period, on the newborn infant.
4. It provides a means of following sequentially the resolution of abnormal neurological signs and of detecting the appearance of new abnormalities.
5. It might provide some guide for prognosis.

Items were intentionally not quantitated collectively to give a single total score because this might mask individual deviations within the comprehensive assessment. The charts will readily define a consistent pattern for the normal infant at varying gestational age, and any deviations in individual parameters readily become apparent. It is also likely that the "normal" pattern may vary from one neonatal unit to another under the influence of aspects of management such as the use of drugs or even the posture in which the baby is nursed. Since the examination can be repeated frequently on the same infant, the evolution of various deviant features can be objectively recorded and followed.

The system has also enabled documentation and evaluation of the progression of certain neurological parameters longitudinally in the preterm infant during postnatal maturation outside the uterus and direct comparison of these parameters with those of the newborn infant of corresponding postconceptional age. This has resulted in a new interpretation on some of the observations documented by earlier authors concerning preterm infants reaching term. Thus, this author believes that some of the neurological signs looked upon by How-

ard and Parmelee as "immature" are probably normal for developing preterm infants because, first, they never develop the mature responses shown by full-term newborn infants (possibly due to the posture in which they are nursed and also the absence of the intrauterine restraint producing the flexed posture in the full-term infant), and second, because of the frequency with which these "immature" responses occur in preterm infants who subsequently have normal or even advanced motor development at follow-up. These results suggest that one ought to probably draw up a completely separate series of norms for preterm infants and not utilize the same criteria on which full-term infants are assessed at follow-up.

Authors in the past have tried to predict the future neurological status of the infant some years later with limited success. The main objective of the author and her colleagues has been to identify and document neurological abnormality in the newborn period. In view of the plasticity of the developing nervous system, the long-term prognosis is likely to be influenced by many factors including the management of the infant, apart from the initial abnormalities themselves, but it would appear that infants who were normal at 40 weeks PMA have a very good chance of remaining normal later.

While the actual interpretation of data will always remain difficult and depend to an extent on experience, the present scheme does provide a means whereby the inexperienced observer can objectively and accurately record meaningful criteria of neurological function in a standardized way. It is hoped that this will provide a useful baseline for the study of the developing nervous system and the factors that influence it.

REFERENCES

Amiel-Tison, C. Neurological evaluation of the maturity of newborn infants. *Archives of Diseases in Childhood,* 1968, *43,* 89–93.

Andre-Thomas, C.Y., & Saint-Anne Dargassies, S. The neurological examination of the infant. *Clinics in Developmental Medicine,* No. 1. London: SIMP/Heinemann, 1960.

Brazelton, T.B. Neonatal behavioral assessment scale. *Clinics in Developmental Medicine,* No. 50. London: SIMP/Heinemann, 1973.

Dubowitz, L., & Dubowitz, V. Neurological assessment of the preterm and full-term newborn infant. *Clinics in Developmental Medicine,* No. 79. London: SIMP/Heinemann, 1981.

Dubowitz, L.M.S., Dubowitz, V., & Goldberg, C. Clinical assessment of gestational age. *The Journal of Pediatrics*, 1970, *77*, 1.

Dubowitz, L.M.S., Levene, M.I., Morante, A., Palmer, P., & Dubowitz, V. Neurological signs in neonatal intraventricular haemorrhage; a correlation with real-time ultrasound. *The Journal of Pediatrics*, 1981, *99*, 127.

Howard, J., Parmelee, A.H., Jr., Kopp, C.B., & Littman, B. A neurologic comparison of preterm and full-term infants at term conceptional age. *The Journal of Pediatrics*, 1976, *88*, 995–1002.

Palmer, P.G., Dubowitz, L.M.S., Verghote, M., & Dubowitz, V. Neurological and neurobehavioural differences between preterm infants at term and full-term newborn infants. *Neuropediatrics*, 1982, *13*, 183.

Parmelee, A.H., & Michaelis, M.D. Neurological examination of the human newborn. In: J. Hellmuth (ed.), *Exceptional infant*, Vol. 2. New York: Brunner/Mazel, 1971.

Prechtl, H. The neurological examination of the full-term newborn infant. *Clinics in Developmental Medicine*, No. 63. London: SIMP/Heinemann, 1977.

Saint-Anne Dargassies, S. La maturation neurologique du premature: [The neurologic maturation of premature infants] *Etudes Neonatales*. [*Neonatal Study*], 1955, *3*, 101.

Saint-Anne Dargassies, S. Neurological development in full-term and premature neonate. Amsterdam: Excerpta Medica, and New York: Elsevier North-Holland, 1977.

Chapter 22

Neonatal Clinical
Neurological Assessment

Paul Casaer, M.D.
Ephrem Eggermont, M.D.
University Hospital, Sint Rafaël-Gasthuisberg, Leuven, Belgium

I N RECENT YEARS, NEONATAL CLINICAL NEURO-
logical assessment has received fresh incentive from two types of studies. First, clinico-
pathological correlations are now possible with
the advent of new brain imaging techniques
such as technetium scanning, computer tomography, ultrasound examination, positron
emission tomography (Volpe, Perlman, Herscovitch, & Raichle, 1982), and nucleic magnetic resonance scanning (Delphy, Gordon,
Hope, Parker, Reynolds, Shaw, & Whitehead,
1982). Second, prenatal behavior can now be
studied with improved ultrasound techniques.
After about 8–10 weeks postmenstrual age,
study of the functional development of the
human nervous system becomes feasible. The
study of behavioral state cycles, posture, and
mobility during the last trimester not only allows assessment of fetal well-being, but also
provides accurate information on the behavior
of preterm infants in the nursery as compared
with *in utero* natural conditions. These two
developments and some new data from prospective studies in the neonatal unit in Leuven

have made it worthwhile to rediscuss neonatal
clinical neurological assessment, including
history, physical examination, and some noninvasive monitoring techniques.

The Neonatal Special Care Unit of the Leuven Children's Hospital has been in operation
since October, 1976. About 910 babies are
admitted each year. Thirty percent of the admitted infants are born in the local department
of obstetrics and 70% of the infants are referred
from regional departments of obstetrics and
pediatrics.

A first prospective study enrolled all babies
(402) admitted from October, 1976 to October,
1979, who had a birth weight of less than 2,000
grams. Follow-up data were obtained from the
outpatient clinic of the department or from
private pediatricians (Eggermont, 1982; Eggermont, Eggermont-Van Den Bossche, Jaeken, DeBisschop, Casaer, & Devlieger,
1977). The second prospective study began in
the autumn of 1979 and enrolled: 1) all infants
born in the local obstetric unit with a birth
weight of less than 2,000 grams, 2) all infants

The authors are grateful to Dr. Hugo Devlieger, neonatologist, and Hans Daniels, experimental psychologist, for their
contributions to the neonatal part of the prospective study as described in this chapter. The authors acknowledge the
obstetricians, pediatricians, and nurses involved in the prospective study. Last but not least, the diligent secretarial help of
Mrs. Paula Trappers is acknowledged.
This research is supported by a grant from the Nationaal Werk voor Kinderwelzijn (National Child Health Organization, Belgium) and by Grant 3.0041 of the Fonds voor Geneeskundig Wetenschappelijk Onderzoek (Medical Research
Council, Belgium).

of diabetic mothers, 3) all infants ventilated from birth not belonging to the previous categories, and 4) a reference group of healthy full-term neonates born in the local obstetric unit. Both in the neonatal period and at the ages of 7 and 18 months (corrected ages), special attention was paid to growth, to nutritional status, and to pediatric or neurological aspects of development by the same small group of researchers with a series of standard protocols (Casaer, Eggermont, Daniels, Devlieger, DeCock, Willekens, & Jaeken, 1982). A study of the neural control of respiration and of developmental aspects of feeding behavior is incorporated in the prospective study (Casaer, Daniels, Devlieger, DeCock, & Eggermont, 1982; Casaer, Devlieger, et. al. 1980; Devlieger, Goddeeris, Moerman, Casaer, & Eggermont, 1982).

ESTIMATION OF GESTATIONAL AGE

Many newborn infants are born after a pregnancy of undetermined duration since their mothers do not know the first day of their last menstrual period. Perinatal pathology is different according to the age of the fetus or the neonate. Therefore, obstetricians and pediatricians developed methods to estimate the gestational age. The relevence of the gestational age for neonatal or follow-up studies cannot be sufficiently stressed; growth and development can only be correctly described if gestational age is taken into account (Gesell & Amatruda, 1947; Parmelee & Schulte, 1970).

Since skin and nervous system maturation are relatively spared during prenatal growth failure, neurological and physical aspects of newborn infants were used to estimate gestational age (Parkin, Hey, & Clowes, 1976; Robinson, 1966). These methods had to be validated on infants of mothers with regular cycles and with a precise knowledge of the first day of their last menstrual periods. The estimation can never be more precise than a variance of ± 2.5 weeks for the 95th percentile range. This variance is due to the biological variation in the time spans between the first day of the last menstrual period, ovulation, fertilization, and delivery (Casaer & Akiyama,

1970). Pseudoaccuracy, therefore, should be avoided in this field (Davies, Robinson, Scopes, Tizard, & Wigglesworth, 1972; Haupt, 1982; Roberton, 1981). A series of studies by Finnström (1972) and by Dubowitz and Dubowitz (1977) resulted in a score combining a series of 10 neurological and 11 external superficial criteria. With this score, the gestational age of relatively healthy newborns can be estimated fairly well. Near term (>37 weeks), the external criteria alone might slightly underestimate the gestational age of small-for-dates (SFD) infants (Ounsted, 1982; Ounsted, Chalmers, & Yudkin, 1978).

Very young and very sick newborns are admitted to neonatal special care units. They are frequently referred from external units without optimal information on maternal and pregnancy history at the moment of their emergency admission. From a series of recent papers, three arguments for not using neurological criteria to estimate the gestational age of these neonates can be derived:

1. In a study of very low-risk premature infants, Prechtl, Fargel, Weinmann, and Bakker (1979) demonstrated that posture is much more an individual than an age-specific characteristic. Furthermore, the variability in posture or the amount of movement resulting in postural changes is so high before a gestational age (GA) of 36 weeks that it is difficult to speak about preference postures when they are only present during 10%–15% of a 2-hour observation period.

2. In sick infants, hypotonia results in lower scores, and hypertonia results in higher scores for the following items: ankle dorsiflexion, leg recoil, head lag in the traction test, and posture during ventral suspension (Ballard, Novak, & Driver, 1979; Hancock, 1973). Therefore, these criteria have been omitted in the Ballard score (Ballard et al., 1979). The remaining neurological criteria (posture in the supine position, square window of the wrist, arm recoil, popliteal angle, scarf sign, and heel-to-the-ear) reflect primarily the visco-elasticity properties of the neuro-

muscular system and, therefore, prenatal postural behavior rather than current nervous system function. It was hoped that the omission of the latter items would improve the Dubowtiz, and even more, the Ballard score (Casaer, Eggermont, Daniels, Devlieger, DeCock, Willekens, & Jaeken, 1982). Studies on infants in neonatal special care units, however, show several shortcomings of the Ballard score, especially of the neurological subscore. The younger the infants, the larger the error in classifying small-for-gestational age (SGA) and appropriate-for-gestational age (AGA) infants. As a rule SGA infants are overestimated. Asphyctic neonates and neonates with severe respiratory distress syndrome (RDS) are underestimated. The errors are significantly smaller if only the external criteria are used (Narayanan, Dua, Guijral, Mehta, Mathew, & Prabhakar, 1982; Vogt, Haneberg, Finne, & Stemsberg, 1981). Dua therefore takes into account only the following external criteria: plantar creases, breast nodule, ear firmness, and a subscore describing the clinical appearance of the anterior vascular capsule in the lens (Narayanan et al., 1982). The

anterior vascular capsule of the lens is a transitory vascular structure that disappears between the 28th and 34th week *in utero*. It can be studied after dilation with direct ophthalmoscopy for the first 48 hours after birth; afterward, it disappears even in the youngest infants (Hittner, Hirsch, & Rudolph, 1977) (see Table 1, item 7). It is interesting to realize that this ophthalmological phenomenon is also the basis for the appearance of the pupil's reaction to light. This last item was selected in 1966 by Robinson as one of the good criteria to differentiate between infants younger than 29 weeks or older than 31 weeks (Robinson, 1966).

3. In a later series of studies, several of the neurological items used for the assessment of gestational age were also used to assess the integrity of the central nervous system of infants during their stay in the intensive care unit (Als, Lester, Tronick, & Brazelton, 1982; Dubowitz & Dubowitz, 1981; Korner, 1980; Ounsted, 1982; Palmer, Dubowitz, Verghote, & Dubowitz, 1982). For infants with known gestational age, this may be a good strategy. In infants with unknown gestational ages, there is obviously a danger of circular reasoning.

Table 1. External characteristics

Criterion	1	2	3	4
1. Breast size Nipple Areola	Below 5 mm Barely visible No areola	5–10 mm Well defined Present; not raised	More than 10 mm Well defined Raised above the skin	
2. Skin opacity (visibility of veins over the abdomen)	Veins, tributaries, and venules clearly seen	Veins and tributaries are seen	A few large vessels are seen	No or very few veins are seen
3. Scalp hair	Fine	Coarse or silky		
4. Ear cartilage	None in the antitragus	Some in the antitragus	Present in the anthelix	Present in the complete helix
5. Fingernails	Do not reach fingertips	Reach the fingertips	Reach or pass the fingertips	
6. Plantar skin creases	Absent	Only anterior transverse creases	Occasional creases on anterior 2/3 of the sole	Whole sole covered with creases
7. Pupillary membrane	Distinct arcades	One or several separate strands	No rests	

$$GA(w) = 21 + 21 \left(\frac{\text{infants score}}{\text{total score}}\right).$$

Adapted from Finnström (1972).

The authors would advocate: 1) putting more effort into obtaining accurate data on maternal and pregnancy history at the moment of transfer of an infant to a neonatal unit; 2) using external criteria as described by Finnström (1972), including the description of the lens, to assess the gestational age (Table 1); and 3) use of neurological assessment to study the normal and abnormal development of preterms in neonatal special care units.

BEHAVIORAL STATES

Close observation of any important variable in the neonate (i.e., transcutaneous oxygen pressure) affords convincing evidence that careful attention to behavioral state cycling is mandatory for sequential clinical evaluation and neonatal monitoring. A comprehensive study of the behavioral state and behavioral state cycling is the most sensitive way to evaluate the integrity of the neonatal nervous system.

Variation in tcP_{O_2} is great in normal neonates. In 2,051 normal neonates during the first week of life, the maximum tcP_{O_2} values varied from 60 to 130 mm Hg, the minimum from 46 to 116 mm Hg (Figure 1) (Huch & Huch, 1981). Hanson and Okken (1980) explain a large part of this variation by sequential studies of tcP_{O_2} taking into account the behavioral states. In normal neonates, tcP_{O_2} is higher in state 1 than in state 2, and is higher in the active awake states (4–5) than in state 2 (Figure 2).

The behavioral states can be described using a simple and lucid four-vector classification

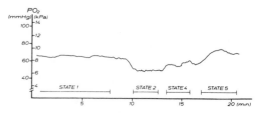

Figure 2. Continuous tcP_{O_2} tracing of a 3,560 g term infant during behavioral states 1, 2, 4, and 5. (Reprinted with permission from Hanson and Okken, 1980).

system (Table 2) (Prechtl & O'Brien, 1982). Meaningful categorization of behavioral and physiological variables (i.e., rate and regularity of heart beat, blood pressure, and several electroencephalographic patterns) is feasible. These variables are listed as state concomitants in Table 3 (Prechtl & O'Brien, 1982). The behavioral state is not only a tool for classification; state is a centrally coordinated mode of neural activity that expresses itself in a variety of variables (Nijhuis, Prechtl, Martin, & Bots, 1982). The lower tcP_{O_2} in state 2 cannot only be explained by cardiorespiratory changes (Hanson & Okken, 1980) but is partly due to a different neural control of respiratory muscle activity and perhaps to a different central reactivity to changes in arterial oxygen and CO_2 tensions. In state 2, there is decreased antigravity muscle activity (Casaer, 1979). A similar decrease in long-lasting intercostal muscle activity during state 2 was found by O'Brien et al. (1982). The resulting loss in thoracic wall stability is at present well documented (Figure 3) (Casaer, Devlieger, Willekens, Daniels, Dereymaeker, Vital-Durand, & Eggermont, 1980; Curzi-Dascalova, 1978, 1982; Henderson-Smart & Read, 1978).

Behavioral States of the Neonate 36 Weeks or Older

State 1   A state 1 interval begins when the respiration becomes regular in an infant who keeps his or her eyes closed. Sighs or short apneic spells occur, but the respiration returns rapidly to regularity (Figure 4). Marked irregularities are always transient and connected with short-lasting gross motor activity. Eye movements under the closed eyelids are not observed. The infant remains in a rather stable posture. Spontaneous clonus can occur in ex-

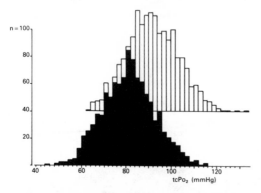

Figure 1.   Probability histogram of the minimal and maximal tcP_{O_2} values in 2051 quiet (awake or asleep) normal neonates during the first week of life. (Reprinted with permission from Huch and Huch, 1972).

Table 2. Vector classification system of behavioral states

	Eyes open	Respiration regular	Gross movements	Vocalization
State 1	−1	+1	−1	−1
State 2	−1	−1	0	−1
State 3	+1	+1	−1	−1
State 4	+1	−1	+1	−1
State 5	0	−1	+1	+1

Signs: +1 = true; −1 = false; 0 = true or false.
From Prechtl and O'Brien (1982).

tremities or at the jaw. Rhythmical mouthing movements appear for a period of seconds lasting to maximum of a few minutes, each burst taking place for 10–20 seconds and the rate increasing to 60 movements per minute. Gross movements are rare but very stereotypic startles do occur and last for a maximum of 1–2 seconds.

State 2 The onset of state 2 after an awake state is determined at the moment the baby closes his or her eyes. If respiration was regular while awake, it becomes more irregular; furthermore, if an antigravity posture was present while awake, this posture will disappear either gradually or stepwise after each body movement during the onset of sleep. The transition from state 1 into state 2 is frequently marked with a startle, gross movements, or at least with a sigh. The respiration is irregular and apneic spells may occur, frequently announced with gross movements. Under closed eyelids, slow eye movements can be observed immediately after the onset of state 2. The typical rapid eye movements appear 1–4 minutes later.

Small twitches are common in state 2; they are visible in the face, hands, and feet. Grimaces, smiles, and rhythmical mouthing are observable at times. Gross movements of one limb or generalized body and head movements are the most characteristic transient events in state 2. Startles do occur, but they are less forceful and less stereotyped than in state 1. The many movements result in frequent changing of postures. In quiet intervals of state 2, the postures are the farthest away from the antigravity postures seen in the awake states and in state 1.

State 3 In state 3, the baby lies still and keeps his or her eyes open. Although there may be moments of staring, most of the time the infant seems to scan the environment with rapid eye movements. The baby frequently shows a stable posture and respiration is regular. State 3 intervals can be very short, lasting only a few minutes. The longest periods can be seen after a feeding. Shorter periods can be observed between two state 2 periods (i.e., awaking during sleep), or as short periods during awake states, preceded or followed by states 4 and 5.

Table 3. Vectors of state concomitants

Variable	State 1	2	3	4	5
Trace alternating EEG	++	−	−	−	−
Low-voltage EEG	−	++	+	++	++
Startles	++	+	−	−	−
Rhythmical mouthing	++	−	−	−	−
Smiles, grimaces	−	++	+	−	−
Gross movements	−	++	−	C	++
Stretch movement	−	++	−	±	−
Antigravity posture	+	−	++	+	+
Slow eye movements	−	++	−	−	−
Rapid eye movements	−	++	++	+	+
Stable heart rate	++	−	+	−	−

Signs: −, absent; ±, rarely present; + and ++, present; O, not applicable; C, a state criterion.
From Prechtl and O'Brien (1982).

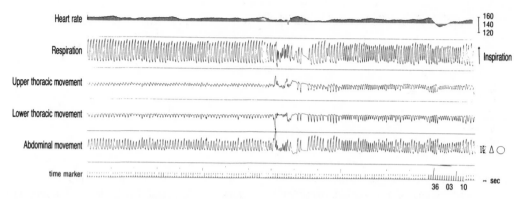

Figure 3. A 3-minute sample of a polygraphic recording of heart rate, respiration, upper and lower thoracic, and abdominal wall movements. The time is marked in seconds. The maximum pen deflection possible for the respiratory movements-recording is 10% of circumferences change. The example shows a transition from State 1 into State 2 in a preterm neonate born at 36 weeks and 3 weeks old at the time of the recording. The changes in the pattern of respiratory movements, the increase in lower thoracic wall retraction at the transition from State 1 into State 2 is clearly displayed.

State 4 The infant in state 4 has his or her eyes open and moves arms, legs, and head. In the prone position, the head lifts and some locomotion does occur; in the supine position, limb movements are frequently less patterned. Periods with large and small movements alternate; respiration is more irregular at moments with large movements. Postures change frequently.

State 5 The major characteristic of state 5 is crying. An infant's cry is a communication signal, and mothers and nurses can discriminate between discomfort, hunger, and pain cries.

Behavioral States of the Neonate Younger Than 36 Weeks

Earlier studies on the ontogeny of behavioral states, mainly based on interval analysis of polygraphic recordings, did not take into account the sequential aspect and came to the conclusion that sleep states gradually emerged from relatively ill-defined and unorganized states into more organized states near term. Up to 36 weeks, 30%–40% of the observed behavior could not be classified in any state. Parmelee and Schulte (1970), among others, used such names as "transitional states." For a review of these early studies, the reader is referred to Casaer and Akiyama (1970).

Prechtl et al. (1979), on the basis of a longitudinal study of very low-risk preterm infants, came to the conclusion that cycles of rest and activity, regular and irregular breathing, and periods with and without eye movements may alternate independently and may accidentally overlap, but often do not coincide at all before 35–37 weeks. After 36 weeks, true behavioral

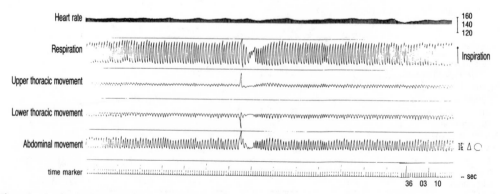

Figure 4. Another 3-minute sample of a polygraphic recording in the same infant as in Figure 3. This sample shows a sigh during State 1.

states could be recognized by the stability of association of parameters for prolonged periods of at least 3 minutes, and by the simultaneous nature of change of parameters at the state transitions. These results could only be found by using the appropriate methodology, namely, a moving window analysis of 3-minute duration, preserving the sequential aspect of the observation.

Behavioral States *In Utero*

With the advent of real-time ultrasonic imaging techniques, it became feasible to study intrauterine mobility, breathing, swallowing, and eye movements of the fetus. Previous studies on rest–activity cycles, on fetal heart rate, and on fetal breathing in the human were inconclusive. Unexplained differences were also found with the common animal model, the fetal lamb. With improved ultrasound techniques, it was demonstrated that human fetuses breathe during parts of REM and non-REM sleep in contrast to fetal lambs, who only breathe during REM sleep (Timor-Tritsch, Dierker, Hertz, Chik, & Rose, 1980; Timor-Tritsch, Dierker, Hertz, Deagan, & Rosem, 1978).

The study of human fetal heart rate as an indicator of fetal well-being was a major advancement because of the recognition of fetal behavioral states. Dawes, Houghton, Redman, and Visser 1982 concluded "the essential feature of normal fetal heart-rate variability in the last trimester is best characterized not by the presence of accelerations, nor absence of decelerations, nor by any overall measure of variability, but by the detection of intermittent episodes of high and low heart-rate variability reflecting changes in fetal state." In Figure 5, the similarity between fetal state cycling and neonatal state cycling is striking (Visser, Carse, Goodman, & Johnson, 1982). Nijhuis et. al. (1982) evaluated the existence of be-

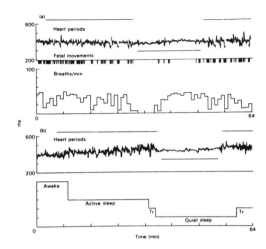

Figure 5. The similarity between fetal state cycling (top) and neonatal state cycling (bottom) is striking. (Reprinted with permission from Visser, Carse, Goodman, and Johnson, 1982).

havioral states and their developmental course in a longitudinal study in 14 low-risk fetuses at 2-week intervals from 32 weeks of gestation until delivery. They defined the fetal behavioral states as follows (see also Table 4).

State 1F: Quiescence, which can be regularly interrupted by brief gross body movements, mostly startles, characterizes state 1F. Eye movements are absent. Heart rate is stable, with a small oscillation band width. Isolated accelerations, strictly related to body movements, occur. This heart rate pattern is called FHRP A.

State 2F: State 2F consists of frequent and periodic gross body movements—mainly stretches and retroflexions—and movements of the extremities. Eye movements are continually present (REMs and SEMs). The heart rate pattern (called FHRP B) shows wider oscillations than FHRP A, and frequent accelerations during movements occur.

State 3F: Gross body movements are absent. Eye movements are continually present.

Table 4. Fetal state criteria represented as vectors

	State vectors			
	State 1F	State 2F	State 3F	State 4F
Body movements	Incidental	Periodic	Absent	Continuous
Eye movements	Absent	Present	Present	Present
Heart rate pattern	A	B	C	D

From Nijhuis et al. (1982).

Heart rate (FHRP C) is stable, but with a wider oscillation band width than FHRP A and no accelerations.

State 4F: Vigorous, continuous activity, including many trunk rotations, is noted. Eye movements are continually present (when observable). Heart rate (FHRP D) is unstable, with large and long-lasting accelerations frequently fused into sustained tachycardia.

Stable constellations and synchronization in the oscillations of state variables only occurred from the postmenstrual age of 36–38 weeks onward, just as it was observed in the low-risk preterms in the nursery. This is a striking example of the possible fruitful interaction between prenatal and postnatal research. The clinical implication of these studies is obvious: "flat" fetal heart rate tracings should only be identified as abnormal when their length exceeds 30 minutes (before 36 weeks) or 40 minutes (near term) (Visser et al., 1982).

Abnormal State, Abnormal State Cycling, and Coma

Nearly every disorder that affects the central nervous system disturbs the level of alertness at some time (Volpe, 1981). Therefore, the first item of the "watch the baby" section of the flow sheet for neonatal intensive care treatment in the neonatal special care unit is related to the behavioral state. In the daily systematic evaluation by means of the Neonatal Special Care Score (see Table 5), item 6 is related to the behavioral state and to increased or decreased activity and reactivity. A baby older than 36 weeks who cannot be classified in one of the five behavioral states is sick or under the influence of medication.

In the full-term neonate, the apathy and coma syndrome are well defined (Prechtl, 1977). A baby is *apathetic* when he or she has a low intensity and high threshold for responses, many absent responses, hypokinesis, and decreased resistance to passive movements. The baby is difficult to arouse. A *comatose* baby is characterized by slow and abnormal respiration, and absent or weak arousal to various stimuli, including pain and vestibular stimulation. Vestibular function can be tested by the vestibulo-ocular responses, and in the not-too-sick baby with the Moro reflex.

To differentiate between normal regular and abnormal regular respiration, attention should be paid to deep breaths or sighs (Figure 4). In a group of 12 normal full-terms, the mean number of sighs during all state 1 intervals of 3-hour observations in the supine position was 1.2

Table 5. Neonatal Special Care Score

Item	3	2	1	
1. Respiration	Ventilator	CPAP	Extra oxygen	Air
2. Circulation	Cardiac shock; bradycardia		Cardiovascular liability	Normal
3. Feeding	Intravenous	Intravenous plus gavage and/or oral	Gavage	Oral
4. Nutritional status	Poor			Good
5. Metabolic homeostasis	Severe deterioration			Good
6. Neurological excitability	Convulsions; coma	Hyperexcitability; apathy	Hyperexcitability on stimulation; lazy	Normal
7. Mobility	Hyperkinetic; hypokinetic			Normal
8. Tonus	Hypertonic; hypotonic			Normal
9. Laterality	Obviously present			Absent
10. Level of care	Intensive	Medium care	Crib	Term infant care

Total score: 30.

Table 6. Levels of alertness in the neonatal period

Level	Arousal response	Motor response	
		Quantity	Quality
Normal	Normal	Normal	Variable
Stupor	Diminished		
Slight	Diminished (slight)	Diminished (slight)	Less variable
Moderate	Diminished (moderate)	Diminished (moderate)	Almost invariable
Deep	Absent	Diminished (marked)	Almost invariable
Coma	Absent	Diminished (marked) or absent	Stereotype

Adapted from Volpe (1981).

sighs in 10 minutes; in the infant seat positioned at 30° from the horizontal the number was 2.7 (Casaer, 1979). Theorell, Prechtl, and Vos (1974) found an absence of sighs in a group of neurologically abnormal infants, several of whom had received anti-epileptic medication.

Although knowledge of spontaneous and elicited behavior in preterms is still very limited, Volpe's (1981) scale describing alertness is applicable to full-terms and to preterms in the author's experience (Table 6). The aspect of quality of movements is very important. Both *in utero* (Prechtl, H. F. R. personal communication, 1982) and in the preterm stereotype, mobility is an indicator of disease and variable mobility is an indicator of health.

The knowledge of spontaneous behavior in state 2 helps in differentiating convulsions from the physiological twitches in the muscles of the face and extremities occurring together with rapid eye movements. This differentiation avoids inappropriate treatment and false risk estimation for the future.

In conclusion, cycles of activity should be present in healthy newborns, in full-terms, and in preterms. After 36 weeks, true behavioral state cycles can be recognized; before 36 weeks, there are more or less independently occurring cycles of activity and quiescence, intervals of regular and irregular breathing, and periods with and without REM movements. These cycles can be recognized from the cardiorespirograms and from the tcP_{O_2} monitoring, especially when they are complemented with good behavioral notes of the nursing staff. Attention to the behavioral state and behavioral state cycling is the single most sensitive way to evaluate the integrity of the neonatal nervous system.

NEONATAL NEUROLOGICAL ALARM SIGNS

There is fair agreement in the literature about neonatal neurological alarm signs. The alarm signs listed in Table 7 are mentioned by many authors (Amiel-Tison & Grenier, 1980; André-Thomas, Chesni, & Saint-Anne Dargassies, 1960; Brown, Purvis, & Forfar, 1974; Joppich & Schulte, 1968; Prechtl, 1980; Saint-Anne Dargassies, 1977; and Touwen, 1978). The occurrence and re-occurrence of respiratory difficulties and apnea as signs of neurological

Table 7. Neonatal neurological alarm signs

1. Persistent fussing
2. Difficult feeding
3. Persistent deviation of head and/or persistent abnormal eye position
4. Persistent asymmetry in posture and movements
5. Imperative opisthothonos
6. Apathy and immobility
7. Floppiness
8. Hyperexcitability, jittery movements
9. Convulsions
10. Abnormal cry
11. Combination of setting-sun sign, vomiting, wide sutures, and/or abnormal increase in skull circumference
12. Occurrence and especially re-occurrence of respiratory difficulties and apnea
13. Loss of variability in physiological parameters such as respiration, heart rate, and transcutaneous oxygen pressure

dysfunction (sign 12) should be stressed in this context (Illingworth, 1957; Miller, 1958; Nelson & Ellenberg, 1979; Schulte, 1974; Volpe, 1977b). To verify the occurrence and reoccurrence of apnea, the effect of gestational age on the incidence and duration of apnea was studied by Henderson-Smart (1981). In his study, recurrent apnea (i.e., three or more episodes of apnea of longer than 20 seconds duration) occurred in 1% of 25,154 live-born babies between 1974 and 1979. In 77% apnea commenced in the first 2 days of life; it was unlikely to commence after 7 days. The gestational age at birth had an enormous impact as to the postnatal age when the last apnea was detected (Figure 6).

As mentioned above, the present authors consider that, in the intensive care situation, the loss of variability in respiratory pattern, heart rate, and transcutaneous oxygen pressure are indicators of severe distress (Table 7, sign 13). Special attention should be paid to decrease or disappearance of sighs (Figure 4).

In conclusion, the alarm signs discussed above may be the first signals of central nervous system damage (e.g., intracranial hemorrhage). More frequently, they result from metabolic disturbances such as hypoxia or hypocalcemia, or from sepsis or meningitis.

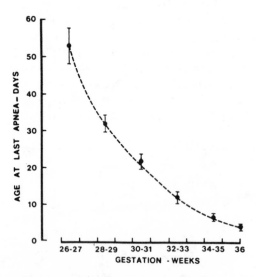

Figure 6. Mean (± standard error of the mean) postnatal age when last apnea was detected versus gestational at birth in 25, 145 infants. (Reprinted with permission of Henderson-Smart, 1981).

The improvement of the neurological condition may be the first sign of appropriate treatment.

SYSTEMATIC NEUROLOGICAL EXAMINATION

Besides these very sensitive but rather nonspecific signs, systematic neurological examination may direct the diagnosis toward specific neurological disorders of the central and peripheral neuromuscular system.

Infants of 36 Weeks Gestational Age or Older

As to methodology, examiners are on solid ground with infants of 36 weeks gestational age or older. The neurological examination devised by Prechtl (1977) is capable of assessing the integrity of the nervous system. The method is sensitive enough to differentiate between central and peripheral muscular system disorders. It allows the description of subsystem dysfunctioning, which can now be correlated with brain imaging techniques. The design and the methodology are discussed in detail elsewhere (Prechtl 1977, 1982). In this section, a few important points are stressed with the help of a flow diagram (Figure 7) from Prechtl (1977).

The term infant is equipped with a variety of transient neural mechanisms. Neurological examination items specific for that age, i.e., the Moro reflex, will therefore never be found in the neurological examination of a 2-year or a 10-year-old child or an adult. Age-specific techniques are essential for any developmental neurological assessment. For standardization factors related to the environment, the infant and the examiner should be specified. Environmental light, temperature, and noise should be taken into account. Bright light makes the baby close his or her eyes although he or she is not asleep. Dull background noise makes the infant sleepy. The behavioral state of the infant and its impact on nervous system functioning has already been discussed. The observed differences in the responses toward various sensory modalities in states 1, 2, and 3 are summarized in Table 8 from Prechtl (1974).

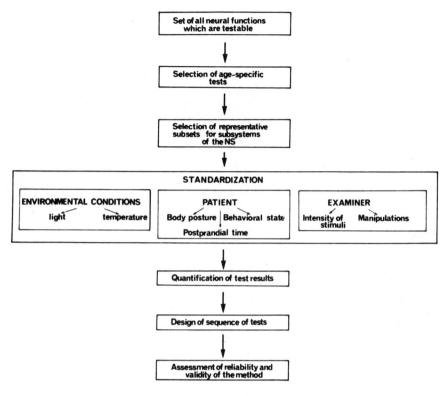

Figure 7. Flow diagram indicating the decision steps for the design of a neurological examination technique. (Reprinted with permission of Prechtl, 1977 and 1982).

The body posture of the baby should be constant and symmetrical if possible since posture has an influence on symmetry and intensity of many spontaneous activites and responses. Food intake also has an effect; therefore, the examination should optimally be carried out 2–3 hours after the last feeding. The examiner should standardize the stimulus in such a way that a good response is elicited. The description of the individual test procedures should be such that interscorer reliability is acceptable. The responses should be quantifiable and quoted as such. Finally, and of utmost importance, the *sequence* of the tests should be standardized. Many responses affect the state and state cycling and may so affect the intensity of following responses.

After working out all these steps, Prechtl made the comprehensive neurological examination available. From a systematic analysis, a short (10-minute) screening procedure was derived. It contains the evaluation of spontaneous posture and mobility in the supine position,

resistance to passive movements, the pull-to-sit procedure, rooting and sucking responses, and the Moro response, and pays special attention to position and movements of the eyes. This short procedure allows evaluators to differentiate between normal and suspect full-terms. The latter should be examined with the comprehensive, 30-minute procedure. This neurological examination is not to be confused with the Neonatal Behavioral Assessment Scale of Brazelton (Brazelton, 1973), which is more "global" but therefore less specific for making a neurological diagnosis.

Preterm Infants of 35 Weeks Gestational Age or Younger

Evaluators are much less confident in their examinations of preterm infants or infants in intensive care situations. The reasons for this insecurity are easily derived following the flow diagram in Figure 7. Knowledge of the ongoing neural mechanisms is much more restrict-

Table 8. Responses to stimulation in different states

	State 1	State 2	State 3
Proprioceptive reflexes			
Knee jerk	+++	±	++
Biceps jerk	+++	±	++
Lip jerk	+++	±	++
Ankle clonus	+++	−	−
Moro tap	+++	−	++
Moro head drop	+++	−	++
Exteroceptive skin reflexes			
Tactile			
Rooting	−	−	++
Palmar grasp	−	+	++
Plantar grasp	−	++	++
Lip protrusion	−	+++	++
Finger reflex	−	+	++
Toe reflex	−	++	++
Tibial reflex	±	++	++
Fibular reflex	±	++	++
Axillary reflex	±	++	++
Pressure			
Babkin	−	+	++
Palmomental	−	++	++
Nociceptive			
Babinski reflex	++	+++	+++
Abdominal reflex	++	+++	+++
Thigh	++	+++	+++
Pubic	++	+++	+++
Inguinal	+++	+++	+++
Auditory orienting	±	++	+++
Visual pursuit	−	−	++
Vestibulo-ocular	−	++	+++

From Prechtl (1974).

ed. The behavioral state concept is not as applicable. Problems of standardization are much more difficult in small infants under intensive care, i.e., imposed position and time since last feeding. One must admit that not enough knowledge is yet available to provide a comprehensive neurological examination for preterm newborns. From several studies of spontaneous activity and from the present authors' study on feeding behavior, it seems that perhaps more than one examination for preterm infants will be necessary. Infants younger than 30 weeks might need another approach than infants 30–34 weeks old and those older than 35 weeks.

Authors with vast experience in a specific area of neurological or behavioral assessment have reported interesting clinical findings on preterms. Dubowitz and Dubowitz (1981), after using various resistance testing maneuvers for the gestational age assessment, reported that increased resistance at the popliteal angle is a good differentiator of normal preterms and preterms with intraventricular hemorrhage. Als et al. (1982) have reported a series of fascinating behavioral descriptions in preterms, but the scale used is not yet accepted as a clinical examination tool. Studies on spontaneous posture and mobility in relation to respiratory patterns and to feeding are currently being carried out by the present authors in the special neonatal care unit to obtain more information on neural functions in those specific age groups (Casaer, Daniels, Devlieger, DeCock, & Eggermont, 1982; Casaer, Daniels, Devlieger, & Eggermont, 1981; and Casaer et al., 1980).

As to clinical diagnosis, the authors have attempted to assess the behavioral state and its "precursors" and to differentiate these states from abnormal states (see Table 6). In the intensive care unit, the sequence of the screening procedure (Prechtl, 1977) was used as a guideline, and the feasibility of test items as well as the responses to test items were noted. In the medium and normal care units, the comprehensive neurological examination of the full-term was used and feasibility and responses were again evaluated in prospective studies. From 34 weeks onward, feasibility was good in the first cohort of 100 infants with a birth weight of less than 2,000 grams.

SPECIFIC CLINICAL NEUROLOGICAL DIAGNOSES

Taking into account the limited knowledge concerning preterm infants of 35 weeks gestational age or younger, a series of specific clinical diagnoses can be made in the intensive and special care units. Some of these are discussed below.

Hyperammonemia in the Preterm Infant

Six infants with transient hyperammonemia and four infants with hyperammonemia secondary to urea cycle defects were recently observed in the neonatal special care unit at Leuven (Eggermont, Devlieger, Marchal, Jaeken, Vandenbussche, Smeets, Vanacker, & Corbeel, 1980; Jaeken, Devlieger, Casaer, & Eggermont, 1982). The clinical picture at the time of severe ammonia elevations can be described as follows: sudden neurological deterioration accompanied by severe hypotonia and areflexia, leading to coma in a few minutes to a few hours. Although the infants were ventilated and although they showed fixed mydriasis and had absent vestibulo-ocular responses, they all responded with stereotypically elicited arm movements on touching the thoracic wall, especially on gently squeezing the lower ribs. The arm movements were always antigravity movements, but the degree of extension and abduction followed by flexion and adduction varied from one baby to the other. On abdominal palpation, they also showed jerky movements of the lower limbs, like a puppet on a string. The segmental imput is very specific, since the movements cannot be elicited by head movements nor by tactile, nociceptive, or proprioceptive stimuli of the extremities.

Neonatal Hypothyroidism

A more gradual deterioration with hypokinesia, hypotonia, and a slowing down of gastrointestinal mobility may point to neonatal hypothyroidism. Prompt institution of therapy may avoid further deterioration requiring intensive care and ventilation assistance (Casaer, Eggermont, Daniels, Devlieger, DeCock, Willekens, & Jaeken, 1982).

Spinal Cord Lesion

Spinal cord lesion is characterized by hypotonia, hyporeflexia, and bladder retention after neonatal asphyxia. It demands a detailed examination of spontaneous motor activity, tonus, and reflexes of upper and lower extremities. The skin reflexes (especially the Galant reflex) are particularly helpful in determining the level of a spinal cord lesion (Bucher, Bolthauser, Friderich, & Isler, 1979).

Neuromuscular Disorders

Orthopaedic malformations of the extremities may reflect nonoptimal intrauterine position and mobility. A detailed family history and neurological examination of the baby and his or her parents may lead to the diagnosis of neuromuscular disease (e.g., Steinert's disease), or to the diagnosis of a caudal regression syndrome (Dubowitz, 1980) or an amniotic band syndrome (Seeds, Cefalo, & Herbert, 1982). A precise diagnosis is not only relevant for the management of the newborn but also for the genetic implications for the family. Feeding difficulties require a detailed examination of the cranial nerves. A hypotrophic tongue, an abducens palsy (no lateral eye movements during the vestibulo-ocular responses), and a facial palsy or paucity of facial expression with absent glabella reflex correspond to a clinical picture of Moebius syndrome. Volpe (1981) provides a detailed and pragmatic discussion of the examination of normal and abnormal cranial nerve functioning.

Hypoxic-Ischemic Encephalopathy and Intracranial Hemorrhage

Among others, Brown et al. (1974), Pape and Wigglesworth (1979), and Volpe (1977a) have described the clinical course of hypoxic-ischemic encephalopathy in detail. The prototype, mostly due to asphyxia occurring *in utero*, occurs between birth and 12 hours of age and results in deep stupor or coma, respiratory irregularities, hypotonia, minimal movement, and seizures. At this stage, pupillary and oculomotor responses are still intact. Between 12 and 24 hours, the clinical features change. The infant becomes less stuporous, has more seizures and apneic spells, and jittery movements occur. A muscle weakness is observed in the hips and shoulders of the full-term infant, while in the preterm infant it is more pronounced in the lower limbs. Between 24 and 72 hours a decisive point is frequently reached. When the situation deteriorates, the infant becomes more stuporous, respiration ceases, and ocular abnormalities occur. The catastrophic deterioration and a bulging fontanel lead to the diagnosis of intraventricular hemorrhage, which is confirmed by lumbar puncture, CT scan, or ultrasound. Infants surviving these 72 hours may evolve toward a clinical picture of diminishing stupor, disturbed sucking, and swallowing, gag, and tongue movements. Hypotonia may turn to hypertonia. Volpe (1981) has explained the dramatic deterioration by the flow of blood through the ventricular system with sequential disturbance of diencephalon, midbrain, pons, and medulla. He has also correlated these clinical syndromes with neuropathological findings and more recently with isotope and CT scans. The parasagittal cerebral necrosis (most frequently observed in the full-term) corresponds with the hip-shoulder weakness in the full-term. This neuropathological correlate precisely fits the topographical representation of the body on the brain surface. The lower limb weakness, more frequently seen in preterm infants, corresponds with periventricular leucomalacia.

In preterm infants, the above described dramatic deterioration may also be observed after 72 hours. In the latter group, a hypoxic-ischemic event frequently occurs 24–48 hours earlier (Pape, Armstrong, & Fitzhardinge, 1976; Papile, Burstein, Burstein, & Koffler, 1978; Volpe, 1981). In a group of 95 consecutively admitted infants born at less than 33 weeks, Thorburn, Lipscomb, Stewart, Reynolds, and Hope (1982) found 36 infants (38%) with periventricular hemorrhage (PVH). The most significant antecedents of PVH were short gestation and the presence of severe respiratory illness, necessitating mechanical ventilation. Pneumothorax was the single most significant antecedent. Convulsions and cardiopulmonary collapse emerged as significant associates but not as antecedents of PVH.

Besides the catastrophic picture of intracranial hemorrhage, a salutary syndrome with a more subtle presentation emerges. It consists of an altered level of consciousness, a change in quantity and quality of spontaneous and elicited movements, hypotonia, and deviations of the eyes (a vertical, mostly downward drift of the eyes, and an incomplete response to the doll's head maneuver). The picture evolves over many hours, and unpredictable improvements and deteriorations may alternate for days. Most of these infants survive. Volpe (1978) states: "the reader should not accept the notion that major periventricular hemorrhage in premature infants is a clinically silent event, but rather accept the challenge to look much more closely at the neurological signs in such infants." In a recent prospective study of 100 preterm infants using independently administered clinical, neurological, and ultrasound examinations, Dubowitz, Levene, Morante, Palmer, and Dubowitz (1981), and Levene, Dubowitz, Palmer, Fawer, and Dubowitz (1981) found that decreased mobility, especially of the lower extremities; increased resistance to passive movements, specifically in the popliteal angle maneuver; and absence of eye-following movements, with presence of roving eye movements, were significantly associated with the presence of blood in the ventricles.

The subsequent evolution toward hydrocephaly of 25%–50% of these infants with blood in the ventricles or in the arachnoidal spaces requires careful clinical follow-up and ultrasound studies, since the classical signs of evolving hydrocephaly (see Table 7, sign 11) may not appear for days and weeks after the ventricular dilatation has occurred (Hill & Volpe, 1981; Korobkin, 1975). In prospective studies combining a detailed and sustained clinical evaluation with the ultrasound examinations, Dubowitz and Dubowitz (1981) found the loss of previously good eye-following movements to be an indicator of evolving hydrocephalus.

In conclusion, a systematic neurological assessment is mandatory for specific clinical neurological diagnoses. Technical investigations such as electroencephalography, electromyography, computerized axial tomography, and ultrasound techniques are valuable diagnostic tools but cannot replace the clinical evaluation.

RISK ESTIMATION OF FUTURE DEVELOPMENTAL ABNORMALITIES

Although the perinatal period is of utmost importance for the developing brain, perinatal hazards are only responsible for 15%–20% of severe developmental handicaps. If learning and behavioral difficulties are included, this percentage may be doubled (Hagberg, 1981; Scheiner & Abroms, 1980). Genetic, environmental, and socioeconomic factors are responsible for the major part of the remaining 80%–85% (Eggermont et al., 1977; Scheiner & Abroms, 1980; Sigman & Parmelee, 1979). Since the growth of the human brain is still marked up to the age of 2 years (Dobbing, 1974), hazards to the nervous system during the early years should not be overlooked.

With a good system for detection and referral of high-risk pregnancies (including genetic and socioeconomic risks), only 5% of all births need to be referred to neonatal special care units. Under these conditions, about 25% of the referred infants have a very high risk and 75% of infants have an increased risk. If for the 25% of high-risk infants a comprehensive neurodevelopmental assessment is assured, 75%–80% of the severely delayed infants will be detected early during the first 2 years; the remaining 20%–25% of severely delayed children should be detected by routine screening in the primary care medical system (DeCock et

al., 1980; Hobel, 1978; Hobel, 1980; Scheiner & Abroms, 1980). Defining risk infants during their stay in a neonatal unit is an important step in early diagnosis.

The Optimality Score

Abnormality, its degree, and duration are hard to define. Therefore, Prechtl (1967) proposed to focus attention on normal events. He made a score of optimal conditions, each point being a well-defined optimal condition that carries the least risk for mortality and morbidity. A comprehensive list of optimality criteria was compiled covering: a) 11 factors related to maternal and obstetrical history including social factors, b) 11 pregnancy factors, c) 10 factors related to parturition, d) 10 perinatal, and e) 10 postnatal factors related to the infant. Examples of such factors are: a) optimal age of the mother, good social class of the family, absence of previous early and late abortion; b) no vaginal bleeding, no hypertension, no drugs; c) cephalic presentation, clear amniotic fluid, no sedation or analgesia; d & e) gestational age, birth weight, Apgar score at 1 minute > 8, Apgar score at 3 minutes > 9.

In the present authors' study, the list of items proposed by Michaelis, Dopfer, Gerbig, Fellerdopfer, and Rohr, (1979) was used. A more recent version was published by Touwen, Huisjes, Jurgens v.d.Zee, Bierman Van Eendenburg, Smrkovsku, and Olingo (1980). A further updating based on statistical analysis of internal consistency is expected soon (H. F. R. Prechtl, personal communication, 1982). Each condition receives one point; thus, a significant decrease of total optimality is only possible if several items are not optimal (Prechtl, 1980). Michaelis et al. (1979) proposed the term "reduced optimality" for the total number of nonoptimal conditions.

It is the authors' experience that if only one condition commanded most of the medical attention during the neonatal period, the optimality score is very useful to avoid overestimation of that condition during neonatal care and follow-up. Huisjes, Okken, Prechtl, and Touwen (1975) showed that maternal hypertension was only associated with an in-

Table 9. Percentile values of the reduced optimality scores in 100 infants with a birth weight of less than 2,000 grams

Optimality criteria	Percentile						
	0	10	25	50	75	90	100
A—Maternal history	−0	−1	−2	−2	−3	−4	−7
B—Pregnancy history	−1	−1	−2	−3	−4	−5	−6
(A + B)	(−2)	(−3)	(−4)	(−5)	(−7)	(−9)	(−13)
C—Parturition	−0	−1	−2	−4	−5	−6	−6
D—Perinatal condition of the infant	−2	−2.5	−3	−5	−6	−7	−8
E—Postnatal adaptation of the infant	−0	−1	−2	−3	−5	−6	−8
(C + D + E)	(−4)	(−7)	(−9)	(−12)	(−15)	(−17)	(−20)
Score total (N = 100)	−8	−11	−13.5	−18	−20	−23	−31
Michaelis et al. (1979) (N = 400)		−3	−4	−5	−7	−10	

creased risk for developmental delay in infancy when the optimal score was low or the reduced optimality was high. Michaelis, Rooschuz, & Dopfer (1980) used the optimality score to show that the hemiparetic type of cerebral palsy is much more related to the prenatal factors of reduced optimality than to delivery or neonatal factors. In the authors' prospective study of infants with a birth weight of less than 2,000 grams, the 25th percentile of the first series of 100 infants had a reduced optimality of −13, the 75th percentile was a −20 (Table 9 and Figure 8). From this analysis, it is obvious that the population in the special care unit in Leuven is at a much higher risk than the reference population of Michaelis et al. (1979) in Tübingen. The 25th and the 75th percentiles of the latter population had a reduced optimality of −4 and −7, respectively. In the special care unit at Leuven, the use of these data displayed in Figure 8 permits a quick evaluation of the risk of a newly admitted infant.

Neurological Events during the Stay in the Neonatal Unit

There are obvious abnormal neurological conditions that carry a high risk for developmental abnormalities. In their analysis of the National Collaborative Perinatal Project (40,057 single births), Nelson and Ellenberg (1979) showed "a more than 20 times increased relative risk for cerebral palsy" for the following situations: neonatal seizures (71), multiple apneic episodes (36), diminished crying for more than 24 hours (21), and gavage or tube feeding required due to feeding difficulties (21). Neurological items such as changes in tone, hypoactivity for more than 24 hours, or marked myoclonic activity resulted in an increased risk of 15–25 times. The more accurate a neonatal neurological etiological diagnosis, the better the risk estimation that can be made. Volpe (1977b, 1981) broke down the percentage of normal development in infancy after neonatal

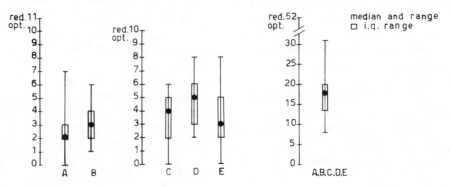

Figure 8. Median, interquartile ranges, and total ranges of the reduced optimality score in the five subcategories, and the total reduced optimality score in 100 infants with a birth weight less than 2,000 grams.

Table 10. Prognosis of neonatal seizures according to the etiological diagnosis

Neurological diagnosis	Percentage of normal development		
Hypocalcemia			
Early onset		50	
Late onset	80	—	100
Primary subarachnoid hemorrhage		90	
Hypoglycemia		50	
Bacterial meningitis	20	—	50
Hypoxic-ischemic encephalopathy	10	—	20
Developmental defect of the brain		0	

Adapted from Volpe (1977b and 1981).

seizures according to their etiology (Table 10). The chance for normal development varies from 0% in an overt developmental abnormality of the brain to 100% in late onset hypocalcemia. Those who expect that computerized tomography and/or ultrasound can solve the problem of individual prediction will be disappointed. Obviously, moderate to severe lesions shown by radiological documentation (large amounts of intraventricular and/or intracerebral blood) will be associated with an enormous increase in risk for severe developmental disorders, taking into account that 50% to 70% of these infants die (Krishnamoorthy, Fernandez, Momose, DeLong, Moylan, Todres, & Shannon, 1977; Papile et al., 1978; Volpe 1979a, 1981). The problem, however, will concern mild to moderate lesions (subependymal lesions or a small amount of intraventricular blood). Of those infants with mild to moderate lesions, only 10% to 25% die. Preliminary follow-up studies during infancy do not show significant differences in motor and mental development of preterms with a birth weight less than 1,500 grams, with or without small or medium sized intraventricular bleeds (Dykes, Lazzake, & Ahmann, 1980; Ment, Scott, Ehrenkranz, Rothman, Duncan, & Warshaw, 1982; Papile, Munsick, & Weaver, 1979).

The prognosis depends on the severity of the hypoxic-ischemic insult that preceded the bleeding, on the severity and length of intracranial pressure increase at the time of the bleeding, on the destruction caused by the bleeding in the periventricular white matter and germinal matrix, and on the evolution toward posthemorrhagic hydrocephalus. Furthermore, the subsequent evolution of the neonate in the neonatal unit, the care he or she will receive in his or her early years of life and his or her genetic make-up will, in a complex, interacting way, determine his or her chances for recovery and compensation.

Neonatal Special Care Score In order to better quantify the course of neonatal events during the stay in the neonatal unit, a Neonatal Special Care Score was developed. The Neonatal Special Care Score (see Table 5) is a day-to-day score reflecting the actual condition of the infant. The items take into account major vital functions such as respiration and circulation, metabolic homeostasis, neurological condition, method of feeding, and level of care required for the baby. The higher the score (with a maximum of 30), the higher the intensity of care needed. Interscorer reliability, calculated on 160 daily scores was 0.89. The score allows a quantification of the day-to-day evolution of the clinical condition of the neonate. The correlation between the daily score (Y) and the corresponding day (X) can be expressed by the equation $Y = aX + b$. The slope a expresses the evolution. In the group of 100 infants with a birth weight of less than 2,000 grams, the 25th percentile for a was -0.50, the median -0.35, and for the 75th percentile it was -0.23. The intercept b reflects the initial peak value. In the group, the 25th percentile for b was 8, the median 11, and the 75th percentile 14 (Casaer, Daniels, Devlieger, DeCock, & Eggermont, 1982). At present, in the neonatal special care unit in Leuven, the individual peak value and the course of an infant can be compared with the data of the first series of 100 infants (Figure 9). Unusual situations can be easily recognized. Similar attempts to describe the neonate and the care he or she receives are

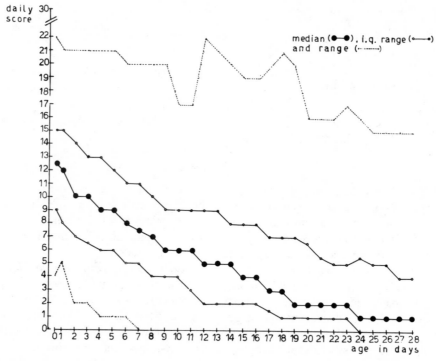

Figure 9. Median, interquartile range, and range of the daily score of the Neonatal Special Care Score in 100 infants with a birth weight less than 2,000 grams.

available in the literature (Haupt, 1982), but a quantification of such a score for the first 28 days in the preterm is, to the authors' knowledge, not yet available. In the prospective study, the initial peak value *b* of the Neonatal Special Care Score was very significantly correlated with the Obstetric Optimality Score (Spearman rank correlation coefficient of 0.42, $p < .001$). The slope *a,* however, had a correlation of zero, indicating that the slope measures other factors in neonatal life. The relation between these neonatal scores and the follow-up data at the corrected ages of 7 months and 18 months are the topic of the authors' ongoing prospective study.

Head Circumferences

Head circumferences of newborns between birth and 38 weeks of postmenstrual age with a birth weight of less than 2,000 grams in Leuven remained between the 25th and 50th percentiles. Catch-up growth is seen in the small-for-dates infants born between 35 and 37 weeks postmenstrual age (Bhavani, 1980). When

head growth can be kept between its initial percentile lines in appropriate-for-dates infants and when catch-up growth is obtained in small-for-dates infants, this has proved to be a favorable indicator for later mental and motor development (Bhavani, 1980; Gross, Oehler, & Eckerman, 1983; Largo, Walli, Duc, Fanconi, & Prader, 1980; Ounsted, 1982; Stave & Ruvalo, 1980).

Feeding Behavior in Preterm Neonates

Although it is well known that feeding difficulties are an early sign of higher or lower neuron disease and that feeding history is of utmost importance in subsequent developmental assessment, few detailed quantitative studies are available. In a recent study, feeding behavior in 100 bottle-fed preterm infants was studied in the authors' unit (Casaer, Daniels, Devlieger, DeCock, & Eggermont, 1982). Feeding efficiency was studied by quantifying the volume of milk intake per minute and the number of teat insertions per 10 ml of milk

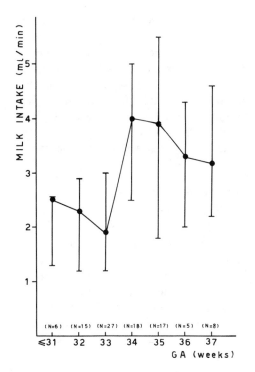

Figure 10. The relation between the volume of milk intake per minute and gestational age in weeks during the first week of oral feeding. Data indicate medians and interquartile ranges.

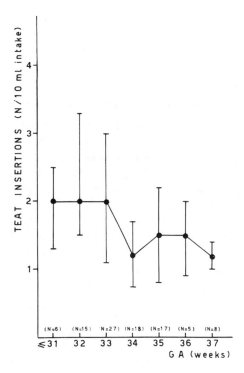

Figure 11. The relation between the number of teat insertions per 10 ml of milk intake and gestational age in weeks during the first week of oral feeding. Data indicate medians and interquartile ranges.

intake. Feeding efficiency was greater in infants above 34 weeks gestational age than in those below this age (Figures 10 and 11). A characteristic adducted and flexed arm posture was observed during feeding. A neonatal feeding score was devised that allowed the quantification of early oral feeding behavior. This score consisted of the two variables describing feeding efficiency as well as a subscore describing the posture of the infant and whether the infant's eyes were open or closed during the feeding. The feeding score obtained during the first week of oral feeding correlated well with some aspects of perinatal assessment. Higher early feeding scores were obtained in those infants who had a normal neurological examination when they were discharged from the unit several weeks later. Significantly, lower feeding scores were found more often in the 13 out of 100 infants who were considered neurologically abnormal at discharge. The feeding score also correlated significantly with the results of the Bayley Mental and Motor Scales at corrected ages of 7 months (Spearman rank

correlation coefficients of .34, $p < .01$, and .25, $p < .05$). These findings are a stimulus to continue study into the relationships between feeding behavior and other aspects of early development, especially of neurological development.

Behavioral-Social Aspects

In the neonatal special care unit in Leuven, the behavioral-social aspects are evaluated in two ways: 1) visits and telephone calls from parents and family to the neonatal special care unit are recorded and analyzed in detail, and 2) the nursing staff is asked to answer a questionnaire on behavioral and social aspects of the newborn during the infant's stay in the unit. The questionnaire is partly based on Brazelton (1973), on Field, Hallock, Dempsey, and Shuman (1978) and on Kronstadt, Oberklaid, Ferb, and Swartz (1979). These aspects are not discussed here. Similarly, the testing of sensory systems is only dealt with briefly. Testing of the sensory systems, especially in the very low birth weight infants ($-$ 1,250 grams) is of utmost importance for their later development and school performances (Vohr & Hack, 1982).

Auditory Screening in the Neonate

Other than the acoustical orienting responses described by Brazelton (1973) (eyes or head turning, or a change in behavior in the response to the sound of a soft bell or to the voice of the examiner who is talking to the baby), no further special investigations are presently carried out in the neonatal special care unit. When a crying newborn can be pacified by the sound of the human voice only, examiners feel reassured as to the newborn's early hearing capacities; follow-up study will have to establish the value of this clinical finding. A series of interesting research questions concerning the acoustical system and brain stem maturation can be studied both by behavioral and physiological techniques. At present, however, a detailed clinical assessment is postponed until a postnatal (corrected) age of 7 months since only at that age can therapeutic measures be taken in Leuven.

Visual Orienting and Visual Testing

Dubowitz and Dubowitz (1981), Miranda and Hack (1979), Morante, Dubowitz, Levene, and Dubowitz (1982), Van Heule (1982), and Vasella, Giambonini, Heits, Kaufmann, Kehrli, & Walti (1979) agree that the newborn as well as the preterm with good visual performance have not only a good prognosis as to the visual system but also as to mental development. The analysis of weak neonatal responses is, however, much more difficult to interpret. Dubowitz and Dubowitz (1981) stress the importance of the loss of previously good visual performance (in the neonatal unit) as an alarm sign. In the authors' neonatal special care unit, the following of a red ball and the following of the face of the examiner (who keeps silent) is tested; furthermore, a drawing resembling a human face described by Goren, Sarty, and Pyck (1975) has proved to be a very efficient stimulus (Daniels & Casaer, in press). Morante

et al. (1982) studied infants at 36 weeks gestational age and noted a significant difference in visual acuity tested with pattern preference between infants with and without intraventricular bleeding. The mandatory ophthalmological follow-up of all infants receiving oxygen therapy is not discussed here, but its importance for the occurrence of retrolental fibro plasia and impaired visual acuity needs to be stressed.

Neurological Examination Before Discharge

As to the predictive value of the neurological examination before discharge, a distinction must be made between follow-up studies in low-risk full-terms and follow-up studies on high-risk neonates. In low-risk full-term infants, there is a low but significant correlation between neonatal neurological evaluation and the follow-up evaluation up to school age (Prechtl, 1980; Touwen 1972; Touwen, Lok-Meijer, Huisjes, & Olinga, 1982). In high-risk preterms, Touwen (1978) found a much higher correlation between neonatal syndromes and follow-up examinations during infancy. The hemisyndrome and hypertonia syndrome have a distinct prognostic value, whereas hypotonia has a poorer one. The hyperexcitability syndrome seems only to correlate with subsequent developmental problems when it persists for more than 6 weeks. However, a hypotonia syndrome that turns into hypertonia is a serious neonatal problem correlating with subsequent neurological disorders (Brown et al., 1974). If, on overall judgment at the end of a stay in the neonatal unit, it is concluded that the baby is definitely neurologically abnormal, taking into account the neurological evaluation and established abnormalities such as macro- and microcephaly, cataracts and seizures, a nearly 100 times increased risk of cerebral palsy does exist (Nelson & Ellenberg, 1979). In the ongoing prospective study in Leuven, the authors are now studying how well the neonatal assessment can detect those infants who will require early intervention programs either in the form of early physiotherapy, or extra help for the optimalization of parent-infant interaction.

CONCLUSION

Risk estimation for future developmental abnormalities cannot be based on one factor, one clinical examination, or one technical examination. It should include careful history-taking of social and maternal variables, pregnancy, parturition, and perinatal and postnatal condition of the infant. In this respect, the optimality score is useful. It should include accurate event recording in the neonatal unit and for this purpose the Neonatal Special Care Score seems to be helpful. During the initial weeks in the special care unit when a comprehensive neurological examiniation is not yet feasible, attention should be paid to vital functions such as feeding and respiration. The evaluation of growth, especially of head circumference, is a simple but objective measurement. The overall judgment of the nursing staff is important and may be summmarized in a quantifiable questionnaire. Finally, an ongoing evaluation of neurological as well as sensory functions with a detailed examination before discharge is meaningful in deciding on the intensity and the quality of the immediate follow-up after the infant is discharged from the neonatal unit.

REFERENCES

Als, H., Lester, B.M., Tronick, E.Z., & Brazelton, T.B. Toward a research instrument for the assessment of preterm infants' behaviour. In: H. Fitzgerald, B. Lester & M. Yogman (eds.), *Theory and research in behavioural pediatrics*. New York: Plenum Publishing Corp., 1982.

Amiel-Tison, C., & Grenier, A. *Evaluation neurologique du nouveau-né et du nourrissoni [Neurological evaluation of the newborn and of the nursing child]*. New York: Masson Publishing USA, Inc., 1980.

André-Thomas, Chesni, Y., & Saint-Anne Dargassies, S. The neurological examination of the infant. In: *Little club clinics in developmental medicine*, No. 1. London: Spastics Society and William Heinemann Ltd, 1960.

Ballard, J.L., Novak, K.K., & Driver, M. A simplified score for assessment of fetal maturation of newly born infants. *The Journal of Pediatrics*, 1979, *95*, 769–774.

Bhavani, S. On nutrition, growth and nutritional status of pre-term infants with birth-weights less than 2,000 gr. Unpublished master's thesis, Katholieke Universiteit Leuven, Belgium, 1980.

Brazelton, T.B. Neonatal Behavioural Assessment Scale. *Clinics in Developmental Medicine*, No. 50. London: SIMP with Heinemann Medical, 1973.

Brown, J.K., Purvis, R.J., Forfar, J.Q. Neurological aspects of perinatal asphyxia. *Developmental Medicine and Child Neurology*, 1974, *16*, 567–574.

Bucher, H.U., Bolthauser, E., Friderich, J., & Isler, W. Birth injury to the spinal cord. *Helvetica Paediatrica Acta*, 1979, *34*, 517–527.

Casaer, P. Postural behaviour in newborn infants. *Clinics in Developmental Medicine*, No. 72. London: SIMP with Heinemann Medical, 1979.

Casaer, P., & Akiyama, Y. The estimation of the postmenstrual age: A comprehensive review. *Developmental Medicine and Child Neurology*, 1970, *12*, 697–729.

Casaer, P., Daniels, H., Devlieger, H., DeCock, P., & Eggermont, E. Feeding behaviour in pre-term neonates. *Early Human Development*, 1982, *7*.

Casaer, P., Daniels, H., Devlieger, H., & Eggermont, E. Upper and lower thoracic and abdominal respiratory movements in pre-term neonates: Effects of position and feeding. *Neuropaediatrics*, 1981, *12*, 424.

Casaer, P., Devlieger, H., Willekens, H., Daniels, H., Dereymaeker, H., Vital-Durand, G., & Eggermont, E. Recording of upper and lower thoracic and abdominal respiratory movements in pre-term neonates. *Acta Paediatrica Belgica*, 1980, *33*, 253–260.

Casaer, P., Eggermont, E., Daniels, H., Devlieger, H., DeCock, P., Willekens, H., & Jaeken, J. The neurological assessment in the neonatal special care unit. *Postgraduate Courses in Paediatrics*, 1982, *55*, 144–166.

Curzi-Dascalova, L. Thoraco-abdominal respiratory correlations in infants constancy and variability in different sleep states. *Early Human Development*, 1978, *2*, 25–38.

Curzi-Dascalova, L. Phase relationships between thoracic and abdominal respiratory movements during sleep. *Neuropaediatrics*, 1982, (13 Suppl.):15–20.

Daniels, H. & Casaer, P. Neonatal leergedrag. Gedragstherapie: English translation, (in press).

Davies, P.A., Robinson, R.J., Scopes, J.W., Tizard, J.P.M., & Wigglesworth, J.S. Medical Care of the newborn. *Clinics in Developmental Medicine*, No. 44/45. London: SIMP with Heinemann Medical, 1972.

Dawes, G.S., Houghton, C.R.S., Redman, C.W.G., & Visser, G.H.A. Pattern of the normal human fetal heart rate. *British Journal of Obstetrics and Gynaecology*, 1982, *89*, 276–284.

Delphy, D.T., Gordon, R.E., Hope, P.L., Parker, D., Reynolds, E.O.R., Shaw, D., & Whitehead, M.D. Non-invasive investigation of cerebral ischemia by phosphorus nuclear magnetic resonance. *Pediatrics*, 1982, *70*, 310–313.

Deonna, T., Payot, M., Probst, A., & Prod'hom, L.S. Neonatal intracranial haemorrhage in premature infants. *Pediatrics*, 1975, *56*, 1056–1064.

Devlieger, H., Goddeeris, P., Moerman, Ph., Casaer, P.,

& Eggermont, E. Some aspects of the anatomy of the anterior muscle wall in the preterm infant. In: M. Thiery, J. Senterre, & R. Derom (eds.), *Proceedings of the 8th European congress of perinatal medicine*. Brussels, 1982.

Dobbing, J. The later development of the brain and its vulnerability. In: J.A. Davis & J. Dobbing (eds.), *Scientific foundations of paediatrics*. London: Heinemann Medical, 1974.

Dubowitz, L.M.S., & Dubowitz, V. *Gestational age of the newborn*. Reading, MA: Addison-Wesley Publishing Co., 1977.

Dubowitz, L.M.S., & Dubowitz, V. The neurological assessment of the preterm and full-term newborn infant. *Clinics in Developmental Medicine*, No. 79. London: SIMP with Heinemann Medical, 1981.

Dubowitz, L.M.S., Levene, M.I., Morante, A., Palmer, P., & Dubowitz, V. Neurological signs in neonatal intraventricular hemorrhage: A correlation with real-time ultrasound. *The Journal of Pediatrics*, 1981, *99*, 127–133.

Dubowitz, V. The floppy infant. *Clinics in Developmental Medicine*, No. 76 (2nd ed.) London: SIMP with Heinemann Medical, 1980.

Dykes, F.D., Lazzake, A., & Ahmann, P. Intraventricular hemorrhage: A prospective evaluation of etiopathogenesis. *Pediatrics*, 1980, *68*, 42–00.

Eggermont, E. Sind intraventrikuläre Blutungen beim Kind mit niedrigem Geburtsgewicht gegenwärtig vermeidbar. In: A. Huch, E. Huch, G. Duc, & G. Rooth (eds.), *Klinisches management des "kleinen" frühgeborenen (> 1500 g)*, Stuttgart and New York: Georg Thieme Verlag, 1982.

Eggermont, E., Devlieger. H., Marchal, G., Jaeken, J., Vandenbussche, E., Smeets, E., Vanacker, G., & Corbeel, L. Angiographic evidence of low portal liver perfusion in transient neonatal hyperammonemia. *Acta Paediatrica Belgica*, 1980, *33*, 163–169.

Eggermont, E., Eggermont-Van Den Bossche, M-M., Jaeken, J., DeBisschop, F., Casaer, P., & Devlieger, H. Levensperspectieven van kinderen met laag geboortegewicht. *Tijdschrift voor Geneeskunde*, 1977, *12*, 653–658.

Farr, V., Kerridge, D.F., & Mitchell, R.G. The value of some external characteristics in the assessment of gestational age at birth. *Developmental Medicine and Child Neurology*, 1966, *8*, 657–664.

Field, T.M., Hallock, N.P., Dempsey, J.P., & Shuman, H.H. Mothers' assessment of term and pre-term infants with respiratory distress syndrome: Reliability and predictive validity. *Child Psychiatry and Human Development*, 1978, *9*, 75–85.

Finnström, O. Studies on maturity in newborn infants. VI. Comparison between different methods for maturity estimation. *Acta Paediatrica Scandinavica*, 1972, *61*, 33–51.

Gesell, A., & Amatruda, C.S. *Developmental diagnosis*. New York: Harper & Row. 1947.

Goren, C.C., Sarty, M., & Pyck, W.V. Visual following and pattern discrimination of face-like stimuli by newborn infants. *Pediatrics*, 1975, *56*, 544–549.

Gross, S. J., Oehler, J. M., & Eckerman, C. O. Head growth and developmental outcome in very low-birth-weight infants. *Pediatrics*, 1983, *71*, 70–75.

Hagberg, B. *Epidemiology and etiology of severe and mild mental retardation*. Ronnie MacKeith Lecture, British Paediatric Neurology Association, Manchester, 1981.

Hancock, B. W. Clinical assessment of gestational age in the neonate. *Archives of Disease in Childhood*, 1973, *48*, 152–154.

Hanson, N., & Okken, A. Transcutaneous oxygen tension of newborn infants in different behavioural states. *Pediatric Research*, 1980, *14*, 911–915.

Haupt, H. *Das neugeborene*. Stuttgart and New York: Georg Thieme Verlag, 1982.

Henderson-Smart, D.J. The effect of gestational age on the incidence and duration of recurrent apnoea in newborn babies. *Australian Paediatric Journal*, 1981, *17*, 273–276.

Henderson-Smart, D.J., & Read, D.J.C. Depression of intercostal and abdominal muscle activity and vulnerability to asphyxia during active sleep in the newborn. In: C. Guilleminault & W.C. Dement (eds.), *Sleep apnoea-syndromes*. New York: Allan R. Liss Inc., 1978.

Hill, A., & Volpe, J.J. Normal pressure hydrocephalus in the newborn. *Paediatrics*, 1981, *68*, 623–629.

Hittner, H.M., Hirsch, N.J., & Rudolph, A.J. The lens in the assessment of gestational age. *The Journal of Pediatrics*, 1977, *91*, 455–460.

Hobel, C.J. Risk assessment in perinatal care. *Clinics in Obstetrics and Gynaecology*, 1978, *21*, 289–295.

Hobel, C.J. Better perinatal health (U.S.A.). *Lancet*, 1980, *I*, 31–33.

Huch, R., & Huch, A. Die variabilität des PO$_2$ in der perinatal medizin. *Gynaekologische Praxis*, 1981, *5*, 649–661.

Huisjes, H.J., Okken, A., Prechtl, H.F.R., & Touwen, B.C.L. Neurological and pediatric findings in newborns of mothers with hypertensive disease in pregnancy. In: Z.K. Stemberra, K. Polacek, & V. Sabata (eds.), *Perinatal medicine*. Stuttgart: Georg Thieme Verlag, 1975.

Illingsworth, R.S. Cyanotic attacks in newborn infants. *Archives of Disease in Childhood*, 1957, *32*, 328–332.

Jaeken, J., Devlieger, H., Casaer, P., & Eggermont, E. Transient hyperammonemia in the pre-term infant. *Neurology*, 1982, *32*, 1070.

Joppich, G., & Schulte, F.J. *Neurologie des neugeborenen*. Berlin: Springer, 1968.

Korner, A.F. Intervention with pre-term infants: Rationale, aims and means. In: V. I. Smeriglio (ed.), *Experiences of newborns and parents*. Hillsdale, NJ: Lawrence Erlbaum Associates, 1980.

Korobkin, R. The relationship between head circumference and the development of communicating hydrocephalus following intraventricular haemorrhage. *Pediatrics*, 1975, *56*, 74–79.

Krishnamoorthy, K.S., Fernandez, R.A., Momose, K.J., DeLong, G.R., Moylan, F.M.B., Todres, I.D., & Shannon, D.C. Evaluation of neonatal intracranial haemorrhage by computerized tomography. *Pediatrics*, 1977, *59*, 165–172.

Kronstadt, O., Oberklaid, F., Ferb, T.E., & Swartz, J.P. Infant behavior and maternal adaptations in the first six months of life. *American Journal of Orthopsychiatry*, 1979, *49*, 3.

Largo, R.H., Walli, R., Duc, G., Fanconi, A., & Prader, A. Evaluation of perinatal growth. *Helvetica Paediatrica Acta*, 1980, *35*, 419–436.

Levene, M.I., Dubowitz, L.M.S., Palmer, P., Fawer, C.L. & Dubowitz, V. Brain ultrasound in pre-term infants. *Lancet*, 1981, *II*, 36.

Ment, L.R., Scott, D.T., Ehrenkranz, R.E., Rothman, S.C., Duncan, C.C., & Warshaw, J.B. Neonates of

−1250 grams birthweight: Prospective neurodevelopmental evaluation during the first year post-term. *Pediatrics*, 1982, *70*, 292–296.

Michaelis, R., Dopfer, R., Gerbig, W., Fellerdopfer, P., & Rohr, M. Die Erfassung obstetrischer und postnataler Risikofaktoren durch eine Liste optimaler Bedingungen. *Monatsschrift für Kinderheilkunde*, 1979, *127*, 149–155.

Michaelis, R., Rooschuz, B., & Dopfer, R. Prenatal origin of congenital spastic hemiparesis. *Early Human Development*, 1980, *4*, 243–255.

Miller, H.C., Behile, F.C., & Smull, N.W. Severe apnea and irregular respiratory rhythms among premature infants. *Pediatrics*, 1959, *23*, 676–685.

Miranda, S.B., & Hack, M. The predictive value of neonatal visual-perceptual behaviors. In: T.M. Field (ed.), *Infants born at risk*. New York: SP Medical & Scientific Books, 1979.

Morante, A., Dubowitz, L.M.S., Levene, M., & Dubowitz, V. The development of visual function in normal and neurologically abnormal pre-term and full-term infants. *Developmental Medicine and Child Neurology*, 1982, *24*, 771–784.

Narayanan, I., Dua, K., Guijral, V.V., Mehta, D.K., Mathew, M., & Prabhakar, A.K. A simple method of assessment of gestational age in newborn infants. *Pediatrics*, 1982, *69*, 27–32.

Nelson, K.B., & Ellenberg, J.H. Neonatal signs as predictors of cerebral palsy. *Pediatrics*, 1979, *64*(2), 225–232.

Nijhuis, J.G., Prechtl, H.F.R., Martin, C.B., & Bots, R.S.G.M. Are there behavioural states in the human fetus? *Early Human Development*, 1982, *6*, 177–195.

Ounsted, M. Basics: Size at birth and its effects on growth and development in the first year of life. In: J. Apley & C. Ounsted (eds.), One child. *Clinics in Developmental Medicine*, N. 80. London: SIMP with Heinemann Medical, 1982.

Ounsted, M., Chalmers, C.A., & Yudkin, P.L. Clinical assessment of gestational age at birth: The effects of sex, birthweight and weight for length of gestation. *Early Human Development*, 1978, *2*, 73–80.

Palmer, P.G., Dubowitz, L.M.S., Verghote, M., & Dubowitz, V. Neurological and neurobehavioural differences between pre-term infants and term and full-term newborn infants. *Neuropediatrics*, 1982, *13*, 183–189.

Pape, K.E., Armstrong, D.L., Fitzhardinge, P.M. Central nervous system pathology associated with mask ventilation in the very low birth-weight infant. *Pediatrics*, 1976, *58*, 473–483.

Pape, K.E., & Wigglesworth, J.S. Haemorrhage, ischaemia and the perinatal brain. *Clinics in Developmental Medicine*, No. 67/70. London: SIMP with Heinemann Medical, 1979.

Papile, L.A., Burstein, J., Burstein, R., & Koffler, H. Incidence and evolution of subependymal and intraventricular haemorrhage. *The Journal of Pediatrics*, 1978, *92*, 529–534.

Papile, L.A., Munsick, G., & Weaver. Cerebral intraventricular hemorrhage in infants < 1500 grams. *Pediatric Research*, 1979, *4*, 528.

Parkin, J.M., Hey, E.N., & Clowes, J.S. Rapid assessment of gestational age at birth. *Archives of Disease in Childhood*, 1976, *51*, 259–263.

Parmelee, A.H., & Schulte, F.J. Developmental testing of pre-term and small-for-date infants. *Pediatrics*, 1970, *45*, 2128.

Prechtl, H.F.R. Neurological sequelae of prenatal and perinatal complications. *British Medical Journal*, 1967, *4*, 763–767.

Prechtl, H.F.R. The behavioural states of the newborn infant. *Brain Research*, 1974, *76*, 185–212.

Prechtl, H.F.R. The neurological examination of the full-term newborn infant. *Clinics in Developmental Medicine*, No. 63. London: SIMP with Heinemann Medical, 1977.

Prechtl, H.F.R. The optimality concept. *Early Human Development*, 1980, *4*, 201–206.

Prechtl, H.F.R. Assessment methods for the newborn infant, a critical evaluation. In: P. Stratton (ed.), *Psychobiology of the human newborn*. New York: John Wiley & Sons, 1982.

Prechtl, H.F.R., Fargel, V.W., Weinmann, H.M., & Bakker, H.H. Postures, motility and respiration of low-risk pre-term infants. *Developmental Medicine and Child Neurology*, 1979, *21*, 3–27.

Prechtl, H.F.R., & Nolte, R. Motility and posture in low-risk and high-risk pre-term infants. In: H. F. R. Prechtl (ed.), *Proceedings of the European brain and behaviour workshop: Neurobiology of development*, 1982.

Prechtl, H.F.R., & O'Brien, M.J. Behavioural states of the full-term newborn. The emergence of a concept. In: P. Stratton (ed.), *Psychobiology of the human newborn*. New York: John Wiley & Sons, 1982.

Roberton, N.R.C. *A manual of neonatal intensive care*. London: Edward Arnold, 1981.

Robinson, R.J. Assessment of gestational age by neurological examination. *Archives of Disease in Childhood*, 1966, *41*, 437–441.

Saint-Anne Dargassies, S. Neurological development in the full-term and premature neonate. New York: Elsevier North-Holland, 1977.

Scheiner, A.P., & Abroms, I.F. *The practical management of the developmentally disabled child*. St. Louis, MO: C. V. Mosby, 1980.

Schulte, F.J. The neurological development of the neonate. In: J.A. Davis & J. Dobbing (eds.), *Scientific foundation of paediatrics*. London: Heinemann, 1974.

Seeds, J.W., Cefalo, R.C., & Herbert, W.H.P. Amniotic band syndrome. *American Journal of Obstetrics and Gynecology*, 1982, *144*, 243–249.

Sigman, M., & Parmelee, A.H. Longitudinal follow-up of premature infants. In: T.M. Field (ed.), *Infants born at risk*. New York: SP Medical & Scientific Books, 1979.

Stave, U., & Ruvalo, C. Neurological development in very low-birth-weight infants. *Early Human Development*, 1980, *4*, 229–243.

Theorell, K., Prechtl, H.F.R., & Vos, J.E. A polygraphic study of normal and abnormal newborn infants. *Neuropaediatrie*, 1974, *5*, 279–317.

Thorburn, R.J., Lipscomb, A.P., Stewart, A.L., Reynolds, E.O.R., & Hope, P.L. Timing and antecedents of periventricular haemorrhage and of cerebral atrophy in very pre-term infants. *Early Human Development*, 1982, *7*, 221–238.

Timor-Tritsch, I.E., Dierker, L.J., Hertz, R.H., Chik, L., & Rose, N.M.G. Regular and irregular human fetal respiratory movement. *Early Human Development*, 1980, *4*, 315–324.

Timor-Tritsch, I.F., Dierker, L.J., Hertz, R.H., Deagan, M.C., & Rosem, M.G. Studies of antepartum behavioural state in the human fetus at term. *American Journal of Obstetrics and Gynecology*, 1978, *132*, 524–528.

Touwen, B.C.L. The relationship between neonatal and

follow-up findings. In: E. Saling & F.J. Schulte (eds.), *Perinatale medizin [Perinatal medicine]*, II: 303–306. Stuttgart: George Thieme Verlag, 1972.

Touwen, B.C.L. Neurological development in infancy. *Clinics in Developmental Medicine*, No. 58. London: SIMP with Heinemann Medical, 1976.

Touwen, B.C.L. Early detection of developmental neurological disorders. In: *Growth and development of the full-term and premature infant. The Jonxis Lectures.* Amsterdam: Excerpta Medica, 1978.

Touwen, B.C.L., Huisjes, H.J., Jurgens v.d.Zee, A.D., Bierman Van Eendenburg, M., Smrkovsku, M., & Olingo, A.A. Obstetrical condition and neonatal neurological morbidity. An analysis with the help of the optimality concept. *Early Human Development*, 1980, *4*, 207–228.

Touwen, B.C.L., Lok-Meijer, T.Y., Huisjes, H.J., & Olinga, A.A. The recovery rate of neurologically deviant newborns. *Early Human Development*, 1982, *7*, 131–148.

Van Heule, R. The visual capabilities of the newborn infant during the first week of life. *Bulletin de la Société Belge d'Ophtalmologie*, 1982, *202*, 1–8.

Vasella, F., Giambonini, S., Heits, B., Kaufmann, R., Kehrli, P., & Walti, U. Development of visual discrimination (pattern preference) in normal infants. *Helvetica Paediatrica Acta*, 1979, *32*, 319–329.

Visser, G.H.A., Carse, E.A., Goodman, J.D.S., & John-son, P. A comparison of episodic heart-rate patterns in the fetus and the newborn. *British Journal of Obstetrics and Gynaecology*, 1982, 50–55.

Vogt, H., Haneberg, B., Finne, P.H., & Stemsberg, A. Clinical assessment of gestational age in the newborn infant. *Acta Paediatrica Scandinavica*, 1981, *70*, 669–672.

Vohr, B.R., & Hack, M. Developmental follow-up of low-birth-weight infants. *Pediatric Clinics of North America*, 1982, *29*, 1441–1454.

Volpe, J.J. Neonatal intracranial haemorrhage. *Clinics in Perinatology*, 1977, *4*, 77–102.(a)

Volpe, J.J. Neonatal seizures. *Clinics in Perinatology*, 1977, *4*, 43–77.(b)

Volpe, J.J. Neonatal periventricular haemorrhage: Past, present and future. *The Journal of Pediatrics*, 1978, *92*, 693–696.

Volpe, J.J. Intracranial haemorrhage in the newborn: Current understanding and dilemmas. *Neurology*, 1979, *29*, 632–635. (a)

Volpe, J.J. Value of neonatal neurological examination. *Pediatrics*, 1979, *64*, 547–548. (b)

Volpe, J.J. *Neurology of the newborn*. Philadelphia: W.B. Saunders Co., 1981.

Volpe, J.J., Perlman, J.M., Herscovitch, P., & Raichle, M.E. Positron emission tomography in the assessment of regional cerebral blood flow in the newborn. *Annals of Neurology*, 1982, *12*, 225–226.

Chapter 23

A Correlation of EEG
with Severity of
Hypoxic-Ischemic Encephalopathy
in Term Newborns

GERALD M. FENICHEL, M.D.
BARBARA J. OLSON, M.D.
DAVID L. WEBSTER, M.D.
RANDALL R. BLOUIN, M.D.
JERI E. FITZPATRICK, B.A., REEGT
Vanderbilt University Medical Center and Children's Hospital, Nashville, Tennessee

B RIEF EPISODES OF PARTIAL ASPHYXIA ARE probably common during the normal birth process, but brain damage due to asphyxia in term newborns is relatively uncommon. The fetal circulation accommodates a reduction in arterial oxygen concentration by maximizing blood flow to the brain and, to a lesser degree, to the heart at the expense of other organs. Asphyxia in the term newborn is almost always an intrauterine event; hypoxia and ischemia occur together. The effect on the brain is a hypoxic-ischemic encephalopathy (HIE).

HIE varies in severity, and three clinical syndromes can be recognized: mild, moderate, and severe. These syndromes are a modification of the stages of HIE suggested by Sarnat and Sarnat (1976). In newborns with mild HIE, consciousness is not impaired except for a brief interval of lethargy after birth. The characteristic feature is jitteriness—a hyperalert state in which there are prolonged periods of wakefulness, irritability, and excessive responsiveness to stimulation. The symptoms are maximal during the first 24 hours postpartum and then progressively diminish. Newborns with mild HIE recover completely and are not at risk for neurological handicaps (Nelson & Broman, 1977).

Newborns with moderate HIE are obtunded for at least the first 12 hours postpartum. Efforts at arousal produce jitteriness. Hypotonia is present at rest, and spontaneous movement of the limbs is decreased. In the period between 48 and 72 hours postpartum, the encephalopathy either worsens or improves. The presence of convulsions, prolongation of the obtunded state, or a progression to stupor is associated with a worsening prognosis.

Newborns with severe HIE are stuporous or comatose immediately after birth. Hypotonia is severe and respirations are irregular or

Dr. Webster was supported in part by a fellowship grant from United Cerebral Palsy. Presented in part at the joint meeting of the American EEG Society and American Epilepsy Society, November 11, 1982, Phoenix, Arizona.

periodic. Apnea and convulsions begin during the first 12 hours postpartum. The convulsions increase in frequency and severity, sometimes progressing to status epilepticus. Mortality is high and those that survive have severe neurological handicaps.

It is now well established that convulsions caused by HIE have a grave prognosis (Holden, Mellits, & Freeman, 1982; Mellits, Holden, & Freeman, 1982). However, the presence of early convulsions is not limited to newborns with severe HIE. Many newborns with a history of perinatal asphyxia have convulsions, but only mild or no HIE. In these infants, the convulsions are probably due to factors other than HIE and the prognosis is better. It is important to quickly delineate the severity of HIE in order to identify those newborns who might benefit from early therapeutic interventions. The authors conducted a study to determine if a single clinical EEG, performed in the first 48 hours postpartum, was a useful tool in helping to define a cohort of asphyxiated newborns for drug trials.

METHODOLOGY

The study cohort consisted of 43 term newborns with historical evidence of perinatal asphyxia (fetal monitor abnormality, passage of meconium, 5 minute Apgar of 5 or less), a clinical syndrome of HIE, and an EEG within 48 hours postpartum. Other term newborns who met the above criteria were excluded if they were dysmorphic or had evidence of intracranial hemorrhage by computerized tomography. The severity of the HIE was graded by one of the authors on the basis of state of consciousness and tone without regard to the presence or absence of convulsions, and the

EEGs were read by others. Among the 43 study newborns, 30 had mild HIE (lethargic, jittery, normal tone); 5 had moderate HIE (obtunded, hypotonia); and 8 had severe HIE (stupor or coma, flaccid).

All EEGs were performed in the intensive care nursery of Vanderbilt University Children's Hospital. Electrophysiological monitoring was performed with an 11-channel Grass EEG machine using standard techniques described elsewhere (Fenichel, Olson, & Fitzpatrick, 1980). Of the 11 channels, six were used for monitoring EEG and five for monitoring noncerebral function. The noncerebral channels consisted of one electrocardiogram, one electromyogram, two electro-oculograms, and one respiratory monitor. A trained observer recorded all changes in clinical state throughout the EEG recording.

Follow-up information on 32 children was obtained from the charts of the Vanderbilt Pediatric Neurology Clinic, and by telephone contact with private pediatricians on those children not followed at Vanderbilt. The duration of follow-up was between 1 and 4 years. Mental retardation was defined as a developmental level of less than 70% of normal. In fact, all of the children reported as mentally retarded were severely retarded.

RESULTS

Table 1 summarizes the EEG findings in relation to severity of HIE, and Table 2 summarizes the EEG findings in relation to outcome.

Among the 30 children with mild HIE, 21 had normal EEGs. One of these had clinical convulsions in the first 12 hours postpartum. Follow-up data were available on 17; 16 were

Table 1. EEG and severity of HIE

EEG	Mild	Moderate	Severe
Normal	21	0	0
Lack of variability	7	2	1
Excessive sharp waves	0	1	0
Discharges, normal background	1	1	0
Discharges, suppressed background	1	1	5
Suppression	0	0	1
Burst suppression	0	0	1
Total	30	5	8

Table 2. EEG and outcome

EEG	Normal	Epilepsy	MR/CP[a]	Died
Normal background	17	1	0	0
Lack of variability	4	1	0	1
Suppression	0	0	4	4
Total	21	2	4	5

[a]Mental retardation, cerebral palsy.

normal including the one with clinical convulsions, and the 17th was developing normally but had developed a focal motor epilepsy. In seven newborns with mild HIE, EEGs demonstrated lack of variability—a background of low amplitude, generally less than 40 μV, and mixed frequencies that varied little with sleep state (Figure 1). Follow-up information was available on four; three were normal and one who had experienced a convulsion on the first day was developing normally but had epilepsy. One other newborn whose EEG demonstrated marked background suppression was lost to follow-up. The last newborn with mild HIE had a clinical convulsion on the first day and the EEG demonstrated rhythmic epileptiform discharges on an otherwise normal background. This child was

considered normal at two months of age and then lost to follow-up.

None of the five newborns with moderate HIE had a normal EEG. In two, the EEGs demonstrated lack of variability; one developed normally and the other was lost to follow-up. The EEG in the third newborn demonstrated excessive sharp wave activity but no epileptiform discharges or background suppression (Figure 2); this child developed normally. The EEG in the fourth newborn demonstrated rhythmic epileptiform discharges on an otherwise normal background. This child had clinical convulsions but was lost to follow-up. The fifth newborn had clinical convulsions and the EEG demonstrated rhythmic epileptiform discharges on a background of voltage suppression. The child has had no further con-

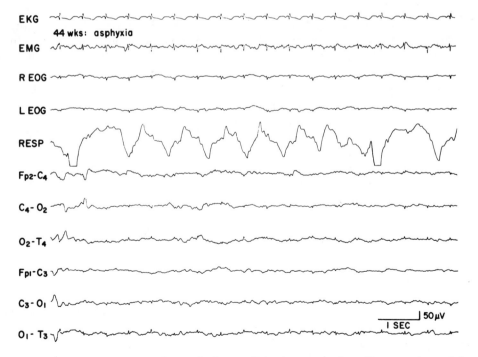

Figure 1. Lack of variability. A background of low amplitude, generally less than 40 μV, and mixed frequencies that vary little with sleep state.

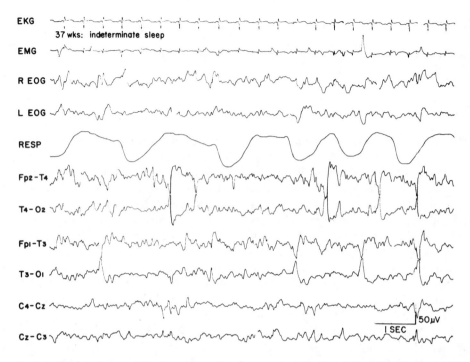

Figure 2. Excessive sharp wave activity. Frequent negative sharp waves at the T_3 and T_4 electrodes without background suppression.

vulsions but is developmentally delayed (Figure 3).

None of the newborns with severe HIE had a normal EEG. In five of the eight, the EEG demonstrated rhythmic epileptiform discharges on a background of voltage suppression. Three died and two survived. The two survivors had clinical convulsions, and both now have severe mental retardation and cerebral palsy; one has epilepsy as well. Of the other three, one EEG demonstrated burst suppression and the child died; one demonstrated severe suppression and the child had clinical convulsions but survived and is now severely retarded and has epilepsy; the last EEG showed lack of variability and the child died.

Nine of the newborns in this study had convulsions during the first 48 hours postpartum. Three had mild HIE, two moderate, and four severe. The EEGs and outcomes are summarized in Table 3. The numbers are too small to draw conclusions and an attempt at correlation is further impaired by the lack of follow-up on the two newborns whose EEGs demonstrated rhythmic epileptiform discharges on a normal background.

DISCUSSION

In 1976, Sarnat and Sarnat described the clinical and EEG findings in 21 term newborns with HIE in order to identify factors predictive of outcome. EEGs were recorded as soon as possible after admission to the hospital, again in 24 hours, and then every 3–5 days until the time of discharge. The children were examined every 3 months during the first year. All of the newborns had at least a moderate encephalopathy, five were severe, and 11 had convulsions. Several EEG patterns were identified that predicted an unfavorable neurological outcome. The important feature of these EEG patterns was amplitude suppression of the background.

Watanabe, Mikazaki, Hara, et al. (1980) performed repeated EEGs on asphyxiated term newborns, including some that were small for gestational age, beginning on the second day. They also noted a relationship between amplitude suppression of the background and an unfavorable neurological outcome. A background of low voltage, irregular activity of less than 50 microvolts, or a burst suppression pattern recorded during the first week predicted

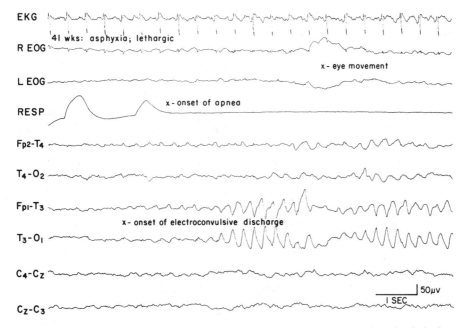

Figure 3. Epileptiform discharges. The discharges are characterized by rhythmic waves at the T_3 electrode. The background is of low amplitude.

brain damage in 64% of cases. If the pattern persisted into the second and third week, the outcome was bad in 100% of cases.

Holmes, Rowe, Hafford, et al. (1982) performed EEGs within 2 weeks of birth, most often on the fourth or fifth day, in 38 term newborns with neonatal asphyxia. They confirmed the association between background suppression and an unfavorable neurological outcome, and noted in addition that rhythmic epileptiform discharges on the EEG were not as reliable at predicting an unfavorable outcome as amplitude suppression of the background.

In contrast to these three studies, Finer, Robertson, Peters, et al. (1983) were unable to demonstrate a correlation between EEGs performed during the first week postpartum and

the neurological outcome in 46 asphyxiated term newborns. It is clear that the EEG, or any other single laboratory test, should not be taken by itself to predict prognosis, but is only one more factor to be considered in the total evaluation of the child.

The focus of the study conducted by these authors was to determine if a single clinical EEG, performed as quickly as possible after birth, was useful in helping to define a cohort of asphyxiated newborns who require therapy. The definition of such a cohort is becoming more important as experimental trials of therapeutic interventions are developed. Therefore, unlike previous studies, the authors included newborns with mild as well as moderate and severe HIE and obtained the EEG as

Table 3. Neonatal convulsions

	EEG	Outcome
Mild HIE	1) Normal 2) Lack of variability 3) Discharge, normal background	Normal Epilepsy Unknown
Moderate HIE	1) Discharge, normal background 2) Discharge, suppression	Unknown Mental retardation
Severe HIE	1) Discharges, suppression 2) Discharges, suppression 3) Discharges, suppression 4) Suppression	Died Cerebral palsy, mental retardation Cerebral palsy, mental retardation, epilepsy Mental retardation, epilepsy

quickly as possible after birth. It is true that later EEGs would have better prognostic significance, but information from early EEGs is needed in order for therapeutic interventions to be tried on the first or second day. Most of the studies were performed in the first 24 hours, but because of a large number of outborns, the EEG was sometimes delayed until the second day.

The results demonstrate a close association between amplitude of the background and severity of HIE as defined by state of consciousness and tone. Of 30 newborns with mild HIE, 22 had a normal background, seven showed mild suppression as characterized by lack of variability, and only one had flattening of the background. Among five newborns with moderate HIE, two had normal backgrounds, two had lack of variability, and one had flattening of the background. Of eight newborns with severe HIE, none had a normal background, one had lack of variability, and seven had flattening of the background. None of the newborns, in any of the groups, with a normal background or lack of variability had a poor neurological outcome. One newborn with severe HIE and lack of variability died shortly after birth. The cause of death was assumed to be myocardial damage.

Clinical convulsions occurred in newborns with mild, moderate, and severe HIE, but a poor neurological outcome occurred only in those whose EEG showed flattening of the background. Two newborns with mild HIE later developed epilepsy. One had no convulsions in the newborn period and a normal EEG, the other had neonatal convulsions and an EEG with lack of variability. Epilepsy in the absence of mental retardation or cerebral palsy is not thought to be a result of HIE (Holden et al., 1982; Nelson & Ellenberg, 1981). It is of interest that 2 of 21 newborns with mild HIE for whom follow-up data are available have later developed epilepsy. It seems likely that the epilepsy was not related to the mild HIE, but no conclusion can be drawn from the data.

It is the authors' conclusion that in selecting term asphyxiated newborns for therapeutic intervention, the presence of marked suppression of the background on an early EEG in association with decreased states of consciousness and hypotonia is the best guide to a poor neurological outcome. Asphyxiated newborns with a normal EEG should either be excluded from research studies or assigned equally to experimental and control groups.

REFERENCES

Fenichel, G.M., Olson, B.J., & Fitzpatrick, J.D. Heart rate changes in convulsive and nonconvulsive apnea. *Annals of Neurology*, 1980, *7*, 577–582.

Finer, N.N., Robertson, C.M., Peters, K.L., et al. Factors affecting outcome in hypoxicischemic encephalopathy in term infants. *American Journal of Diseases in Children*, 1983, *137*, 21–25.

Holden, K.R., Mellits, E.D., & Freeman, J.M. Neonatal seizures: I. Correlation of prenatal and perinatal events with outcomes. *Pediatrics*, 1982, *70*, 165–176.

Holmes, G., Rowe, J., Hafford, J., et al. Prognostic value of the electroencephalogram in neonatal asphyxia. *EEG in Clinical Neurophysiology*, 1982, *53*, 60–72.

Mellits, E.D., Holden, K.R., & Freeman, J.M. Neonatal seizures: II. A multivariate analysis of factors associated with outcome. *Pediatrics*, 1982, *70*, 177–185.

Nelson, K.B., & Broman, S.H. Perinatal risk factors in children with serious motor and mental handicaps. *Annals of Neurology*, 1977, *2*, 371–376.

Nelson, K.B., & Ellenberg, J.H. Apgar scores as predictors of chronic neurologic disability. *Pediatrics,* 1981, *68*, 36–44.

Sarnat, H.B., & Sarnat, M.S. Neonatal encephalopathy following fetal distress: A clinical and electroencephalographic study. *Archives of Neurology*, 1976, *33*, 696–705.

Watanabe, K., Miyazaki, S., Hara, K., et al. Behavioral state cycles, background EEGs and prognosis of newborns with perinatal hypoxia. *EEG in Clinical Neurophysiology*, 1980, *49*, 618–625.

The At-Risk Infant: Psycho/Socio/Medical Aspects
edited by Shaul Harel, M.D., and Nicholas J. Anastasiow, Ph.D.
Copyright © 1985   Paul H. Brookes Publishing Co., Inc.   Baltimore • London

Chapter 24

The Etiology of
Brain Damage in Children

Unusual Dermatoglyphics and
Enamel Hypoplasia as Markers
of Fetal and Perinatal Insult

MICHAEL JAFFE, M.B.Ch.B., M.R.C.P., D.C.H.
Hanna Khoushy Child Development Center, Haifa, Israel

DINA ATTIAS, M.D.

HANNAH DAR, D.Sc.

KURT JAGERMAN, B.D.S.
*Haifa City Medical Centre (Rothschild) and Technion-Israel Institute of
Technology, Haifa, Israel*

ILANA ELI, D.M.D.

HERBERT JUDES, B.D.S. (RAND)
Sackler School of Medicine and School of Dental Medicine, Tel Aviv University, Tel Aviv, Israel

THE ETIOLOGY OF BRAIN DAMAGE REMAINS an enigma in many cases. Hunter, Evans, Thompson, and Ramsay (1980), in a recent study, found that in up to 42% of cases, the cause remained unknown despite adequate investigation. Crome (1960), in his detailed study of the brains of mentally retarded infants, demonstrated developmental abnormalities in 96%. He concluded that in a significant percentage of so-called "idiopathic" brain damage, the cause was due to faulty cerebral development during gestation. This, in turn, was the consequence of genetic or environmental insult to the fetal brain. Holm (1982) utilized historical and clinical criteria in a recent survey on the etiology of brain damage in children. She concluded that at least 50% of cases had their origins during the prenatal period, and that this was probably an underestimation. In many cases, prematurity, difficult labor, or asphyxia were erroneously blamed for the subsequent brain damage, while in fact the fetus had sustained an early insult, and the subsequent difficulties were the consequences thereof.

It is likely that the clinical criteria utilized by Holm to support this contention were probably extreme manifestations, and an examination of other, possibly more sensitive, markers of fetal and perinatal insult might reveal hitherto-unexpected evidence of insult sustained during these periods. The purpose of the study conducted by these authors was to obtain information on the possible occurrence of cerebral insult during two critical stages: 1) gestation, a

Thanks are due to Professor S. T. Winter for invaluable advice during the course of the investigation, and to Hannah Barel for help in preparing the illustrations.

period during which clinical evidence of fetal damage is difficult to detect, and 2) the perinatal period, when the attending clinicians are usually aware of the condition of the fetus or neonate.

As indices of fetal/perinatal injury, markers known to be sensitive to intrauterine and perinatal events were studied: unusual dermatoglyphic/palmar patterns (DGL) and dental enamel abnormalities. By comparing the incidence of these findings in normal controls and in brain-damaged children, it would be possible to assess their value as a source of information regarding the incidence and timing of insults during the critical stages of fetal development.

MATERIALS AND METHODS

Two groups of children were studied: 1) normal, healthy controls, and 2) children with brain damage demonstrating cerebral dysfunction manifesting as mental retardation with or without cerebral palsy. All children were investigated according to the following protocol: a) detailed history of the pregnancy and labor, utilizing medical records where necessary; b) detailed medical history, with specific emphasis on conditions or events likely to be responsible for brain damage; c) psychomotor development history; d) information regarding motor and mental performance in an educational framework (where appropriate); e) family history, with emphasis on hereditary conditions associated with brain damage; f) dermatoglyphic examinations (see description below); and g) tooth examination (see description).

All of the brain-damaged children had undergone a comprehensive medical and educational/developmental assessment including a series of laboratory and other investigations designed to determine the etiology of the disturbance. Some of the more frequently performed special investigations included: blood analysis for amino acids, intrauterine infections, thyroid functions, urine for amino acids, ferric chloride, nitroprusside, dinitrophenylhydrazine; chromosomal studies when brain damage was associated with dysmorphic features; and brain CAT scans and electro-encephalograms as indicated. (These special investigations were selected on the basis of the clinical presentation of the case).

On the basis of the information thus obtained, the children were divided into the following categories: 1) a normal, healthy control group, and 2) a brain-damaged group, subdivided into: a) an idiopathic group (etiology unknown after having undergone the described diagnostic process), and b) a group where the possible etiological factor was identified, including gestational events (uterine hemorrhage, rubella, intrauterine malnutrition, and toxemia of pregnancy) and perinatal events—(asphyxia, and forceps and breech deliveries).

Tooth Examination

Exfoliated or extracted primary teeth from each child were collected, stored in 10% formalin solution, and sent to the School of Dental Medicine of Tel Aviv University for histological examination. The dental investigators were unaware of the diagnosis of the child. Calcified serial sections measuring 100 μm in the buccolingual dimension were obtained using an Isomet machine and examined with a Viso Pan microscope and an ordinary light microscope for the following: 1) identification of the neonatal lines (the normal width of the neonatal line was 5–8 microns; when this line was broader than 15 microns it was interpreted as indicating a complicated birth or perinatal period and was then designated as the perinatal line); 2) identification of any other prominent Retzius' striae as a sign of interference with enamel calcification; and 3) determination of whether the interference occurred pre-, peri-, or postnatally.

Dermatoglyphic Analysis

Finger and palm prints were obtained on each child by the inkless technique (Faurot Inc., New York). The criteria used for defining dermatoglyphic patterns conformed to the *Memorandum on Dermatoglyphic Nomenclature* (Penrose, 1968). Palmar-crease patterns were recorded by direct clinical examination and classified as defined by Dar, Schmidt, and Nitowsky (1977).

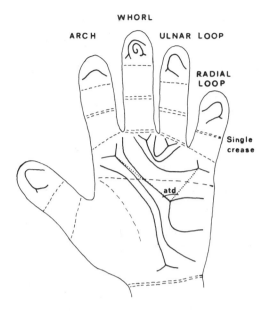

Figure 1. Abnormal palmar prints and dermatoglyphic lines.

DGL patterns and palmar creases defined as abnormal for the purposes of the study were as follows (Figure 1):

1. ATD angle greater than 80° on one or both palms
2. Six or more fingertip arches
3. 10 whorls
4. Radial loop on fourth or fifth digit
5. Simian crease and its variants
6. Unusual palmar creases not conforming to the simian crease or Sydney line classified as Type D by Dar et al. (1977).

Like the dental examinations, the DGL were performed by investigators who were unaware of the diagnosis of the child.

RESULTS

DGL and dental enamel studies (one tooth for each child) were performed on 56 brain-damaged children and 53 controls. The overall distribution and analysis of the cases is presented in Table 1. The table shows a significantly higher incidence of all gestational and perinatal markers of insult in the brain-damaged group. Dental enamel examination also revealed a number of postnatal lines in the brain-damaged group as well as in the controls, thus indicating that the infants had been subjected to various insults after the perinatal period. In contrast to the pre- and perinatal periods, postnatal illness sufficiently severe to cause brain damage (such as meningitis, convulsions, etc.) would have been clinically evident at the time. In all but two cases, a careful history failed to reveal any such potentially brain-damaging episode. It was therefore decided to exclude the postnatal lines from the study, as the causes of these lines are usually minor childhood illnesses and therefore are not related to the etiology of the brain damage. In the control group, 10 teeth demonstrated postnatal lines (18%), and in two cases a possible explanation was obtained (pertussis, failure-to-thrive syndrome). In the brain-damaged group, 14 teeth revealed postnatal lines (24%), and, as mentioned, in only two was a possible etiological association found (neonatal hypoglycemia and neonatal hyperbilirubinemia with convulsions).

Table 1 shows that, in the idiopathic (62.9%) and the possibly identified etiological factor (66.7%) subgroups of brain-damaged children, a similar occurrence of dental-enamel lines was demonstrated. These findings are in marked contrast to the control group, where an incidence of only 7.5% was found.

The markers were demonstrated mainly during the prenatal period, thus indicating that insults were sustained during the second and third trimesters of pregnancy.

Table 2 shows that in 4 out of 53 (7.5 %) of the healthy controls, abnormal dental lines were found (one prenatal, three perinatal). In two of these cases, forceps delivery was performed, which might have been responsible for the perinatal lines.

The DGL findings, as seen in Table 1, show a similar but less dramatic trend. In the brain-damaged group, 13 (22.4%), and in the healthy controls, five (9.4%) children demonstrated unusual dermatoglyphics. This difference is also significant ($p < .05$). In the idiopathic group, of the nine children having DGL findings, seven of these also had prenatal dental lines. (The possible explanation of more than one marker is discussed later.)

Table 1. Unusual dermatoglyphic (DGL) findings and abnormal dental enamel lines in brain-damaged and healthy children

| | Unusual DGL findings | Abnormal dental enamel lines | | | Total number of children with DGL and/or dental enamel abnormalities[a] |
		Prenatal	Perinatal	Total	
Control group (N = 53)	5(9.4%)	1(1.9%)	3(5.6%)	4(7.5%)	9(17%)
Brain-damaged group (N = 56)					
A. Idiopathic brain damage (N = 35)	9[b](25.7%)	19[c](54.3%)	3(8.6%)	21[c](62.9%)	29[c](82.9%)
B. Possible etiological factor identified (N = 21)	4(19%)	11[c](52.4%)	8[c](38.1%)	14[c](66.7%)	17[c](80.1%)
Total brain-damaged group (A + B) (N = 56)	13(22.4%)	30[c](51.7%)	11[c](19.6%)	35[c](62.5%)	46[c](82.1%)

[a]Because some children demonstrated a combination of unusual DGL and abnormal pre- and perinatal enamel lines, the total number of abnormal findings is larger than that of the brain-damaged children.

[b]χ^2 = Differences compared to controls significant at the level of $p < .05$.

[c]χ^2 = Differences compared to controls significant at the level of $p < .001$.

In Table 2, it is seen that of the five healthy controls with unusual DGL findings, only one case was associated with a history of extreme hemorrhage in the fourth month of pregnancy, which conceivably might have been the cause. The correlation between history, DGL findings, and dental markers was poor.

Table 3, which demonstrates the correlation between possible etiology and the markers in the brain-damaged group, shows that 19 abnormal dental enamel lines were demonstrated in 14 children (five teeth had both pre- and perinatal lines). Therefore, 66.7% of the 21 cases demonstrated dental evidence of insult.

In 16 children following pregnancies associated with gestational problems, nine teeth showed corresponding prenatal abnormal den-

tal enamel lines (56%). Of nine cases with perinatal complications, five demonstrated appropriate perinatal lines (55.5%). In the two cases of prematurity (cases 89, 102), it is possible that an unidentified event during gestation was responsible for the prenatal lines and the subsequent premature birth.

DGL findings were less significant. They were demonstrated in four out of 21 cases (17%). A possible etiological relationship was established in two of these cases (fever of unknown origin, and maternal rubella during the third month of pregnancy). As DGL patterns are affected only during the early stage of gestation, the smaller incidence of these changes, when compared to dental enamel findings, was not unexpected.

Table 2. Correlation of significant history with positive DGL and dental enamel findings in the normal controls

| | History | | | Dental lines | |
Case number	Prenatal	Perinatal	DGL	Prenatal	Perinatal
143	Bleeding in first trimester		N	−	−
112	Bleeding in fourth month		A	−	−
86		Forceps delivery	N	−	+
71		Forceps delivery	N	−	+
127			N	−	+
49			N	+	−
30			A	−	−
55			A	−	−
109			A	−	−
113			A	−	−

N = normal; A = abnormal.

+ = pathological line; − = no lines.

Table 3. Brain-damaged subgroup of possibly identified etiology: correlation of etiology, DGL, and dental findings (21 cases)

| Case number | History | | DGL | Dental lines | |
	Prenatal	Perinatal		Prenatal	Perinatal
131	Fever of unknown origin (fourth month)		−	+	−
68	Fever (urine infection) (third month)		+	+	−
139	Bleeding in first trimester		−	+	−
160	Bleeding in first trimester		−	−	−
83	Bleeding in first trimester plus I.U.G.R.[b]		−	+	−
158	Bleeding in first trimester		−	−	−
47	Rubella (third month)		+	−	−
77	I.U.G.R.		−	+	+
67	I.U.G.R.		−	−	+
157	Toxemia of pregnancy		+	−	−
89	Prematurity (28 weeks)		−	+	+
102	Prematurity (28 weeks)		−	+	−
137	I.U.G.R.	Breech delivery	−	−	−
108	I.U.G.R.	Asphyxia	−	−	−
101	Toxemia of pregnancy	Asphyxia	−	+	+
106	Bleeding at 36 weeks	Breech delivery	−	+	+
95		Asphyxia	+	−	−
141		Asphyxia	−	−	+
149		Asphyxia	−	+	−
153		Forceps delivery	−	−	+
156		Asphyxia	−	+	+

[a]Prenatal history only: 12 cases; prenatal and perinatal history: 4 cases; perinatal history only: 5 cases.
[b]Intrauterine growth retardation.

DISCUSSION

This study set out to investigate both the incidence and the timing of fetal and perinatal insults, as registered by abnormal dental enamel markers and unusual DGL patterns, in brain-damaged children. It was hypothesized that, if brain-damaged children demonstrated a higher incidence of the said markers, it would be reasonable to assume that the insults causing them would be etiologically responsible for the brain damage.

The association of DGL alterations and a variety of congenital disorders is well established. These disorders may be of genetic or environmental origin (Holt, 1968), such as viruses, teratogenic agents, or defects in placental function (Achs, Harper, & Siegel, 1966; Jones & Smith, 1973; Milunsky, Great, & Gaynor, 1968). The number of well-defined genetic and chromosomal syndromes characterized by specific DGL patterns is limited. The fingertip and palmar configurations develop during the first trimester and the beginning of the second trimester of pregnancy:

usually DGL variations can serve as nonspecific markers of fetal insult during this period of early gestation. An increased incidence of unusual DGL patterns has been demonstrated in groups of brain-damaged children (Dar, Bolchinsky, Jaffe, & Winter, 1978, Dar et al., 1977).

The second marker studied was deciduous dental enamel development. Deciduous teeth, because of their growth pattern, can provide a permanent record of fetal insults over the period extending from the fourth month of gestation until the age of about 12 months (Levine, Turner, & Dobbing, 1979). Because of the common embryonic ectodermal origin of the tooth and nervous tissue, and the similarity of their embryonic development, it would be logical to conclude that an insult to the developing fetal or infant brain of sufficient magnitude to result in brain damage would be likely to leave its mark on the tooth enamel (McMillan & Kashgarian, 1961). Macroscopic examination of the teeth of brain-damaged children reveals a high incidence of dental enamel hypoplasia (Herman & McDonald, 1963). Kreshover

(Kreshover, 1944; Kreshover, Clough, & Bear, 1953; Kreshover & Hancock, 1954, 1956) was able to verify this association by inducing enamel hypoplasia in rats subjected to artificially produced viremia. This lesion was macroscopically and microscopically similar to that seen in humans. Macroscopic dental enamel hypoplasia is an extreme manifestation, and therefore histological examination might be expected to reveal unsuspected information regarding insults to the developing fetus and infant.

The whole process of dental enamel development takes about 18 months for deciduous teeth, and begins at about 4 months of gestation with the incisors.

A transient, severe metabolic disturbance probably results in a corresponding disturbance to the enamel-forming cells that will manifest as a hypoplastic line or band in the enamel (Levine et al., 1979). The most common fetal "insult" is the birth process, which results in the so-called "neonatal line." Identification of this line enables one to differentiate prenatally formed enamel, which is a register of gestational events, from that formed postnatally (see Figure 2). An abnormally broad neonatal line would indicate an abnormal birth process or perinatal events (perinatal line) (Figure 3).

Of the brain-damaged group, 62.5% ($p <$ .001) showed abnormal dental enamel findings, as compared to 7.5% of normal controls. DGL abnormalities were noted in 22.4% of the brain-damaged group and in 9.4% of the controls. The total incidence of gestational and perinatal markers in the brain-damaged group, 82.1%, as opposed to 17% in the controls, unequivocally supports this hypothesis (Table 1).

The higher yield of abnormal dental enamel markers, compared to DGL patterns, could be explained by the timing of the insult. Dermatoglyphics are affected only during the first 3–4 months of pregnancy, while dental enamel development takes place from the fourth month of gestation until the postnatal age of about 1 year. The other possibility is that tooth enamel development is more sensitive to fetal metabolic upheaval than are DGL patterns.

Table 3 demonstates the concordance of history with appropriate fetal and perinatal markers. This occurred in 55.5% of cases.

An unexpected finding was that in the idiopathic brain-damaged group, the combined total of DGL and dental markers was 82.9%,

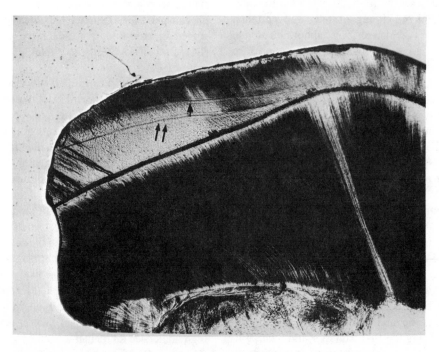

Figure 2. Identification of the neonatal line (one arrow) and the prenatal line (two arrows).

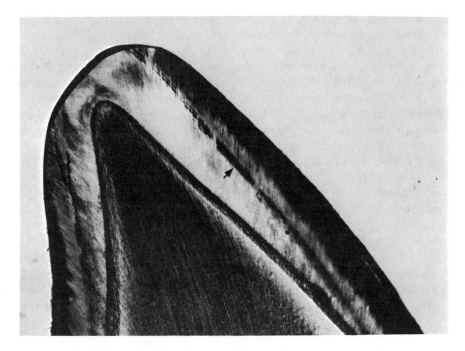

Figure 3.   An abnormally broad perinatal line indicates an abnormal birth process or perinatal events.

which was similar to the incidence in the brain-damaged group of possibly identified etiology. This would indicate that, even though a possible etiological association was noted in the "known etiology" group, the actual relationship to the brain damage is not proved and raises questions concerning either the adequacy of the historical information available or the likelihood of subclinical events being instrumental in causing the brain damage.

The findings from this study, that in 82.1% of the brain-damaged group there was evidence of gestational insult (DGL and dental lines), support the contention of Crome (1960), Holm (1982), and Hageberg, Hageberg, and Olow (1975) that the most critical period in the etiology of brain damage is during pregnancy, even though clinical evidence of the insult might be lacking at the time. This observation can aid the physician in discussing the presumed etiology of the condition with the parents, as well as in assessing the chances of recurrence. For example, in the not-infrequent situation of a baby born with brain damage following a pregnancy associated with maternal fever or uterine hemorrhage, DGL alterations or dental enamel

lines coresponding to the gestational event might be evidence that the said event had resulted in fetal insult and most probably also in the brain damage. Counseling might therefore be based on the etiology of the gestational event.

One of the implications of this study is that, in order to lessen the incidence of brain damage in children, it is necessary to concentrate on the prenatal determinants of fetal development. An increasing list of potentially damaging factors is accumulating, such as maternal infections, alcohol consumption, smoking, drug usage, etc. Intensive education during the school years would probably be beneficial in avoiding such hazards to the developing fetus.

Information regarding the type of gestational insult and the likelihood of its causing brain damage is incomplete. In this study, the most commonly demonstrated associations were with gestational hemorrhage, toxemia, intrauterine growth retardation, abnormal delivery, and perinatal asphyxia. The numbers are, however, insufficiently large to enable definite conclusions to be drawn.

The occurrence of both prenatal and perinatal lines in the same case, or DGL alterations and dental lines, is explainable by the fact that early fetal damage can result in subsequent gestational abnormalities and/or abnormal labor associated with asphyxia. In these situations, the earliest insult would probably be the significant one, while the later events would be merely the secondary consequences thereof.

The results of this study confirm the value of using dental enamel and DGL as nonspecific registers of fetal and perinatal insult. Further studies are required in order to elaborate the nature and severity of the types of insult likely to result in brain damage. Additional information could be obtained in prospective studies correlating modern sophisticated fetal-monitoring techniques with these markers and the subsequent occurrence of brain damage.

SUMMARY

The value of utilizing dermatoglyphic analysis and microscopic dental enamel abnormalities as nonspecific registers of fetal and perinatal insult was investigated.

In 82.1% of a group of brain-damaged children, evidence of gestational or perinatal insult was demonstrated, while only 17% of a group of healthy controls showed similar findings.

It can therefore be concluded that investigation of these markers in the developing child can provide information on the timing and incidence of insults during pregnancy and the perinatal period. Such information is of value in the study of the etiology of brain damage in children, and in certain situations may be of help in the genetic counseling of the parents.

REFERENCES

Achs, R., Harper, R.G., & Siegel, M. Unusual dermatoglyphic findings associated with rubella embryopathy. *New England Journal of Medicine*, 1966, *274*, 148–151.

Crome, L. The brain and mental retardation. *British Medical Journal*, 1960, *1*, 897–899.

Dar, H., Bolchinsky, D., Jaffe, M., & Winter, S.T. Routine analysis of dermatoglyphic and palmar creases in children with developmental disorders. *Developmental Medicine and Child Neurology*, 1978, *20*, 735–737.

Dar, H., Schmidt, R., & Nitowsky, H.M. Palmar crease variants and their clinical significance. *Pediatric Research*, 1977, *11*, 103–108.

Hageberg, B., Hageberg, G., & Olow, I. The changing panorama of cerebral palsy in Sweden 1954–1970. I: Analysis of the general changes. *Acta Paediatrica Scandinavica*, 1975, *64*, 187–192.

Herman, S.C., & McDonald, R.E. Enamel hypoplasia in cerebral-palsied children. *Journal of Dentistry in Childhood*, 1963, *30*, 46–49.

Holm, V.A. The causes of cerebral palsy. *Journal of the American Medical Association*, 1982, *247*, 1473–1477.

Holt, S.B. *The genetics of dermal ridges*. Springfield, IL: Charles C Thomas, 1968.

Hunter, A.G.W., Evans, J.A., Thompson, D.R., & Ramsay, S. A study of institutionalised mentally retarded patients in Manitoba. I: Classification and preventability. *Developmental Medicine and Child Neurology*, 1980, *22*, 145–162.

Jones, K.L., & Smith, D.W. Recognition of fetal alcohol syndrome in early infancy. Lancet, 1973, *2*, 999–1001.

Kreshover, S.J. Pathogenesis of dental hypoplasia: An experimental study. *Journal of Dental Research*, 1944, *23*, 231–234.

Kreshover, S.J., Clough, O.W., & Bear, D.M. Prenatal influence on tooth development: Alloxan diabetes in rats. *Journal of Dental Research*, 1953, *32*, 246–248.

Kreshover, S.J., Hancock, J.A. Vaccinia infection in pregnant rabbits and its effect on maternal and fetal dental tissues. *Journal of the American Dental Association*, 1954, *49*, 549–553.

Kreshover, S.J., & Hancock, J.A. Effect of lymphocytic choriomeningitis on pregnancy and dental tissues in mice. *Journal of Dental Research*, 1956, *35*, 467–470.

Levine, R.S., Turner, E.P., & Dobbing, J. Deciduous teeth contain histories of developmental disturbances. *Early Human Development*, 1979, *3*, 211–220.

McMillan, R.S., & Kashgarian, M. Relation of human abnormalities of structure and function to abnormalities of dentition. I: Relation of hypoplasia of enamel to cerebral and ocular disorders. *Journal of the American Dental Association*, 1961, *63*, 38–48.

Milunsky, A., Great, J.W., & Gaynor, M.F. Methotrexate-induced congenital malformations. *The Journal of Pediatrics*, 1968, *72*, 790–795.

Penrose, L.S. *Memorandum on dermatoglyphic nomenclature. Birth defects. Original article Series 4, No. 3*. New York: National Foundation of the March of Dimes, 1968.

Chapter 25

The Use of Auditory Brain Stem Potentials in Hearing Screening of High-Risk Infants

MORDECHAI Z. HIMMELFARB, M.D.
DANA SCHWARTZ, M.A.
SHAUL HAREL, M.D.
ELIAHU SHANON, M.D.
Tel Aviv University, Tel Aviv, Israel

P UBLISHED STUDIES ON SCREENING OF AUDI-
tory function in high-risk infants with the
help of auditory brain stem potential (ABP)
recordings are scarce and probably do not reflect the true scope of performance in this field.
Schulman-Galambos and Galambos (1979) examined 75 babies discharged from an infant
intensive care unit (ICU) and found hearing
loss greater than 60 dB in one or both ears in
four babies. In a later report (Despland &
Galambos, 1981), 14 of 100 babies in an ICU
were found to have diminished hearing function. The authors identified nine risk factors
associated with hearing loss, the most common
being neonatal asphyxia accompanied by acidosis. Barnet, Weiss, Reutter, and Saumweber
(1981) attempted to classify lower and higher
risk factors for hearing loss. Among the major
risk factors included were gestational age of
26–31 weeks, body weight of less than 1.5
kilograms, Apgar scores of 1–6, assisted ventilation for 5 or more days, intraventricular hemorrhage, and apnea. Of 48 high-risk infants
tested, 12 showed hearing loss (seven bilateral

and five unilateral). The hearing loss was described as mild in six, moderate in three, severe
in one, and profound in two infants. The incidence of diminished hearing was twice as frequent in the higher risk group than in the lower
risk group.

The purpose of this study is to report the
experience of the authors in the use of ABP as
means of hearing screening in high-risk
infants.

MATERIAL AND METHODS

ABPs were recorded in 140 high-risk for hearing impairment infants (76 male and 64 female)
ranging in age from 72 hours to 1 year. The
babies were referred for ABP evaluation by the
maternity hospital and were selected according
to the following high-risk factors: 1) prematurity (46 infants), 2) respiratory distress syndrome (RDS) (32 infants), 3) hyperbilirubinemia (14 infants), 4) deafness in family (14
infants), 5) rubella in pregnancy (eight infants), 6) central nervous system (CNS) dis-

This study was supported in part by a Keren Sapir, Mifal Hapais grant.

Table 1. Hearing loss detected by ABP screening

Type of hearing loss	n	%
Bilateral		
Profound (S/N)[a]	8	5.7
Moderate (S/N)	4	2.9
Moderate (C)[b]	3	2.1
Mild (C)	1	0.7
Unilateral		
Severe-Moderate (S/N)	6	4.3
Moderate (C)	4	2.8

[a]S/N = Sensorineural.
[b]C = Conductive.

eases in family (six infants), 7) cerebral hemorrhage (five infants), 8) small-for-gestational age (SGA) (three infants), and 9) various other diseases (12 infants).

The procedure for recording ABP has been described elsewhere (Shanon, Gold, Himmelfarb, & Carasso, 1979). Hearing threshold for click stimuli was determined by the lowest intensity at which the fifth wave (Jewett V) could be identified. Latency of the first wave as well as otoscopy findings served for evaluation of outer and middle ear function.

RESULTS AND DISCUSSION

The audiological findings are summarized in Table 1. Bilateral sensorineural hearing loss was identified in 8.6% of the infants (5.7% profound and 2.9% moderate hearing loss). An additional 4.3% of the infants were found to have moderate to severe sensorineural hearing loss. Conductive hearing loss was identified in 5.8% of the infants.

The high-risk factors in the 18 infants identified as suffering from sensorineural hearing loss are shown in Table 2. It can be clearly seen that the major high-risk factors in these infants were deafness or CNS disease in the family and rubella during pregnancy.

The high incidence of sensorineural hearing loss among these high-risk factors is further demonstrated in Table 3. Five out of twenty infants referred for testing due to CNS diseases or deafness in their families had bilateral profound sensorineural hearing loss, and in one other, a unilateral sensorineural hearing loss was found. In addition, two out of the eight infants tested as a result of their mothers having rubella during pregnancy were found to have bilateral profound sensorineural hearing loss and two others had unilateral sensorineural hearing loss. Only three of 32 infants with severe respiratory distress had bilateral moderate sensorineural hearing loss.

It should be stressed that follow-up tests of all 2-month-old infants who were identified as having bilateral sensorineural hearing loss were consistent with the initial results. There are no follow-up data on those infants identified as having bilateral moderate sensorineural and unilateral sensorineural hearing losses. All those with conductive hearing loss had normal tracings when retested.

CONCLUSION

Measurement of auditory brain stem potentials seems to be a useful tool in the assessment of hearing function in infants. This is especially so for those at risk for hearing impairment since the incidence of sensorineural hearing loss in such infants is 5–10 times greater than in the

Table 2. High-risk factors in detected sensorineural (S/N) hearing loss

Type of hearing loss	High-risk factor	n
Bilateral profound S/N	Rubella in pregnancy	2
	Deafness or CNS disease	5
	RDS	1
Bilateral moderate S/N	RDS	2
	Hyperbilirubinemia	1
	Pierre Robin syndrome	1
Unilateral severe-moderate S/N	Rubella in pregnancy	2
	Deafness or CNS disease	2
	Prematurity	1
	Cerebral hemorrhage	1

Table 3. Incidence of sensorineural (S/N) hearing loss

High-risk factor	S/N hearing loss	Incidence
Deafness or CNS disease	Bilateral	5/20
	Unilateral	1/20
Rubella in pregnancy	Bilateral	2/8
	Unilateral	2/8
RDS	Bilateral	3/32

general infant population. It appears that, among the high-risk criteria, a distinction can be made between major and minor risk factors. Limited experience suggests that such differentiation may be of practical value in devising hearing screening programs.

REFERENCES

Barnet, A.B., Weiss, S., Reutter, S., & Saumweber, R. *Auditory brainstem and cortical evoked potentials in high-risk premature infants.* Paper presented at the Seventh Symposium of the International Evoked Response Audiometry Study Group, Bergamo, Italy, July, 1981.

Despland, P.A., & Galambos, R. *The auditory brainstem response evaluates risk factors for hearing loss in the newborn.* Paper presented at the Seventh Symposium of the International Evoked Response Audiometry Study Group, Bergamo, Italy, July, 1981.

Schulman-Galambos, C., & Galambos, R. Brain stem evoked response audiometry in newborn hearing screening. *Archives of Otolaryngology,* 1979, *105,* 86–90.

Shanon, E., Gold, S., Himmelfarb, M.Z., & Carasso, R. Auditory potentials of cochlear nerve and brain stem in multiple sclerosis. *Archives of Otolaryngology,* 1979, *105,* 505–508.

Chapter 26

Neurological Assessment from Birth to 7 Years of Age

CLAUDINE AMIEL-TISON
University of Paris V., Paris, France

P ERINATAL BRAIN DAMAGE IS A HETEROGE-
neous entity, and a poor correlation exists
between risk factors and outcome. Gestational,
obstetrical, and neonatal circumstances known
to carry a risk can result in a wide variety of
outcomes; the effects on the neonatal brain
vary from very severe lesions and death, to
moderate and no lesions. Variable factors that
affect outcome in the neonatal brain include the
duration of a hypoxic-ischemic insult, the
chronic or acute nature of the insult, the stage
of maturation at which the insult occurs, and
many other factors that are poorly defined or
completely unknown at the present time. As
the specific risk factors and their effects are not
completely understood in each case, it is important to have objective criteria to evaluate the
individual infant's brain status.

Until recently, the only way to assess an
infant at risk was clinical evaluation. However,
the extensive use of artificial ventilation and
other modalities of newborn intensive care
have made it more difficult to perform this
evaluation properly. Moreover, the smaller
and smaller size of the survivors makes it more
difficult to identify neurological abnormalities;
the normal range for cerebral function in the
population weighing less than 1,000 grams has
not been established. Therefore, clinical evaluation in the intensive care unit (ICU) has been
replaced by new noninvasive techniques.
When bedside ultrasonography (US) became
available as a routine procedure (Pape, Blackwell, Cusik, Sherwood, Houang, Thorburn, &
Reynolds, 1979), the clinical assessment of the
acutely ill neonate became less essential for
immediate evaluation of brain damage. Intracranial hemorrhages and the transient changes
in the periventricular white matter have now
been well documented (Pape, Bennett-Britton,
Szymonowicz, Martin, Fitz, & Becker, 1983;
Partridge, Babcock, Steichen, & Han, 1983).
The next step will be when newer noninvasive
methods such as nuclear magnetic resonance
(NMR), positron emission tomography (PET),
and newer generation CT scans become available. These new methods should be able to
elucidate the cellular lesions that are suggested
clinically but for which objective evidence is
lacking or misleading; more accurate imaging
will give clinicans the ability to differentiate
significant from nonsignificant anomalies observed in the first months of life.

Testing methods have to follow maturation
through infancy and childhood. In clinical
studies, neurological evaluation is complicated
by the rapid maturation process taking place
within the first months and years of life. Defin-

The author thanks Dr. Roberta Goldberg for her expert editing; she patiently transformed schoolhouse English into a decent language.

ing reliable markers of brain dysfunction that change as maturation progresses is essential. One of the major aims of this author's work has been to review and propose guidelines for the clinician, from birth to age 7. Even mild sequelae at age 7 have to be taken into account. Because of the great amount of work involved, questions are frequently asked about children with mild sequelae of perinatal brain damage. Why is follow-up necessary for these children as it might increase the parent's anxiety without providing any real help to the child? Couldn't these mild deviations from the norm be regarded as a further expression of the individuality originating in genetic and sociocultural differences? These difficult questions are addressed in describing the step-by-step approach to the child at risk, according to maturation. The author's answer is that such studies are an absolute necessity for completing the clinical picture and for early detection of learning difficulties so that effective help can be provided for the developing child.

THE NEONATAL PERIOD

Different types of lesions may occur depending on the gestational age (GA) of the newborn. The technical approach to the preterm and term infant is very different as well.

The Preterm Newborn Infant

Intraventricular hemorrhages (IVH) of various degrees of severity can be expected in about 50% of the cohort weighing less than 1,500 grams. Twenty years ago, this diagnosis was a clinical guess (Amiel, 1964) and diagnosed only at post mortem (Larroche, 1964). The frequency of silent IVH was first reported in 1978 by the use of CT scans in infants of under 1,500 grams birth weight (Papile, Burstein, & Koffler, 1978); at the present time, a reliable US can diagnose an IVH which can be classified according to the location and volume of bleeding (Papile et al., 1978). Some neurologists claim that they are able to recognize IVH clinically in a high proportion of cases (Dubowitz, Levene, Morante, Palmer, & Dubowitz, 1981), whereas some do not (Stewart, Thorburn, Lipscomb, & Amiel-Tison, 1983).

The debate is academic, as the most recent data demonstrate that the extent or presence of an IVH is not well correlated with outcome; instead, the newer methods indicate that it is the concomitant leukomalacias that will predict outcome. These white matter ischemic lesions are silent clinically, and unfortunately, at the present time, not reliably detectable by US for several weeks.

This does not mean that clinical observation of sick very low birth weight (VLBW) infants in an intensive care unit is of no value; with little or no manipulations, the neurologist will be able to recognize severe signs such as coma, seizures, gross tone abnormalities, and ocular signs. It may be possible to correlate these abnormalities with outcome. It must be recognized that when severe neurological signs are found, the maturative assessment will often be inacurrate. The estimated GA is not reliable when active tone cannot be tested due to the infant's medical condition, or before 32 weeks when there are no active tone milestones. Confidence based on passive tone only is not reliable for many reasons, among which are "communicated" tone for the first 3 days of life due to the posture *in utero* (Saint-Anne Dargassies, 1977), and fixation of the limbs in relation to the intensive care apparatus. In the immediate neonatal period, when evaluating maturation or looking for neurological signs, one must resist the temptation to use a few nonreliable tests, selected because they are the only ones available at the moment. To go further in the opposite direction, the neurological status of a newborn should not be evaluated if one is unable to test active tone in the axis (Amiel-Tison, 1974).

The Preterm Reaching 40 Weeks

The neurological evaluation is valuable when the VLBW infant reaches the full-term period (40 weeks corrected GA) with satisfactory respiratory function and nutritional status. A full neurological assessment can be done, exploring reactions to the environment, sensorial abilities, tone, and reflexes. Normal findings determined by a careful neurological assessment at the full-term period were not considered in the past as an absolute guarantee of favorable outcome (Amiel-Tison, 1974); a small number of these infants developed neurological sequelae. There is increased confidence, at the present time, that a normal neurological assessment in the full-term period has a high predictive value for good outcome. This has been accomplished by a more comprehensive approach, with the addition of behavioral, organization, and interaction testing (Brazelton, 1973, 1979) of infants who had US in the neonatal period. A recent follow-up by Stewart, Thorburn, Hope, Castello, Goldsmith, Swain, and Reynolds (1983) confirmed the value of neurological assessment in conjunction with US at the full-term period in predicting a good outcome. They concluded that "neurological examination at term improved the recognition of normal infants but not abnormal ones," based on a study of the assessment of 110 very preterm infants.

The best overall prediction of poor outcome has been by the presence of ventricular enlargement identified by US. However, ventricular enlargement is not a simple entity and does not lead to a single therapeutic approach; ventricular enlargement may be the result of two very different events, pathophysiologically easy to understand but not as simple to differentiate clinically. One is the result of a blockage at different levels of the ventricular system with signs of intracranial hypertension (ICH); the other is the result of extensive periventricular leukomalacia, followed by cavitation and sclerosis of the white matter after several weeks. This leads to hydrocephaly *ex vacuo* because the corona radiata shrinks and the lateral ventricles expand, with no increase of intracranial pressure. Clinical assessment plays an important role in making the distinction between these two entities (and therefore determining the necessity of a shunt). Pertinent signs and symptoms include cranial signs (mainly distension of the squamous sutures), tone abnormalities (opisthotonic posture and imbalance between flexors and extensors), and a sunset sign; repeated yawning and lethargy are appearing when the pressure reaches very high levels. The noninvasive procedures to accurately measure intracranial pressure at the fontanel can be very helpful in the neuro-

surgical decision since, during the first weeks of life, a true blockage can stabilize and a hydrocephaly *ex vacuo* can show transient signs of ICH. The question of when to intervene in the child with hydrocephalus and whether early intervention will be effective is being considered by several groups (Chaplin, Goldstein, Myeberg, Hunt, & Tooley, 1980; Hill & Volpe, 1981; Levene & Starte, 1981; Liechty, Gilmore, Bryson, & Bull, 1983). Very little follow-up information is currently available. However, the prognosis appears to be better than in the past, and one group has suggested that only infants with large hemorrhages extending into brain tissue may be neurodevelopmentally abnormal (Lipscomb, Thorburn, Stewart, Reynolds, & Hope, 1983). There is insufficient evidence to conclude that the apparently improved prognosis is due to early intervention, which has been carried out since US was introduced. This conclusion must be tested with large numbers and a multicenter controlled trial.

The Term Newborn

Signs and symptoms of cerebral dysfunction are much easier to elicit in a full-term than a premature newborn. A full assessment is possible in most cases, except when artificial ventilation is necessary very early. Again, a normal overall assessment of neurosensorial function in the first few days of life predicts normal outcome in a full-term with few exceptions, the exceptions being mainly related to cerebral malformations. The following is an approach derived from experience.

Mild Signs Are Often Transient, and, When Transient, Correlate with a Normal Outcome When the neurological assessment is normal within the first 3 days of life, or has normalized after very transient and mild abnormalities of tone and/or excitability (with normal intrauterine growth and normal head circumference), the outcome will be normal; this means that no follow-up is necessary, even if risk factors were present at the time of delivery.

Cerebral Dysfunction of Perinatal Origin Rapidly Changes When neurological signs or symptoms are elicited soon after birth, it is necessary to repeat the assessment at least every other day through the end of the first week, because the signs linked with perinatal difficulties usually change rapidly. The signs can worsen in the first few days and then improve, but rarely remain stable. After the first days, the general tendency is toward rapid improvement.

A Gradation of Signs and Symptoms Is Useful It is very useful to have a clinical classification of signs to correlate with both the adverse causal circumstances and outcome (Amiel-Tison, 1979). It is important to note that there is a hierarchy in the severity of signs, and that the poor correlations observed in many follow-up studies, and more specifically, in multicenter studies, can be linked in part to an absence of gradation of symptoms. A three-stage classification has been used as a clinical routine on all full-term newborns during their first week of life in Port-Royal and Baude-locque Maternity Hospitals in Paris; the gradation is done at the end of the first week, based on the signs that were observed during the whole week of repeated assessments and noted on a grid (Amiel-Tison, 1979).

Mild Signs Hyperexcitability and abnormalities of tone are present, but responsiveness is normal. Primary reflexes are present, and no seizures are observed.

Moderate Signs In addition to disturbances of tone and excitability, consciousness and primary reflexes are also involved. A progressive CNS depression is often seen, with deterioration of alertness and sucking within the first days. Isolated seizures may be observed. The EEG may be normal or show moderate abnormalities (hypoactivity or discontinuous tracing) with rapid changes from one day to the other.

Severe Signs Coma and repeated seizures at short intervals are present. As seizures are often "subtle" and difficult to recognize in a comatose child, the EEG patterns are important to the classification, mainly the inactive or paroxysmal tracings.

Infants with severe or moderate signs are rarely normal at the end of the first week. They should all be included in follow-up studies. Half of the infants with mild signs are normal

by day 7, and are not included in follow-up studies, but are considered as borderline normal.

This clinical gradation was used for years prior to the availability of imaging of the neonatal brain. The evidence provided by US and CT scan has shown this gradation to be valid. Newer imaging methods have given additional information on the nature of the lesions. NMR or CT scan can demonstrate damage that has occurred before delivery. This is not only important for further understanding of etiology, but also gives the obstetrician the ability to differentiate damage directly attributable to the birth process from lesions that predate labor and delivery. Brain damage that is already organized in the first days of life cannot be a consequence of birth trauma but shows how silent prenatal circulatory problems can lead to midcerebral artery area softening or extensive porencephaly. The etiology of these prenatal lesions has been a source of frequent disagreement among obstetricians, pediatricians, and neurologists. Previously, they could only theorize, but not distinguish, prenatal lesions from perinatal damage. It is likely that more objective data will be forthcoming to clearly define the real cause of neurological damage in the neonate. Until then, clinicians should learn to reject easy explanations for pathology that are clearly not pertinent (e.g., a hypoglycemic episode as the cause of severe damage). At the same time, clinicans must remember that a low-risk pregnancy and normal labor and delivery are not a guarantee of a normal newborn.

THE FIRST 3 MONTHS: RECOVERY PHASE

The recovery period extends from 40 weeks to 3 months (corrected age). The necessity of considering this period separately has been recently described by Grenier (1982). During this phase, the VLBW infant or the full-term newborn who has been very sick will often appear different from a normal newborn even if nutritional and cardiorespiratory status have normalized. This is true even if it is subsequently shown that he or she has had no perinatal brain damage. This period is usually spent at home, as most VLBW infants are discharged around the time a full-term birth was expected. It is also the period of maximum anxiety for the parents. They have forgotten about the risk of neonatal death, but not about the possibility of sequelae. They have lost the feeling of security given by an experienced and confident perinatal team. They have to manage by themselves, and take on overwhelming responsibilities. They will begin to compare their child with other children of the same age group. When they go to a follow-up clinic, it is unlikely that they feel reassured about the outcome. The most anxious parents are so afraid of the answers that they don't ask questions about prognosis.

Neurological Characteristics during the Recovery Period

Neurological characteristics during the recovery period most commonly involve the level of excitability (excessive response to noise, manipulations, visceral discomfort, etc.), the level of alertness, and disturbed state regulation. Various types of muscle imbalance are common; during these 3 months of life, significant changes of passive tone are not normally expected and hypertonicity is physiological. Therefore, even a marked hypertonicity in the flexor muscles of the limbs is not a reliable sign; when progressive relaxation of the limbs is observed early, beginning at around 2 months in hands and arms and at around 3 months in lower limbs, these changes are a good index for a normal outcome. Tone imbalance is a worrisome pattern within the first 3 months when excessive hypotonicity in the neck flexors and upper extremities (no resistance to the scarf maneuver) is contrasting with hypertonicity in lower limbs.

As head control is the most significant acquisition expected at 2–3 months, this event should be observed carefully. Most low-risk infants acquire complete head control by around 2 months. The most significant abnormalities for VLBW infants in this period involve imbalance in the development of active tone in neck extensors and flexors, imbalance that is responsible for a delay in head control. When the infant is pulled forward to the sitting position, the neck does not properly follow the axis because of poor active tone in the flexor muscles of the neck. A typical combination of signs and symptoms is poor neck flexors and unlimited scarf movement in a hyperexcitable child.

Usual Evolution of Abnormalities

The course can progress in two different ways with abrupt changes usually occurring in the third month corrected age. In most cases, these deviations from the normal pattern will rapidly vanish, and motor and behavioral normalization will occur, followed by normal motor development within the first year. In a few cases, however, even if head control is acquired between 3 and 4 months, other motor abnormalities will be detected and new markers will have to be recognized (Amiel-Tison & Grenier, 1983).

Differentiation of Normal Infants from Those Who Will Experience New Neurological Signs at Each Step of Maturation
Is it possible to make a reliable prognosis of normal or abnormal outcome? This is the aim of the clinical work of Grenier (Amiel-Tison & Grenier, 1983). The answer is, yes, it is possible to predict normal development early in this recovery phase. This can be done by evaluating not only anteroposterior reactivity as in the classical neurological assessment, but by also exploring lateral reactivity in a state of very high alertness and communication. This is mainly achieved by two maneuvers recently described by Grenier and Amiel-Tison (1983); when the reaction of lateral abduction of the lower limb is present, the absence of cerebral palsy in lower limbs may be affirmed. This may be done as early as the first weeks of life, and the prediction of walking can be made to the parents. When lateral straightening of the trunk with active support by the arms is observed, again, the absence of gross motor impairment may be ascertained as early as the first few weeks of life. The reverse is not true: a negative finding in this difficult clinical assessment does not predict an abnormal outcome.

Further work is needed in this promising clinical evaluation. The neuropediatrician is functioning in two apparently contradictory ways. First she or he wishes to demonstrate good motor function and predict normal outcome; but at the same time, she or he must not overlook any deviations from normal motor development. These two ways of evaluating the same child during one examination should not in fact be considered as contradictory; both types of observations are important for the infant at risk. When normal outcome can be predicted, parents are so obviously encouraged that this in itself is a form of early intervention by its positive effects on parent-infant interaction (Brazelton, 1982). Transient neuromotor abnormalities must not be neglected as they may signal difficulties at school age; the sooner they are identified, the earlier help can be provided.

THE FIRST YEAR: NORMALIZATION OR HANDICAP

Major Neurological Defect: Severe Handicap

For each infant who does not normalize completely during the recovery phase described above, repeated assessments within the first year of life will classify the child. Major defects are easy to recognize, but moderate abnormalities may be persistent or transient and the distinction will not be made before 8–10 months.

The children with major neurological defects are identified within the first year of life. It is unusual for new cases to be discovered after that age (Fitzhardinge, 1980). Hydrocephalus is most often diagnosed during the first 3 months of life, with the therapeutic decisions based on both US and clinical findings. Severe cerebral palsy (CP), diplegia, tetraplegia, or hemiplegia are diagnosed later the first year. In the severe form, spasticity in limbs, hypotonia in the axis, associated gross delay in cognitive functions, and microcephaly are usually evident and stable enough to leave little hope for a partial or total recovery. The US or CT scan findings are well defined in most cases, with signs of localized or generalized cortical atrophy and signs of porencephaly and/or hydrocephaly *ex vacuo*.

Moderate Neuromotor Abnormalities: Persistent or Transient?

The most common dilemma in the first year is to determine if neuromotor abnormalities will be transient when they persist beyond corrected age 3 months. As shown by Hagberg (Hagberg, Hagberg, & Olow, 1982), most of the cases of CP that are perinatal in origin are now mild cases; within the first year, neuromotor abnormalities mimicking spastic diplegia or spastic hemiplegia may be present and will disappear as maturation progresses, usually between 8 and 10 months corrected age. Drillien has demonstrated this phenomenon in low birth weight infants (Drillien, 1972); Nelson has shown the same phenomenon in studying the data of the American Collaborative Project (Nelson & Ellenberg, 1982). Again, the question that the neuropediatrician is asked when he or she is assessing such infants during their first year is how development can be predicted, therefore giving parents an early prognosis. The answer can be summarized as follows: the clinical findings obtained by the classical evaluation of tone and reflexes differ in degree and quality. Table 1 represents the main clinical features differentiating persistent cerebral palsy from transient abnormalities.

Lateral reactivity evaluated by complementary maneuvers gives a guarantee of future motor normalization. When present, the two maneuvers described have the same value at 6 months as at 6 weeks, since this lateral reactivity is part of normal gross motor function all through infancy and adult life.

What help can be expected from US or CT scan during this period? There is little information to be added, as it is quite common not to observe gross modification in moderate as well as transient motor abnormalities; conversely, satisfactory motor development may be observed in cases of moderate hydrocephaly *ex vacuo* or shunted hydrocephaly. At the present time, the prognosis is mainly dependent on clinical findings until new data become available from the most recent noninvasive methods, including NMR spectroscopy. A simple parameter such as head growth has been shown to be well correlated with developmental outcome in VLBW infants (Gross, Oehler, &

Table 1. Main clinical features differentiating persistent cerebral palsy from transient abnormalities

Neuromotor abnormalities indicating cerebral palsy	Neuromotor abnormalities very likely transient
—poor active tone in the axis	—active and passive tone abnormalities are moderate and changing
—strong righting reaction with scissoring	—the stretch reflex is phasic
—no opening of the popliteal angle	—lateral reactivity is normal including lateral abduction of the hip
—tonic stretch reflex in the triceps	

Eckerman, 1983). Developmental scales at one year are poorly related with outcome, as described below (see "The Second Year"). The main sequence of clinical events and testing during the first year of life are summarized in Table 2.

THE SECOND YEAR: EXPLORATION OF COGNITIVE FUNCTIONS

The early evaluation of cognitive function relies mainly on the Bayley Mental Scale or other similar scales. The prediction of a severe mental handicap is possible as early as 6 months, as demonstrated by many observers. The infants who have the lowest scores at 6 months and 1 year (below 70) continue to show problems at later ages. But as observed by Hunt (1979), when the IQ was above 70 at 6 months and 1 year, the potentially normal and abnormal infants could not be differentiated at these ages; by 2 years of age, there is a definitive segregation of scores by outcome category: most who would be normal at ages 4–6 scored above 90 at age 2 whereas most of those who would have problems by ages 4–6 had scores below 90. Fitzhardinge (1980) published comparable data on the reliability of developmental assessments made in the first 2 years of life. A prospective 6-year study was done of 133 chil-

dren with birth weights of less than 1,501 grams; psychometric testing was performed at 6-month intervals for a 2-year period after the term date, using the Bayley Scale of Infant Development and then repeated at 6 years with the Wechsler Intelligence Scale for Children. Although a positive correlation existed between the Bayley scores at all ages and the Wechsler scores at 6 years, the correlation was not highly significant until 18–24 months postterm. At that age, it was possible to predict whether the child would score above or below 85 on the Wechsler test in 80% of the cases. The children who have low scores at 2 years old are candidates for language, fine motor, and behavioral problems and can be helped by early intervention programs.

FROM 2 TO 5 YEARS: PLAYGROUND AGE AND PRESCHOOL TESTING

The Difficulty Involved in Studying Toddlers

The neurological examination of the child aged 2 to 5 closely follows the same pattern as that before 2 or after 5, but it is often impossible to apply in a formal and stereotypical way. The child can no longer be manipulated as in the first year. He or she will not accept clearly structured rules to follow as will the 5-year-

Table 2. Summary of clinical events and testing during the first year of life

Recovery Phase	3–12 Months
—Convalescence at home	—early detection of *severe global handicap* (treatment of hydrocephaly; preventive physical therapy avoiding deformities
—Repeated testing looking for contact, interaction, lateral reactivity	—Separation into two groups when mild to moderate motor abnormalities are present
—Positive findings are noted and parents are given an early prognosis	•*mild* motor handicap very likely *permanent* or
	•*transient* motor abnormalities with normalization as maturation progresses

Recording of any transient abnormalities observed in order to correlate them with outcome at age 7

old. Therefore, observation and game-playing remain the essential method of evaluation. To test motor function, very gross milestones are used; pediatricians expect to see a 3-year-old child jumping in place, standing on one foot, and pedaling a tricycle; they expect to see a 4-year-old hopping on one foot, tiptoeing, and throwing a ball overhand. However, to detect mild abnormalities in fine motricity, a very elaborate set of tests must be standardized; research is being done at the moment in this field and will soon fill this gap present in most of the follow-up studies. An objective and easily reproducible evaluation will allow precise comparisons between groups. An example of this would be observing tasks such as walking backwards, tiptoe walking, heel-toe walking, and hopping on one leg, scoring these on the basis of time and quality of performance. Associated movements are closely related to age and their diagnostic significance varies according to the task the child has been asked to perform (Wolff, Gunnoe, & Cohen, 1983). Behavioral questionnaires are used as well to identify behavioral problems.

Importance of Language Scales in Preschoolers

In addition to motor development, the recognition of language disorders in preschoolers is essential but is complicated by methodological difficulties. The detection of developmental dysphasia is not easy since the limits of normal acquisition of language and those of delay that predict deviance are not clearly defined (Allen & Rapin, 1980). The problems of definition and classification are now in the process of being clarified (Rapin & Allen, 1983) in a practical manner for use by the neuropediatrician in the follow-up clinic. Some fairly simple tests are already available and widely used; developmental language scales such as the one by Reynell (1977) measure expressive language and verbal comprehension independently; in addition, the Symbolic Play Test (Lowe & Costello, 1976) evaluates early concept formation and symbolization.

It appears that there is much more to learn about infants of this age, which will be accomplished if researchers succeed in providing the neuropediatrician with practical tests, particularly fine motricity scores and language scales. This will greatly help the understanding of the children's problems, instead of relying on the caregivers' impressions. The continuity between early motor difficulties and later learning disabilities will then be more clearly established.

SCHOOL AGE: IDENTIFICATION OF MINOR HANDICAPS ASSOCIATED WITH PERINATAL BRAIN DAMAGE

The author's 20 years' experience in the pediatric outpatient department of a Paris maternity hospital has taught her to make reliable guesses about which patients will return between the ages of 8 to 10 due to scholastic difficulties. In general, they are the ones who suffered from transient neuromotor abnormalities during their first year, appeared normal at age 1 year, had a relatively normal experience in kindergarden from age 3 to age 5, and then began to encounter scholastic difficulties.

In order to demonstrate a connection between transient neuromotor abnormalities secondary to perinatal events and difficulties at school age, a sample of 15 full-term newborns was selected who demonstrated neurological symptoms during their first week and neuromotor symptoms within the first year of life (Amiel-Tison, Dube, Garel, & Jequier, 1983); they all appeared normal at 1 year of age. At 5–6 years of age, these 15 children were again evaluated and were compared to controls who had a normal neurological status in the first week of life. Normalization was observed in five out of 15 (33%), i.e., they manifested no overt symptoms and succeeded in all the tests. However, four out of 15 (25%) had abnormal scores on the tests. These four will in all likelihood encounter scholastic difficulties; all manifested problems in fine motor adjustments, and scored less than 85 on the Terman-Merrill IQ test. The remaining six children were intermediate in their symptoms as well as in the predictions that can be made for their future. In the control group, 13 out of 15 children were normal, one was classified as abnormal, and one as intermediate. These results, which must be confirmed in larger groups of infants, verify the proposed hypothesis for the full-term newborn infants. The same link between transient abnormalities of motor development and school performance has been observed in 100 VLBW infants compared to VLBW infants with normal motor development and to healthy-term infants. (Drillien, Thomson, & Burgoyne, 1980). A handicap score, ranging from 0 to 3, was calculated on the basis of school performances, IQ, and motor perceptual difficulties. Generally, those infants with a handicap score of 0–1 were well adapted in school; children with minor problems scored level 2; and a score of 3 was attributed to children with more significant difficulties, all of whom require special schooling. The following results were reported: among the infants with transient abnormalities, 23% had handicap scores of 3; by contrast, only 9% of the VLBW control group had a handicap score of 3, and only 4% of the full-term controls scored 3. It is important to stress the fact that in the group with transient neurological abnormalities, 64% of the children are functioning normally in school (31% scored 0 handicap and 33% scored 1).

Other data are now appearing on learning disabilities. Hunt, Tooley, and Harvin (1982) have described a cohort of infants from a very large group of VLBW infants who were functioning in the normal or borderline range of intelligence but with evidence of significant learning disabilities, defective language comprehension, and/or visual motor integration. Although such learning difficulties may be found throughout the general population (Rutter, 1982), the incidence of 37% of such problems in the group of VLBW infants studied by Hunt et al. (1982) makes it almost twice the highest estimate in the general population. Ellison (1983; Chapter 27, this volume), in her study of infants acutely ill in the newborn period, has shown the same relationship between transient neuromotor abnormalities detected during the first year and poor fine motor skills (finger tapping, finger localization, and grooved pegs) at 4 years.

Thus, neurological abnormalities in infants have been associated with lesser cognitive function, decreased fine motor control, lesser but not markedly abnormal achievement, parental report of learning problems, and some behavioral problems in early school years. Identical conclusions have now been reached by other groups (Gilberg & Rasmussen, 1982).

The data summarized here show how unwise it would be to establish a prognosis for each infant based on transient neuromotor abnormalities observed in the first year, as learning difficulties occur in only one-third of these children. It is of benefit statistically to predict the possibility of difficulties for the high-risk group. This benefit is twofold, first in that scholastic aid programs can be utilized and in that the expense of special education can be concentrated on those with specific need. Second, prediction is beneficial because monitoring of the decreasing number of children in this high-risk group and of the increasing number with normal outcomes each year provides important feedback to obstetricians.

EARLY INTERVENTION FROM BIRTH TO AGE 7 YEARS

The question of what to expect from early intervention arises at each stage of development for an infant at risk for brain dysfunction. Although it may appear very different from the diagnostic approach described here, early intervention is part of any follow-up clinic, and a discussion of its efficacy cannot be overlooked. However, as the data available at the present time are a mixture of objective studies and personal experience, it is not possible to reach a valid conclusion on the value of early intervention for a number of reasons that are summarized below.

The Definition of Early Intervention

Strictly speaking, early intervention suggests providing help to anybody who suffers a physical disease, and is distinct from prevention. However, when applied to the newborn at risk, early intervention is often used as a vaguely defined and very loose concept including medical prevention, psychological prevention, as well as therapy for possible sequelae of anticipated brain damage or dysfunction.

The Level of Action

There are two very different viewpoints as to how early intervention results in improvement in the child with perinatal damage. On one hand, the experimental data recently reviewed on brain plasticity (St. James-Roberts, 1979) suggest that interaction with the environment and motor and sensory stimulation would facilitate the mechanisms involved in brain plasticity to intervene optimally. On the other hand, physical therapy does not act on the brain lesions or cell connections, but affects motor function in many different ways (e.g., maintaining the muscles, the joints, and the bones in good functional status, reducing the effects of transient or permanent tone imbalance, and teaching the young child to use all that is physically available to him or her in the most efficient way). In the first hypothesis, it is suggested that the more immature the fetal brain is at time of insult, the more plasticity (i.e., the greater the opportunity for rebuilding). The second hypothesis does not suggest that there is regeneration, but instead that there are many ways to improve function.

The Absence of Lesional Criteria

The routine use of methods such as US and CT scan has improved the precision of correlations between lesions and outcome; however, this is true only with severe handicap and is not yet so in moderate and mild cases. Even when there is definite lesional evidence of severe damage, preconceived notions and ambiguities still occur. Each pediatrician remembers a few children with extensive destruction of cerebral parenchyma visible on CT scan who have a perfectly normal life and good adaptation to school. Conversely, the same pediatrician may remember newborns who behaved perfectly normally but who turned out to be very poorly adapted children in school for sociofamilial reasons. These puzzling contradictions were questioned by Dr. Fagan in discussing the presentation of an experimental work (Goldman-Rakic, 1980): "It seems to me that having part of your brain taken out is an extreme form of deprivation as opposed to your mother not being so nice to you" (p. 62).

The absence of objective lesional criteria makes it very difficult to effectively measure progress in obstetrical and perinatal prevention. There is again no sharp distinction between the preventive and therapeutic approaches. The epidemiological work of Hagberg et al. (1982) shows that even though a small increase in the number of VLBW infants with CP was observed, there was a relative decrease of severe global handicap, compared to the number of infants with moderate and mild CP and good IQ. Before evaluating the therapeutic approach and judging the value of early intervention, it is first necessary to become more precise in classification of the various types of perinatal brain damage.

Normalization of Function

Normalization of function is frequently related to maturation rather than to plasticity. The transient motor abnormalities in the first year of life are a typical example of normalization. Researchers have learned to recognize certain neurological anomalies and have discovered that the physiognomy of these anomalies differs during the various developmental stages. Some infants may experience transient anomalies, and by the end of the first year it is no longer possible to distinguish such infants from those who have remained normal since birth. However, experience has shown such normalization to be deceptive in that it is attributable only to a certain developmental threshold. Cell damage of perinatal origin is very likely present in both white and gray matter. Given the kind of functioning that cannot, as yet, be explored, white matter deficit can be detected more rapidly than that of gray matter. Therefore, the damage will be manifest again in the following years, typically in the form of behavioral difficulties, fine motor anomalies, or subnormal IQ.

Physical therapy during the first year of life may be useful for the child. It certainly helps the parents by giving them an active role. However, it is likely that motor normalization would have occurred anyway as maturation progressed. Many such cases were observed before physical therapy was commonly used so early. Moreover, using physical therapy before identifying the transient and permanent motor abnormalities may prevent additional articular damage and may result in better function in handicapped infants. These children will have CP anyway, but their motor function can be better preserved (A. Grenier, personal communication, 1983).

Personal Conclusion

At this time, the author completely accepts the opinion expressed by Isabelle Rapin in the preface of her book on children with brain dysfunction:

> Plasticity, the capacity for reorganization after an injury, was assumed until fairly recently to be so great in the immature brain that full behavior recovery was thought to be the rule in young children unless the damage was extensive. We have come to appreciate that plasticity is limited, and that recovery without discernible deficit is in fact uncommon (Rapin, 1982, p. 1).

The author does not consider this statement to be negative or pessimistic; Rapin proposes that brain plasticity has probably been overrated without sufficient evidence, and that perinatal brain damage covers the full spectrum of handicaps.

Limited brain plasticity is not contradictory to the belief that follow-up clinics must include every possible attempt at early intervention in motor function, language, fine motor skills, and finally school adaptation. Any attempt to help the parents to accept their infant and to reinforce interaction is also early intervention, as advocated by Brazelton (1982). The efficacy of much of the therapy is difficult to assess, but intuitively seems good. If the only effect were to decrease the rate of child abuse among children with CP as proposed by Bax (1983), this would indeed be worthwhile.

GENERAL CONCLUSIONS

Follow-up studies are necessary to improve the basic knowledge of perinatal brain damage, to help parents in the difficult recovery period, and to help the child him- or herself to develop his or her abilities optimally. Follow-up studies will also collect data that will give indispensable feedback to the obstetrician. Modern obstetrics has entered a phase of active prevention, resulting in decisions of early delivery of the fetus at risk. The entire spectrum of expected outcome is affected by the obstetricians' decisions. As survival is improving, obstetricians need current data not only on mortality but on all kinds of morbidity in the survivors, mild and moderate handicap as well as severe. The necessity of taking into account "functional ability or the broader spectrum of lesser morbidity seen among VLBW survivors" has been recently stressed by Hack, Rivers, and Fanaroff (in press). This includes the chronic sequelae of immaturity, the need for repeated hospitalizations, the short- and long-term effects on physical growth, and the impact and significance of transient visual, auditory, and neurological abnormalities. A better communication between specialists involved in these surveys will certainly benefit these children at risk.

REFERENCES

Allen, D.A., & Rapin, I. Language disorders in preschool children: Predictors of outcome—a preliminary report. *Brain Development*, 1980, *2*, 73–80.

Amiel, C. Hémorragies cérébrales intra-ventriculaires chez le prématuré: les éléments du diagnostic clinique [Intraventricular hemorrhages in the premature infant: Clinical diagnosis]. *Biologia Neonatorum*, 1964, *7*, 57–75.

Amiel-Tison, C. Neurologic evaluation of the small neonate: The importance of head straightening reactions. In: L. Gluck (ed.), *Modern perinatal medicine*. Chicago: Year Book Medical Publishers, 1974.

Amiel-Tison, C. Birth injury in full-term newborns. In: R. Korobkin & C. Guilleminault (eds.), *Advances in peri-*natal neurology, Vol. 1. New York: Spectrum Publications, 1979.

Amiel-Tison, C., Dubé, R., Garel, M., & Jequier, J. C. Outcome at age 5 of fullterm infants with transient neurologic abnormalities in the first year of life. In: L. Stern, H. Bard, & B. Friis-Hansen (eds.), *Intensive care in the newborn*, IV. New York: Masson Publishing USA, Inc., 1983.

Amiel-Tison, C., & Grenier, A. Neurological evaluation of the newborn and the infant. New York: Masson Publishing USA, Inc., 1983.

Bax, M. Abuse and cerebral palsy. *Developmental Medicine and Child Neurology*, 1983, *25*, 141–142.

Brazelton, T.B. Neonatal Behavioral Assessment Scale.

Clinics in Developmental Medicine, No. 50. London: Spastics International Medical Publications with William Heinemann; and Philadelphia: J.B. Lippincott, 1973.

Brazelton, T.B. Behavioral competence of the newborn infant. *Seminars in Perinatology*, 1979, *3*, 35–44.

Brazelton, T.B. Early intervention, what does it mean? In: H. Fitzgerald, B. Lester, & M. Yogman (eds.), *Therapy and research in behavioral pediatrics*, Vol. 1. New York: Plenum Publishing Corp., 1982.

Chaplin, E.R., Goldstein, G.W., Myeberg, D.Z., Hunt, J.V., & Tooley, W.H. Post hemorrhagic hydrocephalus in the preterm infant. *Pediatrics*, 1980, *65*, 901–909.

Drillien, C.M. Abnormal neurologic signs in the first year of life in low birth weight infants. Possible prognostic significance. *Developmental Medicine and Child Neurology*, 1972, *14*, 575–584.

Drillien, C.M., Thomson, A.J.M., & Burgoyne, K. Low birth weight children at early school age: A longitudinal study. *Developmental Medicine and Child Neurology*, 1980, *22*, 26–47.

Dubowitz, L.M.S., Levene, M.I., Morante, A., Palmer, P., & Dubowitz, V. Neurologic signs in neonatal intraventricular hemorrhage: A correlation with real-time ultrasound. *The Journal of Pediatrics*, 1981, *99*, 127–133.

Ellison, P.H. Neonatal follow-up studies: The predictive value of neurologic abnormalities in the first year of life. In: L. Stern, H. Bard, & B. Friis-Hansen (eds.), *Intensive care in the newborn IV*. New York: Masson Publishing USA, Inc., 1983.

Fitzhardinge, P.M. Current outcome of NICU population. In: A.W. Brann & J.J. Volpe (eds.), *Neonatal neurological assessment and outcome*. Ross Conference on Pediatric Research. Columbus, OH: Ross Laboratories, 1980.

Gilberg, C., & Rasmussen, P. Perceptual, motor and attentional deficits in 7 year old children: Background factors. *Developmental Medicine and Child Neurology*, 1982, *24*, 752–770.

Goldman-Rakic, P.S. Plasticity of the primate telencephalon. In: A.W. Brann & J.J. Volpe (eds.), *Neonatal neurological assessment and outcome*. The report of the Seventy-Seventh Ross Conference on Pediatric Research. Columbus, OH: Ross Laboratories, 1980.

Grenier, A. Diagnostic précoce de l'infirmité motrice cérébrale . . . pourquoi faire? [Why an early diagnosis of cerebral palsy?] *Annales de Pédiatrie* [*Annals of Pediatrics*], 1982, *29*, 509–514.

Gross, S.J., Oehler, J.M., & Eckerman, C.O. Head growth and developmental outcome in VLBW infants. *Pediatrics*, 1983, *71*, 70–75.

Hack, M., Rivers, A., & Fanaroff, A.A. The very low birth weight infant: The broader spectrum of morbidity during infancy and early childhood. *Journal of Developmental Behavioral Pediatrics*, in press.

Hagberg, B., Hagberg, G. & Olow, I. Gains and hazards of intensive neonatal care: An analysis from Swedish cerebral palsy epidemiology. *Developmental Medicine and Child Neurology*, 1982, *24*, 13–19.

Hill, A., & Volpe, J.J. Normal pressure hydrocephalus in the newborn. *Pediatrics*, 1981, *68*, 623–629.

Hunt, J.V. Longitudinal research: A method for studying the intellectual development of high risk preterm infants. In: T.M. Field, A.M. Sostek, S. Goldberg, & H.H. Shuman (eds.), *Infants born at risk: Behavior and development*. London: SP Medical and Scientific Books, 1979.

Hunt, J.V., Tooley, W.H., & Harvin, D. Learning disabilities in children with birth weights ≤1,500 g. *Seminars in Perinatology*, 1982, *6*, 280–287.

Larroche, J.C. Hémorragies cérébrales chez le prématuré: Anatomie et physiopathologie [Intraventricular hemorrhages in the premature infant: Anatomy and physiopathology]. *Biologia Neonatorum*, 1964, *7*, 26–56.

Levene, M.I., & Starte, D.R. A longitudinal study of post hemorrhagic ventricular dilatation in the newborn. *Archives of Disease in Childhood*, 1981, *56*, 905–910.

Liechty, E.A., Gilmor, R.L., Bryson, C.Q., & Bull, M.J. Outcome of high risk neonates with ventriculomegaly. *Developmental Medicine and Child Neurology*, 1983, *25*, 162–168.

Lipscomb, A.P., Thorburn, R.J., Stewart, A.L., Reynolds, E.O.R., & Hope, P.L. Early treatment for rapidly progressive post-haemorrhage hydrocephalus. *Lancet*, 1983, *ii*, 1438–1439.

Lowe, M., & Costello, A. *The Symbolic Play Test (experimental edition)*. Windsor, England: NFER Publishing Co., 1976.

Nelson, K.B., & Ellenberg, J.H. Children who "outgrew" cerebral palsy. *Pediatrics*, 1982, *69*, 529–536.

Pape, K.E., Bennet-Britton, S., Szymonowicz, W., Martin, D.J., Fitz, C.R., & Becker, L. Diagnostic accuracy of neonatal brain imaging: A postmortem correlation of computed tomography and ultrasound scans. *The Journal of Pediatrics*, 1983, *102*, 275–280.

Pape, K.E., Blackwell, R.J., Cusik, G., Sherwood, A., Houang, M.T.W., Thorburn, R.J., & Reynolds, E.O.R. Ultrasound detection of brain damage in preterm infants. *Lancet*, 1979, *i*, 1261–1264.

Papile, L., Burstein, R., & Koffler, H. Incidence and evolution of subependymal and intraventricular hemorrhage: A study of infants with birth weight less than 1,500 g. *The Journal of Pediatrics*, 1978, *92*, 529–534.

Partridge, J.C., Babcock, D.S., Steichen, J.J., & Han, B.K. Optimal timing for diagnostic cranial ultrasound in low-birth-weight infants: Detection of intracranial hemorrhage and ventricular dilatation. *The Journal of Pediatrics*, 1983, *102*, 281–287.

Rapin, I. *Children with brain dysfunction*. New York: Raven Press, 1982.

Rapin, I., & Allen, D.A. Developmental language disorders: Nosologic considerations. In: U. Kirk (ed.), *Neuropsychology of language, reading and spelling*. New York: Academic Press, 1983.

Reynell, J. *Manual for the Reynell Developmental Language Scales (revised edition)*. Windsor, England: NFER Publishing Co., 1977.

Rutter, M. Syndromes attributed to "Minimal Brain Dysfunction" in childhood. *American Journal of Psychiatry*, 1982, *139*, 21–33.

Saint-Anne Dargassies, S. *Neurological development in full-term and premature neonates*. Amsterdam: Excerpta Medica, and New York: Elsevier North-Holland, 1977.

St. James-Roberts, I. Neurological plasticity, recovery from brain insult, and child development. In: H.W. Reese & L.P. Lipsitt (eds.), *Advances in child development and behavior*, Vol. 14. New York: Academic Press, 1979.

Stewart, A.L., Thorburn, R.J., Hope, P.L., Castello, A., Goldsmith, M., Swain P., & Reynolds, E.O.R. Prediction of neuro developmental status at 18 months of age by ultrasound and neurological examination. *Pediatric Research*, 1983.

Stewart, A.L., Thorburn, R.J., Lipscomb, A.P., & Amiel-Tison, C. Neonatal neurological examinations of very preterm infants: Comparison of results with ultra-

sound diagnosis of peri-ventricular hemorrhage. *American Journal of Perinatology*, 1983, *1*, 6–11.

Wolff, P.H., Gunnoe, L.E., & Cohen, C. Associated movements as a measure of developmental age. *Developmental Medicine and Child Neurology*, 1983, *25*, 417–429.

Chapter 27

The Outcome of Neurological
Abnormality in Infancy

PATRICIA ELLISON, M.D.
University of Denver, Denver, Colorado
DAVID PRASSE, Ph.D.
JULAINE SIEWERT, M.A.
University of Wisconsin-Milwaukee, Milwaukee, Wisconsin
CAROL BROWNING, M.D.
Mt. Sinai Medical Center, Milwaukee, Wisconsin

I MPROVEMENT IN NEUROLOGICAL FUNCTION as assessed by the neurological examination has been described in many infants initially treated in the neonatal intensive care unit (NICU) and followed serially after discharge (Ellison, Browning, Larson, & Denny, 1983; Ellison, Browning, & Trostmiller, 1982). Of infants described as abnormal, those with hypotonia were most likely to improve. Hypotonic infants without associated delays in adaptive and personal social skills showed greater improvement than those with global delay. Some infants with a label of cerebral palsy at age 1 year, including those with spasticities (tetrapareses, diplegias, and hemipareses), have reportedly "outgrown" these motor abnormalities by age 7 years (Nelson & Ellenberg, 1982). However, increased percentages of mental retardation, hyperactivity, and emotional immaturity were found not only in infants diagnosed with cerebral palsy at 1 year and outgrowing it, but in infants "suspected" of having cerebral palsy at 1 year and without

cerebral palsy at age 7 (Nelson & Ellenberg, 1982).

The authors hypothesized that the neurological examination in infancy would serve as a "marker" for later abnormalities, specifically lesser cognitive function, motor dysfunction, hyperactivity, emotional immaturity, and learning disabilities. One hundred sixty-four children initially treated in the NICU for 5 days or more in 1975–1976 were assessed at 6 months, 15 months, 4 years, and 6–7 years. Assessment measures at 6–7 years included the McCarthy Scales of Children's Abilities, Wide Range Achievement Tests (WRAT) of Reading, Spelling, and Mathematics, neurological examination, quantified measures of fine motor skills, and three measures of behavior: the Home Situations Questionnaire, the Conners Parent Questionnaire, and the Achenbach Child Behavior Checklist.

Significant correlations ($p < .05$) were found between neurological assessment in infancy and the General Cognitive Index and

The authors thank the Uhrig Foundation of Wisconsin for their financial support; Dr. John Horn, Department of Psychology, University of Denver, for assistance in data analyses; Ralph Mason for his computer skills; the University of Denver for computer use; and the neonatologists who cared for the children in the neonatal intensive care units.

Motor Subtest scores from the McCarthy Scale at both 4 and 7 years. Although correlations between the infancy neurological assessment and the WRAT were significant only for spelling, additional evidence from the Conners Learning Problem subtest showed that learning problems were excessive for these children. The authors concluded that these learning problems were related to neurological abnormality in infancy. The largest correlations were noted between the infancy neurological assessment and fine motor skills at 4 and 7 years (finger tapping, grooved pegboard, maze, and finger localization). Behavior abnormalities correlated significantly with infancy neurological assessment for the Conners Learning Problem ($p < .001$), the Achenbach Boys' Hyperactivity Scale ($p < .01$), and the Achenbach Girls' Somatic Complaints ($p < .01$). Twenty percent of the transiently abnormal infants and 17% of the abnormal children had been assigned to a special class by age 6–7 years.

METHODS

In a comprehensive follow-up study of children initially treated in the NICU, data analyses were directed to the specific question of the relationship of neurological abnormality/ normality in infancy to problems in preschool and early school years. All infants treated for 5 days or more in the NICUs affiliated with the Medical College of Wisconsin in 1975–1976 were entered in the study. Since these were the only Level III NICUs in southeastern Wisconsin, the infants were considered to be representative of neonatal illness and sequelae associated with these illnesses. A large number of variables were recorded and stored in the perinatal data system (Bahr & Grausz, 1980) for the pregnancy, delivery, and neonatal course.

At 6 and 15 months corrected gestational age, infants were assessed developmentally and neurologically. A nurse practitioner obtained anthropometric measures and administered the Denver Developmental Screening Test; a social worker obtained further medical and social history; a physical therapist assessed

neurological status with a quantified scoring system for the Milani-Comparetti and Gidoni method. Additional assessments were scheduled at the discretion of the physical therapist. At age 4 years, the McCarthy Scales of Children's Abilities were administered; anthropometric measures were taken, hearing and vision were screened, interim medical and social history were gathered, and one-half of the children underwent a neurological examination by a pediatric neurologist. Quantified assessments were also made of finger tapping, foot tapping, maze, grooved pegboard, and finger localization skills. At 6–7 years, the McCarthy Scales, a neurological examination including quantified measures, and anthropometric measures were repeated. In addition, the Kaufman Assessment Battery, Token Test, Wide Range Achievement Test, Visual-Motor Integration Test, Home Situations Questionnaire, Achenbach Child Behavior Checklist, and Conners Parent Questionnaire were administered.

The development of the scoring system for the Milani-Comparetti and Gidoni (MCG) assessment has been described previously (Ellison et al., 1983). The MCG assessments were administered by the same two physical therapists throughout. Both were experienced in examining infants and both were concerned about interrater reliability. Each MCG was scored separately with 1 to 5 points (1—severely abnormal; 5—normal).

For purposes of data analysis, the MCG scores for each assessment were summed to yield a total score for each infant at each visit. The infants were then subdivided into three groups on the basis of the scores: abnormal, transiently abnormal, and normal. Although the concept of transient abnormality of infancy has recurred in a series of studies (Amiel-Tison, 1976; Amiel-Tison & Grenier, 1983; Drillien, 1972; Knobloch & Pasamanick, 1967), no agreement has been reached on the types of abnormalities or the ages of abnormalities. Some have reported mild abnormalities appearing early in infancy, as from the neonatal period through 3–6 months; other have reported later mild abnormalities that resolved by 15 or 18 months. In this study, cutoff points were decided upon after careful review of the progression of scores on serial examination and from the scores of infants referred for physical and occupational therapy. For the 6-month evaluation, a total score of 81 or more was defined as normal, 70–80 as transiently abnormal, and 69 or less as abnormal. For the 15–16 month evaluation, scores of 126 or more were defined as normal, 115–125 as transiently abnormal, and 114 or less as abnormal. The category of abnormality was based on the lowest score in the series of assessments. The subdivisions of abnormal, transiently abnormal, and normal were used for cross-tabulation analyses and for mean scores for each test and subtest.

Abnormal infants were further divided into four types: spastic tetraparesis/dyskinesia, spastic hemiparesis, spastic diplegia, and hypotonia. Spastic tetraparesis/dyskinesia was defined as a four-limbed involvement that was more than hypotonia; spastic hemiparesis was defined as spasticity of one side, arm generally greater than leg; and spastic diplegia as bilateral leg spasticity, often with some associated neurological abnormality of arms of lesser degree. Assignment to these types was straightforward with the information available. These six categories—spastic tetraparesis/dyskinesia, spastic hemiparesis, spastic diplegia, hypotonia, transient abnormality, and normal—were transitive and were used for the product moment correlations.

For measures of strength of association between variables and levels of statistical significance, product moment correlation r and p values were reported. Many of the cell numbers in the cross-tabulation tables were too small for statistical tests. While categories could have been collapsed, the authors considered that important divisions would be lost. For example, schools tend to place children with scores 2 or more S.D. below the mean on any of a variety of intelligence tests in classes for mentally retarded students, whereas children with scores 1 to 2 S.D. below the mean are often placed in learning disabilities classes. Thus both forms of data analyses are reported.

Finally, the types of problems at 6–7 years were summed for children who were neuro-

logically abnormal, transiently abnormal, or normal in infancy. The types of problems were defined by subnormal scores greater than 1 standard deviation from the mean for cognitive function (General Cognitive Index of the McCarthy Scale), motor function (McCarthy Motor Subtest or two or more tests from the quantified fine motor battery), hyperactivity (Conners hyperactivity index or Achenbach hyperactivity scale), learning problems (Conners learning problem factor or one subtest of the WRAT), and other behavior (two or more subtests for the Conners or Achenbach scales).

RESULTS

The demographic characteristics of the children at age 6–7 years are shown in Table 1. Ninety percent of the children eligible for assessment at age 6 months were brought for evaluation, and 85% of those eligible at age 15 months were re-evaluated. Fifty percent of children eligible for evaluation at 4 years could be located and had families who agreed to re-evaluation. Eighty-three percent ($n = 164$) of these children were brought for re-evaluation at 6–7 years. Twelve children were classified abnormal, 35 transiently abnormal, and the remainder normal in infancy MCG scores in the 4-year sample; eight were abnormal, 28 transiently abnormal, and the remainder normal in the 6–7 year sample.

Table 1. Demographic data

Sex	
Girls	38.7%
Boys	61.3%
Race	
White	88.4%
Black	11.6%
Gestional age	
≤ 28 weeks	8.9%
29–31	17.3%
32–35	42.4%
36–40	29.5%
≥ 41	1.9%
Birth weight	
≤ 750 grams	0
751–100	8.4%
1001–1250	6.5%
1251–1500	13.5%
1501–2000	23.9%
2001–2500	21.3%
2501–3500	19.4%
3501–5000	7.1

Table 2. General Cognitive Index and Motor Subtests (McCarthy) for children with normal, transiently abnormal, and abnormal infancy MCG scores

	MCG infancy score		
	Abnormal	Transiently abnormal	Normal
All 4-year children			
General Cognitive Index			
Retarded (>2 S.D.)[a]	41.7%(5)	5.7%(2)	2.9%(6)
Dull normal (1–2 S.D.)	8.3%(1)	11.4%(4)	5.9%(12)
Normal	50.0%(6)	82.8%(29)	91.0%(90)
Motor Index			
(>2 S.D.)	50.0%(6)	17.1%(6)	4.0%(8)
(1–2 S.D.)	16.7%(2)	40.0%(14)	24.5%(38)
Normal	33.3%(4)	42.9%(15)	70.3%(62)
4-year children seen at 6–7 years			
General Cognitive Index			
Retarded (>2 S.D.)	25.0%(2)	7.1%(2)	4.6%(5)
Dull normal (1–2 S.D.)	0.0%(0)	3.6%(1)	6.5%(7)
Normal	75.0%(6)	89.2%(2)	88.9%(7)
Motor Index			
(>2 S.D.)	25.0%(2)	14.2%(4)	4.6%(5)
(1–2 S.D.)	25.0%(2)	42.9%(12)	27.8%(30)
Normal	50.0%(4)	42.9%(12)	67.6%(73)
6–7 year children			
General Cognitive Index			
Retarded (>2 S.D.)	25.0%(2)	7.1%(2)	5.5%(6)
Dull normal (1–2 S.D.)	25.0%(2)	10.7%(3)	16.7%(18)
Normal	50.0%(4)	80.0%(23)	77.8%(84)
Motor Index			
(>2 S.D.)	37.5%(3)	10.7%(3)	4.6%(5)
(<1 S.D.)	25.0%(2)	25.0%(7)	14.8%(16)
Normal	37.5%(3)	63.3%(18)	80.6%(87)

All S.D. are below the mean.

The percentages of children with normal, transiently abnormal, and abnormal infancy MCG scores for three ranges of cognitive function are shown in Table 2 for the general cognitive and motor scores for ages 4 and 6–7 years (McCarthy Scales). The 4-year sample is shown in two groups: 1) all children evaluated at age 4 years, and 2) only those 4-year-olds who were also evaluated at age 6–7 years. Comparison of scores of the second group at 4 and 6–7 years showed that some children had dropped from normal to dull normal cognitive function in all neurological categories (two in the abnormal group, two in the transiently abnormal, and 12 in the normal group). In the motor scores, improvement occurred in the transiently abnormal and normal groups (6 and 14, respectively). Infancy MCG scores and cognitive function and motor subtests were significantly correlated ($p < .05$) for 4 and 6–7 years (Table 3).

The percentages of children with normal, transiently abnormal, and abnormal infancy

MCG scores for normal and more than 1 S.D. below the mean Wide Range Achievement Test scores and the product moment correlations for each group are shown in Table 4. The percentages of boys and girls with normal, transiently abnormal, and abnormal infancy MCG scores and Conners Learning Problem scores are shown in Table 5. Both abnormal and transiently abnormal boys were described by their parents as having learning problems.

Table 3. Product moment correlations for infancy MCG scores and McCarthy subtests ages 4 and 6–7 years

	r value	p value
All 4-year children		
General Cognitive Index	.31	.001
Memory	.25	.001
Motor	.38	.001
4-year children seen at 6–7 years		
General Cognitive Index	.14	.050
Memory	.08	.147
Motor	.20	.008
6–7-year children		
General Cognitive Index	.19	.025
Memory	.12	.145
Motor	.30	.001

Table 4. Percentages of frequencies and product moment correlations of WRAT scores for children with abnormal, transiently abnormal, and normal infancy MCG scores

	MCG infancy score		
	Abnormal	Transiently abnormal	Normal
WRAT reading			
>1 S.D. below mean	25.0%(2)	14.3%(4)	9.4%(10)
Normal	75.0%(6)	85.7%(24)	90.6%(98)
Product moment correlation: $r = .10, p = NS$[a]			
WRAT spelling			
>1 S.D. below mean	12.5%(1)	10.7%(3)	10.3%(11)
Normal	87.5%(7)	89.3%(25)	89.6%(97)
Product moment correlation: $r = .18, p = .04$			
WRAT mathematics			
>1 S.D. below mean	25.0%(2)	10.7%(3)	7.7%(8)
Normal	75.0%(6)	89.3%(25)	92.5%(100)
Product moment correlation: $r = .14, p = NS$			

[a]NS = not significant.

Product moment correlations between the Conners Learning Problem scores and the Wide Range Achievement subtest scores are shown in Table 6. Parental perception of a learning problem correlated significantly for subtests, with the math subtest having the highest correlation, followed by the spelling subtest and then the reading subtest.

Special class assignment and MCG subgroups are shown in Table 7. Both the abnormal and transiently abnormal groups have larger percentages of children in special classes than the normal group.

No significant differences were shown among the MCG subgroups and the Home Situations Questionnaire or Conners subtests, with the exception of the Learning Problem subtest. For the Achenbach subtests, only somatic complaints (girls) and hyperactivity (boys) correlated significantly ($p < .01$) with infancy MCG scores. The hyperactivity subtest is shown for percentages of infancy MCG categories in Table 8. Both transiently abnormal and abnormal boys had excessive percentages 1 or more S.D. above the mean.

The product moment correlations between infancy MCG scores and the quantified fine motor items at 6–7 years are shown in Table 9. All were significantly correlated with the exception of finger tapping left.

The numbers of problems within the five defined types (cognitive function, motor function, hyperactivity, learning problems, and other behavior problems) for children who had

Table 5. Conners Learning Problem subtest scores for three ranges of infancy MCG scores

	MCG infancy score		
		Transiently	
Conners Learing Problems score	Abnormal	abnormal	Normal
	Boys		
>1 S.D.[a]	50.0%(3)	13.6%(3)	9.1%(5)
1–2 S.D.	0.0%(0)	45.5%(10)	10.9%(6)
Normal	50.0%(3)	40.9%(9)	80.0%(44)
Product moment correlation: $r = .37, p = .001$			
	Girls		
>2 S.D.	0.0%(0)	0.0%(0)	7.1%(2)
1–2 S.D.	0.0%(0)	0.0%(0)	11.9%(6)
Normal	100.0%(2)	100.0%(6)	81.0%(34)
Product moment correlation: $r = .18, p = NS$[b]			

[a]All S.D. are above the mean.
[b]NS = Not significant.

Table 6. Product moment correlations between Conners Learning Problem scores and WRAT subtests

| | Conners Learning Problem | |
	r value	p value
WRAT		
Reading	.18	.03
Spelling	.29	.001
Mathematics	.38	.001

abnormal, transiently abnormal, and normal scores in infancy are shown in Table 10. The percentages of children with two or more problems were increased for the abnormal and transiently abnormal groups.

DISCUSSION

The authors have previously reviewed studies of the neurological examination in infancy and concluded that neurologically abnormal infants can be distinguished from neurologically normal infants, that many infants had transient or mild neurological abnormalities that resolved, and that even some abnormal infants outgrow the types of neurological abnormality in infancy associated with cerebral palsy (Ellison, 1983; Ellison, 1984; Ellison et al., 1982). That experienced clinicians can detect neurological abnormality is supported by evidence that few infants returned with "undiscovered" neurological abnormality unless there had been an intervening event such as a head injury or meningitis. If such a large amount of the neurological abnormalities resolve, are there any other implications for these abnormalities?

At both 4 and 6–7 years, the children who were neurologically abnormal in infancy had the largest percentages more than 1 S.D. below the mean for the General Cognitive Index. This close association of mental and motor (or neurological) abnormality conforms with previous reports (Cruickshank, Hallahan, & Bice, 1976; Hansen, 1960; Hohman & Freedheim, 1958). In earlier work, the authors had reported sig-

nificant differences ($p < .05$) in the Memory subtest of the McCarthy Scale for transiently abnormal and neurologically normal infants at the 4-year evaluation (Prasse, Ellison, & Siewert, 1983). However, when only those children who were evaluated at both 4 and 6–7 years were considered, no significant differences were seen between transiently abnormal and normal groups. Both groups also had a number of children who dropped from the normal range at 4 years to the dull normal range at 6–7 years.

Achievement scores were then examined. The percentages of the abnormal children with scores greater than 1 S.D. below the mean were excessive for reading and mathematics, but not for spelling; transiently abnormal children had increased percentages greater than 1 S.D. below the mean only for reading achievement (see Table 4). The mean scores for each of the three groups were normal for all three achievement tests. The major reading achievement skill tested at ages 6–7 was word recognition. Children with later difficulties in comprehension, a more complex and abstract skill, might not be accurately identified at this age. How, then, could early learning problems be determined?

In a larger telephone survey of abnormal ($n = 52$) and transiently abnormal ($n = 123$) children from this population, parents reported that 77% and 20% had already had speech and language therapy, 79% and 13% had been in exceptional education, and 21% and 17% were considered hyperactive by the parent by age 5–6 years (Ellison, 1983). In this study, parental report was assessed with the Conners Parent Questionnaire, which rates four areas: 1) difficulty in learning, 2) failure to finish things, 3) distractibility or attention span, and 4) frustration in efforts. Significant correlation ($r = .27$, $p < .01$) was found between the Conners Learning Problem subtest and infancy MCG scores. In addition, higher percentages

Table 7. Special class placement for children with three ranges of infancy MCG scores

| | MCG infancy score | | |
Special class placement	Abnormal	Transiently abnormal	Normal
Yes	16.7%(1)	20.0%(6)	7.7%(8)
No	83.3%(7)	80.0%(22)	92.5%(100)

Table 8. Boys' scores from the Achenbach Hyperactivity Scale for three ranges of infancy MCG scores

Achenbach hyperactivity	MCG infancy score		
	Abnormal	Transiently abnormal	Normal
>2 S.D. above mean	33.3%(2)	9.1%(2)	9.1%(5)
1–2 S.D. above mean	50.0%(3)	49.9%(9)	25.0%(14)
Normal	16.7%(11)	50.0%(11)	67.9%(37)
Product moment correlation:	$r = .28, p = .01$		

of the abnormal and transiently abnormal groups had scores more than 1 S.D. above the mean for the Learning Problem subtest (see Table 5). The product moment correlations between the WRAT and Conners Learning Problem were then reviewed and found to be statistically significant (see Table 6). The authors concluded that the parents were probably accurate in their perception of a learning problem and that these learning problems were centered in children who were neurologically abnormal and transiently abnormal as infants. This was further confirmed by the excessive percentages of these two groups in special classes in school (Table 7).

The assignment to a special class could be made for any of several reasons or for a combination of reasons. In particular, combinations of aberrant behavior and learning problems might predispose a child to selection for a special class. Product moment correlations for the subtests of the Achenbach Child Behavior Checklist and infancy MCG scores indicated significance for somatic complaints for girls (a negative correlation) and hyperactivity for boys ($p < .01$). Percentages of boys with scores for hyperactivity greater than 1 S.D. above the mean were excessive (Table 8). The authors concluded that boys with abnormal and

Table 9. Product moment correlations between MCG infancy scores and fine motor performances at 6–7 years

Fine Motor Tests		r value	p value
Finger tapping	—right	.19	.02
	—left	.02	NS[a]
Maze errors	—right	.24	.003
	—left	.18	.03
Maze time	—right	.47	.001
	—left	.44	.001
Grooved pegboard	—right	.31	.001
	—left	.60	.001
Finger localization	—right	.28	.001
	—left	.22	.008

[a]NS = Not significant.

transiently abnormal neurological examinations were at high risk for hyperactivity.

Of the various sequelae, an excess in motor problems would seem most likely in children with an abnormal neurological examination in infancy. This was confirmed by the Motor Subtest of the McCarthy (see Table 2) as well as by the quantified neurological testing (Table 9). All the 6–7-year quantified items except finger tapping (left) were significantly correlated with infancy MCG items. The maze errors, maze time, grooved pegs, and finger localization performances had the largest correlations and may be most useful in pinpointing abnormal motor function at 6–7 years. Others have used maze tests as indicators not only of abnormal motor function but theoretically as measures of frontal lobe function (Horn, 1972). Abnormal function at 6–7 years that could be classified as cerebral palsy was minimal. The abnormality was better described as clumsy movements or prolonged time required to complete fine motor tasks. While these abnormalities should not interfere with many activities of daily life, they may interfere in the school setting in handwriting, art work, physical education, and in participation in many playground activities.

Children who were neurologically abnormal or transiently abnormal in infancy tended to have multiple problems in the early school years. While many definitions of abnormality are based on scores 2 S.D. from the mean, as for mental retardation, the authors have used 1 S.D. in this study in order to define children with school problems. Specifically, few were retarded, but many were having difficulty with school because of dull normal function; few had cerebral palsy, but many had sufficient motor abnormality to complicate their lives. Furthermore, problems tended to cluster such that special classes and remedial services were required (Tables 7 and 10).

Table 10. Number of problems at 6–7 years and abnormal and transiently abnormal MCG scores in infancy

MCG score in infancy		0	1	2	3	4	5
Abnormal	n	2	2	0	1	2	1
	%	25.0	25.0	0.0	12.5	25.0	12.5
Transiently abnormal	n	6	7	3	9	2	1
	%	21.4	25.0	10.7	32.0	7.0	3.6
Normal	n	41	33	21	7	5	1
	%	38.0	30.6	19.4	6.5	4.6	0.0

Cursory examination of children initially treated in the NICU, such as mean scores on testing of intellectual function, might lead to a conclusion that infants with abnormal or transiently abnormal neurological examinations had little residual sequelae in the early school years. More careful examination would suggest that both abnormal and transiently abnormal children are at risk in the school years: for placement in a special class, for hyperactivity in boys, for learning problems, and for motor problems. In previous work, the authors have discussed the conditions in the neonatal unit that preceded motor dysfunction of infancy (Ellison, Horn, & Browning, 1983; Knoboch, Malone, Ellison, Stevens, & Zdeb, 1982). They conclude here that infants with abnormal or transiently abnormal neurological exams deserve special attention in follow-up through the preschool years for identification of specific lags and referral for remedial services.

REFERENCES

Amiel-Tison, C. A method for neurologic evaluation within the first year of life. *Current Problems in Pediatrics,* 1976, *7,* 1–50.

Amiel-Tison, C., & Grenier, A. *Neurologic evaluation of the newborn and the infant.* New York: Masson Publishing USA, Inc., 1983.

Bahr, J., & Grausz, J. The Milwaukee perinatal data system. In: J. Bahr (ed.), *Proceedings: First national conference on perinatal data systems.* Milwaukee: Wisconsin Association for Perinatal Care, 1980.

Cruickshank, W.M., Hallahan, D.P., & Bice, H.V. Evaluation of intelligence. In: W.M. Cruickshank (ed.), *Cerebral palsy: A developmental disability.* Syracuse, NY: Syracuse University Press, 1976.

Drillien, C.M. Abnormal neurologic signs in the first year of life in low birthweight infants: Possible prognostic significance. *Developmental Medicine and Child Neurology,* 1972, *14,* 575–584.

Ellison, P. Neonatal follow-up studies: The predictive value of neurologic abnormalities in the first year of life. In: A.J. Moss (ed.), *Pediatrics update.* New York: Elsevier Biomedical, 1984.

Ellison, P. Neurological development of the high-risk infant. *Clinics in Perinatology,* 1984, *1,* 41–58.

Ellison, P., Browning, C., Larson, B., & Denny, J. A scoring system for the Milani-Comparetti and Gidoni method of neurologic assessment in infancy. *Physical Therapy,* 1983, *63,* 1414–1423.

Ellison, P., Browning, C., & Trostmiller, T. Evaluation of neurologic status in infancy: Physical therapist versus pediatric neurologist. *Journal of the California Perinatal Association,* 1982, *2,* 63–66.

Ellison, P., Horn, J., & Browning, C. A large sample, many variable study of motor dysfunction of infancy. *Journal of Pediatric Psychology,* 1983, *8,* 345–357.

Hansen, E. Cerebral palsy in Denmark. *Acta Psychiatrica Scandinavia, 35, Neurological Supplement,* 1960, *146,* 1–148.

Hohman, L.B., & Freedheim, D.K. Further studies on intelligence levels in cerebral palsy in children. *American Journal of Physical Medicine,* 1958, *37,* 90–97.

Horn, J. L. The Porteus Maze test. In: O. K. Buros (ed.), *The seventh mental measurements yearbook.* Highland Park, NY: Grypon, 1972.

Knobloch, H., Malone, A., Ellison, P., Stevens, F., & Zdeb, M. Evaluating changes in outcome for infants under 1501 gms. *Pediatrics,* 1982, *69,* 285–295.

Knobloch, H., & Pasamanick, B. Prediction from the assessment of neuromotor and intellectual status in infancy. In: J. Zubin & G. Jervis (eds.), *Psychopathology of mental development.* New York: Grune & Stratton, 1967.

Nelson, K., & Ellenberg, J. Children who "outgrew" cerebral palsy. *Pediatrics,* 1982, *69,* 529–536.

Prasse, D., Ellison, P., & Siewert, J. Neurologic integrity and the McCarthy Scale: Research based qualifiers and applications. *Journal of Psychoeducational Assessment,* 1983, *1,* 273–283.

Chapter 28

Changing Criteria in Neonatal Outcome Studies

CARLOS H. LOZANO, M.D., M.P.H.

Instituto Nacional de Perinatologia, SSA Mexico

SOME OF THE EARLY SKEPTICISM REGARDING efforts to decrease neonatal mortality by establishing regional neonatal intensive care centers has been mitigated by evidence that a large majority of at-risk infants surviving the perinatal period have developed normally. Although this information is reassuring, it has limited value in predicting the outcome of current-day survivors because medical care of high-risk infants has improved and the population of infants is different. Premature newborn infants who survived in the late sixty's and early seventy's were generally larger and more mature than the majority of newborn infants surviving neonatal intensive care today (Table 1). In addition to these factors, there are other reasons inherent in the assessment techniques used that need to be considered, both in the performance of the studies as well as in their interpretation.

BACKGROUND CONSIDERATIONS

It is important to illustrate the kind of information that has been obtained with conventional assessment techniques, and draw some conclusions in that respect.

Practice in this author's follow-up clinic has had its basis in two assessment techniques: one is to evaluate the infant's active and passive motor tone, in addition to seven basic reflexes (Amiel-Tison, 1976); the other one is to assess behavioral and cognitive function (Gesell, Harverson, Thompson, et al., 1940) in a modified version (Bernstein, 1976) adjusted for the Mexican population, covering an age range from 4 weeks to 7 years. A group of mechanically ventilated respiratory distress syndrome (RDS) survivors born between January, 1979, and January, 1980, and followed in the author's program with these two assessment techniques during their first 12 months of corrected postnatal age, showed a significant fluctuation in their muscle tone status from one period of assessment to another (Figure 1). Although there seems to be a definite predominance of hypertonia at the initial assessment, as expected, as the infant gets older, normal muscle tone tends to become the dominant factor for the group. In regard to the observed fluctuation, an analysis of the transition probability was used to discover what kind of shifting from a former finding to a current one had taken place. It was found that normal tone is a stable

The author acknowledges the help of Andres G. de Wit Green, M.D., M.P.H. (ISSSTE's Medical Head), and Leo Stern, M.D. (Professor of Pediatrics and Perinatal Medicine), for their support of this program, and for making it possible to present this paper in Jerusalem, Israel (May, 1983).

Table 1. Follow-up programs: results since 1965

| | | | Neuromotor | | Intellectual | |
| | Period births | Birth | | Severe | | Severe |
Groups	occurred	weights	Normal	damage	Normal	damage
Outerbridge, E.W., Ramsay, N., & Stern, L.	1965–1971	1,050–4,360 grams	84%	13%	—	—
Cukier, F., Amiel-Tison, C., & Minkowski, A.	1967–1970	2,500 grams	49%	15%	66%	9%
Cukier, F., Bethmann, O., Rolier, J.P., et al.	1973–1974	2,500 grams	60%	6%	76%	4%
Rothberg, A.D., Maisels, M.J., Bagnato, S., et al.	1973–1976	1,250 grams	46%	29%	—	—
Markestad, T., & Fitzhardinge, P.M.	1974–1977	1,500 grams	—	—	75%	10%
Driscoll, J.M., Driscoll, Y.T., Steir, M.E., et al.	1977–1978	1,000 grams	83%	17%	84	—
Bennett, F.C., Robinson, N.M., Sells, C.J., et al.	1977–1980	800 grams	81%	12%	—	19%

state as opposed to hypertonia, which is unstable with an important tendency to shift (although the shifting is toward normal tone) from the first through the third assessment periods (Lozano, 1983). Between the third and fourth assessment periods, normal tone consolidates its stable state, and hypertonia begins its stabilization, meaning that from here on, it can be expected that any case found with hypertonia has a greater probability of remaining hypertonic than becoming normal (Lozano, 1983). Using the chi-square statistic, it is possible to validate these observations and show that by comparing the transition from the first to second assessment period to that of the second to

third, the transition probability for hypertonia is very similar (Lozano, 1983). When comparing the transition from the second to third assessment period to that of the third to fourth, there is only a suggested difference. That is, transition modifies in the third to fourth period, resulting in a more stable state of hypertonia than that seen before (Lozano, 1983).

Attention should be called to the fact that these unstable states of hypertonia are not a distinctive feature of mechanically ventilated RDS survivors or at least the author and his colleagues have found it in other follow-up groups studied in a similar manner (Lozano, 1983). What does this mean?

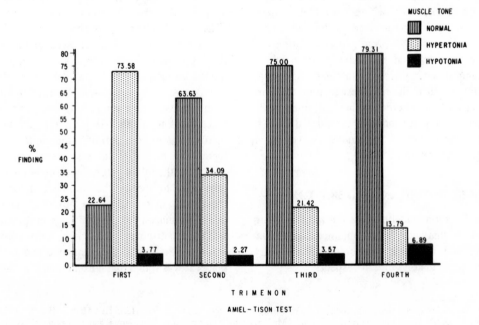

Figure 1. Muscle tone status evaluated in a selected group of mechanically ventilated RDS survivors (Lozano, 1983).

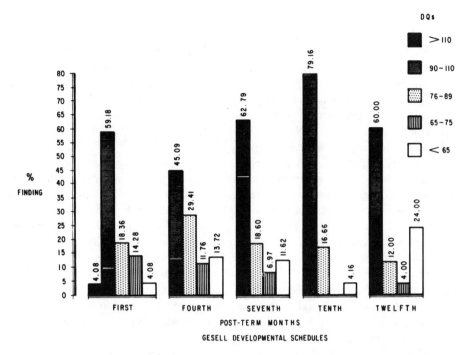

Figure 2. Developmental quotient of the Gesell Developmental Schedules, estimated in a selected group of mechanically ventilated RDS survivors (Lozano, 1983). DQ values over 110 are taken as overstimulation, and below 65 as severe retardation. Between 90 and 110 is normal, 76 to 89 is transitional or mild reversible, and from 65 to 75 is abnormal.

When the developmental quotient (DQ) of the Gesell Developmental Schedules is examined for the same RDS survivors, there is no defined trend; shifting from one DQ to another between assessments is extensive. Nevertheless, normal DQ values predominate (Figure 2). Obtaining the transition probability from the first to the fourth month of assessment, it is evident that there is a tendency toward normal DQ values, but there is no encompassing point (Lozano, 1983). At this early stage, the lowest DQ value might be predictive. Between the fourth and seventh months of assessment, transition probability values continue shifting, demonstrating the infants' developmental instability. Although there is a tendency for normal values to prevail, the lowest DQ value tends to remain static, with no tendency to shift toward more normal levels (Lozano, 1983). The transition probability from the seventh to the tenth month of assessment shows that the tendency toward normal DQ values is more important and is consistent. Shifting continues, but mainly toward normal levels, and the lowest DQ value preserves its degree of significance. Finally, from the tenth to the twelfth month of assessment, the transition probability continues to shift toward normal; no stability has been accomplished up to now, except for the lowest DQ value. Although severely retarded individuals can be identified very early, at 12 months low DQ values seem to reach their point of no return (Lozano, 1983).

There is a need to question criteria under which a follow-up program runs. *What are we seeking through follow-up? Do we wish to find out who is abnormal and who isn't? Do we wish to play with numbers? What are we really up to?* These questions might sound innocent and even trivial, but it appears that follow-up programs have been acquiring facts of historical importance but little practical immediate application. Perhaps it is time to consider a change in the criteria that until now have ruled most follow-up programs.

CLUES FOR IDENTIFYING
CHANGING CRITERIA

One must be observant of changing criteria in the assessment period. First, *all* information developed during the patient's hospitalization should be taken into consideration during follow-up of the "graduates" of the NICU. All that has taken place in the past should remain as historical data, available for future reference.

Second, discrimination between survivors and deaths should continue to the point where the former ones might be considered as follow-up cases and the deaths become closed cases after a mortality discussion, but there is little or no tie established between the deaths and survivors in terms of follow-up.

Third, follow-up, as practiced now, mainly in the outpatient clinic, should be a continuous review link with occurrences in the inpatient state and bolstered with as much information as can possibly be drawn from deaths and other survivors.

We are now in the era of microprocessing, which if applied to patient care, should advance knowledge in terms of outcome. Follow-up could then be reoriented from groups to individuals, and to situations confronted by them. Differences in outcome are governed by circumstances experienced by individual patients during the critical course. These circumstances must be broken down into their composite elements and associated with target units within the individual.

CLINICAL EXPERIENCE

With ultrasound brain scan screening in premature newborn infants of less than 1,500 grams birth weight, a 78% incidence of cerebral hemorrhaging has been found (Udaeta, Felix, Segura, & Lozano, 1982). Approximately 25% of these preterms have a silent course. There is a high percentage of posthemorrhagic hydrocephalus (Figure 3), but there is also a good percentage of arrest. Differences in outcome are guided by circumstances experienced by the patient during the critical course of the bleed.

Currently evoked potential responses have been used with NICU patients. When these infants "graduate" from the NICU, they are followed in the outpatient clinic with brain stem auditory responses at key age intervals when neuromotor and behavioral and cognitive function are assessed. On occasion, brain stem

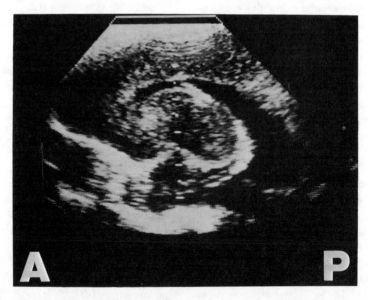

Figure 3.   A premature infant of 31 weeks gestation and birth weight 1,050 grams who suffered birth asphyxia and mild RDS. An ultrasound parasagittal scan 1 week after birth shows moderate dilatation of the lateral ventricle and some areas of periventricular hemorrhage. In an anterolateral scan, the radius of the ventricular was found to show 46% dilatation, and the occipital horn to measure 13 mm. Six months later, the posthemorrhagic hydrocephalus had arrested. The child's development at 1 year is normal.

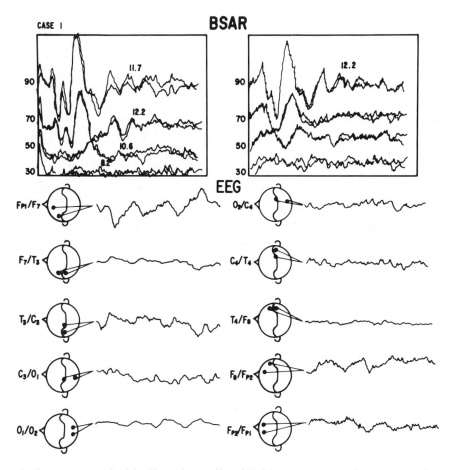

Figure 4. Out-born premature with subdural hemorrhage and hyperbilirubinemia. Brain stem auditory responses (BSAR) recorded at 6 days of age show prolonged latency time for the V wave. The EEG shows generalized suppression in temporal regions. At this early age, it is already possible to predict severe neurological damage.

auditory responses can predict severe neurological damage very early (Figure 4), helping in the decision-making, that is, defining the attitudes to take with a given patient. In addition, by not limiting the use of brain stem auditory responses for the follow-up of NICU "graduates," but also using them as a correlation element of the pathology findings of post mortem studies, a better understanding of the patients' outcome may be obtained.

CONCLUSIONS

Reference to handicapping conditions in the follow-up clinic lists problems such as an abnormal growth pattern, muscle tone abnormalities, a given degree of developmental retardation, and sensory lesions. The individual's specific characteristics, and those particular situations that he or she has confronted that are related to risk factors, cannot be ignored. Some can be anticipated, others not; but, ultimately, they will delineate the outcome.

Outcome should then be explained and not be referred to, i.e., explained in terms of matching individuals, correlating conditions and situations, and confirming the source of the observed effect. With the aid of some special neuropathological studies such as the Golgi staining technique, among others, necessary associations should be able to be made between nonsurvivors and survivors in order to better understand and define degrees of involvement, and in order to relate the meaning of signs and symptoms with outcome.

REFERENCES

Amiel-Tison, C. A method for neurologic evaluation within the first year of life. *Current Problems in Pediatrics,* 1976, *7,* 1.

Bennett, F.C., Robinson, N.M., & Sells, C.J. Growth and development of infants weighing less than 800 grams at birth. *Pediatrics,* 1983, *71,* 319–323.

Bernstein, J. Guía para la aplicación del test de diagnos tico del desarrollo de Gesell. Editorial Paidos, Biblioteca de Psicometría, 1976.

Cukier, F., Amiel-Tison, C., & Minkowski, A. Hyaline membrane disease in neonates treated with artificial ventilation: Neurologic and intellectual sequelae at two to five years of age. In: W.C. Shoemaker (ed.), *The lung in the critically ill patient.* Baltimore: Williams & Wilkins, 1976.

Cukier, F., Bethmann, O., Rolier, J.P. et al. Long term prognosis in hyaline membrane disease. In: L. Stern, W. Oh, & B. Friis-Hansen (eds.), *Intensive care in the newborn II.* New York: Masson Publishing USA, Inc., 1978.

Driscoll, J.M., Driscoll, Y.T., Steir, M.E., et al. Mortality and morbidity in infants less than 1,001 grams birth weight. *Pediatrics,* 1982, *69,* 21–26.

Gesell, A., Harverson, H.M., Thompson, H., et al. *The first five years of life.* New York: Harper & Row, 1940.

Lozano, C.H. Follow-up studies of survivors of the respiratory distress syndrome. In: L. Stern (ed.), *Respiratory distress syndrome.* New York: Grune & Stratton, 1983.

Markestad, T. & Fitzhardinge, P.M. Growth and development in children recovering from bronchopulmonary dysplasia. *Pediatrics,* 1981, *98,* 597–602.

Outerbridge, E.W., Ramsay, N., & Stern, L. Developmental follow-up of artificially ventilated infants with neonatal respiratory failure. *Critical Care Medicine,* 1974, *2,* 23–28.

Rothberg, A.D., Maisels, M.J., Bagnato, S., et al. Outcome for survivors of mechanical ventilation weighing less than 1,250 gm at birth. *The Journal of Pediatrics,* 1981, *98,* 106–111.

Udaeta, E., Felix, I., Segura, M.A., & Lozano, C.H. Diagnóstico de hemorragia intracraneana en recién nacidos de pretérmino porultrasonido. Reporte premiliminar. *Bol Med Hosp Infant (Mex),* 1982, *39,* 812–819.

Section III

INFANCY AND
EARLY CHILDHOOD

ARTHUR H. PARMELEE, M.D.
UCLA School of Medicine, Los Angeles, California

T HE PURPOSE OF THE SECOND INTERNATIONAL workshop on the "at-risk" infant and of this publication is to present and discuss interdisciplinary approaches to "the prevention, diagnosis, and management of developmental disabilities." The word "prevent" is appropriately listed first to focus on the prevention of problems that place infants "at risk." Many of the obstetrical and perinatal problems that place infants at risk for developmental disabilities have been identified and are potentially preventable. The term "risk," however, encompasses an enormous number of unknown factors including all the important and confounding contributions of social circumstances and events, which often play a larger role in determining the degree of risk for developmental disability than the obstetrical and perinatal problems suffered by infants.

In infancy and early childhood, developmental changes are so rapid that it is very important to know how well a child is progressing with or without a known biological problem. One needs to know through appropriate assessment techniques what the child's emotional and cognitive strengths are that make this progress possible. Intervention can then be designed to enhance the child's areas of strength and provide support in the areas of weakness.

In this final section of the book, authors present reviews of special topics related to follow-up surveillance of the development of infants at risk, forms of intervention, and community organization procedures to provide these services. A general review of the issues concerning the assessment of infants and young children at risk for developmental disabilities due to perinatal biological problems is presented by Parmelee and Cohen. The authors believe that, in general, social factors are greatly predictive of outcome, especially intellectual functioning and school performance.

Another factor is identified by Meijer as predictive of outcome. His research suggests that hospitalization in early childhood can serve as a high-risk indicator for behavior and learning problems at school age. The research of Maia, Barbosa, and Gomes directs attention to the significance of including full-term asphyxiated newborns in studies determining intensive care. Michaelis, Haas, and Buchwald-Saal review the issues of neurological evaluations, emphasizing the need for this in addition to the usual behavioral assessments. Their chapter's focus on the value of infant neurology in developmental assessments suggests that the results from neurological examinations are particularly useful in contributing information about causes of delays in development.

Jaffe's research indicates that a definite correlation does exist between excessive weight and motor delay in younger babies, but that before it is concluded that motor delay is associated with obesity, a comprehensive medical and neurodevelopmental evaluation must be performed, because mental retardation, neuromuscular disturbance, or a general medical condition such as hypothyroidism may be the underlying cause.

Data from Leavitt and Ver Hoeve's research suggests that the study of acoustic–cardiac response and its modulation provides an additional dimension in the clinical evaluation of neuromaturation of the premature infant and may result in a useful framework for the assimilation of data obtained noninvasively in the developing infant with those of more molecular physiological investigations. In his review, Bergman presents the importance of early assessment of auditory problems and their relation to language development. Sohmer extends this topic with a detailed discussion of brain stem auditory evoked potentials and their uses in studying audition. His review concludes that the recording of many types of multimodality evoked potentials may serve as a noninvasive diagnostic tool for the early detection of brain dysfunction in at-risk neonates before the appearance of the developmental brain disorder, and may predict the impending disorder.

Oller next provides a detailed discussion of the infant's speech and language development. His review of the myths and clarification of the facts of infant vocal development is valuable for the knowledge it yields to help design intervention strategies for infants expected to show linguistic/phonological impairments. The research of Eillers, Bull, Oller, and Lewis on speech perception with Down syndrome infants showed that DS infants and young children tend to exhibit a similar pattern of discrimination—the most rapid spectral changes were most difficult to distinguish while the least rapid patterns were the easiest to discriminate. Atkinson's chapter provides a detailed discussion of visual assessment in infants and young children. Her review offers some useful advice on the problem of assessing visual acuity in early childhood. The research of Atkinson and Butler showed a marked association of vision problems with other medical problems, twins, and low birth weight. Specifically, the research suggests that most physical or mental disabilities, whether congenital or acquired, are more likely to be associated with sensory problems such as visual defects. The authors emphasize that these children are at an increased risk and thus need careful scrutiny during the preschool years in an attempt to reduce the level of handicap. Holtzman, Harel, and Feinson provide research findings on the phenomenon of the late visual bloomer. Their study revealed that the early recognition of this visual phenomenon is not only imperative for prognostic value, but could also prevent unnecessary and sometimes invasive diagnostic studies.

The results of research by Shapira, Harel, and Tamir justify that the use of the standardized Denver Developmental Screening Test in Israel is necessary in order to avoid both under- and over-referrals of children with developmental abnormalities. In their review, Klein and Feuerstein discuss in detail the importance of parents and caregivers as mediators in the cognitive development of young children. Research by Bromwich suggests that careful observations focused on specific areas of behavior during spontaneous play offer a rich source of information on various aspects of development during infancy. Research by Stevenson, Leavitt, and Silverberg shows that Down syndrome infants and their mothers are less responsive to one another than are nondelayed infants and their mothers. They speculate that the relatively low-responsive environment may contribute to later delays in DS infants. Rabinowitz and Harel review the strengths and weaknesses of educational and child care programs in Israel.

Applications of the neurological, behavioral, auditory, visual, and speech assessments described in this section are necessary during the first months of life in order to identify infants at greatest risk. Further follow-up testing, however, is essential to be more specific in determining the degree and nature of any handicap.

Chapter 29

Neonatal Follow-Up Services
for Infants at Risk

Arthur H. Parmelee, M.D.
Sarale E. Cohen, Ph.D.
University of California at Los Angeles School of Medicine, Los Angeles, California

I N PLANNING NEONATAL FOLLOW-UP PROGRAMS, it is important to recognize the diverse interests of the professionals and the families involved. Obstetricians and neonatologists, community service organizers, and parents each have a somewhat different focus. Frequently, this difference in viewpoint has led to disappointment because follow-up programs have not satisfactorily served any of these interest groups well, a nearly impossible task.

The organization of follow-up programs is further complicated by the inability to identify strong biological determinants of risk for developmental disability. In spite of the common opinion that infants born at biological risk are likely to have problems, in the authors' studies, and in those of others, it has been found that prenatal, perinatal, and neonatal medical problems do not predict the neurological or behavioral outcomes of individual infants. On the other hand, social factors are generally strongly predictive of outcome, particularly intellectual functioning and school performance. Moreover, the largest number of children with neurological, sensory, and mental handicaps come from a population of full-term infants who may not have been identified as at

risk due to perinatal or neonatal problems. These parodoxical statements need to be explained to make them consistent with the usual clinical impressions and logical reasoning.

MEDICAL VERSUS SOCIAL FACTORS AS PREDICTORS OF DEVELOPMENTAL OUTCOME

The results from the authors' follow-up study of preterm infants, as a prototype of infants at risk, illustrate why it is difficult to predict developmental outcome from prenatal, perinatal, and neonatal medical events and why social factors are more predictive (Cohen & Parmelee, 1983; Parmelee, Beckwith, Cohen, & Sigman, 1983). It is known from many studies that preterm infants, as a group, have more neurological and developmental problems than healthy full-term infants, and that the smaller and sicker preterm infants have the greatest number of problems (Kopp & Parmelee, 1979). Nevertheless, since most of the children born preterm develop normally, even the smallest and sickest, it still remains impossible to predict the outcome of individual infants, except for those with immediate and

Research for this chapter was supported by NICHD contract #1-HD-3-2776 and W.T. Grant Foundation Award #B771121

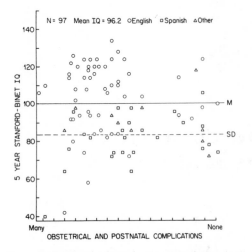

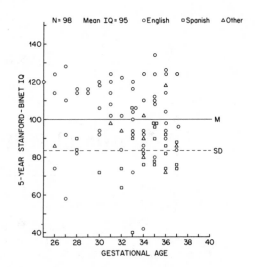

Figure 1. Relationship between obstetrical and postnatal complications and 5-year IQ. (N = 97; mean IQ = 96.2; ○ English; □ Spanish; △ Other.)

Figure 3. Relationship between gestational age and 5-year IQ. (N = 98; mean IQ = 95; ○ English; □ Spanish; △ Other.)

persisting catastrophic neurological problems. Results from the authors' follow-up study are presented in Figure 1. The number of prenatal, perinatal, and neonatal medical problems for each infant is plotted against their 5-year Stanford-Binet IQ scores. It can be seen that most of the infants with IQ scores below 90 also had many perinatal medical problems, which is consistent with other group data reports (Drillien, Thomson, & Burgoyne, 1980). One can also see that the majority of the infants with many perinatal problems have normal intelligence scores and that the correlation between the number of medical problems and 5-year IQ is not significant ($r = -.02$). Figures 2 and 3 illustrate the same lack of significant

correlation between birth weight or gestational age and 5-year IQ scores.

In contrast to the low relationship between perinatal factors and later development, Table 1 illustrates the impact of social factors on the 5-year outcome scores. A family's primary language plays an important role, even though the Stanford-Binet test was given to each child in his or her native language. The authors do not believe that the poor performance of the Spanish-speaking children in this study reflects their native intelligence but rather indicates both cultural biases in the test and the effects of impoverished socioeconomic environments. Children from English-speaking lower SES families were also performing less adequately than those from higher SES backgrounds. Nevertheless, it is clear that the children from Spanish-speaking families are entering school with a strong handicap since the schools, at least in the Los Angeles area, tend to have the same cultural biases as the Stanford-Binet test.

FACTORS IN INTERVENTION

The point the authors wish to make is that by school age, social factors are so dominant in their effect on behavioral outcome that they obscure the impact of perinatal and neonatal medical events. The importance of social factors in determining the behavioral progress of

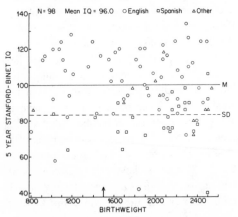

Figure 2. Relationship between birth weight and 5-year IQ. (N = 98; mean IQ = 96.0; ○ English: □ Spanish; △ Other.)

Table 1. Five-year Stanford-Binet scores

	Preterm	Full-term
All subjects	95.7 (N = 97)	103.3 (N = 22)
English-speaking	103.6 (N = 54)	
High SES	108.6 (n = 31)	
Low SES	96.6 (n = 23)	
Spanish-speaking	86.6 (N = 25)	

SES = Socioeconomic status.

healthy newborns has been known for a long time (Broman, Nichols, & Kennedy, 1975). This chapter illustrates the same impact of social factors on infants considered at risk because of neonatal biological problems. That social factors outweigh biological risk for most infants is of significance since the two factors often are compounded. It is more common for socially disadvantaged and immigrant foreign language groups to have more pregnancy problems and more preterm infants because of less access to medical care due to poverty and foreign language communication problems. There is also evidence of a heightened effect when both adverse environmental factors and biological risk are involved (e.g., Drillien et al., 1980; Escalona, 1982; Werner, Bierman, French, Simonian, Connor, Smith, & Campbell, 1968). The fact that social factors play such a dominant role also indicates that, potentially, appropriate intervention services can be provided.

Infants who in the neonatal period may have suffered some central nervous system damage may compensate for this completely, particularly if the insult is minimal. The compensation, however, may require an optimal environment. In this way, advantageous social environments obscure perinatal biological risk. Furthermore, healthy newborns who have suffered no, or minimal, perinatal risks may perform poorly later in life on intelligence tests and in school because of adverse environments. Thus, in this way, too, social factors may confound predictions from the neonatal period based on the absence of biological hazards.

An additional problem for follow-up studies is the fact that the largest number of handicapped children come from neonatal populations not considered at high risk in the neonatal period even though the incidence of problems is much higher in neonatal biological risk populations. For example, there is a much greater occurrence of cerebral palsy among infants born preterm, particularly among preterm infants with birth weights below 1,500 grams, than among full-term infants. However, the incidence of all preterm births is only about 7% of all births and only 1% of all births weighed less than 1,500 grams. Thus, even with a high occurrence of cerebral palsy, perhaps as high as 10%–20%, the actual number of children with birth weights less than 1,500 grams who have cerebral palsy is small. Consequently, a very low occurrence of cerebral palsy, much less than 1%, for full-term infants nevertheless results in at least twice the number of children with cerebral palsy. The same type of statistic is true of most other handicaps, including mental retardation. Nonetheless, in spite of actual numbers of children involved, the greatest concern for the obstetrician and neonatologist is the group of infants with the highest occurrence of cerebral palsy, in this case, preterm infants. The physicians wish to focus on those pregnancy, delivery, and neonatal problems that might be changed to reduce this incidence, a goal with which everyone would agree. To meet this goal, it is appropriate to use a research strategy that concentrates on the group of infants with the highest incidence of handicap in order to maximize the chance of determining etiological factors, even if the total number of cases is small (Saigal, Rosenbaum, Stoskopf, & Milner, 1982).

A further difficulty in satisfying the concerns of obstetricians and neonatologists is the small number of children in the usual follow-up clinic from any individual nursery. Careful and detailed follow-up of the infants with the highest incidence of outcome problems, generally the very low birthweight infants, is possible from a single nursery. However, because the total number of such infants is not large, the value of single nursery follow-ups is limited. The actual number of infants each year with identified handicaps, such as cerebral palsy, is too small to determine perinatal etiological factors that seldom occur singly. It is most likely that each case of cerebral palsy or other neurological handicaps in any one year has a different cluster of possible causal variables. Although follow-up projects from single nurseries do serve important functions such as helping staff morale and providing monitoring of overall morbidity and mortality, it is probable that only very large epidemiological studies involving the follow-up of infants from many nurseries can resolve issues of critical perinatal etiological factors.

Follow-up programs from the point of view of community organizers have a different focus. Public health and education administrators are interested in finding all infants and young children in the community with handicaps as early as possible. They would like to provide early intervention programs for parents and children to optimize the outcome of the child despite the handicap. For this purpose, a follow-up program that only includes the infants with the highest incidence of problems, such as preterm infants of very low birth weight, would not identify most of the infants in the community with handicaps. To achieve this latter goal, a follow-up program that screens the developmental progress of all infants in a community, not just a single-risk group, will be most productive. Since most neurological and developmental problems are difficult to determine early in infancy and begin to express themselves more clearly in the later part of the first year, such massive developmental screening might best be deferred until approximately 9 months from term for practical reasons.

The type of follow-up that is of interest to new parents should be geared to support services. Parents are most interested in medical, social, and educational support services that will help them optimize their infant's health and developmental progress, whether the infant has a disability or not. Parents of all infants are concerned about the possibility of developmental problems but this is particularly so for those infants born preterm and/or sick in the neonatal period. The parents are very apprehensive at the time they take their child home from the nursery and their concerns center on the infant's survival and their own feelings of inadequacy. For them, a follow-up program is most effective if it gives the family immediate social, emotional, and medical support services in the first few days and weeks when the infant is at home. Awareness of specific developmental problems comes lates after the initial adaptation. Parents, of course, also want early identification of problems and specific interventions. Since, however, most of the developmental and neurological problems once identified cannot be cured, the parents are not as concerned with the perinatal causes as are the obstetrician and neonatologist, and are more concerned with what to do for their child from that time forward.

ESTABLISHING PROGRAM PRIORITIES

Given the diverse interests of the various groups in the follow-up studies of newborn infants and infants at risk, it is not surprising that many programs ultimately are not as helpful as they could be to any single group. It is therefore necessary to establish program priorities to make sure the goals of at least one interest group are achieved. It seems most logical to place the parents' needs first and attempt to provide emotional, social, and medical support in the first days and weeks after the child goes home and then plan the additional objectives depending on the specific clinic and community needs.

Each type of follow-up service also needs to consider the most appropriate assessment measures to use to meet their particular objectives. Obstetricians and neonatologists wishing to determine the specific perinatal causes of adverse outcomes of the infants under their care so that they may provide procedures to prevent problems would benefit most from short-term outcome measures. Ideally, assessments should be done in the hospital, prior to the infant's discharge, since long-term follow-up assessments are less likely to answer the questions of primary concern to them. Not only do social factors play an increasing role in the outcome of the infants in later childhood, but obstetric and neonatal care procedures are evolving so rapidly that outcome data obtained several years after birth no longer address current perinatal care.

Community service organizers such as public health administrators and educators, on the other hand, are interested in the identification of all infants and young children who may be having developmental difficulties or are manifesting neurological or sensory handicaps. Thus, tests should be selected that will identify as early as possible infants at potential risk. Although many errors of classification will occur, this study (Cohen & Parmelee, 1983; Parmelee et al., 1983; Sigman & Parmelee, 1979) indicates that if single measures of infant development are selected to identify those infants who will need special help, the most cost-effective strategy is to administer a behavioral developmental assessment such as the Gesell or Bayley assessments late in the first year. This strategy can be applied to the evaluation of all infants, including low birth weight infants and others who have suffered biological hazards and/or social risk.

CONCLUSION

Infant and early childhood assessment procedures and research in this area should be continuously reviewed. This endeavor is greatly aided by all studies of normal development. In the following chapters of the book, thorough descriptions of the applications of neurological and behavioral assessments are presented (Chapter 32), as well as new developments in the assessment of audition (Chapters 35 and 36), speech (Chapter 37), and vision (Chapter 39). Most of these techniques are applicable in the first year. For many of these assessments, their application in the first months of life serves to identify the infants at greatest risk, and further testing in later months is necessary to be more specific in determining the degree and nature of any handicap. It is essential in planning a follow-up program to decide how early to start assessments and how frequently to repeat them and what further surveillance is advisable, as development is plastic, and errors of identification occur, and children shift in their risk classification.

The early identification of infants with problems makes possible the consideration of intervention procedures. These take many forms and can be carried out in a variety of settings as discussed in Chapters 43 and 46.

REFERENCES

Broman, S.H., Nichols, P.L., & Kennedy, W.A. *Preschool IQ: Prenatal and early development correlates.* Hillsdale, NJ: Lawrence Erlbaum Associates, 1975.

Cohen, S.E., & Parmelee, A.H. Prediction of five year Stanford-Binet scores in preterm infants. *Child Development*, 1983, *54*, 1242–1253.

Drillien, C.M., Thomson, A.J.M., & Burgoyne, K. Low-birthweight children at early school-age: A longitudinal study. *Developmental Medicine and Child Neurology*, 1980, *22*, 26–47.

Escalona, S.K. Babies at double hazard: Early development of infants at biologic and social risk. *Pediatrics*, 1982, *70*, 670–676.

Kopp, C.B., & Parmelee, A.H. Prenatal and perinatal influences on infant behavior. In: J. Osofsky (ed.), *Handbook of infancy*. New York: John Wiley & Sons, 1979.

Parmelee, A.H., Beckwith, L., Cohen, S.E., & Sigman,

M. Social influences on infants at medical risk for behavioral difficulties. In: J. Call (ed.), *Frontiers of infant psychiatry*. New York: Basic Books, 1983.

Saigal, S., Rosenbaum, P., Stoskopf, B., & Milner, R. Follow-up of infants 501 to 1,500 gm birth weight delivered to residents of a geographically defined region with perinatal intensive care facilities. *The Journal of Pediatrics*, 1982, *100*, 606–613.

Sigman, M., & Parmelee, A.H. An intervention program for pre-term high-risk infants and their parents. In: T.M. Field, A.M. Sostek, S. Goldberg, & H.H. Shuman (eds.), *Infants born at risk*. New York: Spectrum, 1979.

Werner, E.E., Bierman, J.M., French, F.E., Simonian, K., Connor, A., Smith, R.S., & Campbell, M. Reproductive and environmental casualties: A report on the 10-year follow-up of the children of the Kauai pregnancy study. *Pediatrics*, 1968, *42*, 112–126.

The At-Risk Infant: Psycho/Socio/Medical Aspects
edited by Shaul Harel, M.D., and Nicholas J. Anastasiow, Ph.D.
Copyright © 1985   Paul H. Brookes Publishing Co., Inc.   Baltimore • London

Chapter 30

Hospitalization in Infancy as a Long-Term At-Risk Indicator

ALEXANDER MEIJER, M.D.
Hadassah University Hospital and Hebrew University Medical School, Jerusalem, Israel

R ESULTS OF LONG-TERM FOLLOW-UP AFTER hospitalization in early childhood are less well documented than short-term effects. Rutter (1972, 1976) concluded that single separation experiences at any age rarely have long-term sequelae, unless they are also associated with chronic stresses. Multiple admissions, when the first admission had taken place during the preschool years, are, according to the findings of Quinton and Rutter (1976), associated with an increased risk of both psychiatric disorder and delinquency. Part of this increased risk was attributed to chronic family stresses rather than to the admissions themselves.

In order to compare the late effects of single with multiple hospital admissions of young children, one would have to control for the factor of chronic stress stemming from family interactions, as well as for the reasons for hospital admissions. Douglas (1975) found that short hospital admissions before the age of 5 were statistically significantly associated with later job instability! On the other hand, children whose first hospital admission was after the age of 5 did not have an excess of

adverse ratings in adolescence. It is generally agreed that early hospitalizations are more likely to be associated with later disturbances, particularly when the children come from unhappy or troubled homes (Quinton & Rutter, 1976).

The data on hospitalization in the studies of Douglas and of Rutter were obtained retrospectively from the parents, and this is particularly important with regard to the problem of recall more than 5 years later. Numerous studies have shown, as reported by Rutter (1976), that retrospective recall about events or happenings in the past, even as recently as a year previously, are very subject to inaccuracy and systematic distortion (Brown & Rutter, 1966; Chess, Thomas, & Birch, 1966; Haggard, Brekstad, & Skard, 1960; Robbins, 1963; Rutter & Brown, 1966; Wenar, 1963; and Yarrow, Campbell, & Burton, 1970). One would in particular expect bias among those parents who declared years later that their child had never been hospitalized for a short time at an early age.

Though Douglas checked most of his maternal reports against hospital records, Rutter

The author acknowledges the generous help of Professor Susan Harlap, who made the data of the Jerusalem Perinatal Study available. The author wishes to thank Dr. Helena Kaplan-Feigon for her research assistance with parts of this study, and Dr. Simon Silman for his dedicated editorial help. This study was sponsored by the Natalie Zucker Fund in Child Psychiatry.

was unable to do so, and neither of them was able to check parental statements that their child had never been hospitalized. National and regional figures on hospitalization rates of children at different ages might have cast more light on the validity of their figures.

In the above quoted studies of Douglas and of Quinton and Rutter, the absolute number of cases hospitalized for a short time in the first 2 years of life was very small. With regard to the sex of the children, it is well known that almost all psychiatric disorders and many physical disabilities in childhood are much more common in boys (Meijer, 1976; Rutter, 1976; and Rutter, Tizard, & Whitmore, 1970). In the two quoted studies, sex difference was hardly taken into consideration. Therefore some of the findings may be accounted for by an uneven sex distribution in the various groups of admissions. Boys are much more prone to deviant behavior at the elementary school age than girls.

A suitable population for studying hospitalization would consist of subjects for whom it was known exactly if, when, where, and why they were hospitalized from the time it actually happened. This material was available for the whole of Jerusalem from the perinatal study of Davies, Prywes, Tzur, Weiskopf, and Sterk (1969). Independent of the Davies study, a psychoeducational data pool of cohorts of boys was used.

AIM OF THE STUDY

The aim of this study was to investigate whether a population of boys, hospitalized in the first 2 years of life, was different in behavior and level of functioning at the age of 6 until 10 from a population of boys who were definitely not hospitalized in early childhood. To this end, two independent sets of historical longitudinal data were used, one on early hospitalizations in the whole of the city of Jerusalem, and one on two cohorts of unselected boys who were yearly psychiatrically examined in a standard fashion and who were tested yearly by teacher evaluations on two standard questionnaires.

METHODOLOGY

Subjects

The sample of boys was taken from a data pool of a longitudinal study on high-risk factors in all boys whose mothers visited the well baby clinics of the Hadassah Community Health Center of the Kiryat Hayovel area in Jerusalem and who were candidates for entering two of the biggest schools in the area.

Two cohorts of boys, born in the years 1967 and 1968, were selected for the study because, for those years of birth, hospitalization data were available from the Jerusalem Perinatal Study. This study was conducted by Michael Davies et al. (1969), and later summarized by Harlap, Davies, Grover, and Prywes (1977). One cohort of boys, born in 1967, consisted of 49 subjects, and another, of boys born in 1968, consisted of 65 subjects. A total of 114 boys participated in this study.

Hospital Admissions

Computerized data on hospital admissions in this study originated from the above-mentioned Jerusalem Perinatal Study. This study, originally begun in 1964 in order to study the epidemiology of toxemia of pregnancy, was later extended to survey a wide range of health indices. This included maternal, perinatal, and infant health. In 1965, a prospective surveillance of all birth registrations recorded in Jerusalem was begun. To this basic register was added information, obtained antenatally, on the majority of pregnant women as well as a continuous follow-up of all newborns, with special attention to hospitalization. No hospitalization statistics were available for infants in Jerusalem before the beginning of this study, but the national figures for 1963 showed an admission rate (in episodes) of 22% under the age of 12 months. All pediatric departments in Jerusalem were monitored during 1966–1969, and various birth cohorts were followed up through different ages. Of the births during 1966–1968, 18.1% of babies were admitted to the hospital at least once before their first birthday and the rate of the admission episodes was 26.7%. Admission rates were highest among babies ages 3–5 months, rising with increase in family size and decrease in birth weight, education, and social class. More than one-half of admission episodes were associated with common respiratory tract infections, one-quarter with gastroenteritis, and the remainder were admitted for congenital malformations, other infectious diseases, and other causes (Bentwich, 1970; Harlap & Davies, 1974; and Harlap, Stenhouse, & Davies, 1973).

Longitudinal Study on Boys

The longitudinal study included boys who were registered in the Hadassah Community Health Center in the Kiryat Yovel area in Jerusalem (Meijer, 1977, 1979a, 1981). The study began in 1973 with a cohort of boys who were born in 1967 and who were all registered at the two biggest schools in the area, in which full cooperation with yearly surveillance of these children was assured. Of the four successive cohorts of boys, two could not be used because hospitalization data for those 2 years were not gathered in the Jerusalem Perinatal Study. Furthermore, only anterospective data were to be used in the study.

All subjects were examined annually for 4 successive years. The yearly examinations included the following elements.

The Teacher Classroom Behavior Inventory (CBI)

The CBI (Schaefer, Droppleman, & Kalverboer, 1965) was translated into Hebrew and kept as simple as the original. It consists of 60 questions that cover three bipolar dimensions of classroom behavior. It has been proven to be a feasible, reliable, and valid instrument for collecting data on classroom behavior, useful in cross-sectional and longitudinal research on child adaptation to the classroom. It can also be used in kindergarten. The three main dimensions are: positive-negative task orientation, love-hostility, and extroversion-introversion. For the purpose of the study, six items belonging to the first dimension and to hostility were chosen in advance. These items were: hyperactivity, distractibility, concentration, persistence, irritability, and resentfulness. They represent the main symptoms of the so-called hyperkinetic syndrome (Meijer, 1979b). On each of the six items, five questions had been asked and they were scored on a four-point scale.

Teacher Pupil Evaluation (TPE) Screening Questionnaire

A short 24-question screening questionnaire for lower elementary school grades was devised on the model of the above-described Schaefer CBI questionnaire, but it also included five questions on learning achievement: reading, writing, spelling, arithmetic, and general knowledge. It was scored on a 4-point scale. This questionnaire has been routinely administered yearly to all pupils in the three lowest grades of the above-mentioned two schools since 1976, constituting another data pool on a whole population.

Clinical Questionnaire

The Clinical Questionnaire consists of 64 clinical questions that were presented to the mothers and answered with a yes or no response. The questions relate to the following items: eating, sleeping, bowel and bladder function, habits, antisocial behavior, introverted behavior, and integrative behavior. The final score consists of the sum total of present symptoms. These questions were yearly repeated in every cohort.

Sociodemographic and Developmental Information

The sociodemographic data included: country of origin, years of education, age and type of occupation of the parents, size of the family, and number of rooms in the apartment or home. All data on age, sex, and birth order of the children in the family were registered. The developmental data were not used in this study and neither were the Change Questionnaire data that register yearly which of a series of familial and individual life circumstances had changed, such as change of home or health; death or birth of siblings; or divorce, separation, change of health, or death of parents. The sociodemographic data of the family at the time of the birth of the children were also available from the above-described Davies study, but these were obtained 6 years earlier.

File Linkage

The two independent sets of data in this study were linked on computer by means of the identity card number of the children, which was also the birth registration number. The linkage was checked with the aid of the birth date, which was available in both the Jerusalem Perinatal Study and the Longitudinal Study on Boys. Five children who were not born in Jerusalem were excluded from the study.

Statistical Evaluation

The statistical evaluation was directed toward differences between hospitalized and non-hospitalized children and their families. When no meaningful differences were found between the sociodemographic variables of the hospitalized and nonhospitalized children, it was decided to examine also the differences that may exist between "short" admissions (less than 1 week or once) and "long" admissions (1 week or more, or more than once). This was an attempt to compare the findings with those of Douglas (1975). It could be used as an indicator for the influence of hospitalization as a possible causative factor in behavioral differences between the two groups. The data were examined with the Mann-Whitney-U-test (from the *BMDP* 3S nonparametric statistics package) on the Hebrew University Computer Cyber 70 by the statistician of the Medical Ecology Department who was familiar with the tapes of the Jerusalem Perinatal Study.

RESULTS

The study population decreased during the years of follow-up. Table 1 shows the loss, in absolute numbers and in percentages, of the

initial number of cases for each of the three tests. The average loss in school after 4 years amounted to about one in five of the initial number of cases. This was mainly due to leaving school during the study. Mindful of Rutter's (1977) warning concerning nonresponse bias, the hospitalized group was compared with the nonhospitalized group. One notices a tendency toward greater loss among the hospitalized children, which may have been a cause for fewer differences between the two groups in the course of time. It seems unlikely that the results of this study could have been affected by the loss of cases.

The sociodemographic background of the study population is shown in Table 2.

In general, hospital admission rates increased with family size and birth order (Davies et al., 1969). Table 3 shows differences between short hospitalization (single and up to 7 days duration) and long hospitalization (multiple and/or more than a week). In the latter category were more first born and more only sons. It was of course easier for mothers to be with their child in the hospital when he or she was still a first and only child. Also, these mostly young mothers had less experience in child-rearing and therefore were likely to be more worried when their child was ill. The traveling to, and stay in, the hospital became a burden with increase in the family size. Visiting hours in pediatric wards in Jerusalem are practically unlimited.

Admission rates were highest in the first 6 months of life, as is shown in Table 4. This was also found by Harlap et al. (1977) for all admissions in Jerusalem from their 1966 total population cohort, which they followed over a period of 3 years. In the author's small sample,

Table 1. Number of children and loss of cases in follow-up

Age (in years) at examination	Nonhospitalized in early childhood					Hospitalized in early childhood				
	6	7	8	9		6	7	8	9	
Clin. Q.[a]	84	82	79	67	(20%)	21	21	20	17	(23%)
C.B.I.[b]	92	85	81	79	(14%)	22	22	21	17	(23%)
L. Achiev.[c]				69					17	

[a] Clinical Questionnaire about the child, administered to mothers.
[b] Classroom Behaviour Inventory.
[c] Learning Achievement from the Teacher-Pupil-Evaluation (TPE) Screening Questionnaire.

Table 2. Sociodemographic background variables when children were 6 years old

	Years of education		Ages		Origin			Number of siblings	Crowding
	M[a]	F[b]	M	F		M	F		
Hospitalized (n = 22)									
X̄	9.82	10.14	27.54	30.04	West[d]	59%	77%	3.17	1.87
					East[e]	41%	23%		
S.D.	3.55	2.53	5.04	3.64				1.71	0.95
Nonhospitalized (n = 92)									
X̄	10.3	10.9	28.13	32.80	West	55%	52%	3.31	1.98
					East	45%	48%		
S.D.	3.5	2.7	5.33	6.00				4.50	1.13

[a] Mother.
[b] Father.
[c] Number of persons per room.
[d] Israel, Europe, and America.
[e] Africa and Asia.

59% of the children were hospitalized in the first 6 months of life, of which 36% were hospitalized in the first 3 months of life! Frequency and duration of admissions are by far the highest in the first born sons, 70% of the multiple admissions and 87% of the longer-than-a-week admissions. Of the 19 admission episodes in the "long" hospitalized group, 11 occurred in the first 6 months of life of first born sons. This latter category represented 58% of the multiple admissions. The mothers of the first born sons had an average education of 12.3 years, which is above the average, as can be seen in Table 2. Only one mother, Asian born, had an education that fell under the total sample mean. This indicated that in Jerusalem, the young, well-educated mother, without the burden of additional children, may have her son stay longer in the hospital. In order to substantiate this statement, a larger number of cases and of course the medical diagnoses would be preferred (see Table 5). There were fewer children with low birth weight in the

hospitalized group than in the nonhospitalized group.

Jerusalem statistics on infant death rates per thousand live births (Legg, Davies, Prywes, Sterk, & Weiskopf, 1969) show in the age group of mothers between 20 and 29 years old, a steady increase in death rate in relation to an increase in birth order and a decrease in maternal education. Over one-half of admission episodes in Jerusalem were associated with respiratory tract infections (Harlap et al., 1977). In the sample, the same was found for "short" admissions, but in "long" admissions, other infections also were significant. In both "short" and "long" admission episodes, more than 60% were because of infections. Of these, 59% occurred under the age of 6 months in the "long" admissions and 88% of the infections occurred in the "short" admissions.

Hospital admissions for gastroenteritis, when linked with municipal rating (city tax), served Davies et al. (1968) as a socioeconomic index. In Israel, income differentials between

Table 3. Birth order of admitted children

	Nonhospitalized	Hospitalized	Long	Short
First child	31.6%	40.9%	70%	16.7%
Second child	35.8%	27.3%	20%	33.3%
Third child	20.0%	13.6%	—	25.0%
Four or more children	12.6%	18.2%	10%	25.0%
Only son	29.5%	22.7%	40%	8.3%

Table 4. Age at admission to hospital

Age in months	0–3	3–6	6–12	12–24	Total
Number of boys	8	5	3	6	22

rich and poor are very small by western standards and, therefore, social class cannot be defined easily with the criteria used in western countries. In addition to family size and parental origin and education, a crowding factor, which is the number of people per room (Table 2), was used. All socioeconomic indices showed that the hospitalized children in the sample were certainly not from a lower socioeconomic level than the nonhospitalized children. This is of importance for the interpretation of the following behavioral results, because it is well known that behavioral disorders appear more frequently among boys, and particularly when they come from lower income families (Davie, Butler, & Goldstein, 1972).

Teacher Evaluations

The teacher evaluations were obtained at the end of each academic year, in order that the teacher would be sufficiently acquainted with the pupils. The first evaluation was done in obligatory kindergarten at the age of 6. The next yearly teacher evaluations were made at the end of the first, second, and third grade.

Table 6 shows the differences between children hospitalized in early childhood and those who were not hospitalized in early childhood. Figure 1 and Figure 2 illustrate that the hospitalized children were significantly more hyperactive, irritable, distractible, and resentful and that they also scored significantly lower in concentration and in perseverance at school tasks.

The constant difference during the years of follow-up between hospitalized and non-hospitalized children indicates a real difference in behavioral characteristics between hospitalized and nonhospitalized children. Another teacher evaluation was obtained from the TPE Screening Questionnaire for learning and behavior problems that is administered yearly to all three lower grades in the schools (the boys in this sample were all in these three lower grades). The evaluation contains five questions on learning achievement (LA). Table 6 shows that the hospitalized children were much lower in learning achievement than the non-hospitalized children. This is illustrated in Figure 3, which shows a statistical significance of .007 with the Mann-Whitney U-test.

Clinical Evaluation

On the psychiatric questionnaire that was presented annually to the mothers when the children were 6, 7, 8, and 9 years old, statistically significant differences were found between the scores of the boys who were and who were not hospitalized in early childhood. Table 7 shows a striking consistency of these findings in the first three annual examinations.

"Short" and "Long" Hospitalization

Like Douglas (1975), a hospital admission was classified as "short" if it concerned a single admission of less than a week. Longer single admissions and multiple admissions were classified as "long." Comparison of "long" and "short" hospitalized children was difficult in this study because the number of cases, which ranged from 8 to 11, was small. However, there was a consistent trend in the first three annual examinations of greater differ-

Table 5. Causes of admission episodes

	Hospitalization		
Medical diagnosis	Long (n = 27)	Short (n = 12)	Total (N = 39)
Upper respiratory infection	9 (33%)	7 (58%)	16 (41%)
Gastrointestinal infection	1 (4%)	0 (0%)	1 (3%)
Other infections	7 (26%)	1 (8%)	8 (21%)
Total Infections	63%	66%	65%
Congenital disorders	2 (7%)	0 (0%)	2 (5%)
Accidents	3 (11%)	0 (0%)	3 (8%)
Other	5 (19%)	4 (33%)	9 (23%)

Table 6. Elementary school pupils presenting one or more deviancies in clinical disturbance score, learning achievement score and six school behavior scores in four annual examinations, according to hospitalization and nonhospitalization in early childhood

	Hospitalized	Nonhospitalized
Clinical disturbance		
(Maternal evaluation)		
Children with deviancies	40%	12%
Number of examinations	77	312
Initial number of cases	22	84
Learning achievement		
(Teacher evaluation)		
Children with deviancies	39%	15%
Number of examinations	33	163
Initial number of cases	19	80
School behavior		
(Teacher evaluation)		
Children with deviancies	83%	55%
Number of examinations	79	320
Initial number of cases	22	92

Deviancy = $\overline{X}$ + 1 S.D. of the nonhospitalized.

ences between "long" and "short" hospitalization than between "short" and nonhospitalization in the clinical disturbance scores. The same trend appeared in two of the school behavior items, irritability and resentfulness. These items, which are often present in conduct disorders in childhood and adolescence, point in the same direction as the finding of conduct disorders in the studies of Douglas (1975) and of Quinton and Rutter (1976) after multiple admissions and in those of more than 1 week (Figure 4).

Cumulative Deviancy Figures

As a criterion for deviancy on any of the scores, the mean plus one standard deviation of the

nonhospitalized children was used. The boys with deviancies on any item in each subsequent year of examination were identified in the hospitalized and in the nonhospitalized groups. The findings can be seen in Table 6. The percentage of boys with one or more deviancies in the Clinical Questionnaire was 12% in the nonhospitalized group and 40% in the hospitalized group. By the same criterion, learning achievement was examined. On this measure there were 15% of boys with deviancies in the nonhospitalized group and 39% in the hospitalized group. On the six items of the Classroom Behavior Inventory, 55% of the boys in the nonhospitalized group showed deviancies

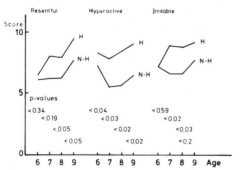

Figure 1. Mann-Whitney-U-test. Kindergarten and elementary school teacher evaluations of hospitalized and nonhospitalized boys in early childhood.

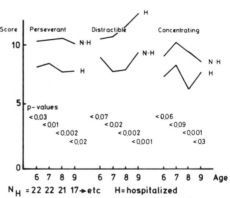

Figure 2. Mann-Whitney-U-test. Kindergarten and elementary school teacher evaluations of hospitalized and nonhospitalized boys in early childhood.

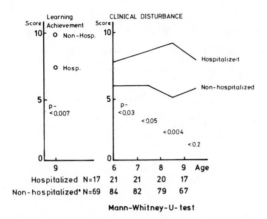

Figure 3. Mann-Whitney-U-test. Learning achievement and clinical disturbance in kindergarten and elementary school of formerly hospitalized and nonhospitalized boys.

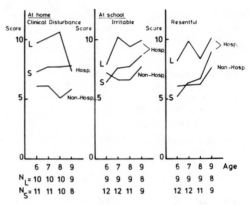

Figure 4. Long- and short-term hospitalized children compared with nonhospitalized children.

as did 83% in the hospitalized group. Comparison of "long" hospitalized and "short" hospitalized boys on the total number of deviancies over a period of 4 years showed no difference between the two categories of hospitalized boys.

In the teacher evaluations of the hospitalized children, one notices more than twice the percentage of learning achievement deviancies in hospitalized than in nonhospitalized children. The difference between the two groups in classroom behavior seems less striking because a composite percentage figure from all six CBI teacher assessment items was presented.

The findings in this study show that boys in the age group 6–10 who were admitted to the hospital in the first 2 years of life were more disturbed at home and at school than children who were not admitted to the hospital in that same period.

DISCUSSION AND CONCLUSIONS

The reasons for the above-described differences in behavior and in learning achievement between boys of early school age who were hospitalized in the first 2 years of life and those who were not admitted to the hospital in that same period are not clear from this study. There could be various reasons. First, it is possible that nonmedical components in the decision and selection for hospital admission will also have later effects. It is known that children suffering from physical disease suffer more frequently from behavior disorders and learning problems than healthy children (Shepherd, Oppenheim, & Mitchell, 1971). However, in this sample, no long-term disabling disease occurred and two-thirds of the children were admitted for ordinary upper respiratory or gastrointestinal infections. Although this could in principle be an indicator of

Table 7. Persistence of differences in four annual assessments of boys who were hospitalized and nonhospitalized in early childhood—p values (Mann-Whitney-U-test)

	Age at assessments			
	6 years	7 years	8 years	9 years
Teacher assessments				
Hyperactivity	.04	.03	.02	.02
Irritability	.59	.02	.03	.20
Resentfulness	.34	.19	.05	.05
Concentration	.06	.09	.001	.30
Perseverance	.03	.01	.002	.02
Distractibility	.07	.02	.002	.001
Learning achievement	—	—	—	.007
Maternal assessments				
Clinical disturbance total score	.03	.05	.004	.20

different psychosocial and demographic backgrounds of the hospitalized children, this was not found in the sample. However, a difference in birth order was noticed. Among the hospitalized children, there were about 1.5 times as many children who were fourth or more in birth order than among the nonhospitalized children, and there were more only sons in the nonhospitalized group. Children of larger families may have a greater chance of being ill and consequently of being admitted to the hospital. There were about 30% more first-born sons among the hospitalized children. Their mothers tended to be younger and less experienced and therefore more tense when their children become ill. By differentiating between short-term hospitalization and long-term and frequent hospitalization, it was hoped that more would be learned about possible influences of the length of hospitalization. There was not much difference in the reasons for admission in these two groups. In the long-term group, there were more than four times as many first-born boys and only sons than in the short-term group. There was no particular reason to assume that these children were more ill, but certainly these mothers had more time at their disposal and, as Rutter (1976), assumed, they may be greater worriers. The availability of a relatively great number of pediatrics beds in Jerusalem, together with a readiness of inexperienced and worried mothers to consult hospital pediatricians, could play a role in this phenomenon.

In Jerusalem, the rate of hospital admission episodes of infants before their first birthday reached 26.7%. In the first 2 years of life, 20% of all Jerusalem-born children were admitted at least once. If it is assumed that maternal worry may have played a role, it could account for more frequent and longer admissions, especially in first and only sons. Also, it would explain the symptoms of the hyperkinetic syndrome, which occurred more frequently in the hospitalized group. Parental tension is considered to be closely associated with these symptoms (Meijer, 1979b). The consistent trend toward more irritability and resentfulness in the long-term hospitalized group could be explained by environmental factors as well as by a temperamental factor from birth, as described by Thomas, Chess, and Birch (1968). Irritable babies and their mothers are likely to suffer more when they are ill. Long-term irritability could account for the finding of Douglas (1975) that early hospitalized children tend to have more job instability in later life.

The limitations of this study were the small sample size, the limited background information on the families, and the lack of information on temperamental characteristics of the children in infancy. Measures of maternal distress might have added an important dimension with regard to the possible role in early childhood hospital admissions and the long-term adverse effects on learning and on behavior at school and at home. The findings indicate that hospital admission in early childhood can be considered a high-risk indicator for behavior and learning problems at school age.

REFERENCES

Bentwich, T. The background of infant hospitalisation in the Jerusalem area with special reference to the social and medical factors involved. Unpublished doctoral thesis, *The Hebrew University in Jerusalem*, 1970.

Brown, G.W., & Rutter, M.L. The measurement of family activities and relationships: A methodological study. *Human Relations*, 1966, *19*, 241–263.

Chess, S., Thomas, A., & Birch, H.G. Distortions in developmental reporting made by parents of behaviorally disturbed children. *Journal of the American Academy of Child Psychiatry*, 1966, *5*, 226–234.

Davie, R., Butler, N., & Goldstein, H. *From birth to seven: A report of the National Child Development Study*. London: Longman, 1972.

Davies, A.M., Prywes, R., Tzur, B., Weiskopf, P., &

Sterk, V.V. The Jerusalem Perinatal Study. 1. Design and organisation of a continuing, community-based, record-linked survey. *Israel Journal of Medical Sciences*, 1969, *5*, 1095–1106.

Davies, A.M., Tzur, B., Prywes, R., & Weiskopf, P. *The Jerusalem perinatal study. Methodology manual*. Jerusalem: The Hebrew University Medical Ecology Department, 1968.

Douglas, J.W.B. Early hospital admissions and later disturbances of behavior and learning. *Developmental Medicine and Child Neurology*, 1975, *17*, 456–480.

Graham, P. Psychosomatic relationships. In: M. Rutter & L. Hersov (eds.), *Child psychiatry—Modern approaches*. Oxford: Blackwell Scientific Publications, 1977.

Haggard, E.H., Brekstad, A., & Skard, A.G. On the reliability of the anamnestic interview. *Journal of Abnormal Social Psychology*, 1960, *61*, 311–318.

Harlap, S., & Davies, A.M. Infant admissions to hospital and maternal smoking. *Lancet*, 1974, *i*, 529–532.

Harlap, S., Davies, A.M., Grover, N.B., & Prywes, R. The Jerusalem Perinatal Study: The first decade 1964–1973. *Israel Journal of Medical Sciences*, 1977, *13*, 1073–1091.

Harlap, S., Stenhouse, N.N., & Davies, A.M. A multiple regression analysis of admissions of infants to hospital: A report from the Jerusalem Perinatal Study. *British Journal of Preventive Social Medicine*, 1973, *27*, 182–186.

Legg, S. Davies, A.M., Prywes, R., Sterk, V.V., & Weiskopf, P. 2. Infant deaths 1964–1966: A cohort study of socioethnic factors in deaths from congenital malformations and from environmental and other causes. *Israel Journal of Medical Sciences*, 1969, *5*, 1107–1116.

Meijer, A. Generation chain relationships in families of asthmatic children. *Psychosomatics*, 1976, *17*, 213–217.

Meijer, A. Child psychiatry in a community health center. *Israel Annals of Psychiatry*, 1977, *15*, 232–244.

Meijer, A. The teaching of child mental health. *Acta Paedopsychiatrica*, 1979, *44*, 269–274. (a)

Meijer, A. Minimal brain dysfunction (Hebrew). *Israel Journal of Psychology and Counseling in Education*, 1979, *11*, 35–42. (b)

Meijer, A. Child psychiatry in the community—The ideal and the reality. In: U. Aviram & Y. Levav (eds.), *Community mental health in Israel*. Tel Aviv: Guma Science Books, Tserikover Ltd., 1981.

Quinton, D., & Rutter, M. Early hospital admissions and later disturbances of behaviour: An attempted replication of Douglas' findings. *Developmental Medicine and Child Neurology*, 1976, *18*, 447–459.

Robbins, L.C. The accuracy of parental recall of aspects of child development and of child rearing practices. *Journal of Abnormal Social Psychology*, 1963, *66*, 261–270.

Rutter, M. *Maternal deprivation reassessed*. England: Penguin Books, 1972.

Rutter, M. Separation, loss and family relationships. In: M. Rutter & L. Hersov (eds.), *Child psychiatry—Modern approaches*. Oxford: Blackwell Scientific Publications, 1976.

Rutter, M. Prospective studies to investigate behavioral change. In: J.S. Strauss, H.M. Babigian, & M. Roff (eds.), *The origins and course of psychopathology*. New York and London: Plenum Publishing Corp., 1977.

Rutter, M., & Brown, G.W. The reliability and validity of measures of family life and relationships in families containing a psychiatric patient. *Social Psychiatry*, 1966, *1*, 38–53.

Rutter, M., Tizard, J., & Whitmore, K. *Education, health and behaviour*. London: Longmans, 1970.

Schaefer, E.S., Droppleman, L.E., & Kalverboer, A.F. *Development of a classroom behavior checklist and factor analyses of children's school behavior in the United States and the Netherlands*. Proceedings of the Conference of the Society for Research in Child Development, San Francisco, 1965.

Shepherd, M., Oppenheim, B., & Mitchell, S. *Childhood behaviour and Mental Health*. London: University of London Press, 1971.

Thomas, A., Chess, S., & Birch, H.G. *Temperament and behaviour disorders in children*. London: University of London Press, 1968.

Wenar, C. The reliability of developmental histories: Summary and evaluation of evidence. *Psychosomatic Medicine*, 1963, *25*, 505–509.

Yarrow, M.R., Campbell, J.D., & Burton, R.V. Recollections of childhood: A study of the retrospective methods. *Monographs of the Society for Research in Child Development*, *35*, No. 5. Chicago: The University of Chicago Press, 1970.

Chapter 31

High-Risk Infants
without Intensive Care
Follow-Up at 9 Months

MARIA MAIA, M.D.
CÉLIA BARBOSA, M.D.
ROSELI GOMES, M.D.
Hospital de Crianças Maria Pia, Porto, Portugal

I T WAS RATHER DISTURBING TO HEAR FROM Hammersmith Hospital (London) that the rate of handicaps has not changed over a 15-year period (Jones, Cummins & Davies, 1979). Kitchen, Richards, Ryan, McDougall, Billson, Keir, and Naylor (1979) found more impairment in infants from intensive care units than from routine care nurseries. Paneth, Kiely, Stein, and Susser (1981) question the role of perinatal care in the outcome.

In light of such findings, it might be of interest to look at the follow-up of high-risk infants from the northern area of Portugal, which still has a very high perinatal mortality rate (Figure 1) and no intensive care nurseries.

METHODS AND DEFINITIONS

The authors' prospective study of high-risk infants from one maternity hospital covers a 12-month period (June 1, 1981–May 31, 1982). Criteria for an infant to be included in the study were: birth weight of less than 2,000 grams, respiratory distress syndrome (RDS) for more than 24 hours in the first days of life, bilirubinemia of 20 mg/dl, and neurological abnormalities in the neonatal period.

All infants were nursed in an intermediate care unit. Incubators were kept at 32°–34° C. with 60%–90% humidity. No pH estimations were available, but in cases with presumed metabolic acidosis (fetal distress or birth asphyxia), perfusions of glucose and sodium bicarbonate were given. For preterms greater than 1,300 grams, feeding with human milk was started 3 hours after birth, giving 35 cal/kg/day in the first 4 days, increased to 60 cal by the eighth day. In preterms less than 1,300 grams, perfusions of 5%–10% glucose solution (60–70 cal/kg/day) were given. Antibiotics were prescribed when necessary.

A form with details of the pregnancy, labor, and neonatal period was devised and filled out by the pediatric staff of the maternity hospital. Gestational age in preterms was determined by the last menstrual period. The infants were followed-up in the Children's Hospital using Mary Sheridan's method (Sheridan, 1975) and a neurological and general pediatric examination.

Cerebral palsy was defined as a disturbance of posture or movement of a nonprogressive kind. In diplegia, the lower limbs are more affected than upper limbs. In quadriplegia, the four limbs are severely affected and mental

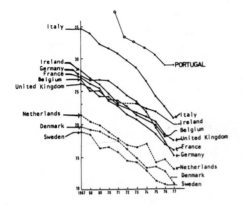

Figure 1. Incidence of perinatal mortality. (Adapted from Breart and Rumeau-Rouquette, 1980.)

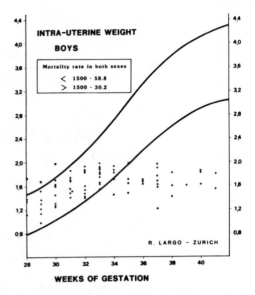

Figure 2. Male newborn distribution for gestational age and birth weight according to Largo et al. (1980) growth standards.

retardation and microcephaly are associated with the cerebral palsy. "Slight delay" in development refers to infants who were not sitting at 9 months but performed well in all other areas. In "moderate delay," the children were not sitting and did not perform some other items in manipulation-vision, hearing-language, or social behavior. In "severe delay," there were severe abnormalities in all areas of development. "Normal variant" was assigned to cases performing well in all areas but showing equinism in the upright position and automatic walking with normal reflexes.

POPULATION

In the study period there were 6,203 live-born infants of which 160 (2.5%) were born elsewhere and were transferred in soon after birth. Three hundred and twelve newborns had a birth weight less than or equal to 2,000 grams but 155 (49.6%) died in the neonatal period. For birth weights of less than 1,500 grams, the mortality rate was 58.8%.

According to the records of the 202 infants who entered the study (23.7% were born outside the maternity hospital), there were 157 with birth weights of less than 2,000 grams, 7 with RDS for more than 24 hours, 8 with bilirubinemia of greater than 20 mg/dl, and 30 with neurological abnormalities. All the infants with the last three diagnoses had birth weights of greater than 2,500 grams. In the low birth weight group, there was just one case with RDS and two with neonatal seizures.

At 9 months corrected age, 182 of 202 infants (90%) were examined. Of the 20 who missed follow-up, there was one cot death at 8 months, another infant died at 1½ months of an unknown cause, one was abroad, and 17 were lost. There were 30 twin pregnancies and three sets of triplets.

In the low birth weight group (Figure 2 and Figure 3), 142 infants were examined (75 were boys). Of these, 94 had a birth weight appropri-

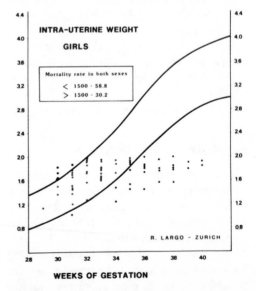

Figure 3. Female newborn distribution for gestational age and birth weight according to Largo et al. (1980) growth standards.

Table 1. Developmental abnormalities of 9-month-old infants with birth weights of less than 2,000 grams

		Delayed development			CP	Doubtful	Variant	Associated pathology
		Slight	Moderate	Severe				
AGA	<1,500		3		2		1	
	>1,500	1	5	1	1	1	1	1 fetal alcohol syndrome
SGA	<1,500	1						1 leprechaunism
	>1,500	3			1	1	4	2 microcephaly plus minor malformation

ate-for-gestational age (AGA) and 48 (33.8%) were small-for-gestational age (SGA) (Largo, Walli, Duc, Fanconi, & Prader, 1980). Birth weight for 37 children was less than 1,500 grams.

Just 21 infants were living in the city of Porto, Portugal; all others were scattered over the northern area of the country, some more than 150 miles away.

Social class was evaluated using the Graffar questionnaire (Graffar, 1961).

RESULTS

The abnormalities in the low birth weight group are shown in Table 1. Excluding the cases with associated pathology of obvious prenatal origin as well as the probable "normal variants" and the doubtful cases, there were definite abnormalities in 13 cases (Table 2). All of the CP cases were boys, and six of the "moderate delay" cases were also boys.

In the RDS group, there was one boy with a hydrocephaly who was operated on at 8 months who was "moderately delayed" at 9 months.

The group with the most severe abnormalities was the group of infants who entered the study with neurological problems (Table 3).

There were 8 out of 25 pathological cases (32%) and half were severe CP cases. These four severe cases were full-term infants with low Apgar scores, prolonged reanimation, and early and multiple fits during the neonatal period (Table 4).

All children with bilirubinemia of greater than 20 mg/dl had exchange transfusion and were well.

A summary of the abnormalities at 9 months in the 182 high-risk infants is shown in Table 5.

According to Graffar's classification (Figure 4), 91% of the total population in the study belongs to classes III and IV; in the low birth weight group, there was a higher proportion from the lowest class (79% coming from classes IV and V).

DISCUSSION

Many studies show that with intensive care, the outcome for low birth weight infants has been improving (Calame, Prod'Hom, & Van Melle, 1977; Fitzhardinge & Ramsay, 1973), with the lowest rate of handicap at 6% (Rawlings, Reynolds, Stewart, & Strang, 1971; Stewart, Turcan, Rawlings, & Reynolds, 1977).

For infants less than 2,000 grams born in

Table 2. Definite abnormalities at 9 months in the low birth weight group

	Birth weight	Delayed development		CP
		Moderate	Severe	
AGA	<1,500	3		2
	>1,500	5	1	1
SGA	<1,500			
	>1,500			1

Table 3. Developmental abnormalities at 9 months in the group with perinatal asphyxia

4 Quadriplegias
1 Diplegia
1 Focal fit at 7 months with hemiparesis
1 Brachial plexus injury (hydrocephalus operation at 5 months)
1 Moderate delay

England in 1946, the mortality was high, but at follow-up the rate of handicap was not different from the control group (Douglas & Gear, 1976), leading the authors to believe that the children with perinatal handicaps would have died.

Although Steiner, Sanders, Phillips, and Maddock (1980) report a handicap rate with routine care similar to that seen with intensive care, the authors' figures are higher: 13.5% (5/37) for infants less than 1,500 grams and 7.6% (8/105) for birth weight of greater than 1,500 grams. The survival rates recorded for birth weights of less than 1,500 grams were 41.2%, in contrast to 64.6% reported by Calame, Homberger, Gamper, Reymondi-Goni, Jaunin, Ducret, Van Melle, & Prod'Hom (1979) and 73% by Rawlings et al. (1971) for similar birth weights.

The most severe sequelae were, however, found in the group with neurological problems who had suffered birth asphyxia. Brown, Purvis, Forfar, and Cockburn (1974) reported 12% of severe handicaps in such infants and Thomson, Searle, and Russell (1977) reported 7%. From Hammersmith Hospital for the period 1966–1971, Scott (1976) reports (2/23) 8.6% with severe quadriplegia.

The authors' figures are much higher—16% (4/25). Such numbers of severe forms of CP in full-term newborns nursed with no assisted ventilation or blood gas estimations point to the importance of intensive care in preventing handicap.

Table 5. Total developmental abnormalities at 9 months in the different groups that entered the study

Birth weight ⩽2,000 grams	13/142 (9.1%)
RDS for more than 24 hours	1/7 (14.2%)
Neurological problems	8/25 (32%)

This high rate of handicaps in full-terms was not surprising because in a survey of 454 CP cases (Maia, 1982), 60% were of perinatal cause (Table 6), mainly birth asphyxia, and there were just 29 preterms and 20 small-for-dates infants in the whole group. Twenty cases of kernicterus (14 of them born after 1970) must still be accounted for in the survey.

From Sweden, Hagberg (1979) reports a slight increase of spastic diplegia in low birth weight infants in recent years. Such cases may represent the price to be paid for saving a great number of normal babies. Those cases of diplegia, however, tend to be only slightly affected from the motor point of view and the children are of normal intelligence. Being a European country that shows perinatal and neonatal mortality rates similar to those of developing countries, most of Portugal's cerebral palsy cases are severe and in full-term infants.

Developed countries take perinatal intensive care for granted and its role is studied only with respect to low birth weight infants (Paneth et al., 1981). It has been suggested in experimental mammals that preterm animals withstand lack of oxygen better than the more mature animal (Mott, 1961). If one of the major roles of developmental studies is the assessment of

Table 6. Causes of cerebral palsy in 454 cases

Prenatal	52 (20 SGA)	11.4%
Perinatal	274 (29 AGA)[a]	60.3%
Postnatal	78	17.1%
Untraceable	50	11.0%

[a]20 kernicterus; 14 born after 1970.

Table 4. Neonatal events in the four cases with severe cerebral palsy

Birth weight	Place of birth	Apgar (1 min.)	Reanimation	Early fits	Stay in (days)
3,350	Out	2	20m	+++	33
3,800	In	?	>20m	+++	29
3,540	In	3	20m	+++	30
3,800	In	?	?	++	20

+++ = multiple fits.
++ = several fits.

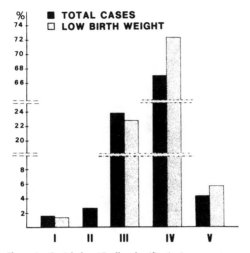

Figure 4. Social class (Graffar classification).

perinatal care, asphyxiated babies and cases with neonatal seizures should not be excluded. In the American National Collaborative Perinatal Project (Niswander & Gordon, 1972), 277 infants with neonatal seizures were 0.5% of the total population but accounted for 21% of the CP cases (only 27 were less than 1,500 grams) (Holden, Mellits, & Freeman, 1982). In judging the role of intensive care in prevention of handicaps, the full-term asphyxiated infant must be included (Brann, Chapter 18, this volume).

The authors are aware that reducing handicaps in Portugal is not just a question of sophisticated neonatal nursing but probably more a question of prenatal care and medical organization.

REFERENCES

Breart, G. & Rumeau-Rouquette, C. Mortalité périnatale et mortalité neonatale infantile [Perinatal mortality and infantile neonatal mortality]. In *Encyclopedie de Pédiatrie [Encyclopedia of Pediatrics]*, p. 4002, F. 50–2, Paris; Editions Techniques S.A., 1980.

Brown, J.K., Purvis, R.J., Forfar, J.O., & Cockburn, F. Neurological aspects of perinatal asphyxia. *Developmental Medicine and Child Neurology*, 1974, *16*, 567–580.

Calame, A., Homberger, C., Gamper, J., Reymondi-Goni, I., Jaunin, L., Ducret, S., Van Melle, G., & Prod'Hom, L.S. Neurodevelopmental outcome of preterm and small-for-date infants. *Perinatal medicine* (Proceedings of the Sixth European Congress, Vienna). Stuttgart: Thieme Publishers, 1979.

Calame, A., Prod'Hom, L.S., & Van Melle, G. Outcome of infants of very low birthweight treated in neonatal intensive care unit. *Revue de Epidémiologie et Santé Publique* [Journal of Epidemiology and Public Health], 1977, *25*, 21–32.

Douglas, J.W.B., & Gear, R. Children of low birthweight in the 1946 national cohort. *Archives of Disease in Childhood*, 1976, *51*, 820–827.

Fitzhardinge, P.M., & Ramsay, M. The improving outlook for the small prematurely born infant. *Developmental Medicine and Child Neurology*, 1973, *15*, 447–459.

Graffar, M. *Étude sociale des echantillons en croissance et développement de l'enfant normal [Samples of social class and development of the normal child]*. Paris, Masson Publishing, 1961.

Hagberg, B. Epidemiological and preventive aspects of cerebral palsy and severe mental retardation in Sweden. *European Journal of Pediatrics*, 1979, *130*, 71–78.

Holden, K.R., Mellits, E.D., & Freeman, J.M. Neonatal seizures. I Correlation of prenatal and perinatal events with outcomes. *Pediatrics*, 1982, *70*, 165–176.

Jones, R.A.K., Cummins, M., & Davies, P.A. Infants of

very low birthweight. A 15 year analysis. *Lancet*, 1979, *i*, 1332–1335.

Kitchen, W.H., Richards, A., Ryan, M.M., McDougall, A.B., Billson, F.A., Keir, E.H., & Naylor, F.D. A longitudinal study of very low-birthweight infants. II Results of controlled trial of intensive care and incidence of handicaps. *Developmental Medicine and Child Neurology*, 1979, *21*, 582–589.

Largo, R.H., Walli, R., Duc., G., Fanconi, A., & Prader, A. Evolution of perinatal growth. Presentation of combined intra and extrauterine growth standards for weight, length and head circumference. *Helvetica Paediatrica Acta*, 1980, *35*, 419–436.

Maia, M.C. Prevenção da Deficiência na criança. A nossa realidade [Prevention of handicap in children. The facts in Portugal]. *Rev. Portuguesa de Pediatria [Portuguese Journal of Pediatrics]*, 1982, *13*, 25a–34a.

Mott, J.C. The ability of young mammals to withstand total oxygen lack. *British Medical Bulletin*, 1961, *17*, 144.

Niswander, K., & Gordon, M. *The women and their pregnancies*. National Institute of Health publication 73-379. United States Department of Health, Education and Welfare, 1972.

Paneth, N., Kiely, J.L., Stein, Z. & Susser, M. Cerebral palsy and newborn care. III Estimated prevalence rates of mortality and impairment of low-birthweight infants. *Developmental Medicine and Child Neurology*, 1981, *23*, 801–807.

Rawlings, G., Reynolds, E.O.R., Stewart, A., & Strang, L.B. Changing prognosis for infants of very low birthweight. *Lancet*, 1971, *i*, 516–519.

Scott, H. Outcome of very severe birth asphyxia. *Archives of Disease in Childhood*, 1976, *51*, 712–716.

Sheridan, M.D. *Children's developmental progress from birth to five years. The STYCAR Sequences*. Windsor, England: NFER Publishing Co., 1975.

Steiner, E.S., Sanders, E.M., Phillips, E.C.K., & Maddock, C.R. Very low birthweight children at school age: Comparison of neonatal management methods. *British Medical Journal*, 1980, *281*, 1237–1240.

Stewart, A.L., Turcan, D.M., Rawlings, G., & Reynolds, E.O.R. Prognosis for infants weighing 1000 g or less at birth. *Archives of Disease in Childhood*, 1977, *52*, 97–104.

Thomson, A.J., Searle, M., & Russell G. Quality of survival after severe birth asphyxia. *Archives of Disease in Childhood*, 1977, *52*, 620–626.

Chapter 32

Neurological Development and Assessment in Infants at Risk

RICHARD MICHAELIS, M.D.
GERHARD HAAS, M.D.
MONIKA BUCHWALD-SAAL, M.D.
Eberhard-Karls University, Tuebingen, West Germany

NEUROLOGICAL EXAMINATIONS ARE NOT ALways believed to be an essential part of a comprehensive developmental assessment in infants at risk. It is of interest to find no chapter about infant neurology in Osofsky's *Handbook of Infant Development* (Osofsky, 1979), nor in Tjossem's *Intervention Strategies for High Risk Infants and Young Children* (Tjossem, 1976), nor in other related books concerned with infants at risk. One of the reasons why neurological examinations are rarely performed or are not even discussed may be the lack of a well-designed and generally accepted procedure. Another reason might be the opinion that information obtained by a neurological examination is of inferior value compared to information from assessments of psychophysiological, cognitive, or socioeconomical behavior and development, since for a long time these kinds of assessments have been proven to be helpful in evaluating developmental profiles. Such profiles are used to decide if an infant should participate in an intervention program. They also provide criteria of developmental progress in an infant. But in most of the affected infants, developmental profiles do not offer information about the factors causing the developmental impairment or retardation.

On the other hand, neurological assessments not only provide details of neurological development, but also yield information about impairment of neural functions. The findings refer to underlying structural or functional defects of the brain, which might explain *why* an infant fails partly or entirely in his or her development. It is the purpose of this chapter to discuss:

1. Which type of neurological examination to use in infants at risk
2. The findings of a neurological examination
3. Which findings of a neurological examination are sufficient to yield reliable information for decisions with respect to diagnosis, prognosis, and therapy
4. Some particular aspects of neurological assessment

THE NEUROLOGICAL EXAMINATION

Over the last 10 years, the rationale of Prechtl's neurology of the newborn has been especially helpful with respect to a neurology of infants (Prechtl, 1977). As with neurology of newborns, the neurology of infants and very young children must be conceived as primarily a neurology of neural functions and, in a much lesser degree, as a neurology of topical lesions of the brain. During infancy and early childhood, the central nervous system is still undergoing a changing and dynamic process of development. Therefore, it is reasonable to accept the rationale of Prechtl's newborn neurology and apply it to a neurology of infants. Nevertheless, it is necessary to admit that a generally accepted design of a neurological examination of infants so far does not exist. Those who employ Prechtl's rationale in respect to infants are using a rather empirical and pragmatic approach. A well-designed neurological examination of infants will, however, be available in the future.

It is not the intention of this chapter to present detailed information about the authors' design of a neurology of infants, but, it will focus on some of the basic aspects. A neurological examination of infants should include evaluation of the following:

Posture in the supine, prone, sitting, and standing positions
Spontaneous motor activity
Resistance against passive movements
Power of active movements (kinetic and static) (Paine & Oppé, 1966)
Deep tendon reflexes
Pyramidal signs
Cranial nerves
Postural reactions like the Landau reaction, asymmetric tonic neck reflex, parachute reactions of the arms, and head control
Neonatal motor responses like the Moro response
Threshold response (excitability)
Vision and hearing

The external conditions at the beginning and during the examination need particular attention, since infants are easily distressed by an inappropriate environment and by insensitive handling during the examination. It is essential to examine infants only in appropriate behavioral states as they were defined by Touwen (Touwen, 1976). The appropriate states are:

State 3: Eyes open, no active movements, relaxed
State 4: Eyes open, active movements, fully cooperative, anticipating

All other states like fussiness, crying, or drowsiness can generate unreliable results.

Infants are no longer newborns. They often vigorously resist examination in the prone or supine positions, thereby shifting out of state 3 and state 4. To keep them in states 3 and 4, infants may also be examined sitting on the lap of their mothers.

The course of the examination should follow a standardized sequence, starting with the least distressing items and concluding with the most intrusive. However, one quite often has to adjust the sequence of the examination to the activities of the infant, trying to catch positions and movements in which valid results can be obtained.

NEUROLOGICAL FINDINGS

Abnormal neurological findings in infants are described best by terms that define deviant neural functions. The same concept was used by Prechtl in his neurology of newborns. Single abnormal neurological findings are of little significance. The significance increases if single findings can be combined with other abnormal neurological findings. Using this concept, most deviant neurological findings might be clustered into different types of neural dysfunctions. These types are:

Abnormal and persistent postural responses
Dysfunction in control of motility (hyper/hypo/dyskinesia)
Dysfunction in control of muscle tone (hyper/hypo/dystonia)
Dysfunction in threshold responses (hyper/hypoexcitability, instability of states)
Abnormal and persistent neonatal motor responses
Dysfunction of cranial nerves
Dysfunction of tendon reflexes (faint, absent, exaggerated)
Asymmetries in motility, posture, muscle tone, and tendon reflexes
Dysfunction in postural responses of head and trunk (Landau response, traction response)

The grouping of deviant neurological findings into specific types of neural dysfunctions seems to be a descriptive one. But only this kind of organization will offer basic information with respect to diagnosis, etiology, prognosis, and therapy in a retarded infant.

NEURONAL DYSFUNCTION AND MENTAL AND MOTOR RETARDATION

In most of the infants suffering from developmental retardation, characteristic combinations 'of specific types of neural dysfunctions will be found. These combinations offer information that is essential to diagnostic decisions. The most important of these neurological categories, from a clinical point of view, is described below in some detail.

The combination of muscular hypertonia and hyperexcitability is found rather frequently in infants at risk. These infants often suffered from perinatal complications and asphyxia. Mild neurological symptoms might be seen up to the age of 6–8 months. In almost all of the infants, the developmental course after the first year of life will be normal. Hypertonia and hyperexcitability as a specific type of neural dysfunction signal some kind of transitory central deficiency in controlling muscle tone and threshold responses (Figure 1).

The combination of muscular hypertonia, dyskinesia, persistent and abnormal postural responses, and exaggerated tendon reflexes are not only found frequently during the first months of life in infants at risk, but also in infants not at risk. If the neurological findings are decreasing during the first year of life, the prognosis will be a good one. If the neurological findings persist or even increase, closer investigations should be started to gain a final diagnosis, which might be a neurodegenerative white matter disease, like orthochromatic leukodystrophy or some kind of cerebral palsy (Figure 2).

In infants presenting muscular hypotonia, the same steps in decision-making should be used. The combination of muscular hypotonia, normal tendon reflexes, and no mental but motor retardation will often be seen in infants with the syndrome of benign, congenital hypotonia described by Dubowitz (1978). The prognosis will be a good one. If the tendon reflexes are found to be faint or absent, neuro-

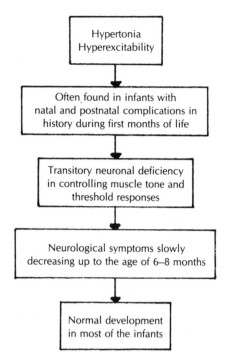

Figure 1. Muscle hypertonia and hyperexcitability in infants at risk.

degenerative diseases with late onset of mental retardation or some kind of neuromuscular or lower motor neuron disorder might again be the final diagnosis. In all of these disorders, genetic counseling is necessary (Figure 3).

The combination of muscular hypotonia, hypokinesia, and normal tendon reflexes will also be found in infants with benign congenital hypotonia. Yet, if mental retardation is also found, chromosomal anomalies, syndromes combined with mental retardation, or primary mental retardation have to be considered. Parents need genetic counseling if they still want to have additional children (Figure 4).

SOME PARTICULAR ASPECTS OF NEUROLOGICAL ASSESSMENTS

Neurological assessment in infants at risk will be especially helpful if used apart from developmental assessment and not only in consideration of motor development. If an infant is found to be retarded in his or her motor development, neurological assessment may provide information as to the cause. Cerebral palsy as well as neuromuscular or neurodegenerative diseases must be considered.

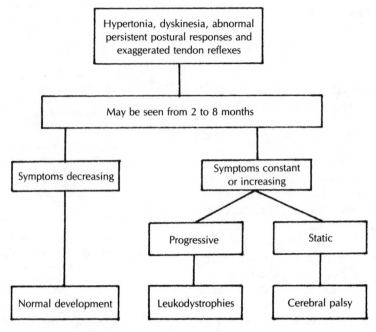

Figure 2. Developmental abnormalities in infants presenting with hypertonia, dyskinesia, and abnormal postural patterns during first year of life.

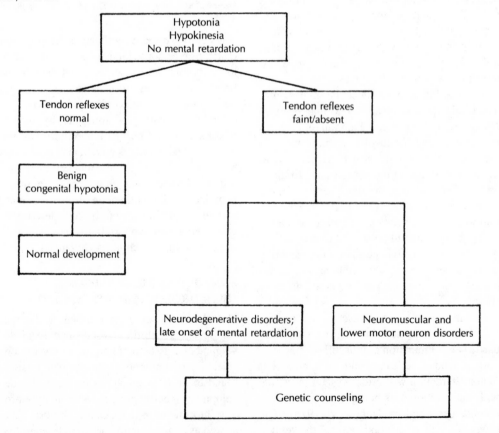

Figure 3. Diagnostic decisions based on tendon reflexes in infants presenting with hypotonia.

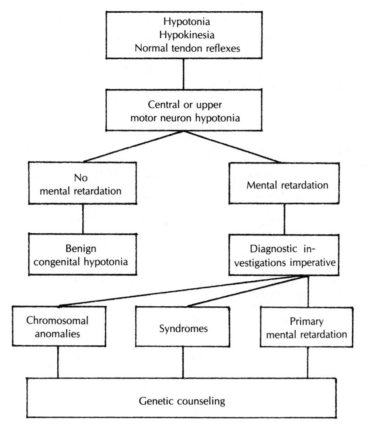

Figure 4. Diagnostic decisions based on abnormalities of mental development in infants presenting with hypotonia.

There are neurological items that are closely dependent on the infant's age. Neonatal motor responses such as the Moro response should no longer be present after the age of 6 months. The same holds true for some postural reactions such as the asymmetric tonic neck reflex or the palmar grasps response (Sheridan, 1981). Some other postural reactions like the Landau response or the head control will improve during the first year of life (Sheridan, 1981). Abnormal neonatal and postural responses will dominate posture and spontaneous motor activities. These kinds of patterns usually are of pathognomonic value, for example, in infants suffering cerebral palsy (Illingworth, 1966). If postural reactions like head control or the Landau reaction are absent, gross motor retardation will be found in infants with muscular hypotonia as well as infants with cerebral palsy.

Diagnostic decisions are especially urgent in infants showing motor retardation due to severe muscular hypotonia (Taft & Barabas, 1982). Muscular hypotonia is known to be a symptom of many different disorders, all needing special diagnostic procedures. One should no longer accept the diagnosis of "hypotonic cerebral palsy" in retarded infants because, with this diagnosis, there is danger that no diagnostic tests will be done and physical therapy will be inappropriately used without the proper diagnosis. The result might be disasterous if another infant is born in the family with the same problem.

Finally, it has been the experience of those who see infants at risk neurologically that many of these infants present serious abnormal neurological findings during their first year, but do not show any developmental abnormalities later in childhood. Plasticity of neuronal functions during the first years of age may account for this very specific and interesting phenomenon of transient neuronal dysfunction.

It has been the intention of this chapter to emphasize the value of infant neurology in developmental assessments. The results from neurological examinations are especially useful in providing information about causes of delays in development.

REFERENCES

Dubowitz, V. *Muscle disorders in childhood*. Philadelphia: W.B. Saunders Co., 1978.

Illingworth, R.S. The diagnosis of cerebral palsy in the first year of life. *Developmental Medicine and Child Neurology*, 1966, *8*, 178–194.

Osofsky, I.D. (ed.). *Handbook of infant development*. New York: John Wiley & Sons, 1979.

Paine, R.S., & Oppé, T.E. Neurological examination of children. *Clinics in Developmental Medicine*, No. 20/21. London: Heinemann; and Philadelphia: J.B. Lippincott, 1966.

Prechtl, H.F.R. The neurological examination of the full term newborn infant. *Clinics in Developmental Medicine*, No. 63 (2nd ed.). London: Heinemann; and Philadelphia: J.B. Lippincott, 1977.

Sheridan, M.D. *From birth to five years: Children's developmental progress*. Windsor, England: NFER-Nelson Publishing Company Ltd., 1981.

Taft, L.T., & Barabas, G. Infants with delayed motor performance. *Pediatric Clinic of North America*, 1982, *28*, 137–149.

Tjossem, T.D. *Intervention strategies for high risk infants and young children*. Baltimore: University Park Press, 1976.

Touwen, B.T. Neurological development in infancy. *Clinics in Developmental Medicine*, No. 58. London: Heinemann; and Philadelphia: J.B. Lippincott, 1976.

Chapter 33

The Motor Development
of Fat Infants

Michael Jaffe, M.B.Ch.B, M.R.C.P., D.C.H.
Celia Cozakov, M.D.
Hanna Khoushy Child Development Center, Haifa, Israel

It may seem logical to assume that a baby will be slow in motor development if he or she is fat. In fact, physicians often make that statement to mothers. There is, however, minimal objective evidence to support this contention. Only two references on the subject have been found in the available literature. Peatman and Higgons, in 1942, found no correlation between weight and motor development in infants. A study by Norval, in 1947, demonstrated a weak correlation between the age of walking on the one hand and birth weight and length on the other. No attempt was made, however, to relate walking age to the parameters of weight and length measured at the time of walking.

This problem was considered by the authors to be sufficiently important to merit further study, using accepted developmental assessment schedules, and criteria of excessive weight.

MATERIAL AND METHODS

The cohort group consisted of 136 healthy infants, ages 6–18 months, attending infant welfare clinics in the Haifa area. Excluded from the study were all low birth weight and premature infants, as well as those who demonstrated specific pathologies, such as Down syndrome, microcephalus, or clinical evidence of neurological damage. Apart from the categories excluded, the group was a random one and resembled the general population with regard to both socioeconomic and ethnic distribution.

The following procedure was performed on each infant:

1. A comprehensive family, gestational, perinatal, and postnatal history was obtained.
2. A general physical examination was conducted, with special emphasis placed on dysmorphic features possibly indicating a specific syndrome.
3. An age-appropriate neurological examination (Paine & Oppe, 1966) was administered.
4. Psychomotor abilities were assessed using the Sheridan Stycar Developmental Assessment Schedules (Sheridan, 1978). This assessment procedure is used extensively in British child development units as well as in infant welfare clinics. Developmental age levels are obtained in four spheres of development: a) posture and gross motor function, b) fine motor (adaptive) function, c) speech, and d) social behavior. Vision and hearing are also assessed at each age level.

5. Should the infant respond to less than one-half of the age-appropriate items in a particular area of development, he or she is regarded as showing a developmental delay. For the purposes of this study, a significant developmental delay was defined as a lag in one of the spheres of development of at least 3 months. This degree of lag was chosen because it is clearly measurable.

6. Supine length was measured, using a stationary headboard with a sliding vertical footpiece on the horizontal board, to which a metal tape measure was attached. Weight was measured using standard infant scales verified as accurate. Tanner weight and height charts were used (Tanner & Whitehouse, 1976). Sveger's index of body weight (Sveger, 1978) was calculated for each infant as follows:

$$\frac{\text{Actual weight}}{\text{Actual height}} = A$$

$$\frac{\text{50th percentile expected weight for age}}{\text{50th percentile expected height for age}} = B$$

$$\frac{A}{B} \times 100 = \text{Sveger's index of body weight}$$

Normal weight was defined as an index of 91–110. Overweight was defined as an index of 111–120. Obesity was defined as an index of above 120.

RESULTS

The 136 babies were separated into two main groups according to their body weight (Sveger's Index) (Table 1). One baby of normal weight who demonstrated general delay was subsequently found to be retarded and was excluded from the study. The remaining 135 normal weight and fat babies were either developing normally or showed only significant gross motor delay; fine motor, adaptive, social, and language development were normal. General medical and neurological examinations performed on all the infants revealed no evidence of systematic disease or neurological damage.

Statistically, using the chi-square test at the level of $p = .05$, the findings (Tables 2 and 3) were as follows. a) The fat babies, for the age range examined, demonstrated a significant delay in motor development as compared to normal weight babies. b) In subdividing the fat babies into an overweight and obese group, it was found that a significantly greater percentage of obese infants had delayed motor development ($p < .05$): of 11 obese infants, four showed motor delay (36%), as compared to 13 of 45 overweight infants (29%). Thus the degree of excess weight was associated with increased incidence of motor delay. Although the numbers in the obese group are small, the differences are statistically significant.

A follow-up general examination and developmental assessment, utilizing the same techniques, was performed on the group of motor-delayed babies 1 year later. (This included both the fat and the normal weight motor-delayed babies.) Of the seven normal weight motor-delayed babies, all were developing normally 1 year later. Fourteen of the 17 fat babies reexamined 1 year later revealed levels of motor development recorded in Table 4. Despite the fact that three overweight babies were lost to follow-up, certain trends were evident 1 year later. a) The majority, 10 (71%), of the fat delayed babies were now of normal weight and developing normally. b) Three (21%) of the babies remained fat and motor delayed (the total number is too small to be

Table 1. Distribution of cohort according to body weight

Body weight	Number of babies
Normal	80[a]
Overweight	56
Obese	11

[a]One baby was found to be retarded and was excluded from study.

Table 2. Relationship of gross motor function to body weight

Body weight	Total infants	Motor development	
		Normal function	Gross delay
Normal	79	72 (91%)	7 (9%)
Fat	56	39 (70%)	17 (30%)
Overweight	45	32 (71%)	13 (29%)
Obese	11	7 (64%)	4 (36%)

Table 3. Age distribution related to motor delay

	Age (months)				
	6,7,8	9,10,11	12,13,14	15,16,17,18	Total
Normal weight group					
Motor delay	2	2	2	1	7
Total number in group	14	34	11	20	79
Fat group (overweight + obese)					
Motor delay	5	1	5	6	17
Total number in group	20	11	11	14	56

statistically significant). c) One baby was still overweight but had caught up in motor development. d) All the originally normal weight motor-delayed infants were now developing normally.

DISCUSSION

From these findings, it is evident that a correlation does exist between excessive weight in babies and gross motor delay (i.e., the greater the degree of excessive weight, the greater the probability of the delay becoming manifest). No attempt was made to elucidate the cause/effect relationship of this observation (i.e., are babies slow in motor development because they are primarily fat, or do certain infants have an inherent predisposition to less activity or slow motor development, and, as a consequence, expend fewer calories and accumulate fatty tissue?).

A survey of the literature revealed observations associating excess weight and decreased motor activity. Mayer (quoted by Passmore, 1963) noted that obese girls playing tennis were stationary on the court for 80% of the time. Kennedy (1957), in attempting to elucidate the possible cause-effect sequence of inactivity and excess weight, was able to induce hypothalamic obesity in rats by artificially restricting their motor activity. Thus, in an experimental situation, motor inactivity caused obesity by disturbing the physiological regulation of body weight. Wenzell, Stults, and Mayer (1962) demonstrated low serum iron levels in obese adolescents with normal hemoglobin levels. They postulated that this may reflect a low myoglobin synthesis, and thus provide a physiological explanation for muscular inactivity.

The longitudinal follow-up of the fat motor-delayed babies indicated a tendency to revert to both normal weight and normal development over the ensuing year. It is not clear from the study whether weight reduction caused the catch-up in motor development or vice versa. The persistence of excessive weight and associated motor delay in three of the 14 fat babies (21%) may indicate a trend, but the numbers are too small to be significant.

It can, therefore, be concluded from this study that a definite correlation does exist between excessive weight and motor delay in younger babies, but that both the body weight and the motor development tend to revert to normal over the ensuing year in the majority of babies. It must be stressed that the majority of fat babies do have normal motor development. In any given infant, therefore, before it is concluded that motor delay is associated with obesity, a comprehensive medical and neuro-developmental assessment must be performed, because mental retardation, neuromuscular disturbance, or a general medical condition such as hypothyroidism may be the underlying cause.

SUMMARY

The motor development of a group of fat babies was compared with that of a group of normal weight babies. A significant correlation was

Table 4. Fourteen fat babies examined 1 year later

Number of fat babies	Reexamination	
	Weight	Motor development
10 (71%)	Normal	Normal
1 (8%)	Overweight	Normal
3 (21%)	Fat	Motor delay
(2 overweight)		
(1 obese)		

found between excessive weight and gross motor delay. Over the ensuing year, both weight and development reverted to normal in the majority of infants. The possible relationship between these observations was discussed, and a plea was made that a comprehensive evaluation of the motor-delayed overweight infant be performed before concluding that the delay is due solely to the excessive weight.

REFERENCES

Kennedy, G.C. The development with age of hypothalamic restraint upon the appetite of the rat. *Journal of Endocrinology*, 1957, *1*, 9012–9014.

Norval, M.A. Relationship of weight and length of infants at birth, to the age of which they begin to walk alone. *The Journal of Pediatrics*, 1947, *30*, 676–678.

Paine, R.S., Oppe, T.E. Neurological examination of children. *Clinics in Developmental Medicine*, No. 20/21. London: Heinemann Medical Books, 1966.

Passmore, R. *IVth International Nutrition Congress*. *Lancet*, 1963, 2, 457.

Peatman, J.G., & Higgons, R.A. Relation of infant's weight and body build to locomotor development. *American Journal of Orthopsychiatry*, 1942, *12*, 234–236.

Sheridan, M. *Sheridan Stycar developmental sequences*. Windsor, Ontario: NFER Publishing Company Ltd., 1978.

Sveger, T. Does overnutrition or obesity during the first year affect weight at age four? *Acta Pediatrica Scandinavica*, 1978, *67*, 465–467.

Tanner, J.M., & Whitehouse, R.H. Clinical longitudinal standards for height, weight, height velocity, weight velocity and the stages of puberty. *Archives of Disease of Childhood*, 1976, *51*, 170–174.

Wenzell, B.J., Stults, H., & Mayer, J. Hypoferremia in obese adolescents. *Lancet*, 1962, 2, 327–328.

The At-Risk Infant: Psycho/Socio/Medical Aspects
edited by Shaul Harel, M.D., and Nicholas J. Anastasiow, Ph.D.
Copyright © 1985   Paul H. Brookes Publishing Co., Inc.   Baltimore • London

A New Technique for the Study of Central Modulation of Sensory-Autonomic Pathways in Preterm Infants

Lewis A. Leavitt, M.D.
James N. Ver Hoeve, Ph.D.
Waisman Center on Mental Retardation and Human Development
Madison, Wisconsin

O VER THE PAST SEVERAL YEARS, DEFICITS IN cardiac and respiratory control have become of increasing concern in the care of preterm infants. Polygraphic studies have shown that even the "healthy" preterm infant is characterized by a high rate of apnea and bradycardia, both of which frequently increase during sleep (Schulte, 1977). Moreover, for a substantial proportion of preterm infants, apnea and bradycardia episodes present more serious problems. These complications include the need for mechanical ventilatory assistance, central stimulants, and resuscitation.

STUDYING CENTRAL AUTONOMIC INSTABILITY

The long-term sequelae of autonomic difficulties during preterm life have not yet been fully determined, although epidemiological studies have shown that preterm infants face a statistically higher risk for succumbing to sudden infant death syndrome (SIDS) (Beal, 1983; Valdes-Dapena, 1980) and are overrepresented in registers of mentally and physically handicapped children (Hunt, 1981). The extent to which central autonomic instability in the preterm infant is directly linked to later problems such as SIDS is problematic. However, it is of interest that the preterm infant shares at least one feature with the SIDS victim, namely, the failure to respond during sleep to powerful sensory stimuli that normally induce arousal and a resumption of normal physiology.

Polysomnograph Study

There have been a number of approaches to the study of autonomic deficit early in life. The foremost of these is the sleep study or polysomnogram, in which heart rate, respiration, and other bioelectric activity are monitored through several cycles of sleep and wakefulness (Guilleminault, 1982). The methods of analyzing sleep records have become increas-

This project received partial support from a NIH Biomedical Research Support Grant to the University of Wisconsin Medical School as well as Waisman Core Grant 5 P30 HD03352. David Sheftel, M.D., performed state ratings and assessed the medical status of the infants in this study. The authors wish to thank the pediatric and nursing staff of Madison General Hospital, Madison, Wisconsin, for their cooperation in the conduct of these studies.

ingly sophisticated in recent years (Guilleminault, Ariagno, Forno, Nagel, Baldwin, & Owen, 1979; Harper, Sclabassi, & Estrin, 1974). These studies have shown small, but statistically reliable, differences in cardiac and respiratory patterns in populations at increased risk for SIDS (Guilleminault, Ariagno, Korobkin, Coons, Owen-Boeddiker, & Baldwin, 1981; Steinschneider, 1977).

The fact that, in increased-risk infants, deficits in cardiorespiratory function are related to the stage of sleep–wakefulness is consistent with the view that SIDS victims have subtle defects in brain stem mechanisms early in postnatal life (McGinty & Sterman, 1980). From a clinical standpoint, although it is possible to distinguish infants who are at increased risk for SIDS, there remains the problem of determining the course of action for the vast majority of infants who hover near the edge of the statistical confidence interval. Indeed, because the autonomic nervous system is a highly regulated feedback system with many levels of redundancy, differences in tonic levels (e.g., basal cardiac and respiratory rate) might be expected to be minimized even in a partially defective system.

Nervous System Response Assessment

Another approach to the study of autonomic deficit has been to assess nervous system responses in increased-risk infants. Infants who have had a "near miss" SIDS episode (i.e., have been resuscitated after presumed pulmonary arrest), have been reported to exhibit abnormal ventilatory responses under hypoxic conditions (Brady, Chir, Ariagno, Watts, Goldman, & Dumpit, 1978; Shannon & Kelly, 1978). Abnormal brain stem auditory evoked responses (BAERs) also have been reported in infants who have had a near miss episode. Orlowski, Nodar, and Lonsdale (1979) reported delayed conduction times in aborted SIDS cases. Although these findings are consistent with the widely held belief that SIDS victims have deficiencies in brain stem function early in life, it has been impossible to determine whether these brain stem abnormalities are secondary to near miss episodes (see also Stockard, 1982).

BRAIN STEM MATURATION ASSESSMENT AND THE PRESTIMULATION EFFECT

The authors have been interested in assessing the maturation of a brain stem mechanism that modulates reflex responsiveness based upon antecedent sensory conditions. The premise of applying this approach to the study of preterm cardiorespiratory control is twofold. First, the *responsiveness* of the autonomic nervous system is considered more likely to exhibit abnormalities than its tonic activity. Second, the prestimulation effect depends upon levels of the brain stem that have global, cross-modal modulatory effects over autonomic activation. This means that the modulatory mechanisms are organized at a higher level in the nervous system and are thus more vulnerable than lower level mechanisms. In addition, due to the cross-modal nature of the prestimulation effect, it is expected that these centers are also activated under hypoxic or other conditions that ordinarily cause an increase in autonomic activity.

The effects of prior stimulation in this context are unlearned and may be facilitatory or inhibitory (Graham, 1975). In the typical procedure, the subject is presented trials of prestimulus-plus-probe and trials of probe-alone. The probe-alone trials constitute a control condition. The effect of the prestimulus is assessed by comparing the prestimulus-plus-probe trials to the probe-alone trials. This prestimulation effect has been studied extensively in adults and animals. In the adult, sensory events presented 30 to about 300 msec prior to a startling stimulus inhibit the amplitude of flexor and cardiac reflexes evoked by the reflex-eliciting stimulus (S2) (Chalmers & Hoffman, 1973; Graham, Strock, & Zeigler, 1981; Hoffman & Ison, 1980). Continuous prestimulation 1 sec or more before S2 often results in a facilitated response (Graham, Putnam, & Leavitt, 1975).

Recent neurophysiological studies indicate that the prestimulation effect depends upon an area of the rostral medial brain stem (nucleus cuneiformis, and nucleus parabrachialis). Leitner, Powers, Stitt, and Hoffman (1981) found that the nucleus cuneiformis, located in the midbrain tegmentum, is crucial for sensory inhibition of the startle flexor reflex. Wright and Barnes (1972) also found that these sub-collicular areas are involved in acoustic inhibition of electrically elicited hindlimb reflexes. These latter investigators found that areas lateral to the inhibitory areas were involved in sensory facilitatory effects. Micro-electrode studies have shown that these mid-brain regions also participate in the initiation and maintenance of sleep states (e.g., Sakai, 1980; Steriade, Oakson, & Ropert, 1982) and may play a role in breathing during sleep (Orem, 1980; Orem & Netick, 1982). It is of interest that this brain stem area, rostral to the medullary centers of pneumotaxis, has been found to evidence fibrillary gliosis in SIDS victims (see, e.g., Becker, 1983; Guilleminault et al., 1979; cf., Pearson & Brandeis, 1983).

Also of interest is the finding that abrupt sensory events preferentially stimulate other centers lower in the brain stem that are endogenously activated during sleep and result in EEG spike activity and powerful neuromuscular inhibition (Glenn & Dement, 1982). It is known that these centers are activated by abrupt stimuli in many modalities and appear to be responsible for startle reflexes (Chan & Barnes, 1972). This is particularly relevant to the study of sleep-related apnea, since several investigators have suggested that life-threatening apnea and bradycardia may result from abnormally prolonged episodes of phasic sleep-related descending inhibition (Iwamura, 1971; Schulte, 1979). Thus, the study of the acoustic-startle response and its modification by prior stimuli during sleep holds the potential for uncovering generalized arousal differences between increased-risk and normal infants and relating these effects to brain stem areas that exert modulatory control over the autonomic nervous system.

AN NICU STUDY
OF PRESTIMULATION

During the course of studies on the development of the prestimulus effect in healthy premature infants, the authors had the opportunity to test several infants, during their stay in a neonatal intensive care unit (NICU), who were experiencing persistent bradycardia and apnea. This chapter presents preliminary data on the effects of prestimulation on the cardiac response of several apneic infants together with age-matched controls.

Procedure

Each subject was tested during active sleep, in order to reduce variability due to state differences, and on the basis that one is more likely to see autonomic deficit in this age group and in this state (Guilleminault et al., 1981). For practical reasons, each subject was tested in the NICU in a closed Isolette (Airshields, Inc.). During a 10-sec period prior to each trial, a neonatologist rated the subject's state according to Prechtl's (1974) classification in terms of gross body movement, eye movements beneath the lids, and twitches of the face and extremities. Testing was halted if, at any time, the infant was not rated as being in State 2 (active sleep). Reliability of the behavioral state ratings was computed to be over 90% (percent agreement).

The stimulus configurations used in the study are illustrated in Figure 1. In the control condition, only S2, a moderately loud abrupt acoustic noise, was presented. In most term subjects, S2 evokes a reliable acceleration of heart rate. In the remaining two conditions, S2 was preceded by the prestimulus (S1). In the 240-msec condition, S1 (40-msec duration)

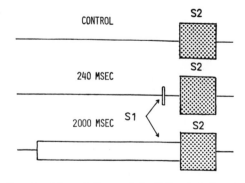

Figure 1. Schematic diagram of stimuli. The stippled box (S2) represents the 88 dB-A 250-Hz square wave tone, and the open boxes (S1), the 75 db-A 1000-Hz pure tone. The three configurations correspond to control (top), 240-msec discrete (middle), and 2000-msec sustained (bottom) conditions.

was presented 240 msec prior to (onset-to-onset) S2. In the 2000-msec condition, S1 was presented 2000 msec before S2 and remained at its steady-state level until the onset of S2. S2 was a 500-msec abrupt complex tone produced by a 250-Hz square wave at 88 dB-A sound pressure level (SPL), referenced to 20 micro Newtons per square centimeter. S2 was 92dB on the C scale, indicating that significant energy was present in the higher frequency ranges. S1 was 75 dB-A SPL, 1000-Hz pure tone. Each infant was presented at least nine trials of each stimulus configuration with a minimum intertrial interval of 30 seconds. Stimuli were delivered through a TDH-49 headphone placed over one ear while the opposite ear was against the mattress in the Isolette.

Cardiac and respiratory activity were measured by the monitors used in the everyday care of these infants and recorded on FM tape along with a stimulus marker. Cardiac activity was converted to 1-sec average heart rate, and nine trials per condition were averaged for each subject.

Case Findings

Figure 2 shows the average change in heart rate (HR) starting at the second prior to S2 onset and continuing for 9 seconds following S2 onset for three preterm subjects (Cases 1, 2, and 3) and some exemplary age-matched controls (Cases 4, 5, and 6).

Case 1 was a female infant born at 31 weeks estimated gestational age (EGA) to a primagravida class C diabetic (diabetes of early age

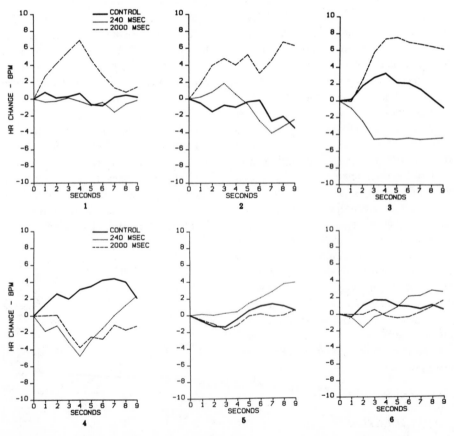

Figure 2. Average changes in heart rate relative to 1 second prior to onset of the square wave stimulus. Response curves for three subjects experiencing persistent cardiorespiratory pauses (top) and three age-matched controls (bottom). (HR = heart rate; BPM = beats per minute.)

onset without evidence of vascular disease). This infant was tested at 34 weeks post-conception. The response of her monozygotic twin (Case 4) is shown below Case 1 in Figure 2. Case 1 had 1- and 5-minute Apgar (1953) scores of 3 and 5, in contrast to her twin who scored 8 and 9. Case 1 experienced persistent episodes of apnea and bradycardia after being removed from the ventilator. Her sister was also on mechanical ventilation shortly after birth but did not experience apnea and brady-cardia upon removal.

Of note in Case 1, as well as the other two cases (2 and 3), is the fact that the facilitatory condition (2000 msec) resulted in a greater heart rate response relative to the control condition, whereas the age-matched controls did not exhibit a facilitatory effect.

Case 2 was a male born at 31 weeks EGA and tested at 35 weeks postconception. This infant was exhibiting an extremely high rate of apnea and severe bradycardia. The acoustic probes were delivered just prior to an atropine regimen. The corresponding graph in Figure 2 (Case 5) is that of a 31-week EGA male also tested 4 weeks after birth in the NICU.

Case 3 was a 32-week EGA male tested at 36 weeks. Shown below his graph in Figure 2 are the responses of an age-matched control (Case 6). Again, the elevated cardiac response in the 2000-msec condition is clearly evident.

Repeated tests were performed on Case 1 and a remarkable consistency was found in the facilitatory effect across a 1-month time period, a finding which was absent in her twin. Several additional subjects with more complicated neurological deficits who were also exhibiting autonomic instability have also shown the facilitatory effect.

Discussion

Taken together, these results are suggestive of a deficit in *central modulation* of arousing sensory signals in a subgroup of preterm infants with autonomic problems. Work by Graham and her colleagues (Graham et al., 1981) has shown that older infants several months of age are very sensitive to facilitatory (sustained prestimulus) manipulations and insensitive to inhibitory prestimulus manipulations. The facilitatory effect is also evident in healthy full-term newborns (Ver Hoeve & Leavitt, in press). The question posed by the present findings is why the preterm infant who is experiencing dysfunction of autonomic regulation exhibits an age-inappropriate response in the sustained prestimulation condition. The present findings suggest several possibilities, which, of course, are speculative at this stage of investigation.

The work of Henderson-Smart, Pettigrew, and Campbell (1983) relates preterm apnea and other perinatal disorders to altered BAER sensory transmission and maturation rates in preterm infants. Specifically, preterm infants experiencing apnea had slower brain stem conduction times yet a faster rate of maturation during postnatal life. Thus, it is possible that stress early in postnatal life may affect precocial development of certain reflex mechanisms. On this basis, it might be argued that the present results reflect accelerated maturation of brain stem mechanisms that modulate the arousal response in stressed infants.

Alternatively, it may be that the facilitatory effect reflects an interaction between chronically activated modulatory centers and the sustained prestimulus. According to this view, the stressed preterm infant is continually receiving sensory signals that impel arousal. This may lower the threshold for the registration of the sustained prestimulus in this group of infants.

Another dimension that may be important for distinguishing the responses of the increased-risk infants concerns the difference between sustained, or long time-constant processes, and phasic, or short time-constant processes. Graham (1975) has suggested that the distinction between neurons capable of following sustained versus transient stimulation is seen throughout the nervous system. These neurons probably are differentially involved in the two types of prestimulus modulaton. The sustained/transient distinction may be relevant for localizing sensory processing deficits in this group. The effect of stimulation of sustained activity pathways may also be involved in the recent reports of facilitation of respiratory rates in kittens during active sleep by continuous slow rocking (McGinty & Hopenbrouwers, 1983) and reduction of apnea in preterms (Korner, 1979).

SUMMARY

These data suggest that the study of the acoustic–cardiac response and its modulation provides an added dimension in the clinical assessment of neuromaturation of the premature infant. The acoustic stimulus technique allows researchers to probe an aspect of central neural control over cardiorespiratory activation by observing responses to well-defined, discrete perturbations. The prestimulus-probe technique bears a number of similarities to techniques used in the domains of neurophysiology and sytems engineering, such as the conditioning-test interval method and the impulse transfer function. The application of such techniques may result in a useful framework for the assimilation of data obtained noninvasively in the developing human with those of more molecular physiological investigations.

REFERENCES

Apgar, V. A proposal for a new method of evaluation of the newborn infant. *Current Research in Anesthesia and Analgesia,* 1953, *30,* 260–267.

Beal, S.M. Some epidemiological factors about sudden infant death syndrome (SIDS) in South Australia. In: J.T. Tildon, L.M. Roeder, & A. Steinschneider (eds.), *Sudden infant death syndrome.* New York: Academic Press, 1983.

Becker, L.E. Neuropathological basis for respiratory dysfunction in sudden infant death syndrome. In: J.T. Tildon, L.M. Roeder, & A. Steinschneider (eds.), *Sudden infant death syndrome.* New York: Academic Press, 1983.

Brady, J.P., Chir, B., Ariagno, R.L., Watts, J.L., Goldman, S.L., & Dumpit, F.M. Apnea, hypoxemia, and aborted sudden infant death syndrome. *Pediatrics,* 1978, *62,* 686–691.

Chalmers, D.V., & Hoffman, H.S. Cardiac and startle responses to acoustic stimuli in the rat. *Physiological Psychology,* 1973, *1,* 74–76.

Chan, S.H.H., & Barnes, C.D. A presynaptic mechanism evoked from the brain stem reticular formation in lumbar cord and its temporal significance. *Brain Research,* 1972, *45,* 101–114.

Glenn, L.L., & Dement, W.C. Motoneuron properties during electromyogram pauses in sleep. *Brain Research,* 1982, *243,* 11–23.

Graham, F.K. The more or less startling effects of weak prestimulation. *Psychophysiology,* 1975, *12,* 238–248.

Graham, F.K., Putnam, L.E., & Leavitt, L.A. Lead stimulation effects on human cardiac orienting and blink reflexes. *Journal of Experimental Psychology,* 1975, *1,* 161–169.

Graham, F.K., Strock, B.D., & Zeigler, B.L. Excitatory and inhibitory influences on reflex responsiveness. In: W.A. Collins (ed.), *Aspects of developmental competence.* Hillsdale, NJ: Lawrence Erlbaum Associates, 1981.

Guilleminault, C. *Sleeping and waking disorders: Indications and techniques.* Reading, MA: Addison-Wesley Publishing Co., 1982.

Guilleminault, C., Ariagno, R.L., Forno, L., Nagel, L., Baldwin, R., & Owen, M. Obstructive sleep apnea and near miss for SIDS: I. Report of an infant with sudden death. *Pediatrics,* 1979, *63,* 837–843.

Guilleminault, C., Ariagno, R., Korobkin, R., Coons, S., Owen-Boeddiker, M., & Baldwin, R. Sleep parameters and respiratory variables in 'near miss' Sudden Infant Death Syndrome infants. *Pediatrics,* 1981, *68,* 354–366.

Harper, R.M., Sclabassi, R.J., & Estrin, T. Time series analysis and sleep research. *IEEE Transactions on Automated Control AC-19,* 1974, *6,* 932–935.

Henderson-Smart, D.J., Pettigrew, A.C., & Campbell, D.J. Prenatal stress, brain stem neural maturation, and apnea in preterm infants. In: J.T. Tildon, L.M. Roeder, & A. Steinschneider (eds.), *Sudden infant death syndrome.* New York: Academic Press, 1983.

Hoffman, H.S., & Ison, J.R. Reflex modification in the domain of startle: I. Some empirical findings and their implication for how the nervous system processes sensory input. *Psychological Review,* 1980, *80,* 175–189.

Hunt, J.V. Predicting intellectual disorders in childhood for preterm infants with birthweights below 1501 gm. In: S.L. Friedman & M. Sigman (eds.), *Preterm birth and psychological development.* New York: Academic Press, 1981.

Iwamura, Y. Development of supraspinal modulation of motor activity during sleep and wakefulness. In: M.B. Sterman, D.J. McGinty, & A.M. Adinolfi (eds.), *Brain development and behavior.* New York: Academic Press, 1971.

Korner, A.F. Maternal rhythms and waterbeds: A form of intervention with premature infants. In: E.B. Thoman (ed.), *Origins of the infant's social responsiveness.* Hillsdale, NJ: Lawrence Erlbaum Associates, 1979.

Leitner, D.S., Powers, A.S., Stitt, C.S., & Hoffman, H.S. Midbrain reticular formation involvement in the inhibition of acoustic startle. *Physiology and Behavior,* 1981, *26,* 259–298.

McGinty, D.J., & Hoppenbrouwers, T. The reticular formation, breathing disorders during sleep, and SIDS. In: J.T. Tildon, L.M. Roeder, & A. Steinschneider (eds.), *Sudden infant death syndrome.* New York: Academic Press, 1983.

McGinty, D.J., & Sterman, M.B. Sleep physiology, hypoxemia, and the Sudden Infant Death Syndrome. *Sleep,* 1980, *3,* 361–373.

Orem, J. Neuronal mechanisms of respiration in REM sleep. *Sleep,* 1980, *3,* 251–267.

Orem, J., & Netick, A. Characteristics of midbrain respiratory neurons in sleep and wakefulness in the cat. *Brain Research*, 1982, *244*, 231–242.

Orlowski, J.P., Nodar, R.H., & Lonsdale, D. Abnormal brainstem auditory evoked potentials in infants with threatened sudden infant death syndrome. *Cleveland Clinic Quarterly*, 1979, *46*, 77–81.

Pearson, J., & Brandeis, L. Normal aspects of morphometry of brain stem astrocytes, carotid bodies and ganglia in SIDS. In: J.T. Tildon, L.M. Roeder, & A. Steinschneider (eds.), *Sudden infant death syndrome*. New York: Academic Press, 1983.

Prechtl, H.F.R. The behavioral states of the newborn. *Brain Research*, 1974, *76*, 185–212.

Sakai, K. Some anatomical and physiological properties of ponto-mesencephalic tegmental neurons with special reference to the PGO waves and postural atonia during paradoxical sleep in the cat. In: J.A. Hobson & M.A.B. Brazier (eds.), *The reticular formation revisited*. New York: Raven Press, 1980.

Schulte, F.J. Apnea. In: J.J. Volpe (ed.), *Clinics in Perinatology*, 1977, *4*(1), 65–76.

Schulte, F.J. Developmental aspects of the neuronal control of breathing. In: F. Falkner & J.M. Tanner (eds.), *Human growth 3. Neurobiology and nutrition*. New York: Plenum Publishing Corp., 1979.

Shannon, D.C., & Kelly, D. Abnormal ventilatory response to CO_2 during quiet sleep in aborted SIDS. *Chest*, 1978, *73*, 301.

Steinschneider, A. Prolonged sleep apnea and respiratory instability: A discriminative study. *Pediatrics*, 1977, *59*, 962–970.

Steriade, M., Oakson, G., & Ropert, N. Firing rates and patterns of midbrain reticular neurons during steady state and transitional states of the sleep-waking style. *Experimental Brain Research*, 1982, *46*, 37–51.

Stockard, J.J. Brainstem auditory evoked potentials in adult and infant sleep apnea syndromes, including sudden infant death syndrome and near-miss for sudden infant death syndrome. In: E. Bodis-Wollner (ed.), *Evoked potentials, Annals of the New York Academy of Sciences*, 1982, *388*, 433–465.

Valdes-Dapena, M.A. Sudden Infant Death Syndrome: A review of the medical literature 1974–1979. *Pediatrics*, 1980, *66*, 597–614.

Ver Hoeve, J.N., & Leavitt, L.A. Neonatal sensory-elicitedcardiac response: Modulation by state and antecedent sensory events. *Psychophysiology*, in press.

Wright, C.G., & Barnes, C.D. Audio-spinal reflex responses in decerebrate and cholarlose anesthetized cats. *Brain Research*, 1972, *36*, 307–331.

Chapter 35

Auditory Development
and Assessment

MOE BERGMAN, ED.D.
Tel Aviv University, Tel Aviv, Israel

THE TERM "AUDITORY" IMPLIES THE COM-
plex activity involving hearing, perception, and processing of acoustic signals.
Audition requires, as a basis, the ability both to
hear a great range of sound intensities and to
perceive sounds discriminatively. Hearing is
therefore but a part, although of critical importance, of auditory activity.

While there are many kinds of acoustic signals worthy of attention, the most compelling
use for infants is in the development of language behavior. This requires the accurate
perception of speech. It is of central concern,
therefore, to understand how auditory perception first occurs in the normal infant and
young child, and how it develops further as the
primary receptive channel for the understanding of spoken language.

While it is clear that a listener's sensitivity to
weak sounds is a function of the peripheral
auditory mechanism, the ear, the conveying of
meaning to a sound or combinations of sounds
encompasses a highly complex array of psy-
choacoustical and, for speech, linguistic discriminations, recognitions, associations, and
interpretations that are distributed throughout
the auditory and associational systems in a way
only barely comprehended today.

THE AUDITORY PROCESS

The auditory process leading to an understanding of a spoken message begins with the
reception by the peripheral ear of the acoustic
characteristics of a sound. In order for this
sound to eventually have a unique meaning, the
peripheral ear must perform a complex analysis
of it into frequency, intensity, and time, which
is then transformed into a neural pattern that
represents appropriately the original acoustic
pattern reaching the ear. It is now known that
there is real possibility for this to be disturbed
even when a sound is heard. Whether pathology of the end organ (the cochlea) results in a
hearing loss or not, there can be poor cochlear
mechanics that will distort the frequency and
intensity relationships of the incoming signal.

For example, in sensorineural hearing loss,
there is inferior ability to discriminate sounds
of close but different frequency. A disturbing
result of this is that noise has a great masking
effect on the sounds of speech, rendering them
more difficult than normal to discriminate even
when they are heard. Another by-product of
such hearing loss is the contraction of the
dynamic range of useful intensities between the
less sensitive threshold and the reduced level of
tolerable sound.

Once the preliminary analysis of the acoustic
(physical) properties of speech sounds occur, it
is necessary to hold that auditory information
in a momentary store, requiring some form of
memory, while the higher linguistic centers of
the brain recognize the sound patterns as belonging to specific speech sounds. That is, the

309

next step is analyzing the sounds in categories, which are called phonemes. Thus, in an early stage of the processing of a speech message, a person differentiates between the sounds of speech through an interaction between the peripheral and central systems. As is shown later in this chaper, there may actually be biologically specialized mechanisms for such phoneme differentiation that are present at birth.

Assuming that accurate neural patterning occurs in the cochlea, there are as yet only dimly understood functions in the brain stem that affect the message. It is known that the first interaction between the information going up the system from the two ears takes place there. Researchers believe that the localization of the source of sound in space depends significantly upon this interaction. It is possible that failure to fuse the signals from the two ears (that is, binaural hearing) or to separate competing messages appropriately may be due in part to dysfunction in the brain stem. Discrepancies in the latencies and morphology of the resulting waves have been reported by those who are doing brain stem auditory evoked potentials studies on children with learning disorders. This raises the possibility of distortion of the neurally encoded signal from the periphery on its way up the central auditory system.

Disturbances on a cortical level have long been suspected of interference in the accurate perception and understanding of speech as well as of visual language—reading and writing.

IDENTIFYING INFANTS AT
RISK FOR AUDITORY IMPAIRMENTS

In brief, attention must be focused on the efficiency of the entire system, from the reception and neural encoding of a message by the cochlea through the timing and interaction activities of the brain stem, to the linguistic functions of the cortical auditory-associational interactions.

How should one begin to evaluate the function of such an ensemble of physiological and psychological activities? Perhaps a prior question is "Where should one look for infants at risk for disorders in this primary human function—oral communication?" Classically, the initial search was for failure of basic hearing sensitivity in infants falling under a list of risk criteria, such as that suggested by the Joint Committee on Infant Hearing Screening Statement of 1982 (Joint Committee on Infant Hearing Screening, 1983). (The Joint Committee consisted of representatives from the American Academy of Pediatrics, Academy of Otolaryngology—Head and Neck Surgery, American Nurses Association, and American Speech-Language-Hearing Association.)

Factors that identify those infants who are at risk for having hearing impairment include the following:

1. Family history of childhood hearing impairment
2. Congenital perinatal infection (e.g., cytomegalovirus, rubella, herpes, toxoplasmosis, syphilis)
3. Anatomical malformations involving the head or neck (e.g., dysmorphic appearance including syndromal and nonsyndromal abnormalities, overt or submucous cleft palate, morphological abnormalities of the pinna)
4. Birth weight of < 1,500 grams
5. Hyperbilirubinemia at level exceeding indications for exchange transfusion
6. Bacterial meningitis, especially Hemophilus influenzae
7. Severe asphyxia in infants with Apgar scores of 0–3, in infants who fail to institute spontaneous respiration by 10 minutes, and in those with hypotonia persisting to 2 hours of age

The goal of screening tests of hearing in infants and young children is to determine whether the hearing is: a) grossly normal (within 30 dB hearing level); b) mildly to moderately subnormal (30–50 dB HL) and the loss is conductive, sensorineural, or mixed; c) severely impaired (50–85 dB HL); or d) profoundly impaired (more than 85 dB). It is not essential to have a threshold audiogram, that is, a precise determination of the weakest sounds the infant can hear, but it is important to know whether the hearing for high tones is worse than for low tones.

It is tempting, of course, to approach the task of identifying infants at risk for hearing disorders hierarchically, beginning with the simplest evidence of hearing—the startle response to sudden sharp sounds. Thus, for example, an infant's hearing is "tested" by noting reflex reactions such as the Moro response to a hand clapping or to other impact sounds. More recently, testers have begun to employ sensitive equipment to note *any* recordable change in an infant's state or activity, from quiet to restless or the reverse, and to print out a permanent record of it together with the details of the stimulus used. Such equipment is still relatively cumbersome and expensive and is therefore mainly recommended for application to infants at risk for hearing problems.

An example of a screening test that monitors a newborn's change of state in response to a relatively strong sound is the "CRIB-O-GRAM." It employs a motion-sensitive transducer below the mattress of a crib or bassinet, and a small loudspeaker placed near the infant. Periodically throughout the day and night a 1-second 92 dB noise pulse centered at 3,000 Hz is sounded by the loudspeaker, and the baby's activity is monitored 10 seconds before, during, and 2.5 seconds after. The presentation schedule and recording of response are computer controlled and a print-out record is available for scoring according to microprocessor algorithms. Pass or referral recommendations are derived from a sequence of 30 trials according to statistical criteria.

The false positive rate was 8% for the well babies and 21% for babies in the intensive care nursery (ICN). The false negative rates reported were 0.001% for the well babies and 0.31% for the ICN babies (McFarland, Simmons, & Jones, 1980).

Results of tests with the CRIB-O-GRAM on over 12,000 babies at The Stanford Hospital in California several years ago (McFarland et al., 1980) yielded rates of confirmed hearing loss of 1 in 954 well babies and 1 in 56 infants in the ICN, a difference of 17 at-risk infants to 1 well baby. This rate, for ICN and high-risk babies, is supported by other reports, such as those by Galambos and Galambos in 1979, who reported an incidence of 1 in 50 such babies.

A somewhat similar screening test of infants, originating in England, is the Linco-Bennett Auditory Response Cradle, in which a multichannel recording is made of such reflexive behavioral responses as head jerk, head turn, and respiration changes, once again avoiding direct contact with the infant through such devices as electrodes on the skin (Bennett, 1979, 1980; Shepard, 1983; Tucker, 1983). This test presents stimuli at moderate and relatively high levels intermittently through ear tips sealed in the external auditory canals. Responses are recorded through transducers built into the crib headrest and mattress, while respiration activity is detected by a 1-inch disc of carbon-impregnated foam pad contained in a waist band around the child or his or her clothing. It is reported to require only 5–10 minutes of testing time.

NONLINGUISTIC TESTS OF HEARING IN INFANTS AND YOUNG CHILDREN

Nonlinguistic tests of hearing in infants and young children fall into the following categories, with examples of each:

1. *Behavioral*
   Reflex responses: Moro, auropalpebral, stilling, etc.; alerting responses to noises, toy sounds, tones; eye or head localization movements
   Rewards: The Peep Show, conditioned orienting reflex (COR), visual reinforcement audiometry (VRA), tangible reinforcement by operant conditioning audiometry (TROCA)
   Play audiometry
2. *Acoustic:*
   Impedance audiometry
       a. Tympanometry
       b. Acoustic reflex
3. *Physiological:* (After Fulton & Lloyd, 1969, p. 245)
   Heart: Heart rate, heart rate variability, pulse rate, pulse volume
   Sweat gland: Electrodermal responses, skin temperature

Eye: Pupil dilation and constriction, blinking
Lungs: Respiration rate, respiration amplitude
Muscle: Post auricular myogenic response

4. *Neural:*
Evoked auditory potentials (electrical response auditory); action potentials (cochlear audiometry), brain stem ("early") responses, middle latency responses, "late" responses, "very late" responses, CNV, etc.

Behavioral Tests:
Reflex and Orienting Responses

In 1961, Wertheimer reported consistent appropriate eye movements to the click of a toy "cricket" activated to the right and left of the neonate at 3 minutes after birth. The infant girl, who had been crying with eyes closed, stopped crying, opened her eyes and turned them in the direction of the click. Reflex responses, such as an eye blink, Moro reactions, and kicks continue during the early weeks, and by the 6th to 8th week, the baby frowns, smiles, cries, or stops his or her activity in response to a moderately strong sound. Finally, after 4 or 5 months, orienting movements such as head turns to the sound if it is close by are present. It is important to know the frequency spectrum of the test sounds that provoke such reactions in order to rule out the possibility of a high-tone hearing loss, so common in babies with hearing problems.

Unless the test noises have been filtered electronically, they will in all likelihood contain a broad range of frequencies that can mislead the tester in deciding that the child hears relatively normally when he or she may in fact be hearing only the low frequency portion of the test toy's sound.

Reward or reinforcement tests provide the baby with incentive to look at something, such as a colored light flashing to his or her side from where a test noise is sounded by a loudspeaker. Such tests have been called conditioned orientation reflex (COR) (Suzuki & Ogiba, 1961) or visual reinforcement audiometry (VRA) (Liden & Kankhunen, 1969; Moore,

Thompson, & Thompson, 1975; Moore, Wilson, & Thompson, 1977). For slightly older babies or retarded children, there are tests in which a visual or other reward is given if the child learns to bang a large button when he or she hears a test tone. Examples of such tests are the "Peep Show" (Dix & Hallpike, 1947) and tangible reinforcement by operant conditioning audiometry (TROCA) (Lloyd, 1968).

Impedance Audiometry

The automatic response of the stapedius muscle in the middle ear to a high-level sound has been studied as a means of deducing hearing sensitivity in infants and young babies. The impedance audiometer, which also reveals the mobility of the eardrum, and through that the condition of the middle ear when suspected for otitis media, permits evaluation of the ear's loudness responses to a broad band of noise in comparison with the response to levels of a pure tone stimulus. The many methods for analyzing the findings of such measurements are neatly summarized by Popelka (1981).

Other Measurements

Measures of changes in the heart rate, in respiration rate and depth, in the electrical resistance at the skin and in the eyes have been reported repeatedly over the years, but without further acceptance by clinicians or researchers. More recently, some success has been reported with the postauricular myogenic response (Flood, Fraser, Conway, & Stewart, 1982; Fraser, Conway, Keene, & Hazell, 1978). In this test, electrodes are placed on the skin in front and in back of the ear, with a ground electrode on the back of the neck or on the arm. As the child sits on the mother's lap, clicks are presented at 60 dB hearing level, and if no myogenic response is seen, additional clicks are presented at 80 dB hearing level. The test is machine scored and is automatically stopped when a positive result is scored or after 2,000 clicks.

In a limited series of follow-ups, Flood et al. report very good figures on false positives and negatives (Flood et al., 1982).

The majority of recent research and clinical activity, of course, has been in the auditory stimulation of neural responses and in their analysis. Historically, the attention, in auditory evoked potentials, has moved from the so-called late responses, in which the waves occurring 150 to 300 msec following a click stimulus were examined for systematic changes, to the "early" responses of 0 to 10 msec latency, and more recently to the "middle" latencies, lying between the early and late waves. Other latency periods lie in wait for future exploration.

The present status of evoked response audiometry is discussed in Chapters 34 and 36.

Which of the various tests give the most accurate information about a child's hearing? The only safe answer at present is that when the child is old enough to cooperate consistently during a pure tone audiometer test (usually from 2½ to 3½ years), this is by far the most useful test of hearing for diagnosis and management, and remains the reference against which all other tests, particularly those performed at an earlier age, must be validated.

AUDITORY PERCEPTION AND COMPREHENSION

Once an infant's ability to hear sounds of an intensity and frequency range has been established, ensuring the reception of speech, normal development of the mechanisms for speech's perception and processing must still be determined.

These mechanisms require at least the following:

1. Threshold sensitivity within near-normal limits
2. Appropriate cochlear mechanics for the discrimination of the sounds of speech by frequency, intensity, and time
3. Integrity of the brain stem and the auditory neural pathways
4. Integrity of the auditory cortical areas
5. Proper functioning of the related cortical areas for linguistic function (e.g., association, memory, etc.)

Two methods for learning about the development of auditory perception from birth on have originated. First, an evolving approach to its study on the physiological level is through

auditory evoked response audiometry. For example, it seems promising to compare the very late responses (over 300 msec latency) with the early brain stem responses, in an attempt to expose relative deviations in children with known central disorders such as mental retardation. Second, it is now possible to study auditory perception behaviorally in infants.

The ability of infants in their first weeks and months of life to differentiate speech-like sounds has received increasing attention, and provocative reports have been published indicating reliable early discrimination of speech phonemes that are generated artificially and exquisitely controlled and varied by microprocessors.

With such a powerful tool to explore the perception of speech, it is possible to monitor the infant's ongoing activity (e.g., heart rate) or a contrived activity, such as having the infant suck on a nonnutritive nipple that has a pressure sensor secreted in it while, through the techniques of operant conditioning, his or her changes in sucking in response to variations in the stimulus are charted (Kuhl, 1980). In this technique, called high amplitude sucking (HAS), the stimulus, such as the sound /da/, is presented through a small loudspeaker in immediate response to the child's sudden increase in sucking amplitude. The number of sucks per minute that exceed a criterion of ongoing sucking activity is the measure of the effect of changing the speech-like stimulus. Such changes are compared to the sucking rates in control infants exposed only to the one unchanging sound. The experimental infant's change is interpreted as his or her recognition of the change in the frequency components of the sounds. In fact, accurate frequency discrimination has been demonstrated through such measures in 6- to 7-week old infants.

Similar reports provide evidence that young infants distinguish duration, intensity, intonation, and the location in space of various speech sounds. The remarkable thing, in such studies, is the observation that speech and nonspeech auditory stimuli are processed differently by infants just as they are by adults, suggesting that there may actually be a built-in ability for the perception of speech. A need for caution arises from reports that chinchillas and cats show almost identical discrimination abilities, but it can also be argued that this might reflect "the general psycho-acoustic predisposition of the mammalian auditory system" (Kuhl, 1976, p. 273).

The existence of biologically specialized mechanisms for the perception of speech has further support from dichotic listening experiments with their now firmly accepted right ear advantage (REA). In such studies, the listener hears competing words presented simultaneously to the two ears. In most persons the right ear (left cerebral hemisphere system) tends to dominate, in this right–left ear competition.

It is remarkable that even if the area of the brain normally dominant for the perception of speech, the left hemisphere, is damaged before or soon after birth, the specialized function can move to another area, the right hemisphere.

Using the dichotic listening technique, 28 children with hemiplegia at or soon after birth were studied, comparing their performance with the same number of normal children of the same ages. Figure 1 shows the results of the normal children, the left hemisphere damaged (LHD) children, and the right hemisphere damaged (RHD) children.

The bars extending above the midline represent the average superiority of the right ear over the left ear in the dichotic listening task, while the bar below shows the amount of left ear advantage, where that occurs. Thus, the normal children showed the usual REA in this test, while the RHD children showed abnormally great REAs due to the reduced ability of the left ear–right hemisphere combination to compete successfully with the healthy right ear–left side of the brain. By sharp contrast, when the child is born with a damaged left hemisphere, is the clear shift of the usual dominance for speech perception on that side to the undamaged right hemisphere.

Why is it important to explore infant auditory perception? There are increasing reports that relate auditory processing disabilities to various language dysfunctions. For example, studies of hemiplegic children on the dichotic listening task showed that both the RHD and LHD children performed significantly more poorly than their normal siblings of the same mean age (Bergman, Costeff, Koren, Koifman, & Reshef, in press).

In another application, Tallal (1980) showed that aphasic children have difficulty in distinguishing two rapidly successive sounds, but they do better when the interval between the stimuli is lengthened. She feels that such findings suggest that the problem in aphasic children may be in auditory processing rather than in higher order linguistic disabilities.

Further tests of auditory perception have been applied to children with delayed speech and others with learning disorders. A particularly revealing test is one in which the child is given simple commands, such as "Put the apple on the box," first in a quiet setting, then over noise that is not as strong as the speech signal. The children with linguistic or learning disorders do as well as the normal children in the quiet situation but break down significantly when acoustic interference, such as a babble of talkers, is added. It is suggested that such inferiority in selective listening may be an important factor in their problem.

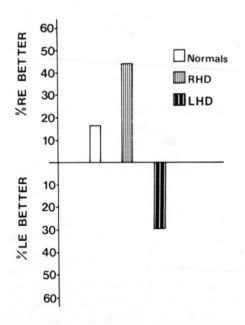

Figure 1. Average differences between right ear and left ear scores for two-word sets on a dichotic listening test given to 28 normal children to 16 children with right hemiplegia (LHD) and 12 with left hemiplegia (RHD). (Ages, 3–12; mean, 7.1 years.)

SUMMARY

It is clearly desirable to discover as early as possible the existence of defects in auditory reception, perception, and processing. Tests of auditory sensitivity are already being applied in the screening of infants at risk and in intensive care nurseries, as well as in well baby centers. The accelerating application of new technology both in the precise generation of auditory stimuli and in the monitoring of physiological and behavioral responses moves us into a new era of sophistication about the development of auditory function. It remains now to learn how to prevent communication disorders in the infant and young child and how to begin effective treatment early when such disorders occur.

REFERENCES

Bennett, M.J. Trials with The Auditory Response Cradle, Part 1. *British Journal of Audiology,* 1979, *13*(4), 125–134.

Bennett, M.J. Trials with The Auditory Response Cradle, Part 2. *British Journal of Audiology,* 1980, *14*(1), 1–6.

Bergman, M., Costeff, H., Koren, V., Koifman, N., & Reshef, A. Auditory perception in early lateralized brain damage. *Cortex,* in press.

Dix, M.R., & Hallpike, C.S. The Peep Show: A new technique for pure tone audiometry in young children. *British Medical Journal,* 1947, *2,* 719–723.

Flood, L.M., Fraser, J.G., Conway, M.J., & Stewart, A. The assessment of hearing in infancy using the post-auricular myogenic response. *British Journal of Audiology,* 1982, *16,* 211–213.

Fraser, J.G., Conway, M.J., Keene, M.H., Hazell, J.W.P. The post-auricular myogenic response: A new instrument which simplifies its detection by machine scoring. *Journal of Laryngology and Otology,* 1978, *92,* 293–303.

Fulton, R.T., & Lloyd, L.L. *Audiometry for the retarded.* Baltimore: Williams & Wilkens, 1969.

Galambos, C., & Galambos, R. Brainstem evoked response audiometry in newborn hearing screening. *Archives of Otology,* 1979, *105,* 86–90.

Joint Committee on Infant Hearing Screening. Joint committee on infant hearing screening statement of 1982. *Ear and Hearing,* 1983, *4*(1), 3–4.

Kuhl, P.K. Speech perception in early infancy: The acquisition of speech-sound categories. In: S.K. Hirsh, D.H. Eldredge, I.S. Hirsh, & S.R. Silverman (eds.), *Hearing and Davis:* Essays honoring Hollowell Davis. St. Louis: Washington University Press, 1976.

Kuhl, P.K. Infant speech perception: Reviewing data on auditory category formation. In: P.J. Levinson & C. Sloan (eds.), *Auditory processing and language.* New York: Grune & Stratton, 1980.

Liden, G., & Kankhunen, A. Visual reinforcement audiometry. *Acta Otolaryngology,* 1969, *67,* 281–282.

Lloyd, L.L. Operant conditioning audiometry with retarded children. In: *Differential diagnosis of speech and hearing problems of mental retardation.* Washington, DC: Catholic University of America Press, 1968.

Lloyd, L.L., Spradlin, V.E., & Reid, M.J. An operant audiometric procedure for difficult-to-test patients. *Journal of Speech and Hearing Disorders,* 1968, *33,* 236–245.

McFarland, W.H., Simmons, F.B., & Jones, F.R. An automated hearing screening technique for newborns. *Journal of Speech and Hearing Disorders,* 1980, *45*(4), 495–503.

Moore, J.M., Thompson, G., & Thompson, M. Auditory localization of infants as a function of reinforcement conditions. *Journal of Speech and Hearing Disorders,* 1975, *40,* 29–34.

Moore, J.M., Wilson, W.R., & Thompson, G. Visual reinforcement of head-turn responses in infants under 12 months of age. *Journal of Speech and Hearing Disorders,* 1977, *42,* 328–334.

Popelka, G.R. *Hearing assessment with the acoustic reflex.* New York: Grune & Stratton, 1981.

Shepard, N.T. Newborn hearing screening using the Linco-Bennett Auditory Response Cradle: A pilot study. *Ear and Hearing,* 1983, *4*(1), 5–10.

Suzuki, T., & Ogiba, Y. Conditioned orientation reflex audiometry. *Archives of Otolaryngology,* 1961, *74,* 192–198.

Tallal, P. Auditory processing disorders in children. In: P.J. Levinson & C. Sloan (eds.) *Auditory processing and language.* New York: Grune & Stratton, 1980.

Tucker, S.M. Hearing screening in the newborn using the auditory response cradle. Paper presented at the 2nd International Workshop on the "At-Risk" Infant. Jerusalem, May, 1983.

Wertheimer, M. Psychomotor coordination of auditory and visual space at birth. *Science,* 1961, *134,* 1962.

The At-Risk Infant: Psycho/Socio/Medical Aspects
edited by Shaul Harel, M.D., and Nicholas J. Anastasiow, Ph.D.
Copyright © 1985   Paul H. Brookes Publishing Co., Inc.   Baltimore • London

Chapter 36

The Use of
Auditory Evoked Potentials in the
Assessment of the At-Risk Infant

HAIM SOHMER, PH.D.
Hebrew University—Hadassah Medical School, Jerusalem, Israel

E VOKED POTENTIALS (EP) IN GENERAL, AND auditory evoked potentials in particular, have made great contributions to audiological and neurological diagnosis. Optimal use of EP in diagnosis can only be achieved if the EP practitioner is familiar with the neuro-physiological and technological bases of the recordings, and their problems, limitations, and pitfalls. The purpose of this chapter is to outline these bases and then to survey the chief uses of EP in assessment of the at-risk infant.

PROBLEMS OF EVOKED
POTENTIAL RECORDINGS

The electroencephalogram (EEG) is a measure of the ongoing, spontaneous electrical activity of the cerebral cortex. In contrast, evoked potentials represent electrical activity that appears only in response to a stimulus (i.e., it is not spontaneous), usually sensory (auditory, visual, or somatosensory). The electrical activity from which the EP is isolated is recorded in the clinical situation by electrodes on the skin. The sensory stimulus, e.g., a light flash, a tap on the skin, or a sound stimulus, is transduced by the appropriate sensory receptor into nerve impulses that ascend the relevant sensory pathway from the receptor up to the cerebral cortex.

Recording of
Auditory Evoked Potentials

Since the recording electrodes have been placed on the skin, the desired "signal" (the EP) is small in amplitude, while the same skin electrodes also record undesired electrical activity such as the EEG and the ECG (electrocardiogram) that are considered "noise" and are often much larger in amplitude than the "signal." This poor signal-to-noise ratio must be improved in order to distinguish the EP from the ongoing "noise."

Separating the signal from the noise can be achieved in several complementary ways, the first of which is to choose a sensory stimulus that will excite many nerve fibers synchronously so that a large number of nerve fibers discharge nerve impulses within the same time interval (latent period) following the stimulus, leading to summation of simultaneous nerve impulses in many nerve fibers and to the gener-

This chapter was supported in part by Mr. A. Leitman of New York.

The author would like to express his sincere gratitude to Professor G. Szabo, Ms. L. Tell, and Ms. H. Levi for the fruitful discussions with them that lead to several of the concepts expressed in this chapter.

ation of a large amplitude compound action potential. The stimulus that leads to maximal synchrony of nerve fibers is an electrical stimulus delivered to a bundle of nerve fibers. This is the stimulus of choice when eliciting the somatosensory evoked potential. This chapter concentrates on the auditory EP and, in particular, the auditory nerve-brain stem evoked response (ABR). Synchrony of firing of auditory nerve fibers is best achieved by using a repetitive (10–20 per second) click acoustic stimulus that is generated by delivering a short (50–100 μsec) square electrical pulse to an earphone. The resultant acoustic click has a duration of less than 1 millisecond.

The electrodes record both the desired response ("signal") elicited by the click stimulus and the ongoing "noise." Electronic filtering of this recorded electrical activity can contribute to the separation of the signal from the noise. To achieve this, advantage is taken of the fact that the signal (nerve impulses) can be assumed to approximate a sinusoidal waveform with a duration of about 1 msec and a dominant frequency of about 1,000 Hz. Alternatively, one of the chief components of the noise is the EEG, the dominant frequency of which is about 10 Hz (alpha rhythm). Therefore, a filter that passes electrical activity with a frequency band of 200–3,000 Hz will remove the EEG from the recording. Other sources of noise can be reduced by averaging. This involves the presentation of repetitive clicks (between several hundred to a thousand) and averaging the electrical activity recorded following each click by means of a signal averager. Such an instrument divides up the electrical activity following each of the thousand clicks into small time intervals (40 μsec in this case) and averages the first 40 μsec following each of the clicks, then the second 40 μsec following the clicks, and so on until about 256 such time intervals following each click have been averaged. In this way, the 10 msec (256 intervals or points multiplied by 40 μsec per point = 10.24 msec) following the clicks have been averaged. By this procedure, recorded electrical activity that is time-locked to the stimulus (always appears with the same latency following the click) is added while randomly occurring activity is canceled out even if the time-locked activity (signal) is smaller in amplitude than the random activity (noise). These stimulus and recording parameters (10–20 clicks per second, frequency bandpass filtering of 200–3,000 Hz, 40 μsec per point, 10–15 msec poststimulus "window") are appropriate for recording ABR only. When using 40 μsec per point, a signal with a duration of 1 msec (a compound action potential) will be portrayed by 25 points giving good waveform representation. These parameters are completely inappropriate for recording most other types of evoked auditory responses such as the cortical auditory evoked response.

Wave Measurement

When these instruments and their parameters are incorporated into the recording system, the response to click stimuli about 70 dB above the normal threshold (70 dB hearing level) is made up of 5–6 waves with amplitude of less than 1 μV (see Figure 1). The first wave has a latency of 1.3–1.5 msec and the succeeding waves follow at intervals of about 1 msec. The first wave is the compound action potential of the auditory nerve resulting from the fact that many auditory nerve fibers discharge their impulses in response to the click synchronously.

In order to determine which nerve fibers fire synchronously in response to the click stimulus, the latent period between the click and each impulse, and the frequency of pure-tone acoustic stimulus to which each nerve fiber responds best, must be determined for many auditory nerve fibers. This can be achieved by observing the poststimulus time (PST) histogram and the characteristic frequency of many fibers as determined by microelectrode recordings from individual nerve fibers in the experimental animal. The PST histogram is a measure of the number of times that particular latent periods appear in response to repetitive click stimuli. Therefore, a peak in the PST histogram indicates that a nerve fiber responds with more or less uniform and constant latencies to repetitive clicks. The characteristic frequency (CF) of a nerve fiber is the frequency of acoustic stimulus to which it responds at the lowest intensity, i.e., the frequency of lowest threshold (see Kiang, Watanabe, Thomas, &

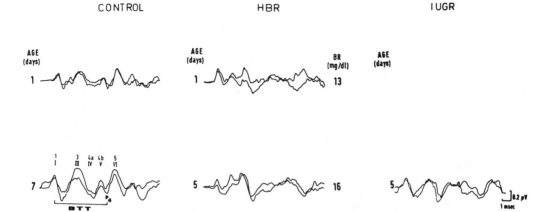

Figure 1. Auditory nerve–brain stem evoked responses (ABR) in several neonates. The waves from a normal neonate have been labeled according to the 2 systems (using arabic or roman numerals) in use. Note that in the case of neonatal hyperbilirubinemia (HBR), wave 4 is absent in the ABR at age 1 day when bilirubin level (BR) was 13 mg/dl. The latency of wave 3 is also prolonged. At 5 days (BR 16 mg/dl), wave 4 may be apparent and the latency of wave 3 has shortened. The final trace is from a 5-day-old neonate born after a full-term pregnancy but with a birth weight of 1.760 kg—that is, there apparently was intrauterine growth retardation (IUGR). The brain stem transmission time (BTT) is abnormally prolonged (6.6 msec compared to 5.9 msec in normal neonates at this age).

Clark, 1962). Nerve fibers with high CF innervate more basal regions of the inner ear and have very short latencies in response to click stimuli as demonstrated by a clear peak in their histogram at about 1.5 msec. Fibers with lower CF innervate more apical regions and have longer latencies—up to 3.5 msec for fibers with CF of 400 Hz. This difference in latency between the first peak in the PST of high CF and low CF fibers is due to the mechanical traveling wave delay along the basilar membrane of the inner ear from base to apex. This leads to the conclusion that the first wave of the ABR response that has a latency of 1.5 msec is made up of the synchronous firing of basal, high CF auditory nerve fibers since only such fibers have the appropriate latencies. Also, all nerve fibers with CF greater than 4 kHz have short, uniform latencies of about 1.5 msec. More apical nerve fibers respond to the click stimulus after the appearance of the compound action potential of the auditory nerve and therefore cannot contribute to this potential.

The ABR waves that follow the first wave (see Figure 1) represent the subsequent activation, by the volley of impulses in the auditory nerve fibers, of the neurons in the brain stem auditory pathway. Each brain stem wave is the compound action potential produced by brain stem neurons that generate their impulses synchronously at that point in time. Even though

there is no unanimity with respect to the exact generator(s) of each wave, there is relative agreement that in the clinical application of ABR, one may assume that the principal component of each wave represents the sequential activation of the ascending brain stem auditory pathway—the second wave generated by axons in the lower brain stem and the later waves in the upper brain stem. In clinical testing, an important measure is the presence or absence of these ABR waves. However, since in normal subjects waves 2 and 5 (sometimes called wave VI) (see Figure 1) are so variable, their amplitude or even absence cannot be taken as a definite sign of abnormality.

Brain Stem Transmission Time An additional wave measure is the ear lobe positive wave following wave 4b (V), (see Figure 1), which is called wave P_4, generated in the rostral regions of the brain stem. Using this and the first wave, one can define brain stem transmission time (BTT) as the time interval between the input to the brain stem—the peak of the auditory nerve response—and the clearest response from the more rostral regions of the brain stem, P_4. BTT is, therefore, the time it takes for impulses to traverse the brain stem. BTT is about 6 msec in neonates (see Figure 1) and reaches adult values of about 4.5 msec in 3-year-olds. This progression to shorter BTT with infant maturation is thought to be due to progressing myelinization of the brain stem axons.

BTT does not seem to change with decreases in the intensity of the click stimulus since the absolute latency of each of the waves increases uniformly. The amplitude of each of the waves decreases, though that of wave 4 changes least. This is probably due to the fact that wave 4 is larger in amplitude at higher intensities as a result of divergence in the ascending pathway. This wave can still be seen at very low stimulus intensities so that the lowest intensity at which wave 4 is still present is considered to be the electrical response threshold and this is approximately equal to the behavioral threshold of the subject at frequencies in the 2–8 kHz range. A threshold elevation is then seen as the absence of ABR waves at click intensities greater than 5–10 dB hearing level.

Amplitude Besides latency, the amplitude of the ABR waves can also be of value in diagnosis. There is variability in the amplitude of the waves, and, in order to overcome this, several groups have suggested the use of amplitude ratio values (4/1) rather than absolute values (Starr & Achor, 1975). This ratio in normal adult subjects is usually greater than one. However, the amplitude ratio may be smaller than one either because the absolute amplitude of wave 4 is reduced or because 1 is augmented in amplitude, or both. It is due to this and the larger standard deviations that amplitude measures are less useful than latency measures.

ABR USE IN AUDITORY ASSESSMENT

The ABR have been successfully used in the auditory assessment of infants and children by providing an electrophysiological, objective measure of hearing threshold. Besides indicating the amount of hearing loss (threshold), the ABR coupled with other types of auditory EP can also contribute to the localization of the lesion responsible for the hearing loss thereby leading to the differential diagnosis of conductive hearing loss (an impairment, usually mechanical, in the external or middle ear leading to attenuation of sound energy on its way to the inner ear), neural hearing loss (absence of

ABR with the sparing of the receptor cell response), sensory hearing loss (absence of both sensory cell response and ABR), retrocochlear hearing loss (a lesion in the auditory pathways of the brain so that some of the brain stem components of the ABR are absent with sparing of the auditory nerve response), and nonorganic hearing loss (in which all auditory EP can be recorded) (see Feinmesser & Sohmer, 1976). Since the ABR is not affected by sleep and by sedative drugs, this test can be used on noncooperative, sedated subjects such as young infants, children, and even retarded individuals. Furthermore, since it has been shown that ABR can be recorded in neonates and even in 1-day-old neonates (Rubinstein & Sohmer, 1982) and in premature babies, such differential diagnosis can be made in neonates at risk for deafness because of factors such as familial deafness, congenital malformations, low Apgar scores, and neonatal hyperbilirubinemia. In fact, these neonatal ABR tests proved to be a more satisfactory indicator of neonatal hearing than a behavioral arousal hearing test (Apriton) (Levi, Tell, Feinmesser, Gafni, & Sohmer, 1983). The follow-up of many of these neonates and others to the age of 3 years, at which time full pure-tone audiograms could be obtained, indicated a limitation of the ABR technique: since the ABR gives an accurate estimate of hearing in the high frequency range (2–8 kHz), it is possible that the ABR would lead to the impression that there is a profound hearing loss in a neonate while his or her audiogram, when obtainable, could indicate a high frequency hearing loss with nearly normal hearing in the lower frequency range (Levi et al., 1983). Research presently being conducted may yield techniques to obtain ABR to lower frequency stimuli, which could also lead to the "reconstruction" of an audiogram.

ABR USE IN EVALUATION OF DEVELOPMENTAL DISORDERS

Following the demonstration that ABR can also contribute to the diagnosis of neurological disorders in adults (Starr & Achor, 1975) due to the fact that the ABR represents the neural activity of a pathway that traverses the brain stem, ABR have also been used in the evaluation of children with developmental brain disorders (Sohmer, 1982). ABR have been shown to be abnormal in autistic, minimal brain dysfunction, and psychomotor retarded children, in adults with Down syndrome and with severe retardation, and in children with borderline retardation. Cortical evoked potentials also show abnormalities in similar cases; visual evoked potentials demonstrate irregular patterns in mental retardation and auditory cortical evoked potentials have been shown to be abnormal in Down syndrome. Many of these patients had suffered from some congenital, perinatal, or neonatal insult (Sohmer, 1982).

ABR USE IN
ASSESSMENT OF NEONATES IN ICU

An additional important use of EP in general and of ABR in particular is for the neurological assessment of neonates in the intensive care unit. The ABR of neonates who suffered asphyxia were abnormal. Hrbek, Karlberg, Kjellmer, Olsson, and Riha (1977) have provided evidence for abnormal visual EP in asphyxiated neonates. The ABR of neonates with neonatal hyperbilirubinemia were initially abnormal (see Figure 1) and showed improvement as the plasma bilirubin levels decreased, though in a way not directly correlated with these levels. ABR abnormalities were also seen in cases of intrauterine growth retardation (see Figure 1) and in neonatal meningitis (Sohmer, 1982).

ABR IN EARLY DETECTION
OF DEVELOPMENTAL DISORDERS

These findings point out the valuable clinical contributions provided by the various types of EP that together can be called multimodality (auditory, visual, and somatosensory) evoked potentials.

These clinical studies have demonstrated abnormal EP in infants and children with de-

velopmental brain disabilities having a history of congenital, perinatal, or neonatal insults. In addition, abnormal ABR can already be recorded in neonates suffering from such insults. Such observations have led to an interesting hypothesis which must be tested. Congenital, perinatal, and neonatal insults, such as asphyxia and hyperbilirubinemia, can induce brain damage (structural or biochemical, focal or diffuse) of varying severity. This brain damage gives rise to abnormal neuronal function and deviant electrical activity. Depending upon the brain region irreversibly affected and depending upon the function of this brain region in the normal subject and the age at which this damaged region "expresses itself," a clinically silent period of varying duration may be followed by the appearance of a developmental brain disorder such as psychomotor retardation, some forms of cerebral palsy, autism, attention deficit disorders, and specific learning disabilities. Therefore, the recording of many types of multimodality EP may serve as a noninvasive diagnostic tool for the early detection of brain dysfunction in at-risk neonates before the appearance of the developmental brain disorder and may predict the impending disorder.

The importance of this as yet untested suggestion concerning the relationship between perinatal events, brain damage, neuronal dysfunction, and the possibility that EP may be able to predict neurodevelopmental deviations derives from the fact that early detection of these impending behavioral deviations by electrophysiological means would lead to close and frequent observation of the infant, proper parental and educational counseling and the early provision of an enriched, stimulating environment for the child in order to enable him or her to reach full developmental potential in spite of the insult suffered at a very early age.

As already stated, this hypothesis must be tested in careful longitudinal studies, including the determination of the cost-benefit ratio, in several laboratories. In any case, this suggested (as yet untested) hypothesis may provide a new use for EP in addition to the already proved contributions to the auditory and neurological assessment of the at-risk infant.

REFERENCES

Feinmesser, M., & Sohmer, H. Contribution of cochlear, brainstem and cortical responses to differential diagnosis and lesion localization in hearing loss. In: S.K. Hirsh, D.H. Eldredge, I.J. Hirsh, & S.R. Silverman (eds.), *Hearing and Davis: Essays honoring Hallowell Davis*. St. Louis: Washington University Press, 1976.

Hrbek, A., Karlberg, P., Kjellmer, I., Olsson, T., & Riha, M. Clinical application of evoked electroencephalographic responses in newborn infants. I. Perinatal asphyxia. *Developmental Medicine and Child Neurology*, 1977, *19*, 34–44.

Kiang, N.Y.-S., Watanabe, T., Thomas, E.C., & Clark, L.F. Stimulus coding in the cat's auditory nerve. *Annals of Otology, Rhinology, and Laryngology*, 1962, *71*, 1009–1026.

Levi, H., Tell., L., Feinmesser, M., Gafni, M., & Soh-mer, H. Early detection of hearing loss in infants by auditory nerve and brainstem responses. *Audiology*, 1983, *22*, 181–188.

Rubinstein, A., & Sohmer, H. Latency of auditory nerve response in neonates one to eight hours old. *Annals of Otology, Rhinology, and Laryngology*, 1982, *91*, 205–208.

Sohmer, H. Auditory nerve-brain stem responses (ABR) in children with developmental brain disorders and in high risk neonates. In: P.A Buser, W.A. Cobb, & T. Okuma (eds.), *Kyoto Symposia (EEG Suppl. 36)*. New York: Elsevier North-Holland, 1982.

Starr, A., & Achor. J. Auditory brainstem responses in neurological disease. *Archives of Neurology*, 1975, *32*, 761–768.

Chapter 37

Infant Vocalizations

Traditional Beliefs
and Current Evidence

D. Kimbrough Oller, Ph.D.
University of Miami, Miami, Florida

T HE SPEECH-LIKE VOCALIZATIONS OF IN-
fants have often been a source of fasci-
nation to parents, educators, physicians, and
scientists. Yet, in spite of general interest, a
number of misconceptions about infant sounds
are widespread. The purpose of this chapter is
to discuss these misconceptions in the light of
current evidence, and to provide a basis for a
more realistic view of infant sounds.

MYTHS ABOUT
INFANT VOCALIZATIONS

The myths about infant vocalizations do not
have a common source, and consequently, they
do not form a coherent position. The list below
provides a topical breakdown of traditional
erroneous beliefs:

1. *The Methodological Myth:* Infant vocalizations are so different from speech that
   they cannot be described as phonetic units.
   The only appropriate description of infant
   sounds is based on instrumental acoustic
   analysis.
2. *Discontinuity Myths:*
   a) Infant vocalizations are composed
      of random sounds, while young-

child speech is highly structured.
   b) All the sounds of all the world's
      languages are heard in infant bab-
      bling.
   c) There is no phonetic relationship
      between infant babbling and
      young-child speech.
3. *Babbling Drift Myths:*
   a) During the first year of life, infant
      sounds gradually come to re-
      semble the sounds of the specific
      language environment.
   b) Research shows that, during the
      first year of life, babies from differ-
      ent language communities babble
      in such a way that adult listeners
      can identify the babies' back-
      grounds just by listening to their
      sounds.
4. *The Myth of Babbling in Deaf Infants:* Deaf babies early in life babble
   just as hearing infants do, but around the
   middle of the first year, the deaf infants
   stop babbling, while the hearing infants
   continue. Hearing is not necessary for
   babbling to occur, but it is necessary for
   babbling to continue.

The preparation of this chapter was supported by the Mailman Foundation and by a grant from NINCDS
(#5RO1NS17604-02). Thanks go to Rebecca Eilers for helpful comments on the manuscript.

5. *McCarthy's Myth:* Early in the first year, infants babble in a substantially passive fashion. Important vocalization features can be attributed to passive response of infant vocal structures with changing orientation of the force of gravity in various body positions.

AN OVERVIEW OF INFANT VOCALIZATIONS BASED ON CURRENT EVIDENCE

The listed myths will be familiar to readers of textbooks in child development and early child language. In general, the traditional beliefs are based upon a dearth of empirical observation and a wealth of armchair philosophy. Yet, some of the beliefs hold a grain of truth that should be preserved in the process of discarding misleading implications.

Scientific myths are often very useful as statements of hypotheses. Research is often inspired by such statements, yielding a clearer view of the facts and the basis for a new set of hypotheses. A part of the task of this chapter is to modify the traditional positions (in some cases drastically) in order to bring them into conformity with current evidence. The new set of statements will imply a new set of hypotheses, to be considered, it is hoped, in further investigations. But prior to addressing the myths and modifications directly, it will be advantageous to review the nature of infant vocalizations in the light of recent investigative reports.

The Focus: Speechiness of Infant Vocalizations

The kinds of vocalizations that are addressed in this chapter are those that appear to have much in common with speech. These vocalization types do not include cries, laughter, coughs, burps, etc. Such vocal sounds are biologically meaningful, and their meanings are largely nonarbitrary and universal and are applied in roughly equivalent ways across ages and cultures. If one coughs, it "means" that the cougher has some obstruction to breathing, irritation of the airway, etc. It cannot within a natural language have a primary meaning of "dog" or "apples." However, a syllable sequence such as [badaga] can be assigned any meaning depending on agreement within a community of speakers without impinging upon biological significance. In the terminology of linguistics, there is an "arbitrary relationship" between the sounds of language (e.g., [badaga]) and possible meanings.

The sounds of interest here are those that *are* potentially arbitrary in meaning, including syllables and syllable sequences. There are, of course, other potentially arbitrary sounds that are not syllables, and infants produce many such nonsyllabic sounds. One major task in the description of infant vocalizations is to assess such sounds and to determine the extent to which they resemble the syllables of speech. Investigation of the "speechiness" of potentially arbitrary sounds produced by infants offers a window through which to observe the emergence of the capacity for speech.

Metaphonology as a Framework for the Assessment of Speechiness

In order to determine the speechiness of a given sound, it is necessary to have a general framework specifying the characteristics of speech, a framework within which to classify sound types with potentially arbitrary meanings. Such a framework is called "metaphonology" or "metaphonetics." A metaphonological system takes account of the acoustic and articulatory patterns that are universal in spoken languages. For example, all languages employ syllables that consist of vowels (requiring an unobstructed vocal tract and normal phonation) and consonants (involving obstruction of the vocal tract), with a transition between the two not to exceed 120 msec duration. All languages string such syllables together in utterances. All languages involve syllables contrasting in quality of vowel, place of articulation of consonants, and manner of articulation of consonants. All languages involve manipulation of the parameters of pitch, loudness, resonance, and timing of articulations in order to cue the relevant contrasts. Such facts are a part of metaphonology.

Concrete phonology, in contrast, involves the specific description of the elements of a given phonological system—the segments, phonetic features, intonation contours, and the stress patterns of, say, English or Arabic. Since each language is different, each concrete phonological inventory has special elements. A metaphonology is directed toward specification of phonological systems in general, and would be capable of verifying that the special elements are indeed potential elements of a spoken language. If one were to make up a language and a corresponding set of sounds, a metaphonological system could be used to determine whether or not the proposed sounds could occur in a real language. The metaphonological approach aims to define the notion "potential phonological system of a natural language."

The power of a metaphonological approach is that it provides the basis for comparison of any sound types against a set of standards of appropriateness for natural, mature speech. The communicative sounds of elephants, whales, or human infants can be compared with those of mature human speech in a metaphonologically oriented description. The framework offers the possibility to specify both the ways in which such sounds are similar to speech and the ways in which they differ.

A metaphonological approach to describing infant vocalizations is different from a concrete phonological approach since the former need not rely on phonetic transcription, nor on the comparison of infant sounds with sounds of a particular language. For example, in a metaphonological approach, one can address the general issue of whether or not an infant sound is a syllable, independent of whether it is a [pa], a [pʰa], or some other syllable. One can assess the extent of the sound's conformity to metaphonological syllabic principles without transcribing it. Similarly, one can assess the infant's manipulation of pitch as a manifestation of metaphonological intonation capabilities without comparing the actual infant utterances with a particular contour, say, English or Italian declarative contour. The approach characterizes infant sounds in terms of their relationship with all possible speech systems rather than with any particular existing system.

SPEECH-LIKE SOUNDS OF THE FIRST YEAR OF LIFE

At 7–8 months of age, a remarkable event occurs in the lives of normal infants. They begin to produce sounds that are so much like speech as to be easily confused with it. Parents, at this point, often think the child has begun to talk, reporting that the baby says "dada" or "mama." In fact, the baby is babbling (producing "canonical babbling"), rather than talking. The onset of babbling is an extraordinary indication of an advancement in the infant's phonological capabilities.

Longitudinal studies suggest that in most cases, the onset of canonical babbling is sudden. Parents and/or investigators can often specify the day on which the babbling began. Prior to this date, babies produce a wide variety of other sounds with arbitrary potential. Although there are a number of different types, these speech-like sounds are collectively referred to as "precanonical."

Precanonical Speech-Like Sounds of Infants

The Phonation Stage (0–1 Months)
During the first 2 months of life, the normal infant produces a large number of sounds that have been referred to as "small, throaty sounds" or "quasi-resonant sounds" (Oller, 1980). Quasi-resonant sounds are produced with a virtually closed vocal tract. Airflow may be largely nasal. Such sounds involve normal phonation (differentiating them from the predominant other sounds of the same period, viz. cries), a feature of vowels in all natural languages. From a metaphonological standpoint, quasi-resonants represent an achievement since they show systematic use of normal phonation. However, quasi-resonant sounds differ from mature speech in that they are made without taking advantage of the vocal tract's resonance potential. The prototypical nucleus of a syllable of speech is not quasi-resonant but fully resonant, involving an open vocal tract. In addition, prototypical syllables involve articulation—both a fully resonant nucleus and a consonant-like gesture (obstructed vocal tract). The quasi-resonant sounds of the phonation stage do not involve these features of speech.

Although quasi-resonant sounds are predominant among sounds with arbitrary potential in the phonation stage, some fully resonant sounds (and other types as well) do occur. The limited frequency of occurrence of the other sounds, plus their lack of repetitive occurrence, suggests that the infant's production of the quasi-resonant sounds is more controlled. In all the stages of infancy, some developmentally progressive vocal types occur, although infrequently, (even canonical syllables occasionally occur in the first months of life), yielding the implication that such sounds are not yet under control. The stage model presented here focuses on sound types that are salient during the stage because they are produced repetitively, and are consequently assumed to be under the infant's control.

The Gooing Stage: Articulation with Normal Phonation (2–3 Months)

During the gooing stage (Oller, 1980), infants produce normal phonation associated with articulatory movements that result in contact of structures at the back of the vocal cavity (tongue dorsum with soft palate, hard palate, or pharynx; or epiglottis with one of the same structures). Because the beginning of gooing represents the onset of one of the requirements of speech systems—articulation during normal phonation—it is metaphonologically significant. The name "gooing" (sometimes "cooing," though the latter term is also sometimes used to refer to vowel-like sounds) results from the fact that adults often identify such infant utterances as involving velar (g- or k-like) articulations. The "oo" (a minimally open vowel) is also more similar to the quasi-resonant nuclei of gooing than any of the other vowels of English. Thus, the term has onomatopoetic validity. It should be noted, however, that quasi-resonant sounds are not exactly like "oo's," and the articulations of gooing often involve frication sounds quite unlike the "g's" and "k's" of English. Furthermore, it should be emphasized that gooing rarely involves sounds that could qualify as canonical syllables. Canonical syllables require fully resonant nuclei and transitions of margin (consonant) to nucleus (vowel) of 120 msec or less.

One or both of these requirements are usually violated in gooing.

The Expansion Stage (4–6 Months)

In the expansion stage (Oller, 1980, or vocal play stage, cf. Stark, 1980), several new sound types become salient, though the order of occurrence has been found to vary from child to child. First, fully resonant nuclei (vowel-like sounds) involve open vocal tracts and normal phonation. These are metaphonologically significant since they are a manifestation of the child's systematic utilization of the resonance potentials of the vocal tract, establishing the basis for vowel quality contrasts. Second, squealing and growling (very high pitched and very low pitched vocalizations) indicate the infant's ability to control pitch, a feature that is involved in many segmental and suprasegmental speech contrasts in natural languages. Third, yelling and whispering (very high intensity and very low intensity vowel-like sounds) indicate infant control of amplitude of vocalization, a feature of major metaphonological significance. Fourth, raspberries (bilabial or labiolingual trills or vibrants) show the infant's control over articulations with the lips, structures involved in speech contrasts in all languages. Finally, marginal babbling (presyllables that involve both fully resonant nuclei and consonant-like articulations, but without the rapid transitions of canonical syllables) signifies the infant's ability to combine many of the key elements of syllables in natural languages.

The expansion stage is filled with periods of repetitive production of new sound types. One day the infant may spend hours producing raspberries, while the next day may be filled with growling. The pattern of occurrence clearly indicates focus on particular sound types during concentrated periods (Oller, 1980; Stark, 1980; Zlatin, 1976).

Canonical Vocalizations

The Canonical Stage (7–10 Months)

Prior to about 7 months of age, infant sounds incorporate many metaphonological characteristics of speech (full resonance, articulation with tongue and lips, pitch control, etc.) but they are still not sufficiently speech-like to be mistaken for words. It is only when canonical stage vocalizations begin that parents and other observers commonly mistake infant sounds for speech. The most salient kind of canonical vocalization, reduplicated babbling (involving sequences such as [baba . . .], [dada . . .], [nana . . .], [mama . . .]), is significant in that its well-timed syllable transitions give evidence of a major metaphonological achievement. In addition, its inherent repetitiveness demonstrates the infant's growing control of speech-like sounds. Reduplicated forms have been incorporated into many languages as nursery terms such as [mama] and [nana] meaning "mother," "grandmother," "father," "grandfather," "bottle," "food," etc. Canonical babbling is not, however, always reduplicated. Infants commonly produce monosyllables or vowel-consonant-vowel (VCV) syllables in the canonical stage.

The Variegated Babbling Stage (11–12 Months) In succeeding months, infants continue to produce predominantly canonical syllables, but with an expanded repertoire including nonreduplicated syllable sequences (Oller, 1980). Variegated babbling, like other infant vocal types, may differ substantially from infant to infant. At one extreme, some infants begin to talk meaningfully soon after the onset of canonical syllables and rarely employ variegated sequences in prespeech. At the other extreme, some infants produce extremely complex variegated babbling (often called gibberish or jargon) prior to meaningful speech. Such complex variegated babbling leaves the impression that the infant is attempting to mimic adult conversational speech.

THE MYTHS REVISITED

The Methodological Myth

The contention that "there is no International Phonetic Alphabet for the utterances of a baby" (Lynip, 1951, p. 226) has fostered a general rejection of the study of infant vocalizations in the light of adult phonetic systems. Such a rejection is shortsighted as was pointed out by Winitz (1960) over 20 years ago. The myth persists despite the fact that it is necessary to compare infant vocalizations with mature speech in order to obtain a clear view of the significance of infant sounds as precursors to speech. The use of instrumental analysis yields the same methodological problems as phonetic analysis, since instrumental analysis of infant sounds must make reference to similar analyses of mature sounds. A *combination* of instrumental techniques and phonetic interpretation methods is needed.

In order to modify appropriately the traditional position on the value of phonetic transcription, it is useful to consider the range of transcribability in infant vocalizations. Canonical syllables are quite transcribable since they obey the syllable timing restrictions of languages and involve fully resonant nuclei. At the same time, precanonical sounds are more difficult to transcribe because they do not manifest the same restrictions. When a parent or investigator asserts that a 3-month-old infant said "aga," it may be quite misleading because the "a's" may not have been fully resonant, the consonant-like element may have been an intermittent friction sound, and the transitions between consonant-like and nucleic elements may have involved excessive durations or voice breaks. An appropriate transcription system for precanonical sequences must take into account such variations from mature speech patterns. A metaphonological framework lays the basis for such transcription while capitalizing on results of instrumental analysis as well.

Conclusion Infant vocalizations can be compared with mature speech within a metaphonological framework. Both instrumental analyses and phonetic transcriptions are useful, but it is necessary to adapt transcription systems to account adequately for metaphonological patterns of precanonical utterances.

The Discontinuity Myths

Random Sounds in Babbling When various authors have referred to infant babbling as "wild," "unformed," "unorganized," or "random" (Gregoire, 1948; Jakobson, 1941;

Lenneberg, 1962; Velten, 1943), they have erred in failing to notice obvious patterns. The random babbling myth was perpetuated by Jakobson's (1941) influential contention that infants "can produce all articulations equally well" during the babbling period (p. 50). In fact, careful observation of infants shows that the babbling sounds of individual infants are quite ordered and that infants consistently produce a common subset of syllable types. Note, for example, that one can list commonly occurring reduplicated babbling sequences ([baba . . .], [dada . . .], [nana . . .], [mama . . .], [wawa . . .], [yaya . . .]) as well as potential syllable sequences that virtually never occur in infant babbling ([stasta . . .], [aldald . . .], [ızız . . .]). The fact that such a list can be constructed indicates a highly ordered activity, and is in sharp contrast with what one would expect if infants produced all sounds equally well.

It is tempting to speculate that references to "random" sounds have not generally been meant to apply to babbling per se, which seems very speech-like and would be easy to recognize as an ordered activity. Rather, the notion of "random sounds" may have been intended for precanonical vocalizations of infants, which are less speech-like and due to their unfamiliarity, more difficult to categorize. Even in the precanonical period, however, the contention of randomness is not borne out. Infants proceed through an orderly sequence of vocalization developments that can be interpreted metaphonologically (as above). Furthermore, examination of the pattern of production of various precanonical vocalization types shows the infant's tendency to produce repetitive sequences of vocal categories (squeals, growls, fully resonant sounds, etc.). This pattern violates the randomness contention.

Conclusion Infant vocalizations are highly ordered both in canonical and precanonical stages. While a total description of production of such sounds by infants may require random factors as well as specific structural restrictions, it would be incorrect to suggest that sounds of babbling are randomly produced.

All Sounds of All Languages in Babbling Perhaps the most persistent myth about infant sounds is that babbling includes all sounds of languages. This idea appears in child development and experimental psychology texts (cf. Biehler, 1981; Osgood, 1953), as well as in the older treatments of child language (Gregoire, 1948; Jakobson, 1941). Although some recent texts have contradicted the myth (cf. Mussen, Conger, & Kagan, 1979), it remains a widespread belief.

Again, an understanding of the origins of the myth may hinge on the distinction between canonical and precanonical vocalizations. Canonical sounds are highly structured and very limited in terms of occurring sound types. It seems likely that the myth developed primarily with reference to precanonical sounds. A variety of rare articulatory gestures do occur in precanonical sounds, including occasional uvular trills, and lingual or labial clicks. Such sounds are not common in the world's languages.

Other sound types, however, do not seem to occur, even in precanonical vocalizations. Among such sounds are lingual trills (tongue tip), retroflex ejectives, lateral clicks, palatalized lateral liquids, and many others. In addition, many infant sound types (including the full volume lingual and labial clicks, and voiced uvular trills) occur extremely rarely.

It is possible that authors of the myth have leaped to the conclusion that occasional occurrence of some rare sounds of the world's languages indicates a total phonetic capacity. Before such a conclusion should be drawn, it would be necessary to conduct a study finding examples of all linguistic sound types in babbling. As far as this author knows, such a study has never even been formally attempted.

Conclusion While a variety of sounds do occur in infant vocalizations, there are some that occur very commonly and others that occur extremely infrequently if at all. Infant vocalizations indicate the tendency to produce certain key sound types to the virtual exclusion of others.

No Phonetic Relationship between Babbling and Young-Child Speech The myth that infant babbling and young-child speech have "nothing in common" is attributable to Jakobson (1941, p. 28). He emphasized the belief by contending that babbling showed "phonetic abundance" while first speech stages showed a "deflation" (p. 25) of sound types to those few sounds that are common to all the languages of the world.

A variety of research studies have discredited Jakobson's view empirically (Cruttenden, 1970; Menyuk, 1968). In fact, the sounds that are mastered earliest in young-child speech are very similar to the preferred (i.e., most frequent) sounds of babbling. Oller, Wieman, Doyle, and Ross (1976) compared the frequency of occurrence of babbled sounds and sounds of young-child speech and found that all the well-documented tendencies of young speech are seen in babbling as well. Such a pattern is consistent with the observation that nursery terms of many languages (e.g., *mama, baba, nana, dada,* etc.) tend to be selected from the inventory of favorite infant babbling sequences. Furthermore, the favorite sounds of both babbling and young-child speech appear to be the sounds that are relatively universal in languages around the world.

Conclusion Infant babbling and young-child speech are extremely similar in phonetic content. Such similarity can be no accident—babbling clearly manifests the emergence of a capacity for speech production, and many of the phonetic restrictions of later speech are foreshadowed in babbled utterances.

Babbling Drift Myths

Gradual Drift in Babbling toward Native Language Sounds The idea that speech-like vocalizations of infants during the first year change gradually to come to resemble those of the language community is based in part upon the reinforcement theory of Mowrer (1954). The inadequacy of the theory is in its failure to conform to the facts. Changes in vocalization systems of infants across the first year of life are often very sudden rather than gradual. Note, for example, that the canonical stage often begins with an explosion of canonical utterances on a single day. Furthermore, the kinds of sounds preferred by infants at the end of the first year of life are clearly the relatively universal sounds (cf. Oller et al., 1975) rather than sounds of the infant's native

language in general. Consider for example that English-learning infants avoid /r/'s, /l/'s, and /s/'s, three of the very common English consonants.

Conclusion Vocal development in the first year of life shows many sudden changes. By the end of the first year, infants tend to produce sounds that are relatively universal.

Audible Differences in Babbling of Babies from Different Communities The belief that babies from different language communities babble differently has been spread on the basis of very preliminary evidence that upon scrutiny proves to be inconclusive (for example, Weir, 1966). Such studies have suggested moderate capabilities to differentiate babies from different backgrounds based upon tape-recorded babbling samples. The studies suffer, however, from crucial methodological problems of sample size (too few infants in each language group can yield discriminations due merely to individual differences), sample matching (socioeconomic factors have not been considered appropriately), and insufficient care in blinding observers. More trustworthy studies (Atkinson, MacWhinney, & Stoel, 1970; Olney & Scholnick, 1976; and Thevenin, Eilers, Oller, & Bull, 1983) have failed to indicate the ability of observers to discriminate among babies of differing language backgrounds. In addition, instrumentally and transcriptionally based studies (Eady, 1980; Eilers, Oller, & Benito-Garcia, 1984; Oller & Eilers, 1982; Preston, Yeni-Komshian, & Stark, 1967) have emphasized dramatic similarities in babbling of infants from differing language backgrounds while finding no convincing differences.

Conclusion The possibility that infants from differing language backgrounds babble differently is still an unproved, though interesting, hypothesis. Because infants babble very similarly regardless of background, it may be difficult to discern differences if they actually occur.

Babbling in Deaf Infants

It is widely believed that deaf infants "babble" in the first year of life and then stop doing so. This belief is primarily attributable to two sources, Lenneberg, Rebelsky, and Nichols (1965) and Mavilya (1969). In fact, these studies offer equivocal information. Neither study employed a categorization system that differentiated between canonical and precanonical sounds as above. What the authors referred to as babbling appears to have been precanonical vocalization of the marginal variety. As indicated in Gilbert's (1982) review of the literature, later researchers misunderstood the import of these studies. More recent work in the University of Miami laboratories with three intellectually normal deaf infants, as well as a survey study by Mykelbust (1957) have suggested that the canonical stage may begin very late (beyond 12 months) in deaf infants, even in those who have early amplification. In addition, the studies suggest a very rich precanonical vocal tendency continuing throughout the first year of life in profoundly deaf children.

Conclusion Deaf infants appear not to reach the stage of canonical babbling in the first year of life. While canonical vocalizations do not appear normally in the deaf, many precanonical sounds occur across the first year.

McCarthy's Myth

McCarthy (1952) supported the view that much of the content of early vocal sounds is attributable to mechanical forces acting upon a passive infant. In her view, the passive infant's velopharyngeal port opens or closes depending on posture (upright or supine), yielding nasal or nonnasal sounds, respectively. In fact, very young infants breathe nasally even in the supine position (cf. Bosma, 1972) and infant crying appears to involve nasality in various postures (Stark & Nathanson, 1973).

The possibility that gooing results from gravitational effects on a passive soft palate and tongue in supine positions is also not supported by evidence. Oller (1981) found that gooing was similarly frequent in upright and supine positions.

Conclusion The contention that gravitational forces impose particular vocal types upon infants is as yet unproved. In fact, infants in the first few months of life show considerble ability to compensate for changes in direction of gravitational force owing to changes in posture.

GENERAL CONCLUSION

The study of infant vocalizations has produced important advances in recent years. It is now possible to outline stages of vocal development across the first year of life in a linguistically significant framework. Metaphonological interpretation of infant sounds indicates that infants progress through several vocal categories, each of which provides the opportunity for the infant to explore a particular parameter or parameters necessary in the maturation of the speech capacity. Recent work has also shown in unambiguous ways that infant babbling and speech are closely related.

Myths about infant vocalizations, such as the myth of randomness or of lack of relation between babbling and young-child speech, are very persistent, but will predictably evaporate in the face of mounting evidence. Some of the other misconceptions discussed above concern as yet unproved hypotheses necessitating further experimentation and observation. Clarification of the facts of infant vocal development is a worthy pursuit both for its pure scientific value and for the information it will yield to help plan intervention for infants expected to show linguistic/phonological impairments.

REFERENCES

Atkinson, K.B., MacWhinney, B., & Stoel, C. An experiment in the recognition of babbling. *Papers and Reports on Child Language Development*, No. 1. Stanford, CA: Stanford University Press, 1970.

Biehler, R.F. *Child development: An introduction.* Boston: Houghton Mifflin Co., 1981.

Bosma, J.F. Form and function of the infant's mouth and pharynx. In: J.F. Bosma (ed.), *Third symposium on oral sensation and perception: The mouth of the infant.* Springfield, IL: Charles C Thomas, 1972.

Cruttenden, A. A phonetic study of babbling. *British Journal of Disorders of Communication*, 1970, 5, 110–118.

Eady, S. The onset of language specific patterning in infant vocalization. Unpublished master's thesis, Department of Linguistics, University of Ottawa, Ottawa, 1980.

Eilers, R.E., Oller, D.K., & Benito-Garcia, C.R. The acquisition of voicing contrasts in Spanish- and English-learning infants and children: A longitudinal study. *Journal of Child Lanugage*, 1984, *11*.

Gilbert, J.H.V. Babbling and the deaf child: A commentary on Lenneberg et al. (1965) and Lenneberg (1967). *Journal of Child Language*, 1982, *9*, 511–515.

Gregoire, A. L'apprentissage du langage [The learning of language]. *Lingua*, 1948, *1*, 162–164, 168–169, 170–172.

Jakobson, R. [*Child language, aphasia and phonological universals*] (A. Keiler, trans.). The Hague: Mouton, 1968. (Originally published in German in 1941.)

Lenneberg, E.H. Understanding language without the ability to speak. *Journal of Abnormal and Social Psychology*, 1962, *65*, 419–425.

Lenneberg, E.H., Rebelsky, G.F., & Nichols, I.A. The vocalizations of infants born to deaf and to hearing parents. *Human Development*, 1965, *8*, 23–37.

Lynip, A.W. The use of magnetic devices in the collection and analysis of the preverbal utterances of an infant. *Genetic Psychology Monographs*, 1951, *44*, 221–262.

McCarthy, D. Organismic interpretation of infant vocalizations. *Child Development*, 1952, *23*(4), 273–280.

Mavilya, M.P. *Spontaneous vocalization and babbling in hearing impaired infants*. Unpublished doctoral dissertation, Columbia University, New York, (University Microfilms No. 70-12879), 1969.

Menyuk, D. The role of distinctive features in children's acquisition of phonology. *Journal of Speech and Hearing Research*, 1968, *11*, 138–146.

Mowrer, O.H. The psychologist looks at language. *American Psychologist*, 1954, *9*, 660–694.

Mussen, P.H., Conger, J.J., & Kagan, J. *Child development and personality*. New York: Harper & Row, 1979.

Mykelbust, H.R. Babbling and echolalia in language theory. *Journal of Speech and Hearing Disorders*, 1957, *22*, 356–360.

Oller, D.K. The emergence of the sounds of speech in infancy. In: G. Yeni-Komshian, C. Kavanagh, & C. Ferguson (eds.), *Child phonology: Perception and production*. New York: Academic Press, 1980.

Oller, D.K. Infant vocalizations: Exploration and reflexivity. In: R.E. Stark (ed.), *Language behavior in infancy and early childhood*. New York: Elsevier North-Holland, 1981.

Oller, D.K., & Eilers, R.E. Similarities of babbling in Spanish- and English-learning babies. *Journal of Child Languages*, 1982, *9*, 565–578.

Oller, D.K., Wieman, L.A., Doyle, W., & Ross, C. Infant babbling and speech. *Journal of Child Language*, 1976, *3*, 1–11.

Olney, R.L., & Scholnick, E.K. Adult judgments of age and linguistic differences in infant vocalization. *Journal of Child Language*, 1976, *3*(2), 145–156.

Osgood, C.E. *Method and theory in experimental psychology*. New York: Oxford University Press, 1953.

Preston, M.S., Yeni-Komshian, G., & Stark, R.E. Voicing in initial stop consonants produced by children in the prelinguistic period from different language communities. *John Hopkins University School of Medicine, Annual Report of Neurocommunications Laboratory*, No. 2, pp. 305–323, 1967.

Stark, R.E. Stages of speech development in the first year of life. In: G. Yeni-Komshian, J. Kavanagh, & C. Ferguson (eds.), *Child phonology*, Vol. 1. New York: Academic Press, 1980.

Stark, R.E., & Nathanson, S.N. Spontaneous cry in the newborn infant: Sounds and facial gestures. In: J.F. Bosma (ed.), *Fourth Symposium on Oral Sensation and Perception: Development in the fetus and infant*. Bethesda, MD: U.S. Department of Health, Education, and Welfare, 1974.

Thevenin, D., Eilers, R.E., Oller, D.K., & Bull, D. *Monolingual and bilingual adults' perception of infant babbling*. Paper presented at the biannual meeting of the Society for Research in Child Development, Detroit, April, 1983.

Velten, H.V. The growth of phonemic and lexical patterns in infant language. *Language*, 1943, *19*, 281–292.

Weir, R.H. Some questions on the child's learning of phonology. In: F. Smith & G.A. Miller (eds.), *The genesis of language*. Cambridge: Massachusetts Institute of Technology Press, 1966.

Winitz, H. Spectrographic investigation of infant vowels. *Journal of Genetic Psychology*, 1960, *96*, 171–181.

Zlatin, M. *Language acquisition: Some acoustic and interactive aspects of infancy*. Final Report, NIE grant, NE-G-00-3-0077, 1976.

Chapter 38

The Discrimination of
Rapid Spectral Speech Cues
by Down Syndrome and
Normally Developing Infants

Rebecca E. Eilers, Ph.D.
Dale H. Bull, Ph.D.
D. Kimbrough Oller, Ph.D.
Diana C. Lewis, M.A.
University of Miami, Miami, Florida

OVER ONE-THIRD OF ALL SEVERELY RE-tarded people are victims of Down syndrome. While individuals affected by Down syndrome (DS) are reported to show general developmental lags, their retardation in the area of speech communication is more severe than would be predicted by mental age alone (Johnson & Abelson, 1969).

SPECIFIC LANGUAGE PROBLEMS OF DOWN SYNDROME CHILDREN

Problems of communication in DS children are most evident in the auditory-vocal channel. Belmont (1971), in his review of the literature on cross-modal perception and sensory integration processes in DS, concluded that the auditory channel is weaker than the visual and that the auditory-vocal channel is particularly deficient. Scheffelin (1968) found poorer per-formance by DS children in experimental tasks that tap the auditory-vocal channel than in tasks that tap the visual-vocal, auditory-motor, or visual-motor channels. Other evidence indicates gestural communication in DS children is superior to their vocal communication (Bilovski & Share, 1965) and that reception of gestural symbols may be better in DS children than reception of spoken words (Oller, Coleman, & Eilers, 1978). Finally, there is considerable evidence that DS children have substantial difficulties in speech articulation (Schlanger & Gottsleben, 1957).

Despite the observations that DS children have particular difficulties in acquiring spoken language, little is known about the nature of the deficits that result in the relative language delay. The audiological and otological litera-ture is replete with reports of conductive hear-ing loss in DS children sometimes complicated

Funding for this project was provided by a grant to the senior author from the National Institutes of Neurological Disease and Stroke (NS 17604). The authors would like to thank the parents of the Down syndrome children who supported their efforts through the period of this research. The authors would also like to express their appreciation to C. Gillman, P. Morse, and the staff of the Waisman Center, University of Wisconsin Computing Center, for their assistance with stimulus preparation.

---

with mild to moderate sensorineural loss as well. Balkany, Downs, Jafek, and Krajicek (1979) and Schwartz and Schwartz (1978) report the incidence of middle ear pathology to be at 60% in a sample of asymptomatic children. In accord with these data, Greenberg, Wilson, Moore, and Thompson (1979) have reported depressed speech reception thresholds in DS. Other research (Walthi, Salvisber, & Auf der Maur, 1973) has suggested that auditory memory deficits might play a role in language-learning difficulties. To date, however, specific speech discrimination abilities of DS infants have not been investigated. Such studies may clarify roles of auditory-specific speech processing mechanisms in the communication problems of DS children.

AUDITORY-SPEECH PROCESSING IN DS CHILDREN

Several kinds of evidence suggest that auditory-speech processing in mentally retarded children may be particularly deficient, especially with regard to dynamic spectral cues (rapid changes in the frequency spectrum of speech sounds). Tallal (1976) and Tallal and Piercy (1974, 1975) have shown that young children with specific language problems prove deficient in discrimination of rapid formant transitions (rapid spectral changes accompanying changes in place of articulation) compared to discrimination of slowly varying or steady formants. Eilers and Oller (1980) have reported that a group of very young retarded children discriminated steady-state speech stimuli (in the Visually Reinforced Infant Speech Discrimination paradigm) comparatively better than rapidly changing speech stimuli. Thus far, no similar research specifically directed toward DS children's discrimination of such stimulus parameters has been performed.

If DS infants do have a particular deficit in processing of rapid spectral cues, the effects of the deficit could be debilitating given the pervasive role played by dynamic spectral change in speech perception in general. Rapid spectral cues embodied in formant transitions account for a wide variety of speech contrasts, including place of articulation of consonants, distinctions of stops, glides, and vowel sequences, and vowel and semivowel quality in rapid speech where steady-state vowel production is virtually nonexistent. Thus, it would seem prudent to begin the exploration of the speech processing capabilities of young DS children and infants by examining their ability to detect rapid spectral change.

METHODOLOGICAL ADVANCES AND THE STUDY OF SPEECH PROCESSING DEFICITS

The dearth of information on speech discrimination skills in young DS children and infants does not result from a lack of interest in the topic, but, rather, research in this area has suffered from a lack of appropriate experimental paradigms to evaluate speech discrimination skills. With the advent of the Visually Reinforced Infant Speech Discrimination (VRISD) paradigm in the mid seventy's (Eilers, Wilson, & Moore, 1977) and its further development (Eilers & Gavin, 1981), it became possible to assess both DS infants and normally developing infants with the same stimulus materials and procedures. Normally developing and DS infants could be matched for mental age with the assumption that both groups would succeed equally well on the VRISD task. Following such a strategy, results could then be interpreted in terms of differences in speech processing rather than differences in intellectual development.

With these tools in hand, it is possible to address DS infants' abilities to process speech-like auditory information in infancy. The authors' study compares the ability of DS infants to discriminate slowly changing versus rapidly changing transitional information. Normally developing infants were tested on the same speech contrasts for comparison.

METHOD

Subjects

Nine full-term normally developing infants (5–11 months old) and nine DS infants were selected for the study. The DS infants were selected from the High Risk Followup Clinic of the Mailman Center for Child Development. Several of the DS infants were tested with the VRISD discrimination procedure for several months before they demonstrated appropriate orientation to the auditory stimuli, a prerequisite for task success. The DS infants were entered in the study at the point at which normal orientation was observed (14–25 months). Normally developing infants had a mean chronological age of 8 months. DS infants had a mean chronological age of 19 months and a mean developmental index score of 53 (a range of 35–64 on the Bayley Scales of Infant Development). All DS infants had hearing within normal limits at the time of testing as assessed by behavioral auditory (VRA) and tympanometry.

Stimuli

Two sets of contrasting stimuli were used in this study: training stimuli and test stimuli. The training stimulus contrast pair consisted of five tokens each of the syllables /bit/ ("beat") and /bɪt/ ("bit") produced by a male phonetician and matched pairwise for overall duration, overall amplitude, peak amplitude, mean fundamental frequency, and peak fundamental frequency. These stimuli differed in the formant structure of the vowel and have been used successfully in the past as a VRISD training contrast (Morse, Eilers, & Gavin, 1982).

The experimental test stimuli consisted of three pairs of syllables, synthesized using the Klatt (1980) routines. The first syllable pair, /ba/ versus /ga/, differed only with respect to the slope of the second formant transition. In natural-speech articulatory terms, the stimuli differed in second formant frequency during the 25-msec transition of consonant to vowel. The second stimulus pair was constructed by lengthening this same transition to 75 msec. This lengthening of the transition duration resulted in stimuli heard as /wa/ and /ya/ by adult listeners. The third pair was made by further lengthening the transition to 225 msec so that the resulting pair sounded like the bisyllabic vowel sequences /ua/ and /ia/. It is important to note that transitions as long as 225 msec rarely

if ever occur in mature syllables. Syllables with lengthy durations have been reported, however, for infants who have not yet reached the stage of canonical babbling (Oller, 1983).

Thus, three stimulus pairs were constructed that differed only with respect to the duration of the second formant transition from consonant to following vowel. The /ba/–/ga/ pair contained rapid spectral changes, while the /ua/–/ia/ pair contained extremely slow spectral changes. The /wa/–/ya/ pair was intermediate in rate of spectral change and the transition duration of this pair was typical of many mature syllables containing semivowels.

For comparison purposes, four adults were presented with the test stimuli for both discrimination and identification testing. Discrimination scores were 100% for all adult perceivers. Adults had no difficulty correctly identifying each of the six stimuli.

Four stimulus tapes were constructed: one for training and three for testing. Stimuli were recorded with each member of the pair on a different channel of a two-track audiotape. The stimulus on a single channel was separated by an interstimulus interval (ISI) of 600 msec. Computer control permitted switching from one member of the pair to the other without clipping stimuli.

Apparatus

The experimental site consisted of a double-walled, sound-attenuated booth equipped with an HPM 100 speaker, four visual reinforcers (housed in a dark plexiglass box), and a response box allowing communication with the computer. The adjoining control room housed high fidelity playback and amplification equipment and a DEC 11/23 laboratory computer for controlling stimulus conditions and reinforcement and for recording and analyzing data.

Procedure

The Visually Reinforced Infant Speech Discrimination (VRISD) paradigm (described in Eilers, Gavin, & Oller, 1982), in which infants are conditioned to turn their heads to a change in a repeating background auditory stimulus, was used to assess infants' speech discrimination. During this procedure, the infant was seated on a parent's lap in the booth and an experimenter attempted to keep the infant in a midline orientation by manipulating a set of quiet toys. Both the parents and the experimenter listened to masking music over headphones during the entire experimental session. As an added precaution, the experimenter wore earplugs. In this artificially "deafened" condition, the experimenter was unable to pass the training criterion set for the infant when the experimenter played the role of subject.

The session began with the continuous presentation at 60 dB sound pressure level (SPL) of the training stimuli on one tape channel (e.g., /bit/). This background stimulus (S_b) remained on throughout the training, interrupted by the presentations of the change stimulus (S_d) on the other tape channel (e.g., /bɪt/).

The experimenter was responsible for monitoring the infants' behavior, initiating trials, and indicating headturn responses. Each test session began with a shaping phase during which the background stimulus (S_b) was changed to the contrasting stimulus (S_d) for approximately 6 seconds at an intensity of 12 dB greater than the background level. If the infant was observed to turn toward the speaker during S_d, the experimenter would activate the reinforcer by depressing a button on the response box. If the infant did not turn on the first trial, on the second trial the reinforcer was activated toward the end of the 6-second period. After a few trials, most infants turned at the presentation of the louder S_d. After two consecutive trials in which the infants responded correctly within the S_d time window, the intensity of S_d was reduced in 4-dB steps until the infant responded correctly on two consecutive trials at each intensity level, after which matched intensity (60 dB) change trials were introduced.

During the matched intensity phase, the change from S_b to S_d occurred on one-half of the trials (change trials). On the remaining trials (control trials), no change from S_b to S_d occurred. During control trials, head turns were recorded but no reinforcement was given. These no-change trials served to control for the infant's spontaneous, random head-turning. On every fifth trial, a probe was presented in

which a change from S_b to S_d was accompanied by a 4-dB increment. These trials were included to maintain the infant's interest throughout the session, but head turns during these intensity-cued trials were not included in the analysis. The order of presentation of the change and control trials was pseudorandom with three possible combinations of change and control trials per block of 10 trials: six change and four control, five change and five control, or four change and six control. The experimenter initiated a trial when the infant was engaged at midline. The pseudorandom order of trial presentation coupled with the absence of auditory information during testing prevented the experimenter from knowing the nature of the test trial. Hence, all observations of head-turning behavior were made free of experimenter bias.

Infants were trained to a criterion of nine out of 10 correct successive equal-intensity test trials with the stimulus pair /bit/ versus /bɪt/. This generally required between one and three sessions, following which the infant returned for testing on the three experimental contrasts. The infants were tested on one contrast each week. At the beginning of each of the subsequent testing sessions, an abbreviated shaping phase was employed in which each infant received only two trials at each of three intensity level differences. This was followed by 30 test trials, approximately half of which were control trials. The three experimental contrasts (/ba/–/ga/, /wa/–/ya/, and /ua/–/ia/) were presented in a counterbalanced fashion. Half of the infants received track-one stimuli for S_b while the other half received track-one stimuli for S_d.

RESULTS

DS infants with developmental ages between 7 and 16 months were able to meet the training criteria for participation in the present study of speech discrimination. DS infants met the criterion in an average of 2.2 sessions, comparable to the normally developing infants who met the criterion in an average of 2.1 sessions.

Performance for each infant on the test pairs was blocked into three groups of 10 test trials each and expressed as a discriminative index

(DI) score for each trial block. The DI score is calculated as the number of hits minus the number of false positives divided by the number of change trials (see Morse et al., 1982 for a discussion of DI scores in VRISD testing). These scores were subjected to both z tests of means to determine whether performance on a contrast differed from chance, and ANOVA to assess differences in performance between groups and contrasts.

Table 1 presents the mean DI scores, averaged across test blocks, for each of the stimulus contrasts within the different subject groups. Since each contrast was tested with nine subjects each receiving 30 trials, the DI scores for the individual contrasts were tested against a population mean of 0, a population standard deviation of 0.198, and a standard error of 0.066 (Morse et al., 1982). The results of the z tests of means are also included in Table 1. These tests indicated that DI scores were significantly greater than chance for DS infants on all three transition duration contrasts. Normal infants failed to show evidence of discrimination of the /ba/–/ga/ pair but did show evidence of discriminating the two pairs with longer transitions. Inspection of Figure 1 indicates that for both groups of infants, performance improved as a function of increased transition duration.

A split-plot ANOVA with one between-subjects factor (normal versus DS) and two within-subjects factors (stimulus contrast and trial block) was performed on the DI scores. This analysis indicated a significant effect for contrast, $F(2,32) = 6.84$, $p < .01$. Main effects for subject group and trial block were not significant, nor were any interactions. Post hoc analyses revealed that performance on the

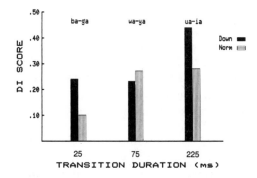

Figure 1. Mean Discriminative Index scores for three transition duration contrasts for both Down syndrome and normally developing infants.

/ba/–/ga/ pair differed significantly from performance on the /ua/–/ia/ pair for both normal and DS infants. There was no significant difference between performance on /wa/–/ya/ and /ua/–/ia/ pairs for normal infants, however DS infants performed significantly better on the longer transition duration pair.

DISCUSSION

The ability to perceive speech accurately and efficiently depends upon the perceiver's ability to process spectral change in relatively rapid time frames. Failure to perceive rapid spectral information has far-reaching consequences for the perceiver, since a large proportion of the speech code is based upon subtle differences in rapid spectral events. Recent research has suggested that some children with language delay have specific temporal processing deficits that have profound effects on their perception of speech. This study was designed to explore the hypothesis that language delayed DS infants also have deficits in temporal processing that affect their ability to perceive rapidly presented spectral information in speech-like stimuli. Accordingly, both DS and normal infants were presented with three syllable pairs for discrimination. Two of the syllable pairs involved formant transition durations (25 and 75 msec) common in speech while the third involved a long transition duration (225 msec) typically found in precanonical vocalizations of infants but not in mature speech syllables.

As expected, both DS and normal infants showed better performance on the longest transition duration stimuli than on the shortest

Table 1. Mean DI scores and z test statistics for normally developing and DS infants

	Mean DI	z test statistic
Down syndrome (intelligence)		
/ba/ versus /ga/	.24	3.63[a]
/wa/ versus /ya/	.23	3.48[a]
/ua/ versus /ia/	.44	6.66[a]
Normal development		
/ba/ versus /ga/	.10	1.66
/wa/ versus /ya/	.28	4.24[a]
/ua/ versus /ia/	.29	4.39[a]

[a]$p < .01$.

transition pair. Moreover, the DS infants discriminated the most rapid spectral transition (25 msec) while normal infant performance did not exceed chance on this pair. Although there was no significant interaction between infant group and transition duration, the two groups showed a different pattern of performance as a function of the test contrasts. As can be seen in Figure 1, a shift in normal infant performance occurs between the 25- and 75-msec transition pair, whereas DS infant performance showed a corresponding improvement between the 75- and 225-msec transition duration. Thus, the slopes of the two discrimination functions appear different for the two infant groups. This difference in the discrimination functions of normal and DS infants is suggestive of a temporal processing deficit in Down syndrome. Confirmation of such a deficit, however, will require discrimination testing with additional stimulus pairs chosen from the continuum of formant transition durations.

Although there was no significant main effect for the infant group, the superior performance of DS infants on both the longest and shortest duration pairs seems surprising. It is possible that this superior performance might be accounted for by language experience. The older DS infants had the opportunity to hear spoken language for up to 20 months longer than the normally developing infants. It is possible that during this period, the ability to track spectral changes developed as a function of auditory experience. This hypothesis could be tested directly only by examining speech discrimination in much younger DS infants. Experience, however, indicates that task demands of the VRISD paradigm preclude testing infants who have not attained a developmental age of 7–10 months.

An interesting, but serendipitous, finding of this study was the failure of normally developing infants to provide evidence of discrimination of the /ba/–/ga/ stimulus pair. This may seem contrary to the literature that suggests that the /ba/–/ga/ contrast is discriminable by infants (Moffitt, 1971; Morse, 1972). The apparent contradiction may be resolved by considering the fact that previous /ba/–/ga/ stimuli contained longer second formant transitions (40–50 msec). It would appear, therefore, that the perceptual boundary for detection of the direction of second formant transitions in stop consonants may lie somewhere between 25 and 40 msec for infants. This boundary is apparently shorter for adults since adult performance was perfect for the 25 msec pair. The fact that DS infants, but not normally developing infants, showed evidence of discrimination of the /ba/–/ga/ stimulus pair may suggest that early language experience (increased period of listening during infancy) results in a shift of the perceptual boundary toward the adult value.

This investigation suggests that the VRISD paradigm is an effective method for investigating the speech perception skills of young DS infants and children. Down syndrome infants with mental ages as young as 7–10 months can be trained as easily as normally developing infants and can be tested on a variety of speech perception questions. The age necessary for successful testing of DS infants is somewhat younger than the minimum age of 20 months reported by Greenberg et al. (1979) for success in a similar but somewhat easier task (visual reinforcement audiometry). Of course, it is possible that Greenberg et al. did not sample young enough infants. Some of the successfully trained DS infants in this study had chronological ages as young as 14 months and developmental ages of roughly 7–8 months. Moreover, it is important to note that both DS infants and the normally developing infants required the same average number of sessions to reach the training criterion. The ease of training and these test results provide a confirmation of the applicability of the VRISD paradigm as a tool for future speech perception research with Down syndrome and other special infant populations.

REFERENCES

Balkany, T., Downs, M.P., Jafek, B.W., & Krajicek, M.J. Hearing loss in Down's syndrome. *Clinical Pediatrics*, 1979, *18*, 116–118.

Belmont, J.M. Medical behaviorial research in retardation. In: N.R. Ellis (ed.), *International review of research in mental retardation*, Vol. 5. New York: Academic Press, 1971.

Bilovski, D., & Share, J. The ITPA and Down's syndrome: An exploratory study. *American Journal of Mental Deficiency*, 1965, *70*, 78–82.

Eilers, R., & Gavin, W. The evaluation of infant speech perception skills: Statistical techniques and theory development. In: R. Stark (ed.), *Language behavior in infancy and early childhood*. New York: Elsevier-North Holland, 1981.

Eilers, R.E., Gavin, W.J., & Oller, D.K. Cross-linguistic perception in infancy: The role of linguistic experience. *Journal of Child Language*, 1982, *9*, 289–302.

Eilers, R.E., & Oller, D.K. A comparative study of speech perception in young severely retarded children and normally developing infants. *Journal of Speech and Hearing Research*, 1980, *23*, 419–428.

Eilers, R.E., Wilson, W.R., & Moore, J.M. Developmental changes in speech discrimination in infants. *Journal of Speech and Hearing Research*, 1977, *20*, 766–780.

Greenberg, D.B., Wilson, W.R., Moore, J.M., & Thompson, G. Visual reinforcement audiometry (VRA) with young Down's syndrome children. *Journal of Speech and Hearing Disorders*, 1979, *44*, 80–90.

Johnson, R.C., & Abelson, R.B. Intellectual, behavioral, and physical characteristics associated with trisomy, translocation and mosaic types of Down's syndrome. *American Journal of Mental Deficiency*, 1969, *73*, 852–855.

Klatt, D.H. Software for a cascade/parallel formant synthesizer. *Journal of the Acoustical Society of America*, 1980, *67*, 971–995.

Moffitt, A.R. Consonant cue perception by twenty- to twenty-four-week-old infants. *Child Development*, 1971, *42*, 717–731.

Morse, P. The discrimination of speech and nonspeech stimuli in early infancy. *Journal of Experimental Child Psychology*, 1972, *14*, 477–492.

Morse, P.A., Eilers, R.E., & Gavin, W.J. The perception of the sound of silence in early infancy. *Child Development*, 1982, *53*, 189–195.

Oller, D.K. Infant babbling as a manifestation of the capacity for speech. In: S. Gerber & G. Mencher (ed.), *The development of auditory behavior*. New York: Grune & Stratton, 1983.

Oller, D.K., Coleman, D., & Eilers, R.E. A comparative study of discriminability of signed and spoken vocabulary. Paper presented at the Southeastern Conference on Human Development, Atlanta, April, 1978.

Scheffelin, M. Comparison of four stimulus-response channels in paired-associate learning with Down's syndrome children. *Dissertation Abstracts*, *28 (12-B)*, 5220–5221, Ann Arbor, MI: University Microfilms, 1968.

Schlanger, B., & Gottsleben, R.H. Analysis of speech defects amongst the institutionalized mentally retarded. *Journal of Speech and Hearing Disorders*, 1957, *22*, 98–103.

Schwartz, D.M., & Schwartz, R.H. Acoustic impedance and otoscopic findings in young children with Down's syndrome. *Archives of Otolaryngology*, 1978, *104*, 652–656.

Tallal, P. Rapid auditory processing in normal and disordered language development. *Journal of Speech and Hearing Research*, 1976, *19*, 561–571.

Tallal, P., & Piercy, M. Developmental aphasia: Rate of auditory processing and selective impairment of consonant perception. *Neuropsychologia*, 1974, *12*, 83–93.

Tallal, P., & Piercy, M. Developmental aphasia: The perception of brief vowels and extended stop consonants. *Neuropsychologia*, 1975, *13*, 69–74.

Walthi, U., Salvisber, H., & Auf der Maur, P. *Schweizesische Zeitschrift für Psychologie und ihre Anwendungen [Swiss Journal for Psychology and its Applications]*. *Separatakzug aus*, 1973, *32*, 132–158.

The At-Risk Infant: Psycho/Socio/Medical Aspects
edited by Shaul Harel, M.D., and Nicholas J. Anastasiow, Ph.D.
Copyright © 1985   Paul H. Brookes Publishing Co., Inc.   Baltimore • London

Chapter 39

Assessment of Vision
in Infants and Young Children

JANETTE ATKINSON, PH.D.
University of Cambridge, Cambridge, England

O VER THE PAST 10 YEARS, AN INTEREST IN DE-
veloping procedures for assessing vision
in infants and young children has evolved,
stimulated by research on adult vision (for
example, Campbell & Robson, 1968; reviewed
by Braddick, Campbell, & Atkinson, 1978),
and research on animal models of the functioning of the visual system (Hubel & Wiesel,
1962; Wiesel, 1982; reviewed by Aslin, Alberts, & Petersen, 1981). This chapter discusses various methods for visual assessment
that are currently in use in the Visual Development Unit at the University of Cambridge and
in a number of other laboratories and clinics. It
briefly discusses the author's experience with
these methods and the range of cases for which
they were found to be usefully applicable over
a period of 18 months in 1981–1982.

These assessments of vision serve two somewhat different functions and fall into two types:
1) clinical assessment of vision, and 2) vision
screening program. A clinical assessment of
vision is a detailed evaluation of visual function in cases where a visual problem is already
suspected or likely. In the vision screening

program, the assessment of vision is in a
"screening" context where the majority of the
children who are screened will be expected to
have normal visual development, and the task
of the screening program is to identify the small
group with a manifest visual problem and those
"at risk" for developing a visual problem.
Where possible, the second at-risk group
should be treated to prevent the later onset of a
visual problem.

CLINICAL ASSESSMENT OF VISION

Accurate information on functional vision
makes an important contribution to the treatment and rehabilitation of infants and children
with a visual problem. However, such an assessment is not a substitute for the assessments
and examinations already made by ophthalmologists and pediatricians, but a supplement
to them, giving a more complete picture of the
visual perceptual functioning of each child.

Over the review period, 75 children were
newly referred to the Visual Development Unit
for detailed clinical assessments. Infants and

This work is supported by the Medical Research Council. The author's thanks are due to the ophthalmologists and
pediatricians of Addenbrooke's Hospital, Cambridge, for their clinical collaboration, particularly Mr. P.G. Watson, Mr. J.
Keast-Butler, and Dr. M. Prendergast. The author gratefully acknowledges the cooperation of the Community Health
Department, Cambridge Health Authority, and the Orthoptic Department, Addenbrooke's Hospital, in the setting up and
operation of the refractive screening program. This work would not be possible without the collaboration of other members
of the Visual Development Unit: Oliver Braddick, Elizabeth Pimm-Smith, Carol Evans, Jackie Day, John Wattam-Bell, and
Kim Durden.

young children were referred from three sources:

1. Referrals from ophthalmology ($n = 25$; 33%). The purpose of most of these referrals was to ascertain the levels of visual function either binocularly (e.g., in cases of bilateral cataract or suspected "cortical blindness") or monocularly (e.g., in cases of ptosis, amblyopia, unilateral cataract, strabismus). Ages ranged from birth to 3 years.

2. Referrals from pediatrics for children with developmental problems ($n = 49$, including 3 also referred from ophthalmology; 65%). Most of the children in this group had marked pediatric problems (e.g., cerebral palsy, hemiparesis, hydrocephalus) as well as a suspected visual defect. The age range was 3 months to 12 years, although most were between 1 and 4 years. Most suffered some degree of developmental delay, so the problems of visual testing were generally those usually associated with younger children. However, the level of sensory and motor development, and the relation between these, was extremely varied.

3. Referrals from general practitioners and health visitors (i.e., community nursing staff). Only 4 infants were referred with suspected total blindness or very severe visual handicap. In two cases, no evidence of functional vision could be found, and since these children showed a more general developmental delay referral to a pediatrician was suggested. The other two children were found to have normal vision for their age.

A larger group of children ($N = 80$) was referred by general practitioners and health visitors over much the same 18-month time period, with suspected strabismus or visual anomalies, but no fear of blindness. These children were included in the screening program (see below).

The aim of each assessment was to find out as much as possible about the child's visual capabilities using a battery of tests carried out by scientists, medically qualified staff, and

paramedics. The procedure used is outlined in Table 1. Each part of the test procedure is briefly described below, together with a reference, where appropriate, to other methods that, although not used regularly at present, could be used in such assessments. Many of the tests are based on research techniques developed in the Visual Development Unit; they are described more fully in the references cited.

Medical/Family History of Vision

It is important to discuss with the parents the child's vision in relation to his or her general perceptual development and to discuss the tests that will be used in the assessment and what they mean in terms of the child's visuoperceptual world. Also helpful is an accurate history of any family eye problems.

General Visuo-Motor Behavior

The period spent by children in the Unit allows extended observation of their visually guided actions in playing with a wide range of toys and responding to the people around them. This is supplemented by informal testing of visually guided reaching and grasping, visual attention to distance (e.g., awareness of parent entering the room, or response to "peek-a-boo" at 2 meters around the edge of a screen) and informal field testing (visually conspicuous, but silent toy or Stycar ball brought in from the peripheral field). In cases of hemiparesis or apparent field loss, it is particularly important to test for field asymmetries. When perceptual rather than sensory defects are suspected, the child's level of object permanence and visual recognition is informally assessed.

Table 1. Clinical assessment of vision

1.	Discussion of child's medical history/family history of visual problems
2.	Observation of general visuo-motor behavior
3.	Orthoptic tests
4.	Acuity assessment (forced-choice preferential looking (FPL), Stycar, Sheridan-Gardiner, "Crowding")
5.	Photorefraction and retinoscopy
6.	Binocular vision Monocular optokinetic nystagmus (MOKN) Binocular visual evoked potentials (BVEP)
7.	Discussion of results

Orthoptic Tests

Four tests can be routinely used:

1. Hirschberg test: assesses symmetry of corneal reflexes, using a penlight
2. Visual tracking: tests for abnormal eye movements in tracking a penlight or small toy
3. Cover/uncover test
4. Ability to overcome 20 diopter base-out prism

Both the third and fourth tests are used to test for phoria and latent or manifest strabismus.

Acuity Assessments

Acuity has usually been tested binocularly or monocularly using a forced-choice preferential looking procedure, abbreviated to FPL (for example, see Atkinson & Braddick, 1981a, 1983a; Atkinson, Braddick, & Pimm-Smith, 1982; Teller 1979). The method depends on "preferential looking" where the infant prefers to look at a striped pattern rather than a blank screen of matched mean luminance (see Figure 1). A staircase procedure to adjust the stripe width and hence determine an acuity threshold is used, with observations being recorded by a "blind" observer (who does not know which of the two screens is displaying the striped pattern). The full staircase procedure works well for infants under 1 year (or children of mental age under 1 year) but can be used on older infants and children in an abbreviated form giving a valuable estimate of acuity. In a few cases where motor control is very poor (for example in a child with choreoathetotic syndrome), and for a number of older children with very limited attention span, it has been possible to gain only a qualitative idea of acuity using the mounted Stycar balls at 1, 2, or 3 meters. Tracking tests such as Catford Drum (Catford & Oliver, 1973) and Stycar balls (Sheridan, 1976) suffer from some shortcomings in target design and procedure (Atkinson, Braddick, Pimm-Smith, Ayling, & Sawyer, 1981), which make them unsuitable for accurate acuity measurement, but they do give the tester an indication of when a marked acuity deficit is present.

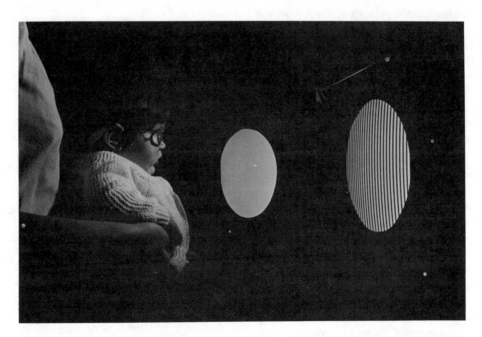

Figure 1. Assessment of acuity using the forced-choice preferential looking procedure (FPL). The child fixates a striped pattern rather than a blank screen matched in mean luminance. The screen sizes are identical, although in this figure they appear to look different because of the camera angle.

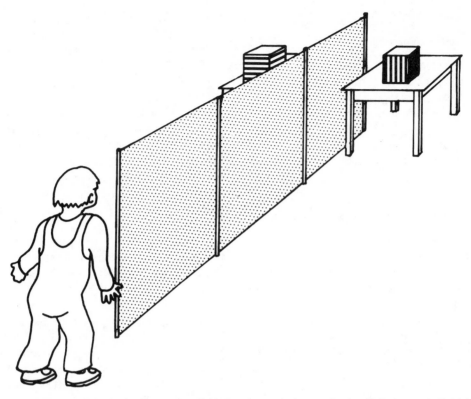

Figure 2a. Assessment of acuity in the alley-running task. The barrier separates the two cubes that display the stimuli. The child has to choose between the vertical stripes and the horizontal stripes.

With some children of over 3 years mental age, an operant alley-running technique (Atkinson, French, & Braddick, 1981) can be used, where the young child has to choose between two gratings of different orientations and find a reward hidden under a consistent orientation of grating, e.g., a sweet always under the cube with the vertical grating on it (see Figure 2a). As well as grating targets, modifications of Sheridan-Gardiner letter optotypes can be used in this test (see Figures 2b and 3). In this task, the child must always pick the cube with the letter "O" on it. This allows the assessment of visual "crowding" (Atkinson, Pimm-Smith, Evans, Harding, & Braddick, in preparation), which may reveal visual problems that are not apparent from a grating or single optotype test.

In a previous publication, Atkinson et al. (1982) discussed clinical assessments using FPL. In the group of 75 children assessed, FPL was used successfully in 60 children, Stycar balls for nine children (some of whom had FPL

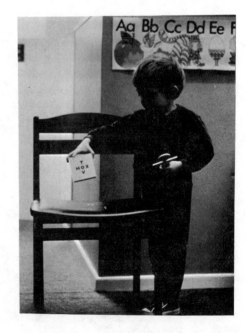

Figure 2b. When the child has made a choice he or she looks under the cube for the reward. For the cubes shown here, a particular central letter has to be selected.

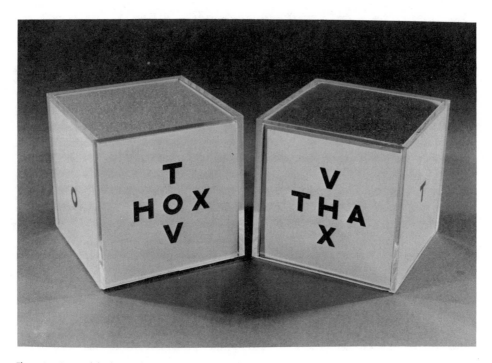

Figure 3. Types of display used to assess visual "crowding."

assessment also), and alley running in four children.

In two infants, no evidence of visual behavior was seen in either the child's general behavior, in preferential looking, or in the Stycar balls test. In such cases, particular emphasis is placed on testing for optokinetic nystagmus (OKN) with a visual stimulus of moving randomly spaced dots. The infant is seated close to the screen of moving dots. The dots are made up of a film loop of Letratone texture that moves in front of a small projector and is back projected onto a large screen (see Figure 4). For the stimulus to be effective, the field has to cover a wide area (approximately 120° visual angle) so that the child is unable to inhibit OKN by fixating an edge or stationary contour. The speed of movement can be varied, but a velocity of around 20–30 deg/sec is usually used with infants and young children. OKN for binocular viewing can be taken as an indicator of at least a functioning subcortical visual system. Both of the infants tested in this manner showed binocular OKN, although neither of them showed any visual awareness or spontaneous shifts of visual attention. Both children

were thought to have extensive cortical damage.

It is also possible to estimate visual acuity and contrast sensitivity using measurement of visual evoked potentials or VEPs (for example, Atkinson, Braddick, & French, 1979; Harris, Atkinson & Braddick, 1976; Marg, Freeman, Peltzman, & Goldstein, 1976; Pirchio, Spinelli, Fiorentini, & Maffei, 1978; Sokol & Jones, 1979; Spekreijse, 1978; Tyler, 1982). Either latency or amplitude measurements can be made. Phase reversing grating patterns with high temporal reversal rates (between 2 Hz and 10 Hz) have been used to measure the amplitude of the VEP which is time-locked to the contrast reversal of the visual stimulus. In general, estimates of visual function by means of the VEP have not been used routinely for these clinical assessments because of the requirement for rapid testing procedures and the need for good cooperation on the part of the child for electrode attachment and noise-free recordings. Nine cases from this clinical group were tested for pattern-reversal VEPs and the positive result was used as an indication of some cortical functioning. The test has proved

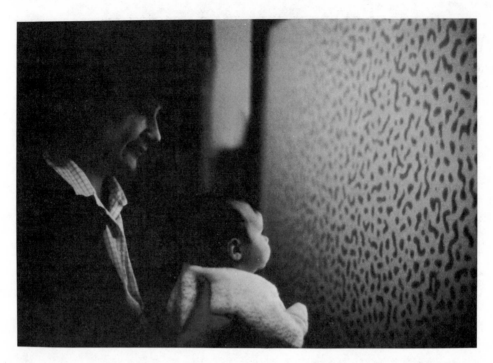

Figure 4. Infant looking at a large field of randomly arranged blobs that move laterally by means of a motorized film loop, to elicit OKN.

particularly useful in cases where motor functions (and in particular head and eye movements) are very restricted or lack coordination.

Photorefraction and Retinoscopy

Isotropic photorefraction (Atkinson, Braddick, Ayling, Pimm-Smith, Howland, & Ingram, 1981) is a technique developed from the original method of Howland and Howland (1974) for photographically observing the plane of focus of the two eyes. In clinical use of the procedure at the Cambridge Visual Development Unit, photographs are taken with a flash delivered through a fiber-optic light guide centered in the camera lens. Three different settings of focus are used on a wide aperture lens, attached to either a single lens reflex camera or a video camera. In the first photograph, the camera is focused on the child at a 75-cm distance; Figure 5 shows the illuminated pupils and corneal reflexes. In the second photograph, the camera is focused behind the infant (150 cm), and in the third, the camera is focused in front of the infant at 50 cm. From the relative size of the blur circles in the second and third photographs (where the light returning

from the infant's eyes has been deliberately blurred), one can tell whether the infant is focused in front or behind the camera and whether both eyes are focused in the same plane. Figure 6 shows an infant with a large difference in focusing between the eyes (anisometropia).

Photorefraction has been calibrated against conventional retinoscopy (Atkinson & Braddick, 1983b; Atkinson, Braddick, Ayling, Pimm-Smith, Howland, & Ingram, 1981; Atkinson, Braddick, Durden, Watson, & Atkinson, 1984) so that the method can be used to measure refractions. It is a particularly useful method for cases where little cooperation is given by the child because the procedure only requires the child to look at the camera for very brief intervals of time. Photorefraction is routinely used to assess the accuracy of active accommodation (Braddick, Atkinson, French, & Howland, 1979), which provides a valuable measure of visual attention as well as a pointer to refractive errors.

In most clinical assessments at the Unit, the child is photorefracted under cyclopentolate cycloplegia (Atkinson & Braddick, 1983b) in conjunction with a retinoscopic refraction

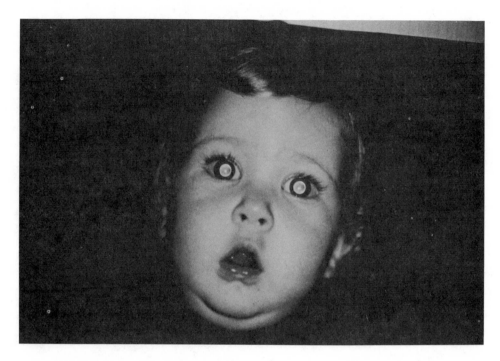

Figure 5. Focused illuminated pupils, using the photorefractor. Note the symmetrically placed corneal reflexes in each pupil, indicating that the child is *not* strabismic.

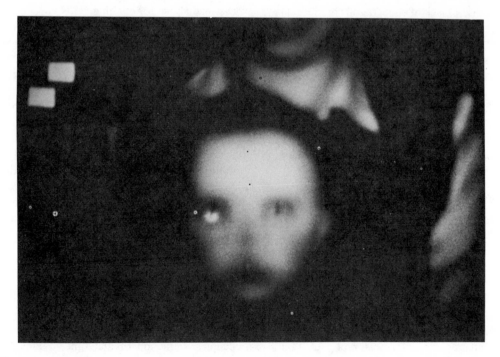

Figure 6. Deliberately blurred photograph using photorefraction, showing an infant with a difference in focusing between the eyes. The bright blur circle in the right eye shows a smaller refractive error than the completely blurred-out image in the left eye.

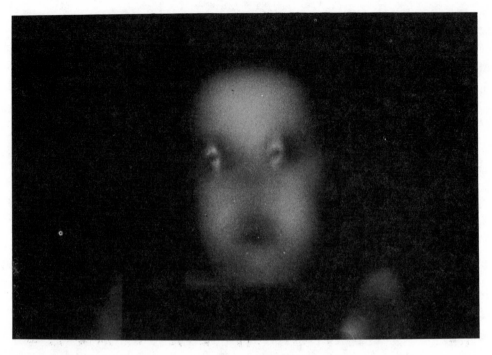

Figure 7. Deliberately blurred photograph, using photorefraction, showing an infant with an astigmatic refractive error. Each eye shows a blurred elipse, the long axis (close to vertical) of which has a larger refractive error than the short axis.

when possible. Of 73 children photorefracted, no retinoscopy was feasible in 15 of them because of lack of cooperation. In most cases, the two techniques of refraction provide valuable complementary information. Conventional retinoscopy is essential for an accurate assessment of very large refractive errors (greater than 5 diopters), whereas photorefraction allows an accurate measurement of the angle of astigmatism. An astigmatic refractive error is shown in Figure 7, where the blur is elongated to an ellipse along the axis of astigmatism.

Tests of Binocularity

Besides the orthoptic checks for phoria and strabismus, there are two specific tests used as indicators of cortical binocularity: symmetrical monocular optokinetic nystagmus and binocular visual evoked potentials.

Symmetrical Monocular Optokinetic Nystagmus (MOKN) Asymmetries of OKN in the two directions with monocular stimulation are an indicator of lack of binocularity (Atkinson, 1979; Atkinson & Braddick, 1981b); directional asymmetries found in

one eye only may be a sign of lateralized occipital cortical damage. The same stimulus described above for eliciting OKN is used for testing MOKN. Thirty-three infants in the review period were assessed for binocular and monocular OKN.

Binocular Visual Evoked Potentials (BVEP) A VEP specifically related to binocular vision can be elicited in infants with normal visual development after the age of 3 months (Braddick & Atkinson, 1983; Braddick, Atkinson, Julesz, Kropfl, Bodis-Wollner, & Raab, 1980). This method (or the psychophysical analogue) has not yet been used in the Visual Development Unit for clinical assessment, but similar behavioral tests are being developed and used in a number of laboratories (Fox, 1981).

Requirements for Visual Assessment In general, a visual assessment such as that described in the preceding pages requires that each child be in the Unit between 30 minutes and 1½ hours, although actual testing only occupies a fraction of that time. While demanding in resources (techniques, personnel, and time), it provides information on children's visual capabilities that is important to parents and to the clinical team. Accurate information on vision makes an important contribution to their treatment and rehabilitation.

In the author's experience, success in these assessments depends on several factors besides the technical facilities and experience in infant vision testing. Among these factors are: 1) a position separate from, but in close contact with, both pediatricians and ophthalmologists; 2) an atmosphere rather different from that of a busy clinic which is oriented principally to adult patients or school-age children (this includes flexibility in scheduling to fit the changing state of young infants and sufficient time and close contact to allow observation of the child's visual behavior in an informal setting); 3) an attitude of concern for informing parents of the nature of the tests and the implications of the findings, and an attempt to answer any queries or problems that the parents may have.

Case Studies

The three case studies below are representative of the type of assessments conducted by the Visual Development Unit.

1. Referral from Ophthalmology

Case HB was found to be a congenital myope and anisometrope at 6 months of age. The assessment revealed the following:

Refraction (corrected for working distance):

$$-6.0D \qquad\qquad -11.0D$$
$$\underset{}{+}\; -4.0D \qquad\qquad \underset{}{+}\; -9.0D$$

HB was given spectacle correction, and was seen for first time 2 weeks after receiving spectacles which were worn all the time.

Tested at 7 months:

Orthoptic check: No strabismus or nystagmus.

General visual behavior: Normal; reaches for toys, passes toys from hand to hand and hand to mouth.

Acuity: Preferential looking at distance of 75 cm revealed the following results: RE = 7c/deg, RE without correction = 3.1c/deg; LE = 7c/deg, LE without correction = 1.2c/deg. No amyblopia was detected at 75-cm testing distance. Attention for preferential

looking could not be gained adequately at distances beyond 1 meter, so Stycar balls were used at 2.5 m. HB was able to detect binocularly the 6-mm ball but not the 3-mm ball wearing spectacles. These results suggested poor distance vision and possible amblyopia for distance.

Binocularity: Symmetrical monocular OKN. Normal binocularity.

Conclusion: No amblyopia was detected at a near distance, but poor distance vision was a possibility. A retest was deemed necessary as the child tired by this point in testing. There was no lack of binocularity.

2. Referral from Pediatrics

Case JC was diagnosed as having cerebral palsy, a heart murmur, and severe deafness. He was 2.3 years of age and had not been seen as an infant because he had just moved to the area.

Visual behavior: JC tracked binocularly a bright toy at close distance. However, there was no reaching or movement of the hands. JC smiled to the peek-a-boo game around the Stycar screen with active face at 2 meters.

Orthoptic test: No strabismus.

Acuity: Preferential looking at 100 cm revealed the following results: binocular acuity = 8c/deg., and left eye acuity = 8c/deg. Although JC was in extreme distress and offered no cooperation when his right eye acuity was tested, he eventually tracked a large toy with RE.

Field test: Data from the field test showed the left side normal to 80°–90°. There was no response on the right side until virtually at midline.

Free accommodation: Large anismetropia, right eye hyperopic, left eye focusing on targets and camera.

Cycloplegic retinoscopy and photorefraction (corrected for working distance):

$$+5.0D$$
$$\underset{}{+}\; +3.0D \qquad \bigoplus \quad \text{plano}$$

Spectacle correction was ordered, but no further testing has been done as yet. A check for amblyopia will be made using monocular preferential looking with the child wearing correction. Effects of any treatment will be monitored.

Conclusion: Amblyopia resulting from anisometropia. Vision normal in left eye.

3. Health Visitor Referral Case SB was 6 months old. A health visitor suspected that the child had a squint and was "blind."

General visual behavior: No reaching for toys, no smiling, no unaided sitting, rather poor tone, and floppy.

Orthoptic test: Alternating intermittent convergent strabismus.

Fields: Very brief tracking of large bright toy from midline position out laterally only to approximately 40°; interest and attention then lost. No field asymmetry.

Free accommodation: No attention was gained beyond a short distance. This was confirmed by a photorefractive finding of myopic accommodation.

Acuity: Preferential looking 6c/deg (normal range for age).

Binocularity: Monocular OKN only for temporal to nasal direction in both eyes suggests a lack of binocularity and an age of visual maturity of less than 4 months.

Cycloplegic retinoscopy and photorefraction (corrected for working distance):

$$
\begin{array}{cc}
+1.5D & +1.0D \\
\underset{\displaystyle +4.0D}{+\!\!\!-\!\!\!-} & \underset{\displaystyle +4.0D}{+\!\!\!-\!\!\!-}
\end{array}
$$

Large hypermetropic refraction, child in "at-risk" refractive group for strabismus and/or amblyopia.

Conclusion: The refractive error may be contributing to the manifest strabismus. However, behavior in all spheres is very delayed, and from visual performance, would be estimated at 2–4 months.

(SB was referred to both the Pediatric and Opthalmology Departments at Addenbrooke's Hospital. She was later confirmed to have cerebral palsy.)

VISION SCREENING PROGRAM

The most common preschool vision problems at the present time are strabismus and amblyopia (irreversible loss of functional vision that cannot be reversed by refractive correc-

tion). Estimates vary as to their occurrence, with the average being around 5% of the population in Britain. This is a far higher incidence than that of more handicapping visual problems such as infant cataract, retinal pathologies, and central nervous system disorders, which affect less than 1% of the population.

It has recently been suggested that infants with a refraction of +2.5D or more hypermetropia at age 1 year are 20 times more likely to develop strabismus and amblyopia than children with a more nearly emmetropic refraction (Ingram, Trayner, Walker, & Wilson, 1979). This raises the possibility that refractive screening of the population in infancy could identify the group of children "at risk" of developing strabismus and amblyopia, and that preventative measures (partial refractive correction) might be possible to reduce the risk of the development of the disorders. Early refractive screening can also detect anisometropia (differences of refraction between the eyes) and any myopic errors that might significantly impair children's vision. The method of photorefraction under cycloplegia (described in the previous section) is one suited to population refractive screening in that it can be used by paramedical personnel, after a brief training session, with apparatus and procedure that is rapid, reliable, and relatively inexpensive.

Programs for refractive screening using photorefraction are underway in the Cambridge and Avon areas. The results of the first 18 months of the Cambridge program have recently been described (Atkinson et al., 1984).

Of the first 1,096 infants photorefractively screened, 5% were found to be hypermetropic (over +3.5D), 4.5% myopic (although less than 1% with myopia exceeding 3D) and 1.3% anisometropic (over 1D). These refractive errors were confirmed on retinoscopic follow-up. Those identified with refractive errors are being followed up to study the course of their refraction and a controlled trial of the preventive value of spectacle correction of large hypermetropic refractive errors is underway. Several general findings are emerging from these results to date:

1. The average cycloplegic refraction for 6–9-month-olds is around 1D hypermetropic.

2. Approximately 50% of the infants in the population show 1.0D or more of astigmatism under cycloplegia at ages between 6 and 9 months. In the Cambridge and Bristol population, these astigmatisms are divided approximately with half being with-the-rule and half against-the-rule, but there may be population differences in these proportions (Atkinson & Braddick, 1983b).

3. Almost all of those children with large astigmatic refractive errors at 6–9 months show a reduction in the level of astigmatism by age 18 months to 2 years, irrespective of whether they are wearing a partial spectacle correction or not. Some of these children show transient anisometropia as the refractions in each eye change at differing rates.

4. Most of the children who show some degree of myopia at 6–9 months become more emmetropic over the first 2 years. A very small group of infants have become more markedly myopic or have stayed myopic over the first 2 years.

5. A very small percentage of infants show manifest strabismus before 18 months of age.

It is hoped that from the analysis of the results of this program a better understanding of the etiology of a number of common childhood visual problems may be possible and that a screening procedure may be established for vision testing at the appropriate time in a child's life to identify the precursors of visual problems and take useful preventative steps. It is further hoped that eventually the photorefractive method will be in widespread use for refractive screening and will help to eliminate a number of cases of common visual defects.

In conclusion, it should be emphasized that the goals and requirements of a screening procedure and an assessment procedure are very different. A procedure tl . is to be used for general screening of a population must be very rapid and economical. It must also yield useful results on the vast majority of individuals tested from a standardized procedure. These requirements are met by photorefraction but not by any of the methods currently available for testing infant acuity or binocularity. Since any case picked up in a screening procedure will undergo more extensive testing at follow-up, a proportion of false positives may be tolerated, but the outcome must be vigorously evaluated in terms of the costs and benefits. These include both the costs associated with each test and the costs in the broadest sense to both patient and service associated with positive and negative errors. The benefits of early detection may be considerable even if a proportion of problems are missed or not predicted, but they are only genuine if a value in terms of efficacy of prevention or of early treatment can be positively demonstrated. Hence, any new screening method such as infant photorefraction must be accompanied by a full evaluation, the trial of refractive correction being an essential part of this.

The organization and evaluation of screening must take into account the fact that the majority of the children passing through the program are normal. In assessment, on the contrary, a child is taking part because of a known or strongly presumed disorder. A much more intensive study is therefore justified, with tests being selected from a wide battery to choose those appropriate for the individual's capabilities and the particular clinical issues raised. The aim is to provide the most accurate picture of the individual child's vision and the investigators must be flexible and persistent to achieve this end. Refraction, monocular and binocular acuity, binocularity, and perceptual capacities in a wider sense, are all practical issues that may require answers.

REFERENCES

Aslin, R.N., Alberts, J.R., & Petersen, M.R. (eds.). *Development of perception, Vol. 2, The visual system.* New York: Academic Press, 1981.

Atkinson, J. Development of optokinetic nystagmus in the human infant and monkey infant: An analogue to development in kittens. In: R.D. Freeman (ed.), *Developmental neurobiology of vision.* New York: Plenum Publishing Corp., 1979.

Atkinson, J., & Braddick, O. Acuity, contrast sensitivity, and accommodation in infancy. In: R.N. Aslin, J.R.

Alberts, & M.R. Petersen (eds.), *Development of perception, Vol. 2: The visual system.* New York: Academic Press, 1981. (a)

Atkinson, J., & Braddick, O. Development of optokinetic nystagmus in infants: An indicator of cortical binocularity? In: D.F. Fisher, R.A. Monty, & J.W. Senders (eds.), *Eye movements: Cognition and visual perception.* Hillsdale, NJ: Lawrence Erlbaum Associates, 1981. (b)

Atkinson, J., & Braddick, O. Assessment of visual acuity in infancy and early childhood. *Acta Ophthalmologica,* Suppl. 157, 18–26, 1983. (a)

Atkinson, J., & Braddick, O. The use of isotropic photorefraction for vision screening in infants. *Acta Ophthalmologica,* Suppl. 157, 36–45, 1983. (b)

Atkinson, J., Braddick, O.J., Ayling, L., Pimm-Smith, E., Howland, H.C., & Ingram, R.M. Isotropic photorefraction: A new method for refractive testing of infants. *Documenta Opthalmologica Proceedings Series,* 1981, *30,* 217–223.

Atkinson, J., Braddick, O.J., Durden, K., Watson, P.G., & Atkinson, S. Screening for refractive errors in 6–9 month old infants using photorefraction. *British Journal of Ophthalmology,* 1984, *8,* 105–112.

Atkinson, J., Braddick, O., & French, J. Contrast sensitivity of the human neonate measured by the visual evoked potential. *Investigative Ophthalmology and Visual Science,* 1979, *18,* 210–213.

Atkinson, J., Braddick, O., & Pimm-Smith, E. 'Preferential looking' for monocular and binocular acuity testing of infants. *British Journal of Opthalmology,* 1982, *66,* 264–268.

Atkinson, J., Braddick, O., Pimm-Smith, E., Ayling, L., & Sawyer, R. Does the Catford Drum given an accurate assessment of acuity? *British Journal of Ophthalmology,* 1981, *65,* 652–656.

Atkinson, J., French, J., & Braddick, O. Contrast sensitivity function of pre-school children. *British Journal of Ophthalmology,* 1981, *65,* 525–529.

Atkinson, J., Pimm-Smith, E., Evans, C., Harding, G., & Braddick, O. Visual crowding in young children. In preparation.

Braddick, O., & Atkinson, J. The development of binocular function in infancy. *Acta Ophthal.,* Suppl. 157, 27–35, 1983.

Braddick, O.J., Atkinson, J., French, J., & Howland, H.C. A photorefractive study of infant accommodation. *Vision Research,* 1979, *19,* 1319–1330.

Braddick, O., Atkinson, J., Julesz, B., Kropfl, W., Bodis-Wollner, I., & Raab, E. Cortical binocularity in infants. *Nature,* 1980, *288,* 363–365.

Braddick, O., Campbell, F.W., & Atkinson, J. Channels in vision: Basic aspects. In: R. Held, H. Leibowitz, & H.L. Teuber (eds.), *Handbook of sensory physiology, Vol. VIII: Perception.* Heidelberg: Springer-Verlag, 1978.

Campbell, F.W., & Robson, J.G. Application of Fourier analysis to the visibility of gratings. *Journal of Physiology,* 1968, *197,* 551–566.

Catford, G.V., & Oliver, A. Development of visual acuity. *Archives of Disease in Childhood,* 1973, *48,* 47–50.

Fox, R. Stereopsis in animals and human infants. In: R.N. Aslin, J.R. Alberts, & M.R. Petersen. *Development of perception: Psychobiological perspectives, Vol. 2: The visual system.* New York: Academic Press, 1981.

Harris, L., Atkinson, J., & Braddick, O. Visual contrast sensitivity of a 6-month-old infant measured by the evoked potential. *Nature,* 1976, *264,* 570–571.

Howland, H.C., & Howland, B. Photorefraction: A technique for study of refractive state at a distance. *Journal of the Optical Society of America,* 1974, *64,* 240–249.

Hubel, D.H., & Wiesel, T.N. Receptive fields, binocular interaction and functional architecture in the cat's visual cortex. *Journal of Physiology,* 1962, *165,* 559–568.

Ingram, R.M., Trayner, M.J., Walker, C., & Wilson, J.M. Screening for refractive errors at age 1 year: A pilot study. *British Journal of Ophthalmology,* 1979, *63,* 243–250.

Marg, E., Freeman, D.N., Peltzman, P., & Goldstein, P.J. Visual acuity development in human infants: Evoked potential measurements. *Investigations in Ophthalmology,* 1976, *15,* 150–153.

Pirchio, M., Spinelli, D., Fiorentini, A., & Maffei, L. Infant contrast sensitivity evaluated by evoked potentials. *Brain Research,* 1978, *141,* 179–184.

Sheridan, M.D. *Manual for the STYCAR vision tests.* Slough: NFER Publishing Company Ltd., 1976.

Sokol, S., & Jones, K. Implicit time of pattern evoked potentials in infants: An index of maturation of spatial vision. *Vision Research,* 1979, *19,* 747–755.

Spekreijse, H. Maturation of contrast EPs and development of visual resolution. *Archives Italienne de Biologie,* 1978, *116,* 358–369.

Teller, D.Y. The forced-choice preferential looking procedure: A psychophysical technique for use with human infants. *Infant Behavior and Development,* 1979, *2,* 135–153.

Tyler, C.W. Assessment of visual function in infants by evoked potentials. *Developmental Medicine and Child Neurology,* 1982, *24,* 853–855.

Wiesel, T.N. Postnatal development of the visual cortex and the influence of environment. *Nature,* 1982, *299,* 583–591.

Chapter 40

Vision Problems in Under 5's
Data from Child Health and
Education in the Seventies

Sue Atkinson, B.Sc., M.A., M.B., B.Chir., D.C.H.
Bristol & Weston Health Authority, Bristol, England
Neville R. Butler, M.D., F.R.C.P., F.R.C.O.G., D.C.H.
University of Bristol, Bristol, England

Information on the prevalence of vision problems in preschool children is scarce and the available data are often on small or selected samples (Amigo, 1973; Kripke, Dunbar, & Zimmerman, 1970; Sturner, Funk, Barton, Sparrow, & Frothingham, 1980). Child Health and Education in the Seventies (CHES), a national study of all children born in 1 week in England, Wales, and Scotland, provided data on vision problems and allowed the investigation of associated factors in the preschool years.

SUBJECTS AND METHODS

The Child Health and Education in the Seventies study collected data on all children in England, Wales, and Scotland born during 1 week of April, 1970. Data were collected by means of structured parental questionnaires administered by health visitors (community nurses working in the field of prevention; they carry out child health surveillance, developmental checks, etc. on preschool children) with added information from health visitor, child

health clinic, and, where available, general practitioner records. The information covered health, social, and education factors. The data presented here were collected when the children were 5 years old. The questionnaire included three items relating to visual disorder: 1) "vision problems" (excluding squint), 2) "glasses," and 3) "squint" with specific information on treatment.

The total birth cohort comprised 16,000 children and at the age of 5 years full information was obtained on 13,135 (82%). Analysis of the data was carried out using SPSS (statistical package for the social sciences [computer package]) for cross-tabulations. Chi-square analyses were used as indicated in the text to test significance levels.

RESULTS

Prevalence

Overall, 1,270 individuals (9.7% of the cohort) were reported as having some sort of visual disorder before the age of 5, but there was

This study was mainly financed by the Medical Research Council with contributions from other agencies. The authors would like to thank S. Dowling, B.C. Howlett, and A. Osborn for their work on C.H.E.S. and other colleagues for their support and help.

Table 1. Prevalence of visual defects

	Number	Percentage
Children in cohort	13,135	100.0
Children with any visual defect	1,270	9.7
Children with squint	973	7.4
Children with glasses	473	3.6
Children with other vision problems	187	1.4

overlap among these children between the three items in the questionnaire. The break-down of different visual disorders is shown in Table 1. Of the children in the cohort, 7.4% were reported as having or having had a squint, 3.6% as being prescribed glasses, and a further 1.4% were described as having other vision problems. This latter group included some serious visual problems such as congenital nystagmus and cataract, refractive errors not requiring treatment or associated with a squint (e.g., anisometropia, hypermetropia) (Ingram, 1977), and minor eye complaints such as conjunctivitis and excessive blinking.

In particular, there was overlap between the individuals reporting both squint and glasses ($n = 363$). Figure 1 demonstrates the overlap between the categories of individuals. More than a third (37.3%) of the children with squint had been prescribed glasses at some stages during their preschool period, although it was in a slightly smaller proportion (34.5%, $n = 336$) that these were considered as "treatment" for the squint. The majority (76.7%) of children with glasses also reported squint.

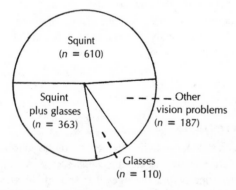

Figure 1. Relationship between squint, glasses, and other vision problems. (Total number of children with any vision problems equals 1,270 [9.7% of the whole cohort].)

Of the 973 children with squint, 541 (55.6%) (4.1% of the whole cohort) had received treatment; 370 (38.0%) (2.8% of the cohort) had been told no treatment was needed, and a further 62 (6.4%) (0.5% of cohort) had never gone for any advice or treatment (Table 2). Of those receiving treatment, combinations of occlusion, glasses, exercises, and operation were reported in various proportions as seen in Table 2. Glasses were prescribed as treatment for 34.5% of the children having squint. Operative treatment was required by 172 children (1.3% of the whole cohort) for their squint before the age of 5 years.

Demographic Factors

The sex distribution among children in the cohort with squint, glasses, and vision problems did not differ from that in the cohort as a whole. However, more boys were reported as having squint before the age of 4 years ($p < .01$). Information on severity of squint and, hence, possible earlier detection was not available.

Trends in social class distribution between those children with vision problems, squint, or glasses, and those without, were not apparent. However, more children in social class V (unskilled workers) of the Registrar General's Social Class rating (Registrar General, 1960) were reported as having squint ($p < .02$). Social class was also related to those children who never went for treatment. The trend was linear with proportionately more children of poorer socioeconomic circumstances not going for treatment or advice.

Regional and ethnic differences may indicate differences in access to services (Black, Morris, Smith, & Townsend, 1980). Fewer children in rural areas had glasses ($p < .02$) although they reported vision problems and squint as frequently as other children. Similarly, fewer Asian children had glasses (1.2%) compared with non-Asian children (3.6%) ($p < .05$), while their reports of vision problems and squint were the same. Cultural effects and/or language difficulties may be of relevance here in relation to the accessibility of health services to Asians.

Table 2. Treatment for squint

	Number	Percentage of children with squint	Percentage of whole birth cohort (N = 13,135)
All children with squint	973	100.0	7.4
Received treatment	541	55.6	4.1
No treatment advised	370	38.0	2.8
Never went for advice or treatment	62	6.4	0.5
Type of treatment			
Occlusion	223	22.9[a]	1.7
Glasses	336	34.5	2.6
Exercises	150	15.4	1.1
Operation	172	17.7	1.3

[a]Figures do not add to 100% due to multiple types of treatment in individuals.

Severe Visual Handicap

Nineteen children in the cohort (0.14%) were reported as having severe visual handicap, including those who were blind and partially sighted. Ten of these children (62.6%) also reported squint, and six had multiple or associated severe handicaps such as hydrocephalus, cerebral palsy, and congenital rubella syndrome. These children were excluded from subsequent analyses.

Associations with Other Medical Conditions

Children with mental and severe sensory handicap (excluding visual handicap), i.e., developmental delay, educational subnormality, and hearing and speech problems, were more likely to have glasses, as well as squint and vision problems ($p < .001$). The increased risks for these children are shown in Table 3. For example, the association between glasses and mental or sensory handicap means that a child with such a handicap is 3.7 times as likely as a child without such a handicap to require glasses. Similarly, it can be seen that children with other major medical conditions, such as cerebral palsy, Down syndrome, hydrocephalus, and tumors, have significantly increased chances of requiring glasses or having a squint or vision problem ($p < .001$).

Significantly more children with convulsions reported squint ($p < .001$). This held true even when children with other cerebral problems that could be regarded as precipitating both squint and convulsions were excluded. If a child had convulsions, then he or she had a 50% greater chance of also having a squint.

Congenital defects (excluding those specifically affecting the eyes), e.g., cleft palate, congenital dislocated hip, endocrine problems, talipes, and congenital heart defect, were also significantly associated with glasses ($p < .001$) and squint ($p < .01$), with increased risk factors as shown in Table 3.

Emotional problems and child abuse were associated with increased reports of visual defects.

Twins and Low Birth Weight

In the whole cohort, there were 125 pairs of twins and an additional 17 individuals who were twins. Of these 267 children, 35 (13.1%) reported having squint, nearly twice the proportion of singletons (7.3%) ($p < .001$). Similarly, the proportions of twins requiring glasses and reporting vision problems showed them to be at about twice the risk of singletons ($p < .001$) (Table 4).

Many twins are of low birth weight, and in comparing the children of low birth weight (≤ 5 lb) with those of higher birth weight, there were significantly more prescriptions for glasses, and squint and vision problems reported ($p < .001$) among the lower birth weight children (Table 4). However, even among twins of higher birth weight, there was still more than twice the chance of squint ($p < .01$).

Multiple pregnancy and low birth weight are known to be associated with birth trauma and hence could be associated with handicapping

Table 3. Increased risk factor[a] of visual problems with associated medical conditions

	Mental or sensory handicap	Major medical condition	Congenital abnormality
Squint	3.9	3.5	1.7
Glasses	3.7	2.6	1.8
Other vision problem	6.0	3.8	3.1

[a]Risk of the visual anomaly in the group compared with children with no medical problem.

conditions. Even when excluding children with handicaps, there was still a marked association between twins and low birth weight, and squint and glasses.

DISCUSSION

The data for this study are a combination of parental reportage, health visitor observation, and available nursing and medical records on children contacted at the age of 5. Specific vision testing or screening was not carried out on the children. The data therefore cover the visual history of children up to the age of 5 and may have some unquantifiable reportage error. In particular, there was a degree of overlap and possibly some inconsistency between the answers to the three questions on the questionnaire relating to vision; hence, squint and glasses are considered primarily in this report and the proportion of children with other vision problems (1.4%) represents a variety of conditions. However, the large database allows an investigation of the association between various factors that would not be possible in other studies due to small numbers of children with particular conditions.

Visual defects were reported by 9.7% of the CHES cohort, which represents the period prevalence up to the age of 5 years (i.e., all cases occurring between the ages of birth and 5 years). Various preschool vision screening programs have taken place during recent years

with the prevalence of visual defects being reported as between about 6% and 15% of the population. These studies were, however, carried out at various ages and some were on selected samples. For example, Amigo's (1973) study screened 3–5-year-olds in four selected nurseries around Sydney and reported 6.2% of the sample to have refractive errors and 2.5% to have strabismus; Köhler and Stigmar (1973) carried out total population screening on 4-year-olds with 15% having a visual defect, of whom only 2.8% were already known. Thus, the prevalence figure of 9.7% from CHES could be regarded as comparable with these studies, although it may also be interpreted as being only the "already known" proportion.

Where squint is concerned, 7.4% of the CHES cohort reported this visual abnormality. From the screening studies, strabismus was reported as occurring in between 1.3% (Friedman, Neumann, Hyams, & Peleg, 1980) and 5.0% (Cameron & Cameron, 1978) of the population. It is again difficult to compare the CHES data with these figures because the CHES data represent period prevalence, i.e., all cases occurring between the ages of birth and 5 years, whereas screening studies detect a point prevalence, at whatever age the screening is performed. Even the large study by Mac-Lellan and Harker (1979), which covered children of all ages up to 5 years and reported 3.5% with strabismus and 4.3% refractive errors, is

Table 4. Twins and birth weight in relation to children with squint or glasses

	Twins		Singletons		Low birthweight (≤ 5 lb)		Normal birthweight (> 5 lb ≤ 9 lb)		High birthweight (> 9 lb)	
	N	%	N	%	N	%	N	%	N	%
Squint	35	13.1[a]	938	7.3	107	12.1[a]	780	7.2	54	5.6
Glasses	20	7.5[a]	453	3.5	53	6.0[a]	380	3.5	28	2.9
All children	267	100.0	12,868	100.0	883	100.0	10,898	100.0	974	100.0

[a]$p < .001$.

not really comparable, as they saw referred children at whatever age they appeared.

In the National Child Development Study (NCDS) (Kellmer-Pringle, Butler, & Davie, 1966), a similar longitudinal study contacting children at 7 years of age, manifest squint was found in 3.1% of the cohort and there was a further 2.9% with latent squint. It is difficult, then, to be precise about the prevalence of strabismus, but it would appear to be about 5% of the preschool and early school-age population.

Over a third of the CHES children with squint were advised that no treatment was necessary for their squint, perhaps suggesting that these may have been infants with pseudo-strabismus and not true squint. Unfortunately, it is not possible from the data available to verify this hypothesis, but if it were true, then the prevalence of true strabismus in the CHES cohort could be regarded as 4.7%, which may be considered closer to estimates from the other studies mentioned.

The majority of children who received treatment for squint received more than one type of treatment, with only 20% of them receiving a single treatment, most commonly glasses. Conservative treatment was frequently inadequate as indicated by the fact that 17.7% of the children with squint required an operation. It would appear that true congenital strabismus was not common, with only 15 children (1.5% of those with squint) requiring operative intervention before the age of 1 year.

The proportion of children in the cohort wearing glasses at 5 years was 3.2%, with a further 0.4% having had glasses previously but not at the age of 5. In the National Child Development Study (Kellmer-Pringle et al., 1966), 6.0% of children were reported as wearing glasses. It seems unlikely that the number of children requiring glasses should double between the ages of 5 and 7 years, and the data therefore suggest that a substantial proportion of children requiring glasses are unknown until they are recognized by the school medical screening services. This may then indicate the usefulness of preschool vision screening programs.

The association between squint and poor socioeconomic circumstances confirms previous similar studies' findings (Kellmer-Pringle et al., 1966; Miller, Court, Walton, & Knox, 1960). The utilization of services was also worse in those with poorer socioeconomic circumstances, in that proportionately more of them had never sought advice about their child's squint. This may also suggest that there could be an even greater proportion of unreported and unrecognized vision disorders among this group. Poorer access to medical services could also explain the discrepancies between the proportion of children with glasses in rural and urban areas, and the low proportion of children of Asian origin with glasses. Specific information on inequalities in provision of services was not available, however.

It has been shown in the Isle of Wight study (Rutter, Tizard, & Whitmore, 1970) that there is an increased incidence of squint and decreased visual acuity in educationally subnormal children and those with neurological problems, and NCDS supported the association between physical incoordination and squint. These CHES data support the association between squint/glasses and mental or sensory handicap, and indicate that there is a markedly increased risk (3.9-fold) of squint in these children. However, children with other medical conditions, not necessarily only those with neurological sequelae, also were shown to be at much higher risk of developing squint (3.5 times), and children with convulsions were 1.5 times more likely to have squint compared with children who had not had convulsions. Perhaps an even more surprising finding was that children with congenital abnormalities that would not normally be associated with vision problems also showed increased risks of visual abnormalities by 1.7 to 3.1 times. Overall, then, it appears that most physical or mental disabilities, whether congenital or acquired, are more likely to be associated with sensory problems such as visual defects. This emphasizes the necessity for careful assessment of vision in children with other conditions by personnel with special skill in testing such children.

The large cohort database allowed investigation of a population of 267 twin births, and of an unselected general population–based sample of children of low birth weight. Both of these conditions, twinning and low birth weight, showed a marked association with squint, glasses, and vision problems and indicated that these two groups of children are at increased risk of visual defects and should be under particular surveillance for visual anomalies.

CONCLUSIONS

The prevalence figures for squint and glasses indicate that squint is the most common preschool vision problem, affecting about 7% of 0–5 year olds, but the data may also suggest that only a proportion of the children with visual problems are already known by the age of 5. The (CHES) survey shows the marked association between children with medical problems of many types, both congenital and acquired, and visual defects. In particular, twins and children of low birthweight are twice as likely as singletons or children with a birth weight of more than 5 pounds to develop squints or other vision problems, or to require spectacle correction. The need, then, is for children in all these categories and with other medical conditions to be scrutinized carefully to ascertain their visual status in an attempt to reduce their level of handicap. As squint is the most common preschool vision problem, then any preschool vision screening and preventive programs should address this condition, but detection in itself without appropriate intervention and treatment would be inadequate.

REFERENCES

Amigo, G. Preschool vision study. *British Journal of Ophthalmology*, 1973, *57*(2), 125–132.

Black, D., Morris, J.N., Smith, C., & Townsend, P. *Inequalities in health*. London: Department of Health and Social Security, 1980.

Cameron, J.H., & Cameron, M. Visual screening of preschool children. *British Medical Journal*, 1978, *2*, 1693–1694.

Friedman, Z., Neumann, E., Hyams, S.W., & Peleg, B. Ophthalmic screening of 38,000 children, age 1 to 2½ years, in child welfare clinics. *Journal of Paediatric Ophthalmology and Strabismus*, 1980, *17*(4), 261–267.

Ingram, R.M. Refraction as a basis for screening children for squint and amblyopia. *British Journal of Ophthalmology*, 1977, *61*, 8–15.

Kellmer-Pringle, M.L., Butler, N.R., & Davie, R. *11,000 seven-year-olds*. First report of the National Child Development Study (1958 Cohort). London: Longmans, 1966.

Köhler, L., & Stigmar, G. Vision screening in 4 year olds. *Acta Paediatrica Scandinavica*, 1973, *62*, 17–27.

Kripke, S.S., Dunbar, C.A., & Zimmerman, V. Vision screening of preschool children in mobile clinics in Iowa. *Public Health Reports*, 1970, *85*, 41–44.

MacLellan, A.V., & Harker, P. Mobile orthoptic service for primary screening of visual disorder in young children. *British Medical Journal*, 1979, *1*, 994–995.

Miller, F.J.W., Court, S.D.M., Walton, W.S., & Knox, E.G. Growing up in Newcastle-upon-Tyne: A continuing study of health and illness in young children within their families. Oxford: Oxford University Press for the Nuffield Foundation, 1960.

Registrar General. *Classification of occupations*. London: Her Majesty's Stationery Office, 1960.

Rutter, M., Tizard, J., & Whitmore, K. *Education, health and behaviour*. London: Longmans, 1970.

Sturner, R.A., Funk, S.G., Barton, J., Sparrow, S., & Frothingham, T.E. Simultaneous screening for child health and development: Visual/developmental screening in pre-school children. *Pediatrics*, 1980, *65*(3), 614–621.

Chapter 41

The Late Visual Bloomer

SHAUL HAREL, M.D.
MOSHE HOLTZMAN, M.D.
Tel Aviv Medical Center, Tel Aviv University, Tel Aviv, Israel
MOSHE FEINSOD, M.D.
Hadassah Medical Center, Jerusalem, Israel

MATURATIONAL DELAY IN SEVERAL AREAS of development (for example, motor and language) is a well-known phenomenon (Illingworth, 1961). Delay in visual maturation is less known to pediatricians, pediatric neurologists, ophthalmologists, and psychologists. Illingworth was the first to focus special attention on this phenomenon (Illingworth, 1961). In his paper on delayed visual maturation, he wrote:

> Having studied the visual development in two such children, I searched the literature for information on the matter. The search included all volumes of the *Quarterly Cumulative Index Medicus* and standard textbooks on ophthalmology. I found very few references to the subject.

The authors, too, searched the literature, and were amazed at the paucity of available information. Little has been published on the subject (Doggart, 1957; Doyne, 1930; Harel, Holtzman, & Feinsod, 1983; Illingworth, 1958; 1961; Law, 1960; Mellor & Fielder, 1980.) This chapter attempts to reinforce Illingworth's findings on delayed visual maturation by reporting on six children with such delay whom the authors call "late visual bloomers." All children were referred by competent physicians to a pediatric neurology clinic for evaluation of blindness and possible

psychomotor retardation. The follow-up of these children after more than 2 years showed normal vision and development. A possible etiology is suggested by data from electroretinograms (ERG) and visually evoked responses (VER) performed at the time of referral and on follow-up. The early recognition of this condition is imperative for prognostic reassurance for parents.

CASE REPORTS

Six infants (five males and one female), ages 3–4 months, were referred to the authors by pediatricians and ophthalmologists as blind and possibly retarded. Each had a strikingly similar history. They were born to healthy, unrelated families after normal pregnancies and deliveries. Their parents had remarked that the infants did not follow faces and objects with their eyes, did not focus, and were unresponsive to visual stimuli, while they readily reacted to voices and touch. The parents were extremely anxious about the possibility that their child was blind, but felt that otherwise he or she was completely normal.

Physical and neurological examination showed no abnormalities except a mild roving nystagmus. Diagnostic studies, including electroencephalograms and brain computerized

359

tomography, were normal. Ophthalmoscopic examinations were normal. Visual electro-diagnostic studies were performed on referral and at 3-month intervals.

Methods

The patients were examined with dilated pupils (Mydriacyl 12) in a darkened room. One hundred, one per second flashes at 20 cm from the eyes were delivered by a xenon discharge lamp activated by a Grass photostimulator PS-22 at intensity 4. Grass gold-plated electrodes were affixed to the scalp with electrode paste. The visually evoked response was recorded between the active O_1 and O_2 electrodes, and the linked ears served as reference (10–20 international nomenclature). The resistance between the active and reference electrodes was 2,000–5,000 Ω. The scalp electroencephalogram was amplified and averaged by a Nicolet CA-1000 instrument. The averaged evoked responses to uniocular stimulation were displayed by an x–y plotter.

Results

At referral, the electroretinograms were normal. The visually evoked responses are of prolonged latency, and only the first negative deflection could be identified (Figure 1, trace 1). Repeated visually evoked responses at 3-month intervals showed constant improvement in the latency and wave forms.

Clinical Follow-Up

At 6–8 months respectively, the babies showed improvement in vision, following objects, focusing, and responding to visual stimuli. The roving nystagmus gradually disappeared. At age 2–2½ years, both eyesight and psychomotor development were normal.

DISCUSSION

Doyne was the first to report that the development of sight is delayed in some children (Doyne, 1930). He described a child who showed no signs of vision by the age of 3 months, but began to develop signs of sight by

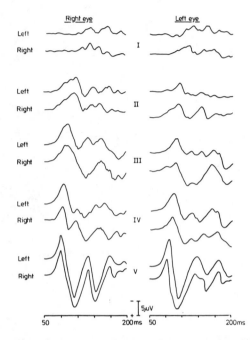

Figure 1. Visually evoked responses taken at 3-month intervals demonstrating the improvements in the brain response to photic stimuli. In the first tracing (1), there is evidence for prolonged latency of the first negative wave. This delay becomes shorter with time until it reaches normal values (50 msec) after a year (tracings IV and V). Concomitantly, there is a gradual development of the W-shape wave that follows the initial negative deflection, which may correlate with processing of visual information. Recordings are made from over the left and right hemispheres.

7 months, and had normal vision at the age of 18 months. The author stressed the common relationship between delay in sight development and mental retardation or albinism. Doggart also reported that some children showed no signs of vision in the early months of life but subsequently developed normal vision (Doggart, 1957).

Illingworth was the first to draw attention to the problem, which he termed "delay in visual maturation" (Illingworth, 1961). He described in detail two children who were regarded as blind during the first months of their lives. At approximately 6 months, they showed early signs of vision, and later had normal vision and psychomotor development. Ophthalmoscopic examination was entirely normal in both children. The authors' clients were almost identical with the children described by Illingworth. Each of them had a normal perinatal history and normal neurological and ophthalmoscopic examinations (Harel et al., 1983). Each initially had a roving nystagmus that gradually disappeared with visual improvement. Illingworth mentioned the absence of roving nystagmus as an important negative feature, but this was not the case in the author's clients. The authors believe that the roving nystagmus suggests that the children were unable to see, rather than unable to interpret what they saw (visual agnosia). All children had a normal psychomotor development, indicating a diagnosis compatible with a pattern of developmental dissociation (Illingworth, 1958). They all seemed to have compensated through other channels such as adequate social responses to voices and touch. The clients were referred to the clinic for evaluation by senior, competent physicians. The parents were all extremely anxious about the possibility of their child being blind and retarded. Because the authors were unaware of the "late visual bloomer" phenomenon, complete diagnostic studies were performed in order to rule out the possibility of a central nervous system disorder. Since that report, the authors have diagnosed another three such children.

Visually Evoked Responses

The special contribution of these cases to the understanding of a possible etiology of this visual phenomenon is the information obtained from the visual electrodiagnostic studies performed during the period of blindness and after normal vision had developed. During the follow-up period on the clients, Mellor and Fielder published similar clinical and electrodiagnostic data on four infants whom they called "slow to see" (Mellor & Fielder, 1980).

Doggart suggested a possible delay in myelination of the optic nerve (Doggart, 1957). He also referred to the frequency with which optic atrophy (pale discs) in children were wrongly diagnosed. Repeated normal electroretinograms could rule out the possibility of Leber's amaurosis.

The VER provoked by a photic stimulus is an EEG response recorded over the occipital cortex and reflects the integrity of the whole visual pathway. Mellor and Fielder, in their clinical and electrodiagnostic study of four cases, reported that the initial visually evoked response showed impaired and immature waveform rather than delayed latencies (Mellor & Fielder, 1980). They therefore favored an etiology based on delayed dentritic and synaptic formation in the occipital cortex rather than unmyelinated pathways. Initial visually evoked reponses from the authors' clients (Figure 1) clearly demonstrate evidence for prolonged latencies as well as immature waveform responses. These responses became rapidly normal as vision improved. It seems to the authors that a combination of a transient delayed myelination and synaptic development could better explain the delay in visual maturation. The clinical implication from this assumption could be that an early abnormal visually evoked response in a blind infant should not necessarily suggest a poor prognosis for vision, but rather be seen as an immature response of possible good prognostic value.

The condition of the "late visual bloomer" is uncommon but not rare. Illingworth (1961) wrote, "I have, however, discussed the problem with many colleagues, and most of them have seen one or two infants presenting features similar to those described." This has also been the authors' experience when discussing this visual phenomenon with pediatricians, pediatric neurologists, ophthalmologists, and psychologists. Illingworth (1961) has already stressed the importance of early recognition of this visual phenomenon. He felt that in most cases, the normal neurological, ophthalmoscopic, and developmental examinations could differentiate this condition from mental subnormality, eye and fundi abnormalities, or childhood autism. The authors agree with this assumption, but would like to suggest the contribution of noninvasive visual electrodiagnostic studies to reinforce the diagnosis.

The early recogniton of this visual phenomenon is not only imperative for prognostic value, but could also prevent unnecessary and sometimes invasive diagnostic studies.

REFERENCES

Doggart, D.H. Infantile fundus lesions in relation to mental capacity. *British Medical Journal*, 1957, *2*, 933–935.

Doyne, P.G. Amaurosis in infants. *Practitioner*, 1930, *125*, 174–178.

Harel, S., Holtzman, M., & Feinsod, M. Delayed visual maturation. *Archives of Disease in Childhood*, 1983, *58*, 298–309.

Illingworth, R.S. Dissociation as a guide to developmental assessment. *Archives of Disease in Childhood*, 1958, *33*, 118–122.

Illingworth, R.S. Delayed visual maturation. *Archives of Disease in Childhood*, 1961, *33*, 407–409.

Law, F. The problem of the visually defective infant. *Transactions of the Ophthalmological Society U.K.*, 1960, *80*, 3–12.

Mellor, D.H., & Fielder, A.R. Dissociated visual development: Electrodiagnostic studies in infants who are "slow to see." *Developmental Medicine and Child Neurology*, 1980, *22*, 327–335.

Chapter 42

The Standardization of the Denver Developmental Screening Test for Israeli Children
Demographic and Socioeconomic Implications

YEHUDA SHAPIRA, M.D.
Hadassah-Hebrew University Medical School, Jerusalem, Israel
SHAUL HAREL, M.D.
Tel Aviv University, Tel Aviv, Israel
DOV TAMIR, M.D.
Department of Health Care, Jerusalem, Israel

T HE DENVER DEVELOPMENTAL SCREENING Test (DDST) (Frankenburg & Dodds, 1967) was recently translated into Hebrew and standardized for Israeli children (Shapira & Harel, 1983). The DDST was introduced as an effective measure for mass screening of pediatric populations for the early detection of developmental disabilities (Frankenburg & Dodds, 1967). Its validity was tested by the original authors (Frankenburg, Camp, & Van Natta, 1971) and by others (Bryant, Davies, & Newcombe, 1974; Ueda, 1978). The DDST has acquired worldwide recognition and was standardized in several countries (Barnes & Stark, 1975; Bryant et al., 1974; Bryant, Davies, & Newcombe, 1979; Cools & Hermanns, 1976; Flehming, Schluun, Uhde, & Van Bernuth, 1973; Jaffe, Harel, Goldberg, Rudolph-Schnitzer, & Winter, 1980; Ueda, 1978). In each of these studies, significant differences were found between the performances of the

local sample of children as compared to the Denver sample.

The development of preschool children of different social and ethnic groups has been discussed in relation to developmental screening (Frankenburg, Dick, & Carland, 1975; Super, 1976). In the Israeli standardization, differences had been found, too (Shapira & Harel, 1983). In addition, the age range between the 25th and 90th percentile in many of the items in the Israeli sample was greater than in the Denver sample. The reason for that difference is still unknown and it was assumed that it results from the heterogeneity of the Israeli population. A high percentage of that population had immigrated to Israel since 1948, about half from North Africa and the Middle East, and the other half from Europe and America (Central Bureau of Statistics, 1981) (Table 1).

This chapter reports on the differences of

This study was generously supported by grants from Henry J. Leir, Esq., and by the Chief Scientist, Ministry of Health, Government of Israel.

Many thanks to Miriam Bobrow, the study coordinator.

Table 1. Demographic characteristics of the subjects in the standardization sample according to the birthplace of the father, compared with the Jewish population

Birthplace of father	Israel (%)	Sample (%)
Israeli born	55	58
Asia-Africa	20	26
Europe-America	25	16

child development norms in the Israeli population, comparing ethnic and socioeconomic characteristics.

THE SAMPLE

Examined in the sample were 2,248 children between the ages of 2 weeks and 6.5 years (1,140 males and 1,108 females). Sampling was based on the population of children coming for visits to well-baby clinics for routine examinations or immunizations, children in nursery schools, and children in kindergartens. The sample selection had to consider stratification according to five criteria: 1) age group, 2) sex, 3) ethnic origin, 4) socioeconomic level, and 5) geographic location. The ethnic origin of the subjects using the father's place of birth was compared with that of the Israeli-Jewish population (Table 1) (Central Bureau of Statistics, 1981). The socioeconomic background of the subjects based on father's occupation was compared with the socioeconomic distribution of the Israeli-Jewish population as detailed in Table 2 (Central Bureau of Statistics, 1981; Kark, Peritz, Shilo, & Sloane, 1964). The sample included the cities of Jerusalem and Tel Aviv, the rural town of Beit Shemesh, agricultural settlements in the Judean mountains, as well as kibbutzim.

Table 2. Socioeconomic characteristics of the sample subjects compared with the Israeli general population

Occupation of fathers	Israel	Sample
Category 1—Higher professions, Larger employers, Managers	14%	16%
Category 2—Lower professions, Owners of medium-sized businesses	62%	12%
Category 3—Skilled workers		40%
Category 4—Semiskilled workers	21%	6%
Category 5—Unskilled workers		6%
Category 6—Kibbutz	3%	10%
Category 7—Others	—	10%

The population sampled represents approximately one-third of the Israeli/Hebrew-speaking population. Children were excluded if they were born prematurely, were twins, if another sibling was already tested, or if they had a major neurological or physical handicap.

METHODS

The DDST manual and test sheets were translated into Hebrew and the test material kits were obtained from LADOCA Publishing Foundation, Denver. All of the 105 items of DDST were used and no changes were made.

Six testers were given a course in the administration of the DDST. The training included the viewing of special DDST 16-mm films, and a practical section where each tester would examine a child with the others observing and scoring independently. All the testers achieved intertester reliability of above 95% before the study was started, and also periodically during the 10 months of testing.

The data obtained were analyzed using the Probit statistical analysis method (Finney, 1971). The results were expressed in percentiles—the percentage of children in each age group that had passed the test item. The age at which 25%, 50%, 75%, and 90% of the children had passed an item was determined.

RESULTS

Range of Time

A comparison of the range of time between the ages equivalent to the 25th percentile and that equivalent to the 90th percentile for each of the 105 items of the DDST is given in Table 3. It can be clearly seen that in three sections: personal/social, fine motor/adaptive, and gross motor, the Israeli sample showed a wider range while in language it showed the reverse tendency when compared to the Denver population.

Performance of Ethnic Groups

The three main ethnic groups in Israel were compared to distinguish differences in when 50% of the population passed items. Only items reached earlier by more than 10% differ-

Table 3. Range of time from the 25th to the 90th percentiles of the DDST items comparing the Israeli and Denver populations

	Personal/ social	Fine motor/ adaptive	Language	Gross motor
Israeli wider	15	22	9	20
Denver wider	6	6	12	9
No difference	1	1	1	3

ence were included. The items, divided into the four categories of the DDST and the three ethnic groups, are presented in Table 4.

It can be noted that in the personal/social section, in 14 out of 23 items there was no significant difference between the ethnic groups, and the rest of the items were passed earlier by the Israeli and Asian-Afro group. In the fine motor section, 15 items out of 30 were passed with no significant difference between the groups. Many of the items in early infancy were passed earlier by the Asian-Afro and Israeli groups, while many of the items in early childhood and preschool age, such as tower building, figure copying, and drawing, were passed earlier by the Euro-American group. In the language section, only nine items out of 22 showed a difference of more than 10% between the ethnic groups. Four items, all in early childhood, were passed earlier by the Israeli group. Only one language item was passed

earlier by the Asian-Afro group. In the gross motor section, eight items showed a significant difference, four of which were reached earlier by the Euro-American group and two each by the other ethnic groups.

Comparison of Socioeconomic Class

The findings of the comparison between the performance of children from high socioeconomic classes (SES) (categories 1 and 2 in Table 2) to that of children from lower SES (categories 3–5), are presented in Table 5. The main difference between the two groups is seen in the fine motor and language areas. In the fine motor area, out of 30 items, children from lower SES performed earlier in six items, most of which were in the first year of life. Children from higher SES passed 14 items earlier, four of which were in the earlier period of development and the other 10 were later in childhood. In the language section, the lower SES children passed three items earlier, all of which were in the first year of life. The children of higher SES reached 13 items earlier, most of which were in the preschool age.

The differences between the two groups in the personal/social and gross motor areas are much smaller, and the trend shows almost equal rates of development for both groups.

Table 4. Comparison of the performance of ethnic groups in Israel for differences when 50% of the population passed items (Only items reached earlier by more than 10% difference were included)

	Israel	Asia-Africa	Europe-America
Personal/social	Indicates wants Uses spoon Removes garment Separates from mother easily	Smiles responsively Helps in house Plays interactive games	Regards face Initially shy with strangers
Fine motor/adaptive	Rakes raisin Dumps raisin, demonstrated Dumps raisin, spontaneously	Hands together Grasps rattle Transfers cube Reaches for object Scribbles spontaneously	Builds tower—two cubes Builds tower—eight cubes Copies 0 Copies + Draws man, three parts Draws man, six parts Picks longer line
Language	Combines two different words Gives first and last name Comprehends cold, etc. Follows directions	Points to one named body part	Turns to voice Dada, mama, nonspecific Recognizes three colors Describes composition of object
Gross motor	Gets to sit Jumps in place	Prone—chest up Walks well	Stands momentarily Walks holding on Catches bounced ball Walks heel to toe

Table 5. Comparison of the performance of socioeconomic classes in Israel for the differences when 50% of the population pass items (Only items reached earlier by more than 10% difference were included)

	Higher socioeconomic classes (categories 1,2)	Lower socioeconomic classes (categories 3,4,5)
Personal/social	Works for toys Indicates wants Uses spoon Removes garment Washes and dries hands	Smiles spontaneously Feeds self cracker Plays pat-a-cake Imitates housework Puts on clothing Plays interactive games
Fine motor/adaptive	Follows past midline Sits, looks for yarn Rakes raisin, attains Thumb-finger grasp Tower of two cubes Tower of four cubes Tower of eight cubes Dumps raisin from bottle (dem.) Imitates bridge Copies + Copies square (dem.) Copies square Draws man, three parts Draws man, six parts	Follows 180° Reaches for objects Sits, takes two cubes Transfers cubes, hand-to-hand Neat pincer grasp Scribbles spontaneously
Language	Vocalizes, not crying Turns to voice Combines two words Names one picture Follows directions Uses plurals Gives first and last name Comprehends cold, etc. Comprehends three prepositions Recognizes three colors Opposite analogies Defines six words Composition of objects	Laughs Squeals Dada, mama, nonspecific
Gross motor	Prone, head up 90° Sits without support Gets to sitting Stoops and recovers Walks backwards Walks up stairs Balance on 1 foot—1 second Balance on 1 foot—5 seconds Balance on 1 foot—10 seconds Pedals trike Heel to toe walk	Prone, lifts head Prone, head up 45° Pull to sit, no head lag Walks holding on to furniture Walks well Kicks ball forward Throws ball overhand Broad jump Hops on one foot Catches bounced ball

Comparison of Life-Style

The comparison between kibbutz and non-kibbutz children revealed differences mainly in the language area, where six out of 22 items, mostly in the preschool age, were passed earlier by the kibbutz children (Table 6). In the fine motor area, five out of 30 items were achieved earlier by kibbutz children, four of which were in using block cubes. In the other two modalities, the kibbutz children achieved faster only in two items each; in personal/social, two items of dressing, and in gross motor, two items of balancing. No items were passed earlier by the nonkibbutz children.

DISCUSSION

The standardization of the DDST for Israeli children was carried out due to the recognized influence of the environment on child development (Shapira & Harel, 1983). The results of that study had justified the preliminary

Table 6. Comparison of the performance of kibbutz versus nonkibbutz children, for differences when 50% of the population passed items (Only items passed faster by more than 10% difference were included)

Personal/social	Fine motor/adaptive	Language	Gross motor
Dresses with supervision	Tower of two cubes	Names one picture	Balance one foot—
Dresses without supervision	Tower of four cubes	Uses plurals	1 second
	Tower of eight cubes	Comprehends: cold, etc.	Balance one foot—
	Imitates bridge	Recognizes three colors	10 seconds .
	Picks longer line	Follows directions	
		Opposite analogies	

assumption that the use of the standardized DDST in Israel is necessary in order to avoid both under- and over-referrals of children with developmental abnormalities. A surprising finding in that standardization was the wider range of time between the 25th and the 90th percentiles of many items in the new Israeli version of the DDST. This was explained as stemming from the ethnic heterogeneity of the Israeli population. This finding prompted the authors to analyze further the data of the standardization and to examine the extent of the interethnic differences in the Israeli-Jewish population. Comparing the development in the three main Jewish ethnic groups in Israel, one can observe several trends: faster fine motor development of Asian-Afro infants in the first year of life, and of Euro-American children in skills such as cube building and drawing. In language development, children of Asian-Afro parents achieved earlier in one item only, compared to four items reached faster by each of the other two groups. In the other DDST modalities, the interethnic differences were less remarkable.

These interethnic differences can be explained by the fact that despite the diversity of the population, the living conditions in Israel act as a melting pot that causes rapid assimilation of immigrants into a newly formed western-oriented society, including the child-rearing habits. Facilitating this process is the very high attendance at the well-baby clinics that provide mother guidance in child development, in addition to training in the common functions of hygiene, vaccinations, and nutrition.

On the other hand, there seem to be more remarkable differences on a socioeconomic basis in Israel. These are mainly seen in language and fine motor/adaptive sections, mostly beyond 2 years of age. An almost identical finding was seen in the Cardiff study (Bryant et al., 1979), which found that children from social classes 4 and 5 were slower in items on the fine motor and language scales. These findings are useful as guidelines for future planning of intervention programs, both preventive and therapeutic.

The performance of kibbutz children parallels clearly with that of the higher SES children on the socioeconomic scale. The achievements of this group of children are probably the result of a combination of social welfare and the practice of communal child-rearing and early education starting at birth.

REFERENCES

Barnes, K.E., & Stark, A. Denver Developmental Screening Test: Normative study. *American Journal of Public Health,* 1975, *65,* 363–369.

Bryant, G.M., Davies, K.J., & Newcombe, R.G. Denver Developmental Screening Test. Achievement of test items in the first year of life by Denver and Cardiff infants. *Developmental Medicine and Child Neurology,* 1974, *16,* 474–484.

Bryant, G.M., Davies, K.J., & Newcombe, R.G. Standardization of the Denver Developmental Screening

Test for Cardiff children. *Developmental Medicine and Child Neurology,* 1979, *121,* 353–364.

Central Bureau of Statistics. *Statistical abstract of Israel, 1981, No. 31.* Jerusalem: Sivan Press Ltd., 1981.

Cools, A.T.M., & Hermanns, J.M.A. *Denver Developmental Screening Test.* Amsterdam: Handleidung Swetz en Zeitlinger, 1976.

Finney, D.J. *Probit analysis.* Cambridge: Cambridge University Press, 1971.

Flehmig, I., Schluun, M., Uhde, J., & Van Bernuth, H.

Denver-Entwicklunsskalen [Denver Developmental Scales]. Stuttgart: Thieme Verlag, 1973.

Frankenburg, W.K., Camp, B.W., & Van Natta, P.A. The validity of the DDST. *Child Development,* 1971, *42,* 474–485.

Frankenburg, W.K., Dick, N.P., & Carland, J. Development of preschool-aged children of different social and ethnic groups: Implications. *The Journal of Pediatrics,* 1975, *87,* 125–132.

Frankenburg, W.K., & Dodds, J.B. Denver Developmental Screening Test. *The Journal of Pediatrics,* 1967, *71,* 181–191.

Jaffe, M., Harel, J., Goldberg, A., Rudolph-Schnitzer, M., & Winter, S.T. The use of the Denver Developmental Screening Test in infant welfare clinics. *Developmental Medicine and Child Neurology,* 1980, *22,* 55–60.

Kark, S., Peritz, E., Shilo, A., & Sloane, C. Epidemiological analysis of the hemoglobin picture in parturient women of Jerusalem. *American Journal of Public Health,* 1964, *54,* 947–960.

Shapira, Y., & Harel, S. Standardization of the Denver Developmental Screening Test for Israeli children. *Israeli Journal of Medical Science,* 1983, *19,* 246–251.

Super, C.M. Environmental effects on motor development. The case of South African infant precocity. *Developmental Medicine and Child Neurology,* 1976, *18,* 561–567.

Ueda, R. Standardization of the Denver Developmental Screening Test on Japanese children. *Developmental Medicine and Child Neurology,* 1978, *20,* 647–656.

Chapter 43

Environmental Variables and Cognitive Development
Identification of the Potent
Factors in Adult-Child Interaction

PNINA S. KLEIN, ED.D.
Bar-Ilan University, Ramat Gan, Israel
REUVEN FEUERSTEIN, PH.D.
Hadassah-WIZO-Canada Research Institute, Jerusalem, Israel

S CIENTISTS TODAY ARE WELL AWARE OF THE complexity of environmental variables affecting the course of children's cognitive development. It is quite clear that the determining factors, i.e., genetic, physiological, cultural, and economic, interact with each other and their effect cannot, most commonly, be determined in isolation from the effects of other factors. It has also been suggested that the effects of every one of these factors is either amplified or circumvented by the kind and amount of human interaction to which a child is exposed.

It is therefore surprising that very little is known about the potent processes within the interactive experiences between the child and his or her environment that determine differential cognitive development.

The objective of this chapter is to suggest an outline of an empirical and theoretical framework for the identification of these processes.

Close to 6,000 published studies reported from 1970 to date were reviewed through the Psychological Abstracts and ERIC databases. Since the major objective of this search was to identify the characteristic processes within

parent-child interactions that lead to differential cognitive development, the search has focused primarily on studies in which observational data were collected. Of the 6,000 identified studies, only 300 met the latter criterion, confirming the relative scarcity of observational studies within the general body of research on child development. It should be noted that observational research on the second and third years of life was especially scarce (see review by Carew, 1980). The authors' search does not exhaust all attempts to summarize the available data on the subject; yet, it is reasonable to assume that it represents a fairly reliable sample of the general state of the art.

Based on this sample of studies, it was rather difficult to answer the basic question about how differences in young children's cognitive development emerge. Many of the studies since 1970 were designed to explore precedents or correlates of differences between groups of children on the basis of variables such as age, SES, ethnicity, or sex. Most researchers focused their studies or reported on specific elements of cognitive performance (e.g., Beckwith, Cohen, Kopp, Parmelee, & Marcy, 1976; Belsky, Goode, & Most, 1980; Bradley & Caldwell, 1977; Cohen & Beckwith, 1976). Cognitive performance was assessed in most studies by conventional measures of IQ, DQ, or other measures including observations of specific abilities mostly focusing on an end product rather than on the process leading up to it.

One of the most common limitations of research on the effects of various child-rearing practices has been the danger of reaching faulty conclusions of cause and effect based on correlational data. Furthermore, with lack of a theoretical conceptual framework, some of the *ad hoc* conclusions based on this type of study led to overgeneralization and misleading conclusions.

Several comprehensive studies involving naturalistic observations were carried out in order to answer the basic question of how differences in cognitive development of young children emerge (i.e., Carew, 1980; Schachter, 1979; White, Kaban, & Attanucci, 1979). White et al. (1979), for example, identified the basic differences between competent and less competent children as related to their ability to please adults, to gain their attention, and procure their services. In addition, they found that competent children displayed more focusing behavior related to gaining information from concentrated looking or listening to "live" language directed at them. One would thus be led to conclude that environments that teach children how to gain adults' attention, how to please adults, and how to focus visual and auditory attention are environments that promote a child's competence.

Of all environmental variables, the central role of the adult caregiver in affecting children's cognitive development is well beyond dispute. Carew (1980) summarized observational studies indicating that mothers of competent infants were found to spend more time teaching the infants, stimulating them intellectually, and facilitating their activities. However, Carew's report inspired additional questions. What does teaching an infant imply? What are intellectually stimulating activities?

Various criteria of maternal behavior, i.e., attentiveness, warmth, responsivity, and non-restrictiveness have been repeatedly isolated in research as variables most indicative of infants' cognitive development (e.g., Beckwith, 1971a, 1971b; Beckwith et al., 1976; Belsky et al., 1980; Bradley, Caldwell, & Elardo, 1979; Clarke-Stewart, 1973; White et al., 1979; Yarrow, Rubenstein, & Pedersen, 1975).

Recent studies (see review by Carew, 1980) demonstrate that experiences involving an infant's interaction with another person, especially experiences in which the adult reacted *to* the child or prestructured experiences for him or her, correlated with measures of development earlier, more highly, and more consistently as compared to intellectual experiences that were created by the child himself or herself and that he or she experienced individually.

Most available data, although indirectly supporting the role of an adult mediator between infant or child and his or her environment, have not as yet presented a universal rather than specific content-related theoretical conceptualization of the characteristics of mediation, interaction, or teaching.

WHAT IS A MEDIATED LEARNING EXPERIENCE (MLE)?

This chapter emerges from Feuerstein's basic theoretical orientation of mediated learning experience (Feuerstein, 1979, 1981; Feuerstein & Hoffman, 1982). According to this orientation, there are two basic ways in which an individual is modified through interaction with his or her environment. The first is modification that occurs as a result of direct exposure to stimuli, i.e., direct contact or exposure to stimuli perceived or experienced through the sensory channels. Direct exposure does not explain differential development. Only a few mature persons actually reach the levels of cognitive functioning that are called by Piaget and Inhelder (1969) formal operations. If formal operations could have been explained solely by biological dispositions (maturation in relation to direct exposure to stimuli), then there should have been no reason why more people would not have reached formal operations in a normal population.

A second process is needed to explain cognitive development; this process has been defined by Feuerstein (1981) and Feuerstein and Hoffman (1982) as mediated learning experience. Whereas the direct exposure modality can be expressed as a stimulus-response process (S-R process), this second modality is one that involves an active human mediator who goes between the organism and the environment and mediates the experience to the organism. Piaget's theory proposes an S-O-R sequence, that is, stimulus-organism-response, in which the organism itself takes an active role in selecting and processing the information presented by the environment. But even the S-O-R sequence deals with direct exposure, since the organism cannot serve as a mediator between the environment and himself or herself.

In view of Piaget's theory, the role of mediated learning is rather limited, and when the organism is biologically mature, he or she will learn from direct exposure to stimuli and through active involvement in the processes of assimilation and accommodation. However, as stated before, these direct learning experiences and maturation do not explain why so few people achieve formal operations and why there is horizontal decalage within individuals.

The process of mediated learning experiences explains development and its multifaced manifestations in different individuals. It is the process of learning that occurs when another person serves as the mediator between the child or learner and the stimuli. The mediation is an active process. The mediator acts upon the stimulus before it enters the organism. The mediator selects, accentuates, frames, and locates the stimulus in time and space, and schedules groups. The mediation enables the individual to benefit from experience; it actually prepares him or her to learn, to become modified.

The concept "culturally deprived," or "culturally disadvantaged," reflects a condition characterized by the low ability of individuals to be modified through direct exposure to stimuli, a condition caused by lack of or deficient MLE.

Limited modifiability is often manifested in a series of restrictions on processing information. If one's perception is blurred, if one has no systematic way of obtaining accurate information through the senses, if one has sweeping exploration, lack of need for precision, inappropriate use of temporal and spatial dimensions, lack of perception and projection of sequences, lack of spontaneous comparative behavior and the need for logical evidence, how is one going to benefit from direct exposure to stimuli? One acquires the need for adequate functioning of these processes through mediated learning experiences.

MLE begins with interactions on a preverbal level and is not specifically related to a modality, language, or content. It is a universal phenomenon. There are two basic components of MLE. One relates to components which, were it not for MLE, could never have reached the consciousness of a person. The other component relates to structures, to the form of processing information.

Through the MLE, the child can benefit from experiences that he or she has not perceived directly. The transmission of the past is made possible only through mediational processes that enlarge the temporal spheres available to the child. The awareness of the past, coupled with anticipation of the future, which is also mediated, enables the child to expand his or her understanding and learning of time and space.

The more mediation the child receives, the more he or she grows capable of learning from future experience and being modified by it. The child who receives MLE develops a set of *needs* to seek mediation in order to expect events to have meaning, to search for relations to go beyond the information provided by the senses at any given moment. There is an optimal level of MLE that is best for cognitive development. Too much mediation may be deleterious to development since it may leave no time for the child to apply his or her newly acquired modified schemata in new learning situations.

In sum, the MLE is one of the two basic modes of learning from experience. It is universal, not specific to one culture, not content related. It enables further change of the individual through direct exposure to stimuli, and allows a child to acquire basic structures that prepare him or her for future learning.

BASIC CRITERIA OF MLE

Five criteria of a MLE interaction have been identified. These criteria are as follows: 1) intentionality, 2) transcendence, 3) meaning, 4) competence, and 5) regulation of behavior.

Intentionality and Mutuality

Intentionality of the mediator is communicated to the child at a very early stage and creates a joint intention, an openness, a readiness to perceive changes and to respond on the part of both parent and child. Both the child and the stimuli are affected and modified, made compatible to each other by the process of mediation. The intention to mediate between the environment and the child has several basic components such as regulating the state of arousal of a child, calling his or her attention to stimuli, and affecting his or her response.

MLE is clearly not accidental; it is a conscious intentional act. It is a dynamic process in which the mediator (most frequently the mother) attempts a series of actions to reach the objective of her mediation. She moves her head toward the infant or away from the infant's face until he or she focuses on her eyes, or moves an object until the infant focuses on it. She may vary her tone of voice or rhythm of speech until the infant responds in line with her intentions.

Intentionality affects the manner in which a stimulus is presented and in which it is attended to by the child. The mother, through modification of her behavior, selects that part of the environment on which she wishes to focus the child's attention and she chooses and regulates the modes of his or her response.

Intentionality affects the basic processes of arousal. The mother may calm the baby before starting to mediate. She will not engage in MLE if the infant is too sleepy. She does it, for example, through introducing body movement or vocalization in accordance with the child's momentary rhythmic behavior and gradually reducing or increasing the pace in the direction intended. Daniel Stern (1977) gives a detailed account of the "atoms" of such interactions. He speaks of the differences in adults' behavior toward infants as compared to their behavior toward others. Components such as exaggeration in facial expressions and variation in rate of speech and vocal tone may be considered as parts of the MLE, as tools of intentionality, although these various components *may not necessarily be consciously directed*. The need to mediate, in itself, is intentional. The component expressions of intentionality are not necessarily consciously controlled. There are intentions that stem from the fact that mothers belong to or are part of a cultural, social, or ethnic group.

The authors have found in one of their recent studies that mothers' behavior toward their premature infant boys differed significantly as compared to their behavior toward premature girls while still in the intensive care unit in the hospital. Mothers explained this difference by expressing their belief that girls are weaker and thereby need more visiting (Klein, Mogilner, Mogilner, Alkon, Halevi, Shriky, & Lamdan, 1982). In several studies comparing groups of immigrants in Israel, it was found that mothers who believed that their children developed slower spoke less to their infants and provided them with fewer objects with which to play (Feitelson, 1954; Goshen-Gottstein, 1975).

What mothers think about their infants, their theories of child-rearing, and their image of what a child should grow up to be, shape their behavior toward the infants and are included and expressed in the mothers' intentionality, affecting both the manner in which stimuli are presented as well as how the learner attends to the stimuli.

Transcendence

The second criterion of MLE is transcendence from the immediate experience, from its immediate precedents and consequences in relation to others remote in time and space. The goal of interaction is transcended. A mediated experience is not restricted to the satisfaction of immediate needs. It is by transcending beyond the immediate that structural changes occur in the child, structural changes in the sense of anticipation of, search for, and need for information beyond the immediate.

White et al. (1979) in their comparison of competent and less competent infants, indicate that the competent children know how to ask for assistance or information and do so. But, how does the child know that he or she can expect more information, that every experience can be viewed as part of other experiences than what meets his or her eyes or other senses? If one asks a child to carry out a chore, such as delivering an object, the command is sufficient to bring about the desired behavior, but not a mediated learning experience. In essence, the mere fact that the child has carried out the chore has achieved the immediate goal of the command. However, it has not served as a mediated learning experience until placed by a mediator in relation to more distant cause, effect, or any other expansion beyond the immediate.

The conceptualization of transcendence is thus different from reinforcement; it is also different from explaining an act or merely labeling it verbally. Saying to the child, "Thank you," or smiling at him or her would reinforce his or her act and perhaps his or her tendency to do what is asked, but telling him or her, for example, what the tool is needed for and what may happen if the tool is not used properly is transcendence beyond the immediate and constitutes an MLE.

In sum, transcendence creates in the child an expansion of the individual's spatial and temporal life space, an expansion of his or her need system, an expansion of his or her structural modifiability.

Transcendence should not be mistakenly understood as a means of verbal enrichment since numerous enrichment programs emphasize the component of verbalization in a child's actions or expansion of his or her expression. In the latter, the focus is on the immediate and on the verbal labeling of it, whereas the conceptualization of MLE focuses on, or draws attention to, the creation of structural changes in the child's expectation and need system, *the need to go beyond the immediate act or behavior*. In the immediate future, he or she will seek more information from the adult and later, provided the child gets enough MLE, he or she will attempt to relate, on his or her own, what he or she perceives to a context of knowledge that goes beyond what he or she experiences through his or her senses. Transcendence expands the child's need system and the means for its achievement.

Meaning

The third attribute of MLE is the establishment of meaning. The mediator endows stimuli with meaning of objects or of relations.

The objects that surround a child have *no* meaning to him or her unless they bear meaning to the mediator, an affective value-oriented connotation that can be transmitted to the child through the mediated LE and cannot be obtained through direct exposure to stimuli. As strange as it may sound to some, one has to learn how to pause to wonder.

A child has to learn to expect relations between what is perceived or experienced and affectual connotations and undertones that may derive from cultural values or other parental experiences. Through mediation, the child learns that things and events have meaning beyond what he or she has directly experienced, for example, "This is not just an ordinary cup; it was your father's when he was a baby," or "Oh, look at that beautiful sunset." It was there before this was said and it is possible that through direct exposure the child could have seen it. But, seeing it without the mediation of its value or the effect it arouses in the adult might not have brought about the effect of wonder or attachment and thus would not enable the child to form similar relations with future experiences that would present other meaningful objects or relations.

Since the MLE is not content related, it does not matter if what is transmitted through the act of mediation is true to reality in the "objective" mind, or whether it is correct according to cultural sets. The important aspect of this criterion is the fact that someone attaches meaning with an experience for the child.

In a country such as Israel, in which cultural diversity is one of the highest in the world, one has to stress the fact that, rather than teaching a mother new ways of instructing her infant or young child (i.e., conveying the message that what she is able to contribute to her infant without new information or an expert's opinion is not enough), all cultural background is viewed as equally beneficial in mediation of experience. Since the process is mediated, regardless of content, it is only through experiences of mediated meaning that other experiences gain meaning. Parents do this all the time; they are, however, not aware that they mediate meaning. Meaning is mediated verbally when a parent says, for instance, "Look at that tiny, little, soft kitten." It is mediated in a nonverbal way, for example, by making a surprise sound and raising brows or by indicating empathy through sighing and making a sad facial expression. Mediation of meaning includes mediation of effect. Meaning is mediated partially through endowing the object with affect. The child may experience affect. He or she may feel content, angry, or fearful, but if it is not mediated, it is an isolated experience.

Mediation of Feelings of Competence

The fourth criterion of MLE is mediation of a feeling of competence. Through mediation of a feeling of competence, the child acquires a sense of mastery, a feeling that he or she is capable and successful, which contributes, no doubt, to a willingness to explore the new and attempt to apply oneself to new and challenging endeavors. If one wants to encourage curiosity and active exploration, one must encourage MLE of the feeling of competence.

The existing theories of child or personality development relate to the accumulation of successful experiences, to the end product, to the sum. The MLE focuses not only on the direct exposure to the success or failure, but to its interpretation by a human agent as to the place of these experiences in relation to other actions of the child, to other parts of the same activity, to possible events that could have led to the outcome, and to possible consequences. Merely saying to the child, "This is very good!" reinforces his or her efforts, but by focusing on the processes that led to success and on the mental process that preceded it, this enables him or her to use future experiences to construct a realistic picture of success or of failure. There are many adults who do not have a frame of reference for success, who consider themselves as failures, who do not dare to attempt a new task predicting failure. Educational psychologists frequently tend to interpret this as a result of the accumulation of failure experiences.

Success and failure are learned to a large extent through MLE. In those areas of functioning in which people have less mediated learning experiences, they are less capable of learning from direct exposure to successes, and are more vulnerable to criticism and more unsure of themselves.

For MLE to produce feelings of competence, an adult may wait patiently for the child to complete a task or he or she may design situations in which the child may have a good chance to succeed and gain competence. The adult then points out the child's actions as a success, interprets its basic component, gives the reasons why the action was successful, and relates it to other successes or failures. An example can be seen in a boy learning to tie his shoelaces. His mother lays out the laces in a position that requires only one single step before the knot is tied. The child who has previously pulled one loop too hard succeeds this time and receives a warm, enthusiastic smile from the mother followed by a remark, such as, "Very good, you did it carefully; you did not pull too hard on the shoestring." The child not only learns that he did well, but he learns that doing it carefully, not pulling hard, contributed to his success.

This example leads to the fifth criterion of MLE. In order for feelings to gain meaning, a child needs an adult to mediate them for him or her, to relate the experience to preceding events and to consequences, to other occasions in which similar feelings were felt by himself or herself, and by others including the mediator himself or herself.

Regulation of Behavior

The adult, by modeling or by scheduling objects or events in time and space, introduces a pattern (plan) of activities for the child, thus regulating the pace and reducing the child's impulsiveness in perception, elaboration, and expression. Mediation of regulation of behavior results in a learned awareness of the possibility to regulate one's own behavior and enables one to use experiences and to learn from them to improve this control. Regulation of behavior entails *matching* the characteristics of the task to be performed with the characteristics of one's own level of functioning both in terms of cognitive skills and level of efficiency. This match will result in the adaptation of the pace of the work in order to reach an adequate balance between the rapidity and the required precision in performing a task.

All five criteria of the mediated learning experience can be transmitted both verbally and nonverbally, including meaning, which is commonly believed to depend on verbal expressions. For example, meaning of a certain sight or musical tone is mediated when the mother stops what she is doing, closes her eyes, and with a facial expression of content, rocks with her child to the sound of the music.

When an experience with an adult contains any one of the criteria of MLE, that experience is an experience of mediated learning. A child, however, *needs all five criteria* mediated to him or her in order to enable him or her to benefit from future experience and to allow his or her social, emotional, and intellectual growth.

Parents naturally provide their children with MLE. This is, as was said, universally true. Parents may, however, differ as to the amount or quality of one component of mediation as opposed to the others. It is almost possible to refer to a profile of mediation. A child may receive mediation of intentionality, meaning, transcendence, and regulation of behavior in abundance, but little, if any, experiences of mediated competence. He or she may then know how to relate and place objects and events in their place in space and time. He or she may feel for events, for people, for things around him or her. Yet the child may not dare express himself or herself, become an active participant, or encounter new challenges. The reverse is possible, too, i.e., in the case of a

nonrealistic, overemphasized mediation of competence, when meaning, transcendence, and regulation are rarely experienced.

RECENT EMPIRICAL DATA

In a longitudinal study carried out at Bar-Ilan University, 40 first-born infants were followed up from birth (the infants are now 3–4 years old). Home observations during the first year of the study were based on Yarrow et al.'s (1975) time sampling observational method and during the second and third years on an evaluation of each of the basic criteria of MLE rated on a 6-point scale. Cognitive performance of the children in the study at the age of 3 could be predicted based on an evaluation of the kind and level of MLE they were exposed to at 13–16 months of age. Based on ratings of MLE, three children (all girls) were identified: two had been identified as recipients of high levels of MLE (rated 5–6 on the 6-point scale) and one child was identified as receiving significantly low MLE (1–2 on the rating scales). It is of interest to note that observations based on Yarrow et al.'s time sampling observational technique did not yield significant differences between the three children identified through the MLE ratings and the other children. In other words, these children, for example, were not noted to be deprived or overstimulated visually, auditorially, kinesthetically, or played with less than others. Similarly, no significant differences were found between these infants and others in the sample of the Uzgiris-Hunt Ordinal Scales of Psychological Development and on the Gesell Developmental Schedules.

At the age of 3, the two children identified at 1 year of age as receiving high ratings of MLE scored an equivalent of over 130 IQ, based on the Illinois Test of Psycholinguistic Abilities (ITPA). The child identified as receiving low ratings of MLE gained an IQ of 90 based on the same measure.

All three of these children received similar ratings of maternal warmth and no significant differences were noted between the amount of visual, auditory, and kinesthetic stimulations they had received. Some differences were found between these children on Yarrow et al.'s observational categories of social mediation.

In sum, it may be concluded that infants' cognitive development can be better predicted when the type of interaction with the adult caregivers is taken into consideration. More specifically, ratings of the five criteria of mediated learning experience were powerful predictors of cognitive development of young children.

In a currently ongoing study carried out in collaboration with Tel-Hashomer Hospital, the authors have evaluated cognitive performance of 2- and 3-year-old children born prematurely and weighing less than 1,500 grams at birth. The evaluation included the Illinois Test of Psycholinguistic Abilities, Beery Test of Visual Motor Integration, and the Peabody Picture Vocabulary Test. In addition, the interaction between the parents and their children was observed throughout the testing session and during 20 minutes of waiting prior to testing. Although the final analysis of the data has not been completed, it appears that cognitive performance of the subjects in the study could not be determined by the severity of their condition at birth, independently of the kind of mediation to which they had been exposed. One of the children in the sample was one of the lowest birth weight infants reported to survive in Israel. She was born after an eventful pregnancy weighing 540 grams. When evaluated at the age of 3, she scored significantly above average on several cognitive measures (specifically on measures of abstract reasoning, i.e., visual and auditory association tests on the ITPA) and on an average level on measures requiring

sequential memory and continuous attention. Another example is a boy, born weighing 800 grams with an Apgar score of 2 at birth, who at the age of 3 functioned on a level equivalent to the high normal expected for his age.

One can hardly draw conclusions based on two examples only. However, even these two examples are sufficient to conclude that high physiological risk at birth is not sufficient to produce retardation of cognitive functioning. Furthermore, and most importantly, ratings of the parents' mediational processes during the testing sessions, their educational philosophy, and attitudes were found strongly related to the level of the children's ability to cope with situations requiring new adaptations, new learning, and problem-solving.

Questions such as 'What kind of MLE are given to the child?'' ''How does he or she respond?'' ''What opportunities does he or she get for learning through MLE and consequently through direct exposure?'' are questions no less important than ''What is the size of the child's vocabulary?'' ''Can he or she classify or solve puzzles?'' if the objective of an assessment is to provide assistance or guidance directed toward the promotion of the child's development. It is necessary to evaluate processes through which cognitive growth occurs. Thus, there is a growing need to add to the child-oriented assessment an observation of the relationship between mother and child or primary caregiver and child. The criteria of MLE can serve as guidelines in the assessment of these experiences in a content-free and process-oriented manner.

REFERENCES

Beckwith, L. Relationships between attributes of mothers and their infants' IQ scores. *Child Development*, 1971, *42*, 1083–1097. (a)

Beckwith, L. Relationships between infants' vocalizations and their mothers' behaviors. *Merrill-Palmer Quarterly*, 1971, *17*, 221–226. (b)

Beckwith, L. Relationships between infants' social behavior and their mothers' behavior. *Child Development*, 1972, *43*, 397–411.

Beckwith, L., Cohen, S.E., Kopp, C.B., Parmelee, A.H., & Marcy, T.C. Caregiver-infant interaction and early cognitive development in preterm infants. *Child Development*, 1976, *47*, 579–587.

Belsky, J., Goode, M.K., & Most, R.K. Maternal stimulation and infant exploratory competence: Cross-sectional, correlational, and experimental analyses. *Child Development*, 1980, *51*, 1163–1178.

Bradley, R.H., & Caldwell, B.M. Early home environment and changes in mental test performance in children from 6 to 36 months. *Developmental Psychology*, 1977, *12*, 93–97.

Bradley, R., Caldwell, B., & Elardo, R. Home environment and cognitive development in the first two years: A cross-lag panel analysis. *Developmental Psychology*, 1979, *15*, 246–250.

Carew, J.V. Experience in the development of intelligence

in young children at home and in day care. *Monographs of the Society for Research in Child Development,* 1980, *45* (6–7, Serial No. 187).

Clarke-Stewart, K.A. Interactions between mothers and their young children: Characteristics and consequences. *Monographs of the Society for Research in Child Development,* 1973, *38* (6–7, Serial No. 153).

Cohen, S.E., & Beckwith, L. Maternal language in infancy. *Developmental Psychology,* 1976, *12,* 371–372.

Feitelson, D. [Education of the small child amongst the Kurdish community.] *Megamot,* 1954, *5,* 95–109. (Original in Hebrew.)

Feuerstein, R. Ontogeny of learning in man. In: M.A.B. Brazier (ed.), *Brain mechanisms in memory and learning: From the single neuron to man.* New York: Raven Press, 1979.

Feuerstein, R. Mediated learning experiences in the acquisition of kinesics. In: B.L. Hoffer & R.N. St. Clair (eds.), *Developmental kinesics, the emerging paradigm.* Baltimore: University Park Press, 1981.

Feuerstein, R., & Hoffman, M.B. Intergenerational conflict of rights: Cultural imposition and self-realization.

Journal of the School of Education. (Indiana University), 1982, *58,* 44–63.

Goshen-Gottstein, E.R. Potentially harmful child-rearing practices. *Israel Annals of Psychiatry and Related Disciplines,* 1975, *3,* 85–104.

Klein, P.S., Mogilner, B.M., Mogilner, C., Alkon, S., Halevi, E., Shriky, S., & Lamdan, D. The relationship between maternal visiting patterns and the development of premature infants. *Journal of Psychosomatic Obstetrics and Gynaecology.* 1981, *1*(3/4), 124–127.

Piaget, J., & Inhelder, B. *The psychology of the child.* New York: Basic Books, 1969.

Schachter, F. *Everyday mother talk to toddlers: Early intervention.* New York: Academic Press, 1979.

Stern, D. *The first relationship.* London: Open Books, 1977.

White, B.L., Kaban, B.T., & Attanucci, J.S. *The origins of human competence.* Lexington, MA: Lexington Books, 1979.

Yarrow, L.J., Rubenstein, J.L., & Pedersen, F.A. *Infant and environment.* New York: John Wiley & Sons, 1975.

The At-Risk Infant: Psycho/Socio/Medical Aspects
edited by Shaul Harel, M.D., and Nicholas J. Anastasiow, Ph.D.
Copyright © 1985   Paul H. Brookes Publishing Co., Inc.   Baltimore • London

Chapter 44

Play Behavior of Handicapped and Nonhandicapped Infants between 9 and 24 Months

ROSE M. BROMWICH, ED.D.
California State University, Northridge; Northridge, California

P LAY IS AN IMPORTANT MEDIUM FOR THE IN-
tellectual, emotional, and social development of infants. It is also the most natural
spontaneous activity of infants, and therefore
lends itself readily to the study of behavior.
Infants behave quite differently and show different strengths when they are engaged in independent play than when they are asked to
follow directions or imitate the adult's behavior, as in a testing situation. Careful observations focused on specific areas of behavior
during spontaneous play offer a rich source of
information on various aspects of development
during infancy.

Since the mid seventies, infant play has been
studied by a number of scholars. Their studies
have focused on the cognitive development of
infants through observations of their play at
different ages, for example, manipulation and
play of 7½- and 11½-month-olds (McCall,
1974), analysis of the effects of social and
inanimate environments on 5- and 6-month-
olds (Yarrow, Rubenstein, & Pedersen, 1975),
cognition and motivation of 5- and 6-month-
olds (Yarrow & Pedersen, 1976), manipulative

play in the first 2 years (Fenson, Kagan, Kearsley, & Zelazo, 1976), functional play in
12-month-olds (Zelazo & Kearsley, 1977),
developmental trends in the play of infants
(Rosenblatt, 1977), the analysis of pretend
play to assess symbolic maturity (McCune-
Nicolich, 1977), the antecedents of cognitive
functioning in infancy (Kagan, Lapidus, &
Moore, 1978), spontaneous play and imitation
in infants between 9 and 30 months (Largo &
Howard, 1979), and the representation of objects in symbolic play from 18 to 34 months
(Ungerer, Zelazo, Kearsley, & O'Leary,
1981). The subjects in these studies have been
normal, and at times, highly competent infants. In contrast, half of the sample of the
study reported on in this chapter consisted of
handicapped infants.

PURPOSE OF THE STUDY

The purpose of the Study of Play-Associated
Behaviors of Handicapped and Non-Handi-
capped Infants[1] was threefold: 1) to examine
play-associated behavior longitudinally be-

[1]The study was carried out at UCLA in the Department of Pediatrics, School of Medicine with Arthur H. Parmelee as
the principal investigator; Judy Howard as the coprincipal investigator; Rose M. Bromwich as the research director; Suzanne
Fust as the administrative assistant and research associate; and Ellen Khokha as the research associate. The 3-year study was
funded by the Easter Seal Research Foundation, Grant No. R 7711.

tween 9 and 24 months of age; 2) to compare the behaviors, during independent play, of handicapped and nonhandicapped infants at different development ages; and 3) to develop and refine a tool that could serve to organize and structure observations of behavior associated with the spontaneous play of infants. Some of the more intriguing findings of this 3-year study are presented here.

METHOD

The method used in the study is summarized briefly. Only three of the variables of the study are discussed below.

Subjects

The sample of the study included 23 handicapped and 23 nonhandicapped infants (henceforth referred to as "normal" infants, for the sake of brevity) who were matched by developmental age, based on scores obtained on the Bayley Mental Scale. The infants in both groups were from predominantly middle class families in which both parents had had some education beyond high school. From among the 23 handicapped infants, 11 had cerebral palsy (some were also delayed), six had Down syndrome, and the remaining six infants had various combinations of sensorimotor and emotional problems. In the handicapped group (henceforth referred to as the H group), nine subjects obtained developmental quotients (DQs) of 50 or below (on the Bayley Mental Scale); five, between 51 and 69 DQ; seven, between 70 and 89 DQ; and four, between 90 and 110 DQ. All the subjects in the normal group (henceforth referred to as the N group) scored above 90 DQ on the Bayley Mental Scale. The H group had an almost equal number of males and females (11 and 12, respectively), whereas the N group consisted of over twice as many males as females (16 and 7, respectively). The handicapped subjects were recruited from a number of intervention programs in the Los Angeles area. The normal subjects were volunteers—children of parents who were interested in participating in the study.

Procedure

The play sessions, lasting 10 or 12 minutes (depending on age), were structured as follows. Carefully selected toys were grouped and placed in a semicircle on the carpeted floor in the middle of a small room. The mother, seated a few feet away from the toys, was given a magazine to read so that she would appear to the child to be occupied. She was asked not to initiate interaction with the child, but to respond in a natural manner when the child initiated contact with her, without unnecessarily prolonging the interaction. The videotaping was done through an aperture in a wall with a large one-way mirror.

Play sessions of infants in the N group were videotaped at 9½ and 12 months and, thereafter, at 3-month intervals. By 9½ months of age, most normal infants engage in some of the activities that fall into the fourth stage of Piaget's sensorimotor period. Play sessions of the infants in the H group were videotaped at 4-month intervals because of the assumption that the infants in that group would show developmental change more slowly than the infants in the N group. The nature of the study required that the handicapped subjects be able to see and grasp a toy, pick it up, and hold it securely enough to explore it visually, manually, and to bring it to their mouths. At the initial videotaping, the handicapped infants ranged in chronological age from 9½ to 22 months. Each videotaped segment was viewed twice, simultaneously by two observers, and scored on the Play Assessment Checklist for Infants (described in next paragraph), especially developed for the study.

Observations of infant play during the pilot phase of the study led to the development of a checklist of behaviors that was used by the observers in the study. The Play Assessment Checklist for Infants (PACFI) was organized into four categories of variables: temperament characteristics expressed behaviorally; social and language behavior; cognitive-motivational behavior, subdivided into motivational-attention span variables and cognitive process variables; and cognitive-social behavior consisting of functional and representational (or symbolic) play.[2] The term "cognitive-motivational," first used by Yarrow et al. (1975), points to the interdependence of these two domains of infant behavior. The activities included in this category are viewed "as expressions of the infant's motivation to learn about and to master the environment, as early manifestations of effectance motivation" (Yarrow et al., 1975, p. 160). The term "cognitive-social" suggests that functional and representational (or symbolic) play have social and cognitive components that are inseparable. The findings discussed below are limited to the cognitive-motivational category and to the cognitive-social category.

Analysis of Data

In order to examine relationships between variables at identical developmental age points, a correlation matrix of all the variables was computed separately for the two groups at each age point. For all the variables, *t* tests of difference between the two groups were computed. Graphs were also plotted that showed the percentage of subjects who obtained high scores at the different age points to illustrate the progression over time of individual behaviors in the cognitive-motivational and cognitive-social category.

RESULTS AND DISCUSSION

The discussion of findings focuses on one variable of special interest in the cognitive-motivational category, and on two variables in the cognitive-social category. The first of these to be discussed is the variable in the cognitive-motivational category: *visual planning/evaluation of effect*. Of particular interest in the pilot phase of the study was the observation that normal infants vary considerably with respect to the age at which they can be observed to plan an act and then follow it up by evaluating its effect. Such behavior, observable first in the infant's manipulative play, has not been the focus of study in infant research.

The Variable:
Visual Planning/Evaluation of Effect

The onset of intentionality during Piaget's sensorimotor stage is considered to be a milestone in intellectual development. Also, the infant's capacity to observe the effect of his or her own actions is emphasized repeatedly in Piagetian theory. More recently, the cognitive and affective consequences of such acts were stated succinctly by Yarrow and Pedersen (1976):

> Being able to do something to an object and to observe the consequences of this action undoubtedly enhances the child's developing sense of mastery and competence, the development of feelings that he can have an impact on his environment (p. 389).

For the purpose of the study, visual planning/evaluation of effect (henceforth referred to as visual plan./eval.) was operationally defined as follows: infants engage in visual planning and evaluation of effect when they search or look for specific objects that they intend to use (often in combination with other objects), proceed to use them purposefully (with apparent intent or goal), and subsequently evaluate or check the results or effects of their own actions. At first, an attempt was made to identify visual planning and evaluation of effect separately, but it was too difficult to do in most cases. The two components of this variable are connected, in fact, intertwined, because the evaluation of the result usually guides the plan for the subsequent action. This composite behavior demonstrates the infant's capacity to plan before using a toy in a particular manner, and then to check the effect of his or her action.

Before summarizing the findings relative to visual plan./eval., the other variables in the cognitive-motivational category are listed and briefly defined: *interest in play* (time spent with toys), *attention span/characteristic* (length of time with one group of objects or with one activity, most typical during the session), *attention span/capacity* (longest time

---

[2]The Play Assessment Checklist for Infants (PACFI) was developed for use in the study, and has been modified since the completion of the study. The checklist and manual are available, at cost of reproduction and mailing, to professionals working with infants in various settings who are interested in trying it with infants between the ages of nine and 24 months developmental age. Feedback from individuals or groups that have used it is more than welcome!

with an activity during the session), *complexity of play* (proportion of goal-directed versus purely exploratory schemata), *number of [different] schemata* (scored only at 9 and 12 months), and *schema sequencing* (number of schemata in a chain or purposeful sequence with a group of objects—scored from 15 months on). Once an infant begins to use a wide variety of schemata, sometime between 13 and 15 months of age, the sheer number of different schemata no longer constitutes a discriminating variable. Therefore, beginning at the 15-month age point, schema sequencing took the place of number of schemata. As in the case of attention span, two separate variables were identified: *schema sequencing/characteristic* (most common during session) and *schema sequencing/capacity* (highest number of schemata per sequence observed).

Findings The correlations between visual plan./eval. and all the other cognitive-motivational variables listed above are shown in Table 1 for the H group and in Table 2 for the N group. The composite variable, *sum*, has been added on the tables to show the relationship between visual plan./eval. and the sum of all the single variables in the cognitive-motivational category. The correlations with sum were significant at all age points in both groups, although at higher levels of significance in the H group at most age points. Significant correlations between visual plan./eval. and other single variables were greater in number and reached higher levels of significance in the H group than in the N group.

Correlations between visual plan./eval. and sum were expected to be significant, based on the assumption that visual plan./eval. incorporates cognitive acts of central importance in infant play. However, this variable was not expected to show more significant correlations with other cognitive-motivational variables and at higher levels of significance in the H group than in the N group.

Another unanticipated finding was the highly significant between-group differences on visual plan./eval. at all but one age point (Table 3). The differences between groups on this variable are also illustrated graphically (Figure 1) by two curves; the percentage of high-scoring subjects is represented by a dot or a circle at each age point. More subjects in the N group than in the H group engaged in this complex behavior at all the developmental age points except at 24 months. The graph also shows the progression of each group on this variable over time. The similarity in the shape of the two curves demonstrates that there was a similar pattern of change over time in spite of the differences pointed out above.

Discussion and Implications The findings suggest that the operations that make up visual planning/evaluation of effect are worthy of note as they seem to bear a close relationship to other cognitive operations and motivational factors associated with play. Although unexpected, it is interesting that more correlations were significant and showed higher levels of significance in the H group than in the N group (Tables 1 and 2). At the

Table 1. Correlations with *visual planning/evaluation of effect* in the handicapped group

	Age points of study				
	9 mo (N = 18)	12 mo (N = 18)	15 mo (N = 21)	18 mo (N = 16)	21 mo (N = 13)
Interest in play	.18	.15	.52^b	.22	.33
Attention span/char.	.51^a	.62^b	.64^b	.52^a	.52
Attention span/cap.	.52^a	.59^b	.68^b	.72^b	.72^b
Complexity of play	.68^b	.48^a	.49^a	.68^b	.84^c
Number of schemata	.58^a	.13			
Schema sequencing/char.			.44^a	.57^a	.68^a
Schema sequencing/cap.			.25	.55^a	.49
Sum^d	.75^c	.75^c	.84^c	.88^c	.90^c

$^a p < .05.$
$^b p < .01.$
$^c p < .001.$
^{d}Sum = Sum of all the cognitive-motivational variables.

Table 2. Correlations with visual planning/evaluation of effect in the normal group

	Age points of study				
	9 mo (N = 23)	12 mo (N = 23)	15 mo (N = 23)	18 mo (N = 22)	21 mo (N = 21)
Interest in play	.23	−.04	.82[c]	−.17	.07
Attention span/char.	.06	.26	.46a	.25	.16
Attention span/cap.	.14	.15	.09	.32	.40
Complexity of play	.46[a]	.35	.42[a]	.65[b]	.69[c]
Number of schemata	−.01	.18			
Schema sequencing/char.			.37	.37	.64[b]
Schema sequencing/cap.			———[d]		
Sum[e]	.63[b]	.51[a]	.71[c]	.52[a]	.54[a]

[a] $p < .05$.
[b] $p < .01$.
[c] $p < .001$.
[d] All subjects in the normal group had achieved the maximum score by age 15 months.
[e] Sum = Sum of all the cognitive-motivational variables.

same time, the operations involved in visual planning/evaluation of effect developed more slowly and were observed later in the H group than in the N group. These play actions that involve cognitive operations as well as motivation may be worthy of consideration in infant intervention programs.

The differences found in the study between the two groups may have implications for intervention methodology. The emphasis in many intervention programs is the direct teaching of skills to the infant. The complex chain of actions, involving the visual searching for objects, planning, executing the plan, and then checking the result of the action, is not likely to occur in activities demonstrated with precision by the adult. Opportunities should be created for infants with developmental disabilities in which a few simple objects are made available with which infants can plan and execute actions of interest to them. When an infant engages in a particular action, the adult might encourage the infant to pause and look at what happened as a result of the action. In some cases, the adult might talk softly, simply, and briefly about the infant's action. In the case of physically handicapped infants within the normal range of intel-

ligence, the infants should be given sufficient time and frequent opportunities to evaluate the results of actions, and to signal their plan or intention to someone who could then execute the actions planned by the infants, if they are physically unable to do so independently.

Functional and Representational Play

Functional and representational play have been identified in this study as variables in the cognitive-social category. The variable *functional play* was defined as the use of objects according to social conventions; e.g., the child puts a cup to his or her mouth. *Representational play* (often used synonymously with "symbolic play") was defined here as involving the act of pretending; e.g., the child "pretends" that the doll is a real baby, and he or she proceeds to feed the doll (the doll 'represents" the baby). The child allows object X to represent object A, and object X becomes the symbol for object A.

Functional play usually begins at around 1 year of age and increases rapidly after that. Representational play generally is not observed until sometime between 15 and 18 months of age. It also increases over time and becomes

Table 3. Between-group differences on the three variables

Variables	9 mo.	12 mo.	15 mo.	18 mo.	21 mo.	24 mo.
Visual plan/eval.	.000[a]	.000[a]	.007[a]	.001[a]	.008[a]	1.0
Functional play		.132	.404	.012[b]	.165	.184
Representational play			.419	.011[b]	.015[b]	.016[b]

[a] $p = .009$ or less
[b] p 5013 between .05 and .01.

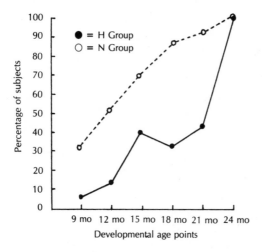

Figure 1. Percentages of high-scoring subjects on the variable *visual planning/evaluation of effect* in each of the two groups across the age points of the study. (Unbroken line connecting dots = handicapped group; Broken line connecting small circles = normal group.)

more complex (sequences of related acts occur later).

Findings Functional play showed significant differences between the two groups only at 18 months. In contrast, differences between the groups were significant for representational play at 18, 21, and 24 months (Table 3). The tabulation of differences (Table 3) begins at 12 months for functional play and at 15 months for representational play. Prior to these age points, the percentage of subjects showing these types of play was too small for differences to be meaningful. As can be seen in Table 4, only 4%, or 1 of 23 subjects in the Normal Group, and no subjects in the Handicapped Group, showed functional play at 9 months. Representational play was observed in only one subject in each group at 12 months, and in none prior to that age point.

One of the intriguing outcomes of the study

was the wide discrepancy between functional play and representational play with respect to between-group differences. Table 4 shows the rate of increase (by percentage of subjects) to be fairly similar for the two groups in functional play; however, in representational play, the rate of increase was much slower for the handicapped group than for the normal group. These differences between groups on both variables are graphically illustrated in Figures 2 and 3.

The wide range of chronological ages of the handicapped subjects, especially at the developmental age points of 18 and 21 months, must be taken into account when interpreting the findings. The handicapped subjects at 18 months developmental age (DA) ranged from 19 to 39 months chronological age (CA), and at 21 months DA, from 21 to 45 months CA. But at the 24-month age point, when some of the low DQ subjects could no longer be included in the data (could not be matched by DA with the normal infants at 24 months), the chronological age range for the handicapped subjects was from 24.5 to only 34 months. Thus, the data of subjects functioning in the low DQ range could not be included at the higher developmental age points, and the data of subjects functioning in the higher DQ range (most of whom became participants in the study sometime in their second year of life) could not be included at the lower developmental age points. As can be seen in Table 1 (N tabulated at all age points), the handicapped group includes the largest number of subjects at the 15-month age point ($N = 21$). At the high and low age points, the number of subjects is smaller; the smallest number of subjects is reflected in the data at the highest age point ($N = 9$ at the 24-month age point).

Table 4. Percentages of subjects with high scores[a]

Developmental age points	Functional play		Representational play	
	H group	N group	H group	N group
9 mo	0%	4%	0%	0%
12 mo	11%	26%	6%	4%
15 mo	62%	70%	19%	17%
18 mo	44%	91%	12%	41%
21 mo	85%	100%	38%	81%
24 mo	78%	100%	44%	100%

[a]A high score was given when two or more instances of the designated type of play were observed.

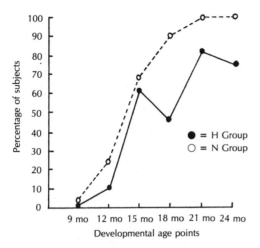

Figure 2. Percentages of high-scoring subjects on the variable *functional play* in each of the two groups across the age points of the study. (Unbroken line connecting dots = handicapped group; Broken line connecting small circles = normal group.

Discussion and Implications Functional and representational play have cognitive and social components. The progression of these types of play shows a relationship to the progression in cognitive or intellectual development. Functional play always precedes representational play. Representational play, unlike functional play, involves symbolic acts. Therefore, verbal language, which also requires the use of symbols, usually increases

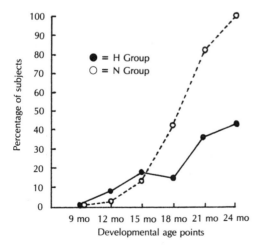

Figure 3. Percentages of high-scoring subjects on the variable *representational play* in each of the two groups across the age points of the study. (Unbroken line connecting dots = handicapped group; Broken line connecting small circles = normal group.)

rather rapidly as representational play progressively replaces manipulative and functional play. The use of symbols, whether in play or in language, represents a milestone in intellectual development. It shows that the child has reached stage six of the Piagetian sensorimotor period.

In the context of what is known about functional and representational play in the development of infants, the findings of this study seem to indicate that there is indeed a considerable difference between these two types of play. Functional play is the act of using objects according to social conventions; it involves imitation. The two groups of infants in the study, matched by developmental age at every age point, did not show wide differences in functional play. The handicapped subjects, chronologically older, had been in the world for a longer period, and therefore were more likely to have been exposed to social models using objects according to social conventions more frequently than the nonhandicapped subjects. More exposure to social models may have partially compensated for lower levels of developmental functioning in some areas. Thus, if functional play is largely dependent on imitation, then the timetable for functional play may be dependent on chronological age to a greater extent than some other activities that require higher levels of cognitive competence.

Although functional play always precedes representational play, the latter may involve more than a simple step forward on the developmental continuum. A cognitive transformation may have to occur before the child can progress from imitating adult models to using symbols that require internal representations.

Representational play, having a close tie with language in that both require the use of symbols, may be a highly effective facilitator for the development of language. Prior to this study, it had been frequently observed that the appearance and increasingly frequent occurrence of representational play tends to be followed by a period of intense interest and rapid progress in language development. As representational/symbolic play becomes more complex, language is increasingly integrated into "pretend" play as that type of play takes on a social character (dramatic play). Representational play and language are likely to be mutually reinforcing, and both enhance cognitive and social development. These interrelationships have major implications for the importance of using sign language early with infants whose verbal/oral language can be expected (for whatever reason) to be delayed. The early acquisition of symbols for objects and actions (through learning sign language), besides fostering cognitive development, also encourages representational play, and allows it to take on an increasingly social character.

In a similar manner as has been suggested for the encouragement of visual planning and the evaluation of the effect of actions in play, the following suggestions might be helpful in encouraging the developmentally delayed infant to bridge the gap between functional and representational play.

Materials should be provided that motivate representational play. The adult could try to identify and, at times, enlarge upon any activity that even approaches the use of symbols in play. The adult could become involved socially with the infant's play without being too directive. After capturing the infant's interest, the adult can engage in the kind of modeling of representational play that will continue to hold the child's interest. The child must, however, be a participant, not an inactive observer of the play.

The child's motivation or interest in what is taking place is of paramount importance in this kind of play. Most "normal" children gradually begin to invite others (adults first, then other children) to participate in their representational play, and to enter the act of "pretending" with them. In the case of the delayed child, when the child has been performing acts regarded as functional play, it may help him or her to be exposed to other children who are engaging socially in representational or "dramatic" play. The child needs to be invited in a sensitive manner to participate in the "pretend play" with the adult, and preferably also with other children, in order to get the maximum benefit from this play.

At first, what appears to be representational play may be strictly imitative play, but gradually, with low-key verbal commentary and social interaction relevant to the content of the play, delayed infants may begin to engage in representational play sooner than if left to themselves. It may also be fruitful to encourage symbolic acts in play and to watch for these to occur before expecting much progress in verbal language. In normal development, symbolic acts in language seem to follow closely upon symbolic acts in play.

In the case of the infant whose primary handicap is neuromotor, the infant may need the hands of a sensitive adult to execute the symbolic acts that the infant is able to generate in his or her mind but cannot, at this time, motorically carry out by himself or herself.

SUMMARY

The findings regarding three variables from a study on play-associated behaviors of normal and handicapped infants between 9 and 24 months developmental age have been highlighted and discussed here. Significant between-group differences were found for *visual planning/evaluation of effect*—a complex variable involving cognitive and motivational factors, and for *representational play,* involving symbolic acts. A third variable, *functional play,* involving primarily imitation, did not show significant differences between the two groups. The differences and similarities between groups with respect to these variables are graphically illustrated in Figures 1, 2, and 3.

The actions and behaviors involved in all three variables are considered to be important in cognitive and social development. Implications for infant development are discussed and suggestions are given for enhancing the behaviors involved in two of the three variables in infant intervention with handicapped young children.

REFERENCES

Fenson, L., Kagan, J., Kearsley, R.B., & Zelazo, P.R. The developmental progression of manipulative play in the first two years. *Child Development*, 1976, *47*, 232–236.

Kagan, J., Lapidus, D.R., & Moore, M. Infant antecedents of cognitive functioning: A longitudinal study. *Child Development*, 1978, *49*, 1005–1023.

Largo, R., & Howard, J. Developmental progression in play behavior of children between nine and thirty months: Spontaneous play and imitation. *Developmental Medicine and Child Neurology*, 1979, *21*, 299–310.

McCall, R.B. Exploratory manipulation and play in the human infant. *Monographs of the Society for Research in Child Development*, 1974, *39*, (2, Serial No. 155).

McCune-Nicolich, L. Beyond sensory-motor intelligence: Assessment of symbolic maturity through analysis of pretend play. *Merrill-Palmer Quarterly*, 1977, *23*, 89–99.

Rosenblatt, D. Developmental trends in infant play. In: B. Tizard & D. Harvey (eds.), *Biology of play*. Philadelphia: J.B. Lippincott, 1977.

Ungerer, J.A., Zelazo, P.R., Kearsley, R.B., & O'Leary, K. Developmental changes in the representation of objects in symbolic play from 18 to 34 months of age. *Child Development*, 1981, *52*, 186–195.

Yarrow, L.J., & Pedersen, F.A. The interplay between cognition and motivation in infancy. In: M. Lewis (ed.), *Origins of intelligence*. New York: Plenum Publishing Corp., 1976.

Yarrow, L.J., Rubenstein, J.L., & Pedersen, F.A. *Infant and environment*. New York: John Wiley & Sons, 1975.

Zelazo, P.R., & Kearsley, R.B. *Functional play: Evidence for a cognitive metamorphosis in the year-old infant*. Paper presented at the biannual meeting of the society for research in child development, New Orleans, April, 1977.

The At-Risk Infant: Psycho/Socio/Medical Aspects
edited by Shaul Harel, M.D., and Nicholas J. Anastasiow, Ph.D.
Copyright © 1985   Paul H. Brookes Publishing Co., Inc.   Baltimore • London

Chapter 45

Mother-Infant Interaction
Down Syndrome Case Studies

MARGUERITE B. STEVENSON, PH.D.
LEWIS A. LEAVITT, M.D.
SUSAN B. SILVERBERG, M.S.
Waisman Center on Mental Retardation and Human Development, Madison, Wisconsin

EDUCATORS AND PSYCHOTHERAPISTS WHO work with the developmentally delayed infant use a variety of formal and informal assessment techniques to evaluate social interactions. The characterization of the dynamic aspects of interaction between infant and caregiver has been of particular interest. While there is agreement that therapeutic advice and intervention should be informed by the patterns of caregiver-infant interaction that occur at home, there is little agreement on instrumental or statistical techniques that may summarize such information in a clinically useful way.

In this chapter, using Down syndrome case studies, the authors present an observational and statistical technique for obtaining and displaying information on mother-infant interaction patterns. The authors believe that this methodology helps characterize in a practical way important aspects of the mother-infant relationships. Moreover, these displays may be visually and statistically compared to detect change over time. The data presented here are part of a longitudinal study conducted on the development of mother-infant communication in families with Down syndrome infants.

The authors were particularly interested in studying the contexts of vocalization in the homes of Down syndrome infants for several reasons. First, the Down syndrome infants in the study have been identified very soon after birth. Second, their diagnosis carries with it a commonly acknowledged destiny of serious developmental delay. Third, their gross physical behaviors during the first several months of life are quite similar to those of the nondelayed infant.

OPTIMIZING THE EARLY ENVIRONMENT

Infant Signals and Maternal Behavior

Early social and cognitive habilitation programs for developmentally delayed infants place great emphasis on optimizing the early

This work was supported in part by a grant from the Graduate School of the University of Wisconsin and NIH grant HD-03352 to the Waisman Center on Mental Retardation and Human Development. The authors would like to thank Drs. R. Pauli and R. Laxova and the staff of the Genetics Clinic of the Waisman Center on Mental Retardation and Human Development for their assistance in recruiting families. Their work was in part supported by the Wisconsin Statewide Genetic Service Network grant AS001. The authors also would like to express their appreciation for the contributions of M.A. Roach and J.N. Ver Hoeve.

environment. One might ask, then, what features can contribute to an optimal environment. There is theoretical and empirical support for the idea that an optimal environment is one that is responsive to infant signals. In Lamb and Easterbrook's (1981) discussion of parental sensitivity, maternal responsiveness is shown as important from four diverse theoretical perspectives. First, psychoanalysts emphasize the role of early maternal sensitivity in later personality development. Second, the ethological-attachment theorists explain that adults' responsiveness to infant signals is innate. This responsiveness then leads to a secure attachment of the infant to its mother. Third, the organismic theorists (e.g., Brazelton, Koslowski, & Main, 1974) emphasize the early capacities of the infant to communicate with the sensitive parent. Fourth, the social learning theorists suggest that the infant's competencies and sense of competency derive from parental behavior that is contingent upon the infant's own behavior. While Wachs and Gruen (1982) argue otherwise, there is considerable empirical support for the importance of adult responsiveness for infants' social and cognitive growth (Ainsworth & Bell, 1974; Lewis & Coates, 1980; Watson & Hayes, 1981; Yarrow, Rubenstein, & Pederson, 1975).

Investigations that examine infant behavior and infant responsiveness serve to complement this research on maternal behavior. In one line of research, the behavior and responsiveness of nondelayed infants has been compared with that of developmentally delayed infants. Findings reveal that the developmentally delayed infant demonstrates fewer behaviors, especially attentional and affective behaviors, than nondelayed infants (Cicchetti & Sroufe, 1976, 1978; Emde, Katz, & Thorpe, 1978). In addition, these infants are less responsive than their nondelayed agemates (Buckhalt, Rutherford, & Goldberg, 1978; Jones, 1980; Terdal, Jackson, & Garner, 1976). For preschool age children, less initiation of behavior and less responsiveness have been shown for mentally retarded (Cunningham, Reuler, Blackwell, & Deck, 1981; Eheart, 1982) and for language delayed children (Siegel, Cunningham, & van der Spuy, 1979) relative to nondelayed children.

Perhaps as a reaction to the child's low level of behaviors and lack of responsiveness, mothers of developmentally delayed infants have been shown to be more frequent initiators of interaction (Eheart, 1982). The methodology used to date, however, has not shown these mothers of delayed infants to be less responsive (Redditi, Stevenson, Lawton, & Ibler, 1982; Terdal et al., 1976; Vietze, Abernathy, Ashe, & Faulstich, 1978). Research does at least suggest less maternal responsiveness by the presence of more child-dependent interaction sequences (Jones, 1980) and more simultaneous mother and infant vocalization (Berger & Cunningham, 1983). Both Jones (1980) and Berger and Cunningham (1983) conclude that interventions should encourage maternal responsiveness and the reciprocal interactions that that implies.

In view of these findings and the crucial role that maternal responsiveness may play in infant development, further research in this area seems warranted. Earlier methods for assessing maternal responsiveness may not have resulted in sufficiently detailed information to capture the possible differences between mothers of nondelayed infants and mothers of developmentally delayed infants. In their study of Down syndrome infants, the authors have used lag-sequential analyses of behavior streams. Extensive experience with these measures of responsiveness (Stevenson & Leavitt, 1983a, 1983b; Stevenson, Ver Hoeve, Leavitt, & Roach, 1982; Ver Hoeve, Stevenson, Leavitt, & Roach, 1981) has informed their use in the present research.

Most therapeutic analysis of behavioral interaction relies on global assessment of interactive patterns. By contrast, laboratory assessment of behavioral interaction commonly records behavior in great detail, but in a setting that may be artificial and constrained. As Bronfenbrenner (1979) has shown, behavior is best studied in its natural context. The research reported here brings the methodology of detailed behavioral analysis to the study of interaction at home. In this chapter, the patterns of vocal exchange between Down syndrome infants and their mothers are compared with those of nondelayed infants and their mothers.

CASE STUDIES

For the Down syndrome case studies presented here, a mother and her 4-month-old baby were observed interacting at home for an hour. Two observers used hand-held keyboards to record the behaviors of each partner during the interactions. These interactions took place in the family's usual living area and the mother was encouraged to engage in her usual activities; she was generally present throughout the hour. The first infant was living in a middle-class home with his mother, father, and 3-year-old brother. For most of the observation period, he played on a blanket placed on the floor near his mother and brother. The Bayley Scales of Infant Development indicated a Mental Developmental Index of 94 for this infant. The second infant was also a later born living in a middle-class home. This infant was fed during the first few minutes of the observation and held for most of the hour. His test performance indicated a Mental Developmental Index of 74.

The observations of the families are in part a reflection of the nature and effects of the clinical advice given to these parents and interventions that have been performed. Both families were visited regularly at home as part of an infant stimulation program available in their community. The home-based intervention program included an initial developmental assessment of the infant to determine the areas for which special attention might prove beneficial. Parents were educated through discussion about their infant's present condition and future potential. An intervention program was then developed based on the information gathered from the initial assessment and discussion. Subsequent weekly visits were made by a staff member trained in early childhood special education.

The specialist's time in the home was used for presenting special materials to the infant and engaging him or her in new activities and exercises. In addition to providing the infant with stimulating experiences, these visits were used to teach parents ways of enriching their infant's everyday environment. Education was achieved indirectly through modeling of the teacher's behaviors, and more directly through the teacher's advice and an activity notebook left in the home each week that recorded the activities presented during the home visits. For example, the parent was shown ways of positioning the infant during parent-infant interaction and how to use items in the home to encourage the development of motor skills. Within the domain of vocalization, the parent was encouraged to talk about the environment surrounding the infant and to respond to the infant's sounds through imitation.

COMPARISON SAMPLE

The data presented below contrast vocal exchange patterns of these two later born Down syndrome infants and their mothers with those of nondelayed later born infants and their mothers. For several years, the authors have been studying the patterns of vocal exchange between 4-month-old nondelayed infants and their mothers at home (Stevenson et al., 1982; Ver Hoeve et al., 1981). Analyses of patterns of behavior were based on the lag-sequential model proposed by Sackett (1979). This model can characterize the patterns of vocal responsivity displayed within mother-infant pairs. When examining, for example, the responsivity of mothers, the focus is on whether the probability of maternal vocalization increases following infant vocalization to a level above that observed in the absence of an infant vocalization. In this example, the criterion behavior is an infant vocalization, and the likelihood of subsequent maternal vocalization is compared with the chance level of maternal vocalization. More generally, the model asks whether, following the occurrence of a selected criterion behavior, the likelihood of another specified behavior increases to a level that is significantly above the chance of that behavior occurring in the absence of the criterion behavior. The lag profile enables one to examine events beyond the first event following a criterion behavior. It is a way of displaying the changes in the probability of a behavior for a series of events (or lags) following a criterion behavior. The $Z(1)$ statistic recommended by Allison and Liker (1982) makes the necessary comparisons between probabilities.

For the comparison sample of nondelayed infants, two visits were made to the homes of 14 later born 4-month-olds. On the first visit, the mother was interviewed about her baby's schedule and the observation system was introduced. Approximately 1 week later, hour-long observations were made in each home by two observers. Mothers were asked to continue their usual activities during the visit. One observer recorded infant behavior, while one recorded mother behavior; the computer later synchronized the records of the two observers. The use of this procedure reduced the attentional demands on the observers while preserving the complexity of the interaction sequence.

Behavior codes requiring minimal observer judgment were selected on the basis of observations in the homes of pilot families. Infant behaviors included nondistress vocalization, fussing and crying, smiling, looking at the mother, mouthing something, and eating. Mother behaviors included vocalization, imitating the infant's sounds, smiling, looking at the infant, holding, rocking, touching, and presenting something to the infant. In addition, the mother's proximity to her infant was continuously recorded.

The solid line in Figure 1 illustrates the information obtained from a lag analysis when the profiles were combined (Cochran's Z) for the 14 later born mother-infant pairs (Stevenson et al., 1982). The criterion was a vocalization of the infant. To obtain this graph, the probability that the mother would vocalize was calculated for the next event, or lag, following the occurrence of an infant vocalization. The $Z(1)$ score was used to measure responsiveness by comparing this probability with the probability that the mother would have vocalized without her infant having vocalized. This procedure was performed for the next nine events following the first criterion event. When the scores exceed the shaded area parallel to the axis at zero, the likelihood that the infant behavior will occur is significantly different from chance. Alpha was set at .0025 to reduce the probability of falsely rejecting the null hypothesis (Type I error).

From the solid line of Figure 1, it is apparent that at event lag one, that is, the first recorded event after an infant vocalization (the criterion event), maternal vocalizations were significantly elevated. By the third lag, the probability of a maternal vocalization was significantly suppressed. This shows the elicitation of a maternal vocalization by a vocalization of the infant and the subsequent suppression of the probability of a maternal vocalization.

RESULTS

An identical methodology was used to study the Down syndrome infant-mother pairs at home. The responsiveness of the mothers of the Down syndrome infants is shown with the two broken lines in Figure 1. For these mothers, there was neither an initial increase in the probability of a vocalization following the infants' vocalization nor a later suppression. For the more developmentally advanced infant (Case 1, dashed line), there was a slight increase in maternal responsiveness at lags six and eight. Overall, these mothers were less responsive than mothers of the nondelayed infants. A chi-square test was used to compare the initial responsiveness (lag one) of these two mothers with the responsiveness seen in the sample 14 mothers of later born nondelayed infants. Their initial responsiveness was significantly less.

The infant's responsiveness can be examined by looking at infant vocalizations following the criterion event of maternal vocalization. The solid line in Figure 2 shows this

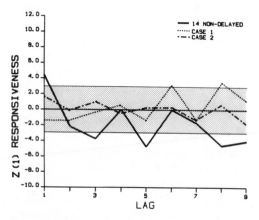

Figure 1. Lag-sequential analysis of maternal vocalizations for the nine events following a criterion event of an infant vocalization.

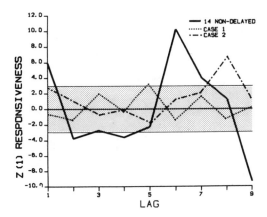

Figure 2. Lag-sequential analysis of infant vocalizations for the nine events following a criterion event of a maternal vocalization.

responsiveness for the 14 nondelayed infants. Note that at lag one (the first event following the maternal vocalization) and at lags six and seven these infants were vocalizing at an above chance level. By contrast, both Down syndrome infants (the dashed lines in Figure 2) showed only the later elevation in the probability of a vocalization. Immediately following their mother's vocalizations, the nondelayed infants responded with a vocalization of their own. Both Down syndrome infants were, however, less immediately responsive to maternal vocalizations than were the nondelayed infants. The chi-square test indicated this difference to be statistically significant. The elevation at lags six and seven for the nondelayed infants indicated a response to a maternal vocalization followed by five events that were not maternal vocalizations. For the Down syndrome infant, there was a later elevation at lag five (Case 1, dashed line) and at lag eight (Case 2, dot/dashed line). Both the nondelayed infants and the Down syndrome in-

fants responded to this period without maternal vocalization with a vocalization of their own.

An alternative to examining patterns of responsiveness is to simply look at the rates of maternal and infant behaviors. Table 1 reports this information for the 14 later born nondelayed infants and their mothers and for both Down syndrome cases. It is interesting to note that the rate of behavior analysis produces a picture of mother-infant interaction that differs from that based on lag-sequential analysis of responsiveness. As can be seen in Table 1, the behavior rates of the Down syndrome infants and their mothers are not statistically different from those of the 14 families of nondelayed infants. All the rates of behavior lie within 2 standard deviations of those displayed in the sample of nondelayed infants and their mothers. The lag-sequential analysis of vocal responsiveness thus was able to detect differences in mother-infant interaction patterns that were not apparent in a simple comparison of behavior rates.

CONCLUSION

Both Down syndrome infants and their mothers are less responsive to one another than are nondelayed infants and their mothers. From the author's work with other populations of nondelayed and at-risk infants, they speculate that the relatively low-responsive environment may contribute to later delays in these infants. The intervention program in which the mothers participated was an infant stimulation program designed to show the mothers ways to enrich their infant's environment. By its emphasis on stimulation, this program could have limited the responsiveness of the infant's environment. Recall that the developmental level of the first

Table 1. Maternal and infant behavior rates per minute

Partner	Behavior	Nondelayed		Down syndrome	
		Mean	S.D.	Case 1	Case 2
Mother	Vocalization	5.00	2.51	1.90	8.26
	Look	1.55	.55	1.07	.82
	Smile	.65	.40	.28	.55
	Touch	1.21	.67	1.25	1.65
	Present	.36	.23	.24	.25
Infant	Vocalization	2.70	1.79	.70	3.56
	Look	.67	.40	.83	.68
	Smile	.22	.23	.23	.02
	Fuss	.66	.67	.60	.32

infant is essentially normal, yet the deviant expectations of the mother, the infants' non-responsiveness, and the training program may combine to suppress the mother's vocal responsiveness. The authors would like to join Jones (1980) and Berger and Cunningham (1983) in suggesting the importance of providing a responsive environment for delayed infants. In an intervention program for mothers of developmentally delayed chilren, Seitz and Hoekenga (1974) showed the feasibility of training mothers to increase their responsiveness.

These two case studies are reported as a first glimpse of a more comprehensive longitudinal study of Down syndrome infants and their families. Information on mother-infant interaction at home when the infants are 4, 8, and 12 months old will be supplemented by laboratory study of mother-infant and father-infant interaction. These case studies are presented as an example of the potential of detailed analysis of parent-infant interaction that may in the future help evaluate and direct modalities of therapy.

REFERENCES

Ainsworth, M.D.S., & Bell, S.M. Mother-infant interaction and the development of competence. In: K.J. Connolly & J.S. Bruner (eds.), *The growth of competence*. New York: Academic Press, 1974.

Allison, P.D., & Liker, J.K. Analyzing sequential categorical data on dyadic interaction: A comment on Gottman. *Psychological Bulletin*, 1982, *91*, 393–403.

Berger, J., & Cunningham, C.C. Development of early vocal behaviors and interactions in Down's syndrome and nonhandicapped infant-mother pairs. *Developmental Psychology*, (1983), *19*, 322–331.

Brazelton, T.B., Koslowski, B., & Main, M. The origins of reciprocity: The early mother-infant interaction. In: M. Lewis & L.A. Rosenblum (eds.), *The effect of the infant on its caregiver*. New York: John Wiley & Sons, 1974.

Bronfenbrenner, U. *The ecology of human development: Experiments by nature and design*. Cambridge, MA: Harvard University Press, 1979.

Buckhalt, J., Rutherford, B., & Goldberg, K. Verbal and nonverbal interaction of mothers with their Down's syndrome and nonretarded infants. *American Journal of Mental Deficiency*, 1978, *82*, 337–343.

Cicchetti, D., & Sroufe, A. The relationship between affective and cognitive development in Down's syndrome infants. *Child Development*, 1976, *47*, 920–929.

Cicchetti, D., & Sroufe, A. An organizational view of affect: Illustration from the study of Down's syndrome infants. In: M. Lewis & L.A. Rosenblum (eds.), *The development of affect*. New York: Plenum Publishing Corp., 1978.

Cunningham, C., Reuler, E., Blackwell, J., & Deck, J. Behavioral and linguistic developments in the interactions of normal and retarded children with their mothers. *Child Development*, 1981, *52*, 62–70.

Eheart, B.K. Mother-child interactions with nonretarded and mentally retarded preschoolers. *American Journal of Mental Deficiency*, 1982, *87*, 20–25.

Emde, R., Katz, E., & Thorpe, J. Emotional expression in infancy: II. Early deviations in Down's syndrome. In: M. Lewis & L.A. Rosenblum (eds.), *The development of affect*. New York: Plenum Publishing Corp., 1978.

Jones, O. Prelinguistic communications skills in Down's syndrome and normal infants. In: T. Field, S. Goldberg, D. Stern, & A. Sostek (eds.), *High risk infants and children: Adult and peer interactions*. New York: Academic Press, 1980.

Lamb, M.E., & Easterbrook, M.A. Individual differences in parental sensitivity: Origins, components and consequences. In: M.E. Lamb & L.R. Sherrod (eds.), *Infant social cognition: Empirical and theoretical considerations*. Hillsdale, NJ: Lawrence Erlbaum Associates, 1981.

Lewis, M., & Coates, D. Mother-infant interaction and infant cognitive performance. *Infant Behavior and Development*, 1980, *3*, 95–105.

Redditi, J.S., Stevenson, M.B., Lawton, J.T., & Ibler, I.M. *Mother-infant interaction in families with infants who are developmentally delayed, developmentally delayed with physical handicaps or developmentally normal*. Paper presented at the seventh biennial meeting of the Southeastern Conference on Human Development, Baltimore, April, 1982.

Sackett, G.P. The lag sequential analysis of contingency and cyclicity in behavioral interaction research. In: J. Osofsky (ed), *Handbook of infant development*, New York: John Wiley & Sons, 1979.

Seitz, S., & Hoekenga, R. Modeling as a training school for retarded children and their parents. *Mental Retardation*, 1974, *4*, 28–31.

Siegel, L.S., Cunningham, C.E., & van der Spuy, H.I.J. *Interaction of language delayed and normal preschool children with their mothers*. Paper presented at the biennial meeting of the Society for Research in Child Development, San Francisco, March, 1979.

Stevenson, M.B., & Leavitt, L.A. *Mother-infant interaction: A Down's syndrome case study*. Paper presented at the Second International Workshop on the ''At Risk'' Infant, Jerusalem, May, 1983. (a)

Stevenson, M.B., & Leavitt, L.A. *Individual differences in mother and infant vocal responsiveness: Low birth weight and normal birth weight infants*. Paper presented at the Second International Workshop on the ''At Risk'' Infant, Jerusalem, May, 1983. (b)

Stevenson, M.B., Ver Hoeve, J.N., Leavitt, L.A., & Roach, M.A. *Lag sequential analysis of mother-infant interactions at home: Low birthweight and full term infants*. Paper presented at the International Conference on Infant Studies, Austin, Texas, April, 1982.

Terdal, L., Jackson, R.H., & Garner, A.M. Mother-child interactions: A comparison between normal and developmentally delayed groups. In: E. Mash, L. Hamerlynck, & L. Handy (eds.), *Behavior modification and families*. New York: Brunner/Mazel, 1976.

Ver Hoeve, J.N., Stevenson, M.B., Leavitt, L.A., & Roach, M.A. *Patterns of mother-infant communication at four months.* Paper presented at the biennial meeting of the Society for Research in Child Development, Boston, April, 1981.

Vietze, P.M., Abernathy, S.R., Ashe, M.L., & Faulstich, G. Contingent interaction between mothers and their developmentally delayed infants. In: G.P. Sackett (ed.), *Observing behavior, Volume I: Theory and applications in mental retardation.* Baltimore: University Park Press, 1978.

Wachs, T.D., & Gruen, G.E. *Early experience and human development.* New York: Plenum Publishing Corp., 1982.

Watson, J.S., & Hayes, L.A. *A new method of infant-environment interaction analysis.* Paper presented at the biennial meeting of the Society for Research in Child Development, Boston, April, 1981.

Yarrow, L.J., Rubenstein, J., & Pedersen, F. *Infant and environment.* New York: John Wiley & Sons, 1975.

Chapter 46

Educational and Health Planning
for Infants and Toddlers
Guidelines for an Ecological
Model for Early Infancy Education

GALYA RABINOVITZ, M.A.
SHAUL HAREL, M.D.
Tel Aviv Medical Center, Tel Aviv University, Tel Aviv, Israel

EARLY CHILDHOOD EDUCATION TODAY IS A process that professionals cannot ignore. In almost every early childhood intervention program, some type of day care is in effect; thus, professionals must consider ways and means to improve these centers and prevent them from becoming another risk factor to the at-risk infant and family.

The pressure to open more day care centers came both from scientific research and social processes, that is, from concern over the at-risk infant and from increasing participation of young women in the labor force. Thus, most of the young children of today and tomorrow will be cared for both in families and in other "homes away from home."

EDUCATIONAL PLANNING

In recent years, there has been increasing concern for early identification of young children at risk for developmental problems. Children at risk for later sensory, motor, mental, and social handicaps may never be able to achieve their full potential as productive citizens without appropriate interventions. Differences be-

tween social groups within a society, the so-called "ethnic" or "social" gap that exists in many countries, may have significant effects upon individual and group levels of cultural, social, and economic achievement. Detection and assessment of infantile developmental defects need to be carried out at the earliest possible age. The prevention and treatment of developmental problems as well as the closing of these "social" gaps are foremost for all professions caring for the child.

There is widespread agreement on the investigation of developmental disabilities prior to their onset rather than after their occurrences. Current knowledge of human development, neurology, biochemical genetics, immunology, obstetrical care, and environmental effects should aid in the establishment of preventive practices. If followed, the emotional and financial impact accompanying the birth and long-term management of a handicapped child could be minimized for the family as well as for the community. Combined with early detection, via screening of an at-risk population, there should also be a program for a more careful follow-up of these children as well as for the early implementation of remedial steps to ameliorate the various handicapping conditions.

In previous years, the major focus of concern was on preschool or school-age children. Many remedial programs yielded disappointing results because of a failure to recognize that children may have reached a "point of no return" for effective intervention. Current knowledge of human brain development has shifted the major focus of concern to intrauterine brain growth and to the first 2 or 3 years of life, a so-called "critical period." This highly critical period of development is especially sensitive and vulnerable to both antenatal and perinatal insults and to neglect. It is also crucial to the timing of early rehabilitation, provided the brain is protected from further injuries. It is now apparent that biological and environmental events in that early period of human development may have a unique and profound impact on the course of subsequent development.

In the context of the influence of the socioeconomic environment on the child, the major role parents can play in causing a child to be at risk became increasingly apparent. It is well known that the infant is totally dependent on his or her parents, especially the mother. This period has been called "second" or "extra-abdominal pregnancy." This link is crucial for the critical transition period from reflex to perceptive and cognitive life. The more competent the parents, the greater the chance for the child to achieve a better social maturation and adaptability. It is also a known factor that parents who were deprived of proper management during their childhood may be inadequately equipped to provide the appropriate care and education for their own children. Based on this approach, the concept of the at-risk parent was derived. Therefore, malfunctioning parents who were themselves at-risk infants usually will have an at-risk child. Not only is it likely that the child at risk is born to a mother at risk, but both mother and infant usually reside in an environment that is less than adequate to meet either the infant's or the parents' needs. Factors found to be detrimental to parental functioning are: poverty, low level of education, single parenthood, teenage parenthood, severe marital conflicts, drug use, and mental illness. Thus, caregiver, infant, and environment transact in a mutually reciprocal manner to either deepen the at-risk factors or to overcome them. Many drug cure centers were planned and opened to counteract some of these risk factors in parent-infant interaction.

The complexity of the interrelationship between the various biological and environmental factors affecting brain development has brought many investigators to look upon clusters of pregnancy, neonatal, and environmental events and factors that may interact cumulatively. These additive factors, combined with repeated assessment, can be significant predictors of later developmental disabilities.

Studies on the influences of alternative environments for children reveal that physical, cognitive, and socioemotional development of infants who visited a day care center is not different from the development of children who stayed only with their mothers. The role of the mother, attachment to her, or interaction with her are quite similar. Those few differences that were found were more prominent when the infant was new at the day center, and disappeared when the child adapted to the new experience. Thus, it can be concluded that there is no evidence of harm caused by early infancy education (Bronfenbrenner, 1979; Caldwell & Richmond, 1968).

In studies that isolated socioeconomic status, it was found that middle-class infants were not harmed by day care experiences while lower-class children actually benefited from them, especially when cognitive development and linguistic skills were measured.

Differences in child behavior were explained better by home environment and mother's behavior than by their experiences in the day care. Some large-scale studies (N.P.C.S.) pointed out the structural characteristics of a beneficial day care environment, that is, defined those variables that enable the day care to better meet the needs of very young children. These characteristics are:

1. High staff–child ratios
2. Low ceiling on group size

3. Staff qualification in child-related education and training, but not necessarily formal education

To summarize, although research on early childhood education lacks in experimental design, and although the ecological processes of decision-making concerning day care were not investigated, day care was not found to be a harmful or risky environment, if certain necessary demands were fulfilled. Educational planning seems to be one of the processes by which the risks and harms of early education can be prevented and the positive contribution to very young children even enhanced.

Planning is a process of clearly stating goals, arranging them in some hierarchy of importance, and choosing between means to achieve these goals. Planning is also a continuous process of feedback concerning how successful one is in achieving these goals. In educational planning for infants, a nonstop measurement of success versus developmental needs of children and their families should be taken into account. These needs of infants and families cannot be contradicted by societal or educational goals. The debate around teaching infants to read, or using computers in day care centers are such contradictory issues.

The National Level

Educational planning should occur on several levels. Planning on the national level should start with legislation concerning infants' rights, family rights and duties, and minimal requirements of an educational environment for infants at home or away from it. At this level of planning, the relative importance of this age group and its needs should be decided. Decisions on the national level should deal with the ministerial responsibilities over infants and families, and how these responsibilities are to be coordinated.

In relating means to ends, decisions should be made on the importance of preparation of professionals in various fields dealing with infants and creating services for infants, families, and alternative caregivers. These services should include prevention, diagnosis, consul-

tation, and treatment of infants' and families' problems and handicaps.

In countries where mass media are nationally controlled, special planning of mass media communication concerning child and family development should occur, and be acted upon.

Of special importance on the national level is the planning of educational environments for the handicapped infant and professional services for the staff in them. Dispersion of services to peripheral areas should be planned to ensure access to information and professional expertise.

Planning on the Regional and Municipal Levels

Regional centers for prevention, follow-up, diagnosis, and intervention should be planned to ensure highly skilled care for infants. These centers should supply supervision and guidance to educational institutes, and will help to prepare suitable caregivers in day care centers. Patterns and processes of communication, coordination, and referral should be allotted to ensure that no educational organization will supply services in a professional vacuum. Regional or municipal centers should also plan parks, libraries, cultural activities, and creativity corners in the areas that meet the needs of infants and young children, including the purchase of toys and books.

Planning on the Community Level

In each community and neighborhood, specific needs of families and infants should be assessed. Creating educational institutes should meet these needs. Day care centers in a depressed urban area should be different from those in middle-class neighborhoods or in underdeveloped remote rural areas. Methods of enrollment and criteria of selection should be defined, and characteristics of caregivers and the daily activities in the day care center should be planned.

Planning of patterns of communication between the day care center and community agencies is very important at this stage. In any community, there are various agencies dealing with family and infants, social and welfare services, health centers, pediatricians, and psychological services; other educational organizations such as schools and kindergartens all exist and should coordinate their efforts to ensure efficiency and continuity. Patterns of interaction with voluntary organizations in the community should also be planned to prevent confusion and harm to the infants. Another focus of planning should be the patterns of participation of other agents and parents in the activity of the day care. Professionals in the community should visit the center regularly to ensure that they are meeting with infants in normal situations and, thus, are able to intervene before continuous damage is done to the infant. Patterns of referral to professionals should be planned, and ways of involving parents should be clearly defined.

Informal support networks in the community of relatives, friends, neighbors, and informal public opinion leaders should be studied specifically and used in planning intervention programs in the community, using the day care center as a natural starting point.

Planning in the Educational Organization

In the educational institute, several processes of planning should occur. One is the planning of activities in the day care center in units of hours, days, weeks, seasons, and special holidays (religious and national). Planning the activities of the infants should be done in reference to a curriculum that fits both infants' needs and cultural values and goals of the community. These plans cannot ignore ways to recognize individual needs, temperaments, and developmental processes of infants.

Planning of the physical environment to fit infants' developmental needs, and planning of toys, games, and materials to promote infants' ability to experiment and experience, are very important. Patterns of adequate communication between staff members, with parents, and with community agents should be structured. Built-in mechanisms of feedback and problem-

solving in the day care center should be planned. Participation of caregivers in ongoing in-service training programs should be ensured by careful planning for trained substitutes. Continuity of relations with caregivers and the other infants in the group should be ensured by careful placement of infants in their groups, and processes of receiving new members to the group and departure from it should be thought of prior to the occurrence.

Educational Planning on the Family Level

Ways and means to help parents become conscious and efficient educators without damaging the unique emotional atmosphere of the family, and without lessening their satisfaction from interaction with their infants should be carefully planned. Information-giving, sensitivity-training, and efficiency-increasing programs should be planned and open to all families. Ways of increasing parents' participation in planning and enacting such programs should be conceived. As consumers of information and counseling, parents' involvement in their infants' development should be increased in the day care centers. Such planning should take into consideration specific family needs and mold programs to individual families rather than force universal programs to fit a unique family's needs.

CONCLUSION

Educational planning is one of the ways to increase the contribution of professional expertise and knowledge to everyday life. One of the basic roles of a professional is to use his or her ability of rational thinking in areas loaded with emotions and feelings. The state of our knowledge of the child and family today makes such rational thinking both possible and necessary so that early infancy education will not become another high-risk factor.

REFERENCES

Bronfenbrenner, U. *The ecology of human development.* Cambridge, MA: Harvard University Press, 1979.

Caldwell, B.M., & Richmond, J.B. *The Children's Center: A microcosmic health, education & welfare unit.* In: L. Dittman (ed.), *Early child care: The new perceptions.* New York: Atherton Press, 1968.

Index